Anti-Aging Therapeutics
Volume XII
2009 Conference Year

Editors
Dr. Ronald Klatz
and
Dr. Robert Goldman

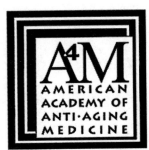 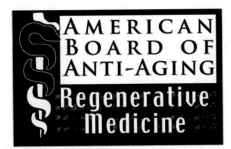 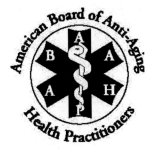

An official educational work published by A4M Publications
1510 West Montana Street
Chicago, IL 60614 USA
TEL: (773) 528-4333; FAX: (773) 528-5390; E-MAIL: a4m@worldhealth.net
WEBSITE: www.worldhealth.net

Visit
The World Health Network, at www.**worldhealth.net**, the Internet's leading anti-aging portal;
And
The A4M's Special Information Center, at www.**a4minfo.net**, the A4M's Publishing and Media Showcase

IMPORTANT – PLEASE READ

The content presented in the *Anti-Aging Therapeutics, volume 12* is for educational purposes only and is specifically designed for those with a health, medical, or biotechnological education or professional experience. *Anti-Aging Therapeutics, volume 12* does not prevent, diagnose, treat or cure disease or illness.

While potentially therapeutic pharmaceuticals, nutraceuticals (dietary supplementation) and interventive therapies are described in the A4M's *Anti-Aging Therapeutics, volume 12*, this work serves the sole purpose of functioning as an informational resource. Under no circumstances is the reader to construe endorsement by A4M of any specific companies or products. Quite to the contrary, *Caveat Emptor*. It is the reader's responsibility to investigate the product, the vendor, and the product information.

Dosing of nutraceuticals can be highly variable. Proper dosing is based on parameters including sex, age, and whether the patient is well or ill (and, if ill, whether it is a chronic or acute situation). Additionally, efficiency of absorption of a particular type of product and the quality of its individual ingredients are two major considerations for choosing appropriate specific agents for an individual's medical situation.

Furthermore, anyone with malignancy should consult their physician or oncologist prior to beginning, or continuing, any hormone therapy program.

Finally, please be mindful that just because a product is natural doesn't mean it's safe for everyone. A small portion of the general population may react adversely to components in nutraceuticals (especially herbal products). A complete inventory of interventions utilized by a patient should be maintained by physicians and health practitioners dispensing anti-aging medical care.

Anti-Aging Therapeutics, volume 12 is, again, designed for those with a health, medical, or biotechnological education or professional experience. It is not intended to provide medical advice, and is not to be used as a substitute for advice from a physician or health practitioner. If you are a consumer interested in any of the approaches discussed in these chapters, it is absolutely essential that you have a thorough discussion with your physician to understand all benefits and risks.

For those individuals interested in the diagnostics and/or therapies described by chapter authors of *Anti-Aging Therapeutics, volume 12*, A4M urges that you consult a knowledgeable physician or health practitioner, preferably one who has been Board Certified in Anti-Aging Medicine. You may find one by utilizing the Online Physician/Practitioner Locator at the A4M's educational website, www.worldhealth.net, or you may call our international headquarters in Chicago, IL USA at (773) 528-4333.

ISBN 978-1-934715-05-5 (print & CD-ROM)

Printed in the United States of America.

Table of Contents

* Denotes speaker at Spring 2009 Session of the Annual World Congress on Anti-Aging Medicine & Regenerative Biomedical Technologies;
** Denotes speaker at Summer 2009 Session;
*** Denotes speaker at Winter 2009 Session.

v

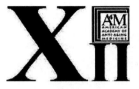

Chapter 1
The A4M Twelve-Point Actionable Healthcare Plan: A Blueprint for A Low Cost, High Yield Wellness Model of Healthcare

Contributing Editors:

Ronald M. Klatz, M.D., D.O., President & Physician Co-Founder, American Academy of Anti-Aging Medicine (A4M); Appointed member, Global Action Council on the Challenges of Gerontology, World Economic Forum; Director, World Anti-Aging Academy of Medicine

Robert M. Goldman, M.D., Ph.D., D.O., FAASP, Chairman & Physician Co-Founder, American Academy of Anti-Aging Medicine (A4M); World Chairman, International Medical Commission; Chairman, World Anti-Aging Academy of Medicine; President Emeritis, National Academy of Sports Medicine

Joseph C. Maroon, M.D., Professor of Neurosurgery, Heindl Scholar in Neuroscience and Vice Chairman of Neurosurgery, University of Pittsburgh Medical Center; Member of the International Editorial Board, Neurological Research and the Journal of Sports Medicine; Past President, Congress of Neurological Surgeons

Nicholas A. DiNubile, M.D., Orthopaedic Consultant to the Philadelphia 76ers Basketball Team and Pennsylvania Ballet

Michael Klentze, M.D., Ph.D., Secretary-General, European Society of Anti-Aging Medicine; Medical Director, Vitalife Wellness Center of Bumrungrad Hospital, Thailand

The American Academy of Anti-Aging Medicine (A4M; www.worldhealth.net), the world's largest professional organization dedicated to advancing research and clinical pursuits that enhance the quality, and extend the quantity, of the human lifespan, unveils an innovative, technology-based fix to healthcare with the potential to:
- Increase the lifespan, or improve the healthspan, of all Americans by 29+ years;
- Slash healthcare costs, saving $3.7 Trillion; and
- Replace the disease-based approach to medicine with a wellness-oriented model

A comprehensive program to reform and advance healthcare in the United States, *The A4M Twelve-Point Actionable Healthcare Plan: A Blueprint for A Low Cost, High Yield Wellness Model of Healthcare* has garnered support from 35 professional medical organizations and educational institutions and was developed with invaluable input from the 24,000 physician, health practitioner, and scientist members of the American Academy of Anti-Aging Medicine (A4M; www.worldhealth.net) who represent 110 nations worldwide.

The contributing editors, authors and endorsing organizations of *The Twelve-Point Plan* submit that the underlying philosophy of healthcare in this nation must be reformed in revolutionary new ways. In place of the disease-based approach that treats people after they exhibit signs of illness, we submit that it is time for the nation to adopt a wellness-oriented model to healthcare. Such a model stresses very early detection of illness and promotes disease prevention, yielding opportunities for the best prognoses and economical treatments. As reported by the Congressional Budget Office, up to one-third of this nation's healthcare spending -- more than $700 billion -- does not improve Americans' health outcomes.

To compound the issue of healthcare reform, the United States is a driving force in a trend of unprecedented global aging. The average age of the world's population is increasing at an unprecedented rate. The number of people worldwide ages 65+ was 506 million as of midyear *2008; by 2040, that number will hit 1.3 billion. Thus, in just over 30 years, the proportion of older people will double from 7% to 14% of the total world population. In the United States, men and women ages 65+ represented 12.4% of the population in the year 2000, with that age bracket projected to swell to stand at 20% of the population by 2030. In 2007 in the United States, six major diseases among Americans ages 65+ resulted in medical and lost productivity costs of more than $196 billion. In the coming years, the cases of these six diseases, namely -- chronic lung disease, ischemic heart disease, stroke, lung cancer, pneumonia and gastrointestinal illness -- are expected to surge as the population ages, potentially sending the costs of age-related diseases skyrocketing. Steps to prepare the nation to address the social, economic, and personal ramifications of a graying society now, are urgently necessary.

The A4M Twelve-Point Actionable Healthcare Plan: A Blueprint for A Low Cost, High Yield Wellness Model of Healthcare provides the following practicable "here and now" solutions to reform and advance healthcare in the United States, while addressing the challenges of global aging:

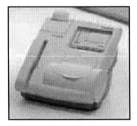
I. Point of Care (POC) Laboratory Testing: We propose funding for development of a comprehensive, all-in-one POC laboratory testing device which will measure a set of standardized medical biomarkers of aging and thus enable the very early detection risk factors for aging-related disease.
Projected Extension in Healthspan / Lifespan: 2 ADDITIONAL YEARS PER PERSON
Projected Savings to Healthcare System: <u>US $6.75 BILLION SAVINGS</u>

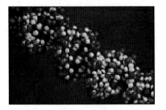
II. Biomarkers of Aging and Health Measurement: We propose the establishment and deployment of a complete, state-of-the-science Biomarkers of Aging and Health Measurement program, to accurately assess biological age. Such data quantitatively demonstrates the benefits of various therapies for lifestyle intervention that may exert a positive effect on slowing or mitigating the degenerative process of aging. Such an Assessment Panel could be deployed across the population, thus making it possible to judiciously allocate resources wisely and efficiently, focusing particularly on those who can benefit most in terms of diagnosis and prevention.
Projected Extension in Healthspan / Lifespan: 5 ADDITIONAL YEARS PER PERSON
Projected Savings to Healthcare System: <u>US $119.5 BILLION SAVINGS</u>

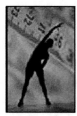 **III. Free Biannual Comprehensive Metabolic Testing (CMT):** We propose the establishment of a Twice-yearly Comprehensive Metabolic Testing program, comprised of specific metabolic parameters. When subsidized by national government, a free biannual Comprehensive Metabolic Testing program minimizes the onset and/or severity of metabolic disorders. Such a population-wide CMT program also greatly augments quality of life by sparing individuals from these life-draining diseases.

Projected Extension in Healthspan / Lifespan: 3 ADDITIONAL YEARS PER PERSON
Projected Savings to Healthcare System: US $154.6 BILLION SAVINGS

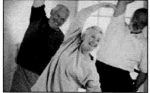 **IV. 24/7 Telemedicine Consultation Access:** We propose the development of a nationwide telemedicine platform for advanced preventive medicine, to include a variety of state-of-the-technology features to promote effective and accurate diagnoses, disease modeling, and teleconferencing.

Projected Extension in Healthspan / Lifespan: 3 ADDITIONAL YEARS PER PERSON
Projected Savings to Healthcare System: US $400 BILLION SAVINGS

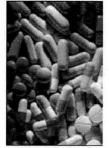 **V. Aging Intervention Drugs:** We urge the nation to (1) Establish a category of drugs under the terminology "aging intervention pharmaceuticals." Doing so will promote directed and focused research into aging intervention, as compared to the serendipitous discoveries on which anti-aging pharmaceutical therapeutics currently relies. And (2) Fast-track the discovery, development, and approval process for aging intervention pharmaceuticals. With projections estimating that by the year 2050, the older population in the United States will account for 21% of the total national population, it is thus critical to expedite the timetable for aging intervention pharmaceuticals.

Projected Extension in Healthspan / Lifespan: 3 ADDITIONAL YEARS PER PERSON
Projected Savings to Healthcare System: US $39.2 BILLION SAVINGS

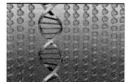 **VI. Stem Cells, Nanotechnology, Genetic Engineering:** We urge national funding to encourage development of clinical applications of stem cell therapies, nanotechnology, genetic engineering, and other biomedical technologies. Additionally, it is imperative to eliminate the regulatory barriers to the widespread utilization thereof. Such encouragement will have a profound effect on the neuromuscular disorders associated with the aging process and deliver dramatic beneficial economic effects.

Projected Extension in Healthspan / Lifespan: 4-12 ADDITIONAL YEARS PER PERSON
Projected Savings to Healthcare System: US $197.1 BILLION SAVINGS

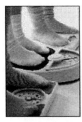

VII. Personalized Genetic Testing and Nutrigenomics: If subsidized by national governments, population-wide personalized genetic testing, will fast-track the field of nutrigenomics, thereby rapidly elucidating novel natural therapeutics that can improve the health of broad segments of the population.
Projected Extension in Healthspan / Lifespan: 2 ADDITIONAL YEARS PER PERSON
Projected Savings to Healthcare System: US $292.3 BILLION SAVINGS

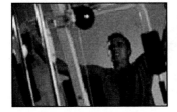

VIII. Free/Subsidized Access to Gym, Spa, Detoxification, and Physical Rehabilitation Facilities: We urge the nation's government to subsidize widespread free access to gym, spa, metabolic detoxification, and physical rehabilitation facilities. Such access promotes self-treatment of musculoskeletal disorders common and ubiquitous to the aging process, such as arthritis, back, knee, and hip pain, and mobility issues, as well as promote the rejuvenation and regeneration of diseased muscle and nerve tissues. As a result, much of the costs associated with aging-related disabilities can be prevented and/or ameliorated. Such services would also dramatically reduce the large proportion of society which now is classified as disabled and would ensure that a large majority of its citizens can remain healthy and able-bodied late into life, far beyond 70 or 80 years of age.
Projected Extension in Healthspan / Lifespan: 2 ADDITIONAL YEARS PER PERSON
Projected Savings to Healthcare System: US $23.4 BILLION SAVINGS

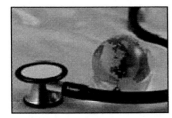

IX. Online Electronic Database on Aging Intervention: We encourage the establishment of an online electronic database on aging intervention. Doing so will enable the worldwide medical community to arrive more expeditiously at innovative approaches to disease. Such large-scale data collection promotes analyses that lead to evidence-based therapeutic successes in treating aging-related disorders, dysfunctions, and diseases.

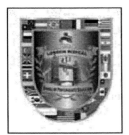

X. Free Online Medical Education: We propose federal support to develop Postgraduate Medical E-Learning and Certification programs. Such an invaluable educational resource serves to (1) Empower patients to serve as their own health advocates; and (2) Educate health professionals to keep them updated on the wide array, and rapidly changing environment, of advanced preventive medicine.

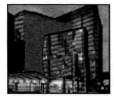

XI.   The World Center for Anti-Aging Medicine: The World Center is envisioned as a world-class, university affiliated research and treatment facility unique in its focus on the investigation and application of diagnostic and treatment protocols that extend the length, and enhance the quality, of the human lifespan. The World Center will be the leading facility established to realize effective interventions that alter the detrimental course and impact of the degenerative diseases of human aging. We urge federal funding for a World Center for Anti-Aging Medicine, at which a coordinated program of research, education, and clinical training will expedite the development and implementation of safe and effective anti-aging therapeutics for all mankind.

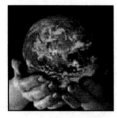

XII. The Leisure Class: The global financial meltdown of 2008 has led to an accelerated adjustment of economic reality for billions of people worldwide. Indeed, automated technologies such artificial intelligence, voice recognition, virtual secretaries/personal assistants, and service industry robotics will become more utilized and thus displace the need to have humans in 7 out of 10 of jobs in the service, administrative, and support sectors. As a result, millions of people will not be needed in the workforce, thus giving rise to The Leisure Class. These early retirees may wish to pursue community-oriented activities such as mentoring, hospice work, and other volunteer activities. The Leisure Class gives rise to a new crop of artists, poets, philosophers, scientists, and similar creative minds to fuel the next Renaissance Age. Forward planning to provide adequate care and living to support The Leisure Class is an emerging societal concern. It will become necessary for nations to establish a Social Contract for The Leisure Class, which subsidizes free education, entertainment, housing, food, and healthcare for this segment of the population and provides incentives for them to still be positive contributors to society at-large.

Points IX – XII: Projected Extension in Healthspan / Lifespan: 5 ADDITIONAL YEARS PER PERSON
Points IX – XII: Projected Savings to Healthcare System: US $2.4 TRILLION SAVINGS

The contributing editors, authors and endorsing organizations of *The A4M Twelve-Point Actionable Healthcare Plan: A Blueprint for A Low Cost, High Yield Wellness Model of Healthcare* urge this nation to adopt a technology-driven, wellness-oriented model to healthcare. Anti-aging medicine is the pinnacle of biotechnology joined with advanced clinical preventive medicine. Seeking to improve the quality and extend the quantity of the human lifespan, anti-aging medicine offers a viable model of specific attainable goals on which a comprehensive and integrated program of healthcare reform may be based. Thus, adoption of the anti-aging medical model delivers the best of advanced preventive medicine to all Americans, not merely our older population.

The elements of *The Twelve-Point Plan* will significantly improve and extend the healthy human lifespan. Each of the points of this Program will also deliver a profound net economic savings via three major mechanisms:
1. Conservation of worker productivity
2. Reduction of disability and hospitalization costs
3. Reduction of the burden of costs associated with chronic long-term medical conditions.

The Twelve-Point Plan provides practicable "here and now" solutions to reform and advance healthcare in the United States, while addressing the challenges of global aging. Indeed, the implementation of *The A4M Twelve-Point Actionable Healthcare Plan: A Blueprint for A Low Cost, High Yield Wellness Model of Healthcare* may **save our society a projected $3.64 Trillion in healthcare costs,** and **extend the healthy lifespan of each of our nation's residents by up to 29 productive, vital years.**

Complete references and supporting data for projections may be viewed in the full version of *The A4M Twelve-Point Actionable Healthcare Plan: A Blueprint for A Low Cost, High Yield Wellness Model of Healthcare.* Request your free copy of this White Paper, at:
www.waaam.org/twelve_points_summary.php.

Chapter 2
Telomerase Activation: The Future of Anti-Aging Medicine

William H. Andrews, Ph.D.
President & Chief Executive Officer, Sierra Sciences (Reno, Nevada USA)

ABSTRACT

In the last three decades, there has been a tremendous upsurge of scientific knowledge of how and why we age. There is a clock that ticks inside every dividing cell of our bodies. This clock operates by telomere shortening. This is an inherent property of DNA replication that makes it impossible for our cells to divide indefinitely, and which research suggests is a primary cause of aging.

Inside every one of our cells is a gene that produces an enzyme called telomerase. Telomerase stops the telomere clock from ticking, and can give cells the potential to divide forever. The gene for telomerase is turned off in most adult cells, but a small-molecule compound should be able to turn it back on.

The first such compound ever proven to increase telomerase activity in adult cells is the nutraceutical TA-65, discovered by Geron Corporation and distributed by TA Sciences. Early results demonstrate that TA-65 has measurable and remarkable benefits.

The aims of this paper are:
1. To educate the reader about telomere biology and the scientific basis for aging.
2. To provide evidence that aging can be reversed or cured and not merely treated.
3. To familiarize the reader with a new approach to anti-aging therapeutics.

INTRODUCTION

In order to live a long and healthy life it is vital to eat a healthy diet, take regular exercise, and to make healthy lifestyle decisions. While following these steps will promote good health, they will not enable us to remain fit and healthy into our 100s.

We have made tremendous gains in lifespan extension in the last 100 years. In 1900, the average lifespan was just 47.3 years, today it is 78.0 years. This dramatic improvement in lifespan is due to numerous factors, including: better sewage systems, vaccines, refrigeration, better diets, cleaner water, antibiotics, improved oral care, antihypertensive medication, coronary artery bypass surgery, and chemotherapy. All of these factors (and many more) have enabled us to extend life, but none of them are going to stop aging.

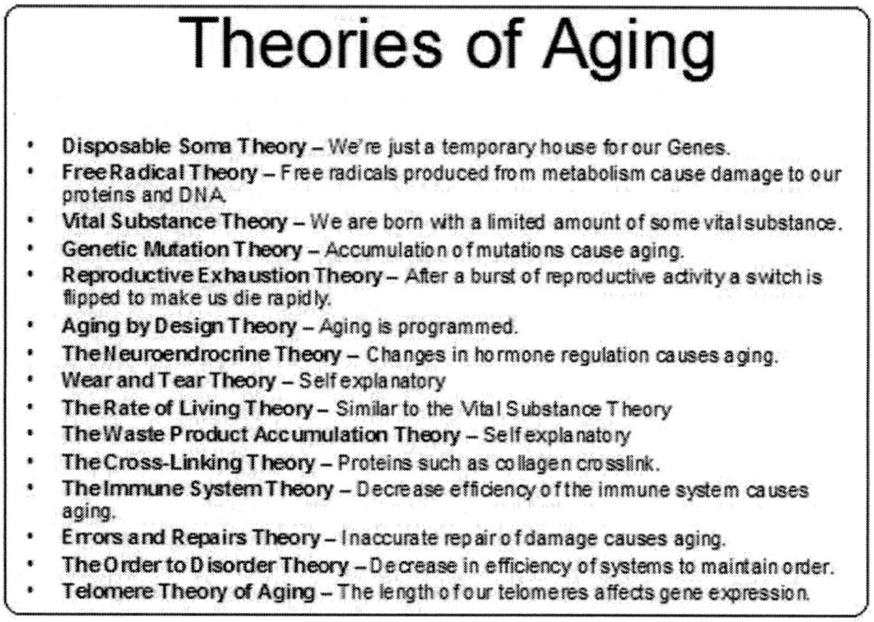

Theories of Aging

- **Disposable Soma Theory** – We're just a temporary house for our Genes.
- **Free Radical Theory** – Free radicals produced from metabolism cause damage to our proteins and DNA.
- **Vital Substance Theory** – We are born with a limited amount of some vital substance.
- **Genetic Mutation Theory** – Accumulation of mutations cause aging.
- **Reproductive Exhaustion Theory** – After a burst of reproductive activity a switch is flipped to make us die rapidly.
- **Aging by Design Theory** – Aging is programmed.
- **The Neuroendrocrine Theory** – Changes in hormone regulation causes aging.
- **Wear and Tear Theory** – Self explanatory.
- **The Rate of Living Theory** – Similar to the Vital Substance Theory.
- **The Waste Product Accumulation Theory** – Self explanatory.
- **The Cross-Linking Theory** – Proteins such as collagen crosslink.
- **The Immune System Theory** – Decrease efficiency of the immune system causes aging.
- **Errors and Repairs Theory** – Inaccurate repair of damage causes aging.
- **The Order to Disorder Theory** – Decrease in efficiency of systems to maintain order.
- **Telomere Theory of Aging** – The length of our telomeres affects gene expression.

Figure 1. Theories of Aging

Numerous scientists believe that the theoretical maximum lifespan of a human being is 125 years.[1-3] Why this is we do not know, however we cannot seem to pass this threshold of 125 years. There are numerous theories on what causes aging (Fig. 1). I like to think of each theory as a stick of dynamite that is burning inside of ourselves, and that when one of the fuses runs out we die of old age. Of course, the stick of dynamite that matters the most is the one with the shortest fuse. So, whilst it is accepted that there are a lot of factors that cause aging, the problem is that we do not know for certain which factor is the most important (the shortest fuse). There are a lot of people trying to identify which theory of aging might be the holder of the shortest fuse. I believe that the shortest fuse is the length of our telomeres.

The aim of this paper is to introduce telomere biology and the telomere theory of aging, and to discover how the ability to maintain the length of our telomeres may enable us to reverse the aging process.

TELOMERASE ACTIVATION: THE FUTURE OF ANTI-AGING MEDICINE
An Introduction to Telomere Biology

The human body contains approximately 100 trillion cells. Every cell contains a nucleus and inside these nuclei there are chromosomes. A chromosome is an organized structure that contains a single coiled strand of DNA. The strand of DNA is approximately 10 million bases long. Each end of a chromosome is capped by a region of repetitive DNA called a telomere.

The DNA in the telomeres of an embryo is approximately 15,000 bases long. However, as soon as cell division begins the telomeres start to shorten and by the time an infant is born their telomeres will have already shortened to approximately 10,000 bases. As cell division continues throughout life the telomeres become shorter and shorter, and when they get as short as 5000 bases, we die of old age. Telomeres cannot get shorter than 5000 bases. We are conceived at 15,000 bases, we are born at 10,000 bases, and we die at 5000 bases. Eating a healthy diet, regular exercise, and getting plenty of sleep may well benefit general health but they will not stop telomeres from shortening.

Probably the best example of how telomeres play a role in aging is the disease progeria. Progeria is a genetic condition that causes a child to be born with very short telomeres. Affected children have a maximum life expectancy of around 20 years and they suffer from all the same age-related ailments that elderly people do. A method of stopping or slowing telomere shortening could provide us with a cure for this disease, and may also provide us with a unique method of combating the normal aging process.

Telomere shortening has been implicated in almost all aspects of normal aging, and has been shown to play a central role in the pathology of two main causes of death – cancer and atherosclerosis. When telomeres get short chromosomes become unstable, this increases the likelihood of genetic mutations that increase the risk of developing cancer. Furthermore, when the telomeres in immune cells get short, immune cells lose their ability to fight cancer. Thus, short telomeres increase the risk of getting cancer and decrease the body's ability to fight cancer. If you examine the blood vessels of someone with atherosclerosis you will find that the telomeres in the endothelial cells and smooth muscle cells surrounding atherosclerotic plaques are shorter than those in plaque-free areas. This is because the cells with shortened telomeres are older and are thus less able to fight against plaque development. So, if we can find a way to prevent telomere shortening it may well provide us with a method of treating or even preventing atherosclerosis. Telomere shortening has also been linked to: Alzheimer's disease, osteoarthritis, osteoporosis, skin aging, macular degeneration, liver cirrhosis, muscular dystrophy, impaired immunity, and numerous other conditions.

Exactly why do telomeres shorten? When a cell divides, the DNA has to replicate. Each strand of the original double-stranded DNA molecule serves as template for the reproduction of the new strand. Thus, two identical DNA molecules are produced from a single double-stranded DNA molecule. The problem is that the cell is unable to replicate the very end of the chromosome. As a result, every time DNA is replicated the telomeres of the duplicate chromosome are slightly shorter than those of the original chromosome.

Again, there is nothing that can be done to prevent telomere shortening. No matter how well you eat, no matter how much you exercise, you cannot stop telomere shortening. On the other hand, there are a number of factors that can accelerate telomere shortening, these include: obesity, lack of exercise, psychological stress, and smoking. So, it is possible to prevent accelerated telomere shortening, but there is currently absolutely nothing that can be done to reduce the basal level of telomere shortening.

Thus, finding a way of preventing telomere shortening could provide us with a unique solution to aging, and that is exactly what we are trying to do.

Telomerase Activation

Reproductive cells have been very useful to us in our quest to discover a method of preventing telomere shortening. This is because reproductive cells do not age. This is a very important property of reproductive cells, because if they did age, our children would be born with aged cells. Studies have shown that reproductive cells do not age because they do not experience telomere shortening, and the reason for this is that they contain an enzyme called telomerase. The function of telomerase is to add specific DNA sequence repeats to the end of DNA strands in the telomere regions, thus lengthening the telomere and preventing telomere shortening.

Could we use telomerase to prevent telomerase shortening in somatic cells? Is it possible to activate telomerase in somatic cells? Unfortunately, somatic cells do not produce telomerase. However, they do contain the gene for telomerase. What this means is that somatic cells do have the ability to produce telomerase, but that the telomerase gene is switched off. Therefore the most sensible strategy is to determine a way of turning the telomerase gene back on again. The telomerase gene is switched off by a repressor molecule binding to a regulatory element. Thus, the ideal solution would be a drug that would bind to the repressor, and therefore prevent the repressor molecule from binding to the regulatory element. Then, if a scenario arose where a patient decided they did not want the telomerase gene to stay switched on, all they would have to do is stop taking the drug. This would free the repressor molecule, and enable it to bind to the regulatory element and switch off the telomerase gene.

Will telomerase activation provide us with a cure for aging? We do not know the answer to such questions yet. The work we have been doing for the last 10 years is all based upon theories. However, results of a number of proof of concept experiments support these theories.

We have around 30 scientists whose job is to search for an anti-aging telomerase activator. We have now been searching for 10 years and have screened approximately 142,000 chemicals. So far we have had 32 hits – that is 32 different chemicals that have turned on the telomerase gene. At present, these drugs are many years away from human use. We have spent the last 10 years in the drug discovery phase, and we are now beginning to enter the drug development phase. In this phase we will closely examine these 32 different chemicals, and then we will begin to design new drugs that are more potent and less toxic. Once the drug development phase is complete we will have something that is safe for human use, and then we can begin clinical trials. What this means is that it could be anywhere between 5 and 20 years until such an anti-aging drug is available for public use.

A drug that would turn on the telomerase gene by binding to the repressor would be the ideal situation; however such a drug does not exit yet. Is there anything else we can do? What we have done in the past is to introduce the telomerase gene through a process called telomerizing. This involves using a virus to insert the telomerase gene into the chromosome. When we do this the telomerase gene is not regulated, and so remains switched on. As can be seen in Figure 2, if you take a normal skin cell and grow it in culture you find that only a limited number of cell divisions occur before cell senescence occurs. This is the Hayflick limit. However, in 1997 we successfully telomerized human skin cells, and in this instance cell division was not limited (Fig. 3).[4] The telomerized cells kept on growing. Furthermore, they had a significantly decreased risk of mutations, including cancer. The real surprise of this experiment was that the telomeres did not just stop shortening as we expected, but that they actually got longer. So, does this mean that we actually made the cells younger?

Funk *et al* transplanted human skin cells onto the back of a mouse. When this was done with young cells, the skin looked young, and when it was done with old cells, the skin looked old. However, when the old cells were telomerized, the old skin cells began to produce young skin, thus suggesting that the cells had become young. Indeed, DNA microarray analysis of the telomerized cells confirmed that the telomerized cells had a gene expression pattern similar to that of the young cells.[5]

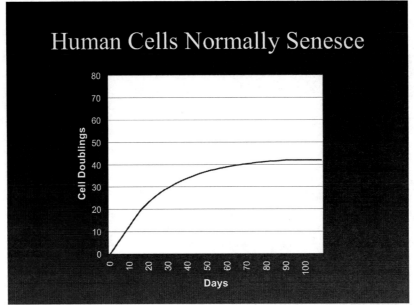

Figure 2. The number of times a normal somatic cell can divide is controlled by the Hayflick limit.

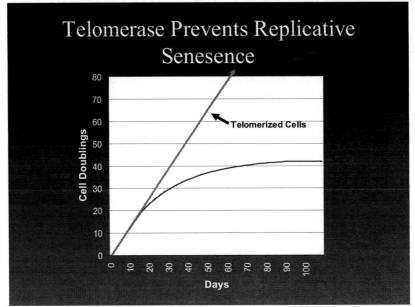

Figure 3. Telomerization removes the Hayflick limit and prevents replicative senescence.[4]

Ruldoph,[6] Samper,[7] and Tomás-Loba[8] provide further proof of concept in their studies on genetically engineered mice. Rudolph *et al* engineered telomerase-null mice in order to study the impact of telomerase deficiency. Results showed that the resulting telomere shortening and accompanying genetic instability were associated with shortened life span, a reduced capacity to respond to stresses such as wound healing, and an increased incidence of spontaneous malignancies.[6] Samper *et al* re-introduced telomerase in late generation telomerase-deficient mice, which have short telomeres and severe proliferative defects. The results of this study showed that the re-introduction of one copy of the telomerase gene in these mice elongated critically short telomeres, rescued chromosomal instability, and prevented severe proliferative defects. The authors concluded: "These results also support the notion that telomerase activity re-introduction in adult somatic cells or tissues could be a potential approach for gene therapy of those age-related diseases triggered by telomere exhaustion, or for premature aging syndromes characterized by a faster rate of telomere shortening."[7] Tomás-Loba *et al* overexpressed telomerase reverse transcriptase (TERT), one of the components of telomerase, in mice engineered to be cancer resistant. Results showed that TERT overexpression delayed aging and increased median life span. The authors concluded: "These results demonstrate that constitutive expression of TERT provides anti-aging activity in the context of a mammalian organism."

It may surprise many people that there is also a proof of concept in humans. There is actually a commercially available nutraceutical that induces telomerase expression. Research shows that telomerase expression is only small, however a little is better than nothing. Even a small amount of telomerase will at least slow telomere shortening. In collaboration with another lab, we took blood samples from people taking this nutraceutical and looked at their telomeres. Even though we could not see the average telomere length increasing, we could see that the shortest telomeres were increasing, which is telling us that this nutraceutical is inducing telomerase and the telomerase is having an effect on the telomeres. Furthermore, tests in people who had been taking this nutraceutical for more than a year showed that they had decreased levels of CD28-T cells, increased levels of naïve T cells, decreased levels of natural killer cells, decreased blood pressure, and increased skin elasticity – all of which suggest that the nutraceutical is having some impact upon the aging process.

CONCLUDING REMARKS

The available evidence suggests that telomerase activation will provide us with a novel anti-aging strategy. However, we still do not know if we will be able to exceed the theoretical maximum lifespan of 125 years. I predict that we will. However, we have to remember that it is likely that telomere shortening is not the only cause of aging.

REFERENCES

1. Carnes BA, Olshansky SJ, Grahn D. Biological evidence for limits to the duration of life. *Biogerontology*. 2003;4:31-45.
2. Hayflick L. "Anti-aging" is an oxymoron. *J Gerontol A Biol Sci Med Sci*. 2004;59:B573-578.
3. Weon BM, Je JH. Theoretical estimation of maximum human lifespan. *Biogerontology*. 2009;10:65-71.
4. Bodnar AG, Ouellette M, Frolkis M, Holt SE, Chiu CP, Morin GB, Harley CB, Shay JW, Lichtsteiner S, Wright WE. Extension of life-span by introduction of telomerase into normal human cells. *Science*. 1998;279:349-352.
5. Funk WD, Wang CK, Shelton DN, Harley CB, Pagon GD, Hoeffler WK. Telomerase expression restores dermal integrity to in vitro-aged fibroblasts in a reconstituted skin model. *Exp Cell Res*. 2000;258:270-278.
6. Rudolph KL, Chang S, Lee HW, Blasco M, Gottlieb GJ, Greider C, DePinho RA. Longevity, stress response, and cancer in aging telomerase-deficient mice. Cell. 1999;96:701-712.
7. Samper E, Flores JM, Blasco MA. Restoration of telomerase activity rescues chromosomal instability and premature aging in Terc-/- mice with short telomeres. EMBO Rep. 2001;2:800-807.
8. Tomás-Loba A, Flores I, Fernández-Marcos PJ, Cayuela ML, Maraver A, Tejera A, Borrás C, Matheu A, Klatt P, Flores JM, Viña J, Serrano M, Blasco MA. Telomerase reverse transcriptase delays aging in cancer-resistant mice. Cell. 2008;135:609-622.

ABOUT THE AUTHOR

Dr. William Andrews leads the scientific research and development function of Sierra Sciences. Under Dr. Andrews direction, Sierra Sciences has discovered and filed patent applications on many previously unknown, key elements of the regulation of telomerase. Dr. Andrews earned his Ph.D. in Molecular and Population Genetics at the University of Georgia in 1981. He was a Senior Scientist at Armos Corporation and Codon Corporation, Director of Molecular Biology at Codon and at Geron Corporation, and Director of Technology Development at EOS Biosciences. As of April 2006, Dr. Andrews name appears on 23+ issued US patents specifically related to telomerase, as well as 10 other patents in molecular biology. He has more than 25 refereed publications and abstracts. At Sierra Sciences he has been responsible for all aspects of research, all of the company's patent applications, and all R&D facility and equipment matters.

Chapter 3
Low-Dose Naltrexone: A Possible Safe Effective Treatment for Autoimmune Disease and Cancer

Paul J. Battle, PA-C
Barolat Neuroscience (Denver, CO USA);
Boulder Longevity Institute (Boulder, CO USA)

ABSTRACT

Naltrexone is an opiate antagonist drug that has been used safely for 25 years in addiction medicine. Research has shown that in addition to its opiate antagonist properties at 50-300 mg per day dosages, it has immunoregulatory properties at dosages as low as 3.0 mg,

Low dose naltrexone (LDN) improves the clinical state of patients with autoimmune diseases such as Crohn's disease, rheumatoid arthritis, and multiple sclerosis. Another impressive property of LDN is its ability to arrest cancer cell growth.

The remarkable fact is LDN can enhance the immune system for these two major disease classifications with little or no side effects. This paper will describe the science behind LDNs physiological mechanisms to reduce the effects of autoimmune disease and inhibit cancer cell growth. The author hopes to generate research interest in these mechanisms of disease modification, which enhance the body's own immune system without side effects.

Keywords: naltrexone, autoimmune disease, low-dose naltrexone, cancer treatment, opiate growth factor, OGF.

INTRODUCTION

Many of the most difficult diseases to treat in modern medicine are those in malignancy and autoimmune categories. We still have not made much headway on curing cancer, with the exception of a few cancers. Cancer therapy with chemotherapy and radiation kill the cancerous cells, but also weaken the cells of the immune system – the very cells that battle infection and control cancer cell growth. Whilst autoimmune diseases are still treated with drugs that are helpful but have long-term risks and side effects.

Naltrexone is an opiate antagonist drug, which was FDA-approved for the management of drug addiction in 1984. Naltrexone has been used in chemical dependency clinics to reduce the euphoric effects of opiates. In addition, some practitioners have used it for alcoholic treatment. It is now a generic drug that can be obtained for $15-40 per month. Research suggests that low-dose naltrexone (LDN) may well be a safe, economic, and effective treatment for autoimmune disease and cancer. LDN modulates the deregulation of the immune system with autoimmune disease and inhibits cancer cell growth to help control malignant disease. The usual dosage of naltrexone used for LDN is between 3.0 mg and 4.5 mg. To date there have been no serious side effects recorded when using these dosages. There are an estimated 70,000 patients around the world who are using LDN. The most common side effect is sleep disturbances during the initial first two weeks of use.

AUTOIMMUNE DISEASE AND LOW-DOSE NALTREXONE

The immune system has several functions. One of them is to fight off infection from viruses, parasites, fungi, and bacteria. Another major function is to suppress the growth of abnormal cells which have uncontrolled growth and develop into malignancies. The delicate balance of these functions is dependant on many check and balance systems, which keep our bodies free of infection and cancer. These systems are regulated by hormones, cytokines, cellular activity, and humoral responses. Imbalances that may occur with these responses lead to autoimmune diseases, including rheumatoid arthritis, Crohn's disease, and systemic lupus erythematosus (SLE).

When activated, the immune system may initiate an inflammatory response that is necessary for tissue repair after injury. Unfortunately, uncontrolled inflammatory responses can lead to dysfunction of that tissue. For example, in Crohn's disease the intestinal lining becomes inflamed, causing malabsorption of nutrients, pain, and fibrosis. Another example is multiple sclerosis (MS), where an inflammatory T cell response destroys oligodendrocytes and demyelinates nerves.

B lymphocytes, T lymphocytes, and natural killer (NK) cells originate from the bone marrow. Lymphocytes are differentiated by the surface marker molecules or cluster of differentiation (CD). For example, CD4 cells are known as helper T cells. CD4 cells are activated when exposed to an antigen. Their function can change dependant on other molecules and cells they interact with. CD4 cells have two broad categories: Th1 or Th2 cell types. Th1 cells are more involved in cell mediated activity. The cytokines that affect Th1 cells are interferon gamma (IFN-γ), interleukin (IL)-2, IL-12, tumor necrosis factor-alpha (TNFα), and TNFβ. Cytokines that affect Th2 cells are IL-4, IL-5, IL-10, and IL-13. Overactivity of the Th1 response generates problems of autoimmunity, such as asthma, because Th1 cells and cytokines upregulate the inflammatory response and the cytotoxic effects of CD8 and NK cells. In contrast, Th2 cytokines have a more inhibitory response to inflammation and suppress the Th1 response. LDN increases IL-10, transforming growth factor-beta (TGFβ), and NK cells, and reduces TNFα and the Th1 response. This favorably changes the Th1/Th2 balance, reducing the inflammatory response, yet still enabling the body to fight infection. Thus, LDN is able to restore the Th1/Th2 balance to a more homeostatic state.

Another group of chemicals that regulate the immune response are the peptides of endorphins and metenkephalins. The endorphins are found in the brain and adrenal gland. Beta-endorphin (β-endorphin) can suppress or increase the immune response depending on the needs of the organism. For example, if the body is free from infection, β-endorphin downregulates the antibody and inflammatory response, however if infection is present, β-endorphin upregulates the antibody response.

Research suggests that there may be a relationship between levels of β-endorphin and autoimmune activity. Dr Maira Gironi, a clinical and experimental researcher in the immunological mechanisms of neurological disease at IV° Universitary Clinic of Neurology of Milan, Italy, has conducted extensive studies on the effects of endorphins on autoimmune disease. She found that patients with Crohn's disease, rheumatoid disease, and MS had low levels of β-endorphin. Results of one study showed that the mean level of β-endorphin in patients with MS was approximately 45 pg/million cells, compared to 100 pg/million cells in the control patients. After treatment with interferon, β-endorphin levels increased to 80 pg/million cells.[1] LDN has been shown to increase β-endorphin levels in MS patients by 200-300%.[2]

Bihari observed that AIDS addiction patients that were taking naltrexone seemed to have less mortality and morbidity.[3] This observation led Bihari to research Dr. Ian Zagon's studies on LDN, whereby he found that 4.5 mg naltrexone would increase β-endorphin levels by 200-300%. Bihari went on to treat hundreds of patients with autoimmune diseases and cancer with LDN. One anecdotal story is that a friend of his with large lymphoma tumors, who had already been unsuccessfully treated with radiation and chemotherapy, decided to try LDN. Within just 9 months of starting treatment with LDN her tumors had shrunk away. She went on to live for another 10 years, until she died of a myocardial infarction.

Knowledge of the relationship between β-endorphin deficiency and autoimmune disease, and LDN's ability to significantly raise β-endorphin levels is of great importance if we are to understand LDN's ability to improve the clinical outcome of these diseases.

LDN and the Treatment of Autoimmune Diseases
LDN and Multiple Sclerosis
Gironi led a study to show the safety of LDN in patients with primary progressive MS (PPMS) – the most aggressive form of MS. Forty patients were treated with 4.5 mg of naltrexone for 6-months. Results showed that the LDN was very well tolerated, with the exception of a few patients who experienced sleep disturbances, such as insomnia and vivid dreams. Results also showed that neurological disability progressed in just one patient throughout the study. β-endorphin levels increased, as was expected by the researchers.[2]

A MS mouse model was studied by Zagon. He induced a MS-like disease state called experimental autoimmune encephalitis (EAE) in mice and then treated them with either LDN or [Met(5)]-enkephalin (which he called opiate growth factor (OGF)), an endogenous opioid peptide neurotransmitter peptide that is elevated by LDN. Results showed that there was no disease progression in any of the treated mice. Spurred on by the positive results of this study, Zagon took the experiment one step further and pretreated the mice with LDN or OGF before inducing EAE. He found that significantly fewer mice developed EAE, and that the mice that did develop EAE had a milder form of the disease.[4]

Studies investigating the biochemical affects of LDN on MS have found that it helps to protect oligodendrocytes (cells that form the myelin sheath on nerve cells) against apoptosis. LDN does this by reducing inducible nitric oxide synthase activity, which causes a decrease in peroxynitrite formation, which, in turn, reduces the glutamate response and thus reduces glutamate's excitatory neurotoxicity.[5] Studies also show that naltrexone reduces inflammation in neurons.[6]

In 2007, Dr Bruce Cree of the University of California, San Francisco began the first (and only known) patient-funded study of the effects of LDN on MS. Since naltrexone is a generic drug, it is very difficult to obtain funding for research, thus this was a very significant study. The object of the study was to see if LDN improved the quality of life. Around 70 patients received either LDN or a placebo for 8-weeks, followed by one week without either, and then a further 8-weeks on the alternate regimen. Results showed that 8-weeks of treatment with LDN significantly improved quality of life indices for mental health, pain, and self-reported cognitive function of MS patients as measured by the MS Quality of Life Inventory (MSQLI). No changes in physical quality of life indices, including bowel and bladder control, sexual satisfaction, fatigue, and visual function, were observed, however it is important to remember that the treatment period was just 8-weeks. Results also showed that the benefits of LDN were independent of disease course, age, treatment order, or treatment with either interferon beta or copaxone. Like with every other study, no significant adverse side effects were noted.[7]

Skip Lenz, Pharm.D. F.A.S.C.P., has conducted numerous random surveys of treatment outcomes in patients using LDN for MS. Results of a survey presented at the 2007 LDN conference revealed that 71% of the 278 patients who took part reported that LDN had increased their quality of life, while 9% reported a complete resolution of symptoms. Furthermore, 83% percent stated they had not had an exacerbation of MS since starting treatment with LDN. With regards to side effects, 20% of patients reported experiencing one side effect (mostly sleep disturbances, as in other studies), while 6% of patients reported experiencing two side effects (sleep disturbances and increased spasms).[8]

Personal Anecdotal Experiences

I have had some personal anecdotal experiences with patients with MS:

- I had a physician assistant coworker who had MS. Her condition was causing fatigue that was limiting her ability to work more than 20 hours per week. I advised her to talk to her neurologist about LDN. Four months after she started LDN and stopped her interferon drug she reported that she had not felt as well in 5 years. The most striking improvement in her condition was the improvement in fatigue. Her neurologist was so impressed with her results that he has now prescribed LDN to at least 10 other MS patients.

- An MS patient in our neurostimulation practice, who had severe thoracic neuritis, required a new spinal cord stimulator system to manage his severe left-sided chest pain. I recommended that he should consider trying LDN. At a follow-up visit several months later, he said he was not using his new stimulator system any longer. When I enquired as to why he was no longer using his stimulator, he told me that within 4-weeks of taking LDN his pain levels had dropped down to a 2/10 pain score. He also reported that his fatigue had improved and was continuing to improve each day (previously he was limited to walking just 100 feet, but he was now able to walk two blocks). He is still doing well seven months later.

- An MS patient I met at the Fourth Annual LDN Conference in 2008 told me about his total body neuritis. He had been suicidal due to the fact that his medicine was not controlling the pain. He was attending the conference to celebrate his 4-year anniversary of being pain-free after starting LDN therapy.

- A woman, well known in the LDN circles, who was left totally disabled and wheelchair dependant by MS, was able to return to work in the fall of 2008 after being treated with LDN.

These accounts are dramatic accounts of LDN use in the treatment of MS – it is important to remember that not all MS patients respond in such a way. However, even if a patient does not have a dramatic reversal of their disease, many of them will not have progression. LDN can give them hope until a potential cure is found. Since there are no significant long-term side effects and it is very economical, the risk-reward ratio for LDN is very low. Other current therapies can cause flu-like sensations, liver toxicity, and infection risks.

LDN and its Remarkable Effect on Crohn's Disease

This topic is what inspired me to research LDN and educate practitioners and patients about LDN therapy. One of my family members was diagnosed with Crohn's disease 6-years ago. He needed 60 cm of his small bowel to be resected initially, and then he continued on azothioprine for 4-years. Despite this therapy he ended up in hypovolumic shock due to an acute exacerbation of Crohn's that involved his entire gastrointestinal tract. He was not recovering until he began taking LDN two months later. Within 2-weeks his color was better and his energy levels had increased. Three months after he began taking LDN, laboratory tests showed that his C-reactive protein level had dropped from 20 down to just 0.5, and his hemoglobin level, which had not been above 12 since he was diagnosed, had risen to over 15.0. In two years he gained 60 pounds in weight and 7 inches in height – when he was diagnosed he had not grown for 2 years. Since he began treatment with LDN, he has not had any change in bowel movements, although he does suffer from the occasional cramp if he eats junk food. He is also fit enough to play hockey on a regular basis.

My rationale to try LDN on my relative was based on the results of a study by Dr. Jill Smith, a gastroenterologist at Pennsylvania State University. She treated 17 patients with active Crohn's disease with 4.5 mg naltrexone/day for a total of 12-weeks. Results showed that 89% of patients exhibited a positive response to therapy and 67% achieved a remission.[9] The rates of positive response and remission seen in this study are far greater than those seen with TNF inhibitors. Furthermore, LDN is not associated with any significant side effects, whereas TNF inhibitors are associated with a 3-4 fold increased risk of developing lymphoma and a 25% increased risk of mortality from systemic fungal infections. Indeed, the results of Smith's study were so promising that she has received additional funds for a follow-up study of LDN therapy in adolescents with Crohn's disease.

There are instances when standard pharmaceutical protocols are not effective or where the treatment is associated with significant side effects – the treatment of Crohn's disease is a good example of such an instance. Fortunately, LDN offers great promise in the treatment of Crohn's disease.

LDN and Fibromyalgia

Fibromyalgia (FM) is notoriously difficult to manage. There are a number of different treatments for FM, although none are 100% effective. The etiology of FM encompasses infection, autoimmune, hormonal, neurological, and psychological factors. Some practitioners still do not believe that FM exists as a separate disease state. As with many disease states that we do not yet fully understand, many practitioners unfortunately label the patient as "crazy" or "depressed". It is most likely that the main reason why FM is difficult to treat is because of its multifactorial etiology (it is thought that an initial viral infection causes an exaggerated immune response, which can cause inflammation of the nerves with coexistent hormonal deficiencies). Treatment of a disease with a multifactorial etiology requires a multidisciplinary approach.

LDN treatment of fibromyalgia may help several aspects of the disease. From prior discussion one can see that LDN may help with the inflammatory response by modifying cytokine activity. Many people who use LDN report a better sense of "wellness and contentment" (most likely due to the fact that it elevates β-endorphin), thus it may also be useful for treating the psychological aspect of FM. If patients have autoimmune thyroid disease it may even help their hypothyroidism – many people with Hashimoto's thyroiditis have reported that they were able to reduce their dose of thyroid replacement after they started taking LDN.

Younger and Mackey tested the effectiveness of LDN in treating the symptoms of FM in 10 women meeting the criteria for FM and were not taking an opioid medication. Results showed a 30% decline in symptoms. This reduction in symptoms included a 20% increase in mechanical sensitivity threshold and an increase of 0.9 C° of heat tolerance. There was no change in cold tolerance. The patients tolerated the LDN better than placebo.[10] Further studies are planned.

LDN AND CANCER

One of the key components to curing cancer is controlling cancer cell growth. Zagon's LDN research on cell growth, including over 700 published studies, will have a tremendous impact on the future understanding and treatment of cancer. His discovery of the peptide [Met(5)]-enkephalin, or OGF, may be one of the most significant discoveries of cancer treatment in modern day medicine. LDN treatment increases the level of both OGF and β-endorphin.

OGF is an autocrine produced peptide that uniquely binds to another peptide called the opioid growth factor receptor (OGFr). The OGFr is found in the nuclear envelope, nucleus, and the perinuclear cytoplasm of the cell. OGF has an affinity for OGFr that is 7-times greater than for other opiate receptors such as gamma, delta, and kappa. When OGF binds to the OGFr the complex interacts with the cyclin inhibitor kinase P21 pathway. This interaction inhibits the G1-S phases of cell division, and thus stops the growth of the cells. When interacting with the head and neck squamous cell carcinomas the OGF/OGFr complexes interact with a different pathway. In those cancers it interacts with the P16 inhibition pathway instead of the P21 pathway.[11] The other difference is that these types of cancers have less OGF/OGFr complexes relative to other cancers.[12] These differences may account for the lower response that these types of cancers have to LDN treatment.

What cancers may be sensitive to this therapy? Zagon examined 31 human cancer cell lines, which represent 90% of the human cancers in the world. Results showed that the OGF-OGFr axis, was a feature of all the cancer cell lines studied.[13]

Zagon implanted human pancreatic cancer cells in mice that went on to develop tumors. They then administered exogenous OGF to the mice and saw a 55% reduction in tumor size. Results also showed that mice pretreated with OGF and inoculated with human pancreatic cells showed slower tumor growth – at the end of the study period (45 days) the average tumor size of OGF treated mice was 70% smaller than that of control mice.[14]

In clinical practice, there has been evidence of LDN and OGF working effectively for pancreatic cancer in Dr. Burt Berkson's clinic in New Mexico. He presented his experiences with pancreatic cancer therapy with 3 or 4 patients at the 2008 LDN conference. The majority of them showed a positive response, but all but one returned to their oncologist with further chemotherapy that ended with fatal outcomes. The remaining patient was diagnosed with pancreatic cancer with liver metastases about 9 years ago. He was in his late forties with pancreatic cancer and large liver metastasis. Eight years later he was still continuing with LDN and alpha lipoic acid treatment. His primary tumor was barely identifiable on CT scans presented at the time [2008].[15] Dr. Berkson has also been using LDN for the treatment of autoimmune disease. At that same conference he presented many cases of rheumatoid arthritis that had improved with LDN therapy.

Hytrek *et al* found that LDN reduced tumorgenicity in mice inoculated with human colon cancer cells. After 10 days all the control mice had developed colon cancer tumors, however just 30% of mice treated with LDN had developed colon tumors.[16]

In addition to slowing or stopping cancer cell growth directly, research suggests that OGF may inhibit angiogenesis. Blebea *et al* exposed chorioallantoic membranes from chick embryos to OGF in order to examine the role of endogenous opioids in the modulation of angiogenesis. Results showed that OGF had a significant inhibitory effect on angiogenesis, reducing both the number of blood vessels and the total vessel length by 35% and 20%, respectively.[17]

CONCLUDING REMARKS

The clinical applications of LDN, and therefore OGF, are many and varied. The changes that LDN induces in the immune response by modifying the balance of Th1 and Th2 cytokines back to a healthy balance can dramatically improve many autoimmune diseases (Crohn's disease, rheumatoid arthritis, systemic lupus erythematosos, ankylosing spondylitis, MS, amyotropic lateral sclerosis). Besides the effectiveness of LDN, the most significant benefit of using it with autoimmune disease is that it lacks significant side effects. When one considers the side effects associated with current treatments for autoimmune disease (prednisone, methotrexate, azathioprine, and TNF inhibitors), which can range from development of cancer to death, a trial of LDN might be a consideration before committing a patient to the risk profile of the agents used in most protocols. Another advantage of LDN is cost. At a cost of $15-30 dollars per month relative to $5000 per infusion with TNF inhibitors, it also makes economic sense for the patient and our healthcare system.

To date, more than 700 studies have investigated the effects of LDN on cancer cell growth. These have included cellular studies, animal studies, and some promising human studies. However, more research is needed to more clearly define LDN's role. Research suggests that LDN may be of use in many situations, from prophylactic treatment of smoldering myeloma conditions to the treatment of metastatic cancer. Again due to the low cost and low risk of LDN in cancer treatment, it should be considered as an option for patients with cancer.

REFERENCES

1. Gironi M, Martinelli V, Brambilla E, Furlan R, Panerai AE, Comi G, Sacerdote P. Beta-endorphin concentrations in peripheral blood mononuclear cells of patients with multiple sclerosis: effects of treatment with interferon beta. *Arch Neurology.* 2000;57:1178-1181.
2. Gironi M, Martinelli-Boneschi, Sacerdote P, Solaro C, Zaffaroni M,Cavarreta R, *et al.* Pilot trial of low dose naltrexone in primary progressive multiple sclerosis. *Multiple Sclerosis.* 2008;14:1076-1083.
3. Bihari B, Plotnikoff NP. Methionine Enkephalin in the Treatment of AIDS-Related Complex. In: Plotkinoff NP, Good RA, Murgo AJ, Faith RE, eds. *Cytokines: Stress and Immunity.* Boca Raton, Fl: CRC Press; 1998:77-92.
4. Zagon IS *et al.* Low-dose naltrexone and opiate growth factor's effects on experimental autoimmune encephalomyelitis. Paper presented at: World Congress on Treatment and Research in Multiple Sclerosis; September 17-20, 2008; Montreal, Canada.
5. Agrawal YP. Low dose naltrexone therapy in multiple sclerosis. *Med Hypotheses.* 2005;64:721-724.
6. Elaine Moore Graves' and Autoimmune Disease Education. The Use of LDN for MS, Crohn's, and Other Autoimmune Diseases. Available at: http://www.elaine-moore.com/MyArticles/LowDoseNaltrexone/LDNUseforMSCrohnsandOtherAIDiseases/tabid/195/Default.aspx. Accessed February 23, 2010.
7. Cree B, Ross M,Violich I, Berry B, Beheshtian A, Kornyeyyeva E, Goodin D. A single center, randomized, placebo-controlled, double-crossover study of the effects of low dose naltrexone on quality of life as measured by the Multiple Sclerosis Quality of Life Inventory. Paper presented at: World Congress on Treatment and Research in Multiple Sclerosis; September 17-20, 2008; Montreal, Canada.
8. Lenz HA. A retrospective survey of low dose naltrexone patients. Paper presented at: The Third Annual LDN Conference; October 20, 2007; Nashville, Tennessee.
9. Smith JP, Stock H, Bingaman S, Mauger D, Rogosnitzky M, Zagon IS. Low-dose naltrexone therapy improves active Crohn's disease. *Am J Gastroenterol.* 2007;102:820-828.
10. Younger J, Mackey S. Fibromyalgia symptoms are reduced by low-dose naltrexone: a pilot study. *Pain Medicine.* 2009;4:663-667.
11. Cheng F, Zagon IS, Verderame MF, McLaughlin PJ. The opioid growth factor (OGF)-OGF receptor axis uses the p16 pathway to inhibit head and neck cancer. *Cancer Res.* 2007;67:10511-10518.
12. McLaughlin PJ, Stack BC Jr, Levin RJ, Fedok F, Zagon IS. Defects in the opioid growth factor receptor in human squamous cell carcinoma of the head and neck. *Cancer.* 2003;97:1701-1710.
13. Zagon IS, Donahue RN, McLaughlin PJ. Opioid growth factor-opioid growth factor receptor axis is a physiological determinant of cell proliferation in diverse human cancers. *Am J Physiol Regul Integr Comp Physiol.* 2009;297:R1154-1161.
14. Zagon IS, Jaglowski JR, Verderame MF, Smith JP, Leure-Dupree AE, McLaughlin PJ. Combination chemotherapy with gemcitabine and biotherapy with opioid growth factor (OGF) enhances the growth inhibition of pancreatic adenocarcinoma. Cancer *Chemother Pharmacol.* 2005;56:510-520.
15. Berkson B, Rubin D, Berkson A. The long-term survival of a patient with pancreatic cancer with metastases to the liver after treatment with the IV alpha lipoic acid/ low dose naltrexone, *Integrative Cancer Therapies.* 2006;5:83-89.
16. Hytrek SD, McLaughlin PJ, Lang CM, Zagon IS. Inhibition of human colon cancer by intermittent opioid receptor blockade with naltrexone. *Cancer Lett.* 1996;101:159-164.
17. Blebea J, Mazo JE, Kihara TK, Vu JH, McLaughlin PJ, Atnip RG, Zagon IS. Opioid growth factor modulates angiogenesis. *J Vasc Surg.* 2000;32:364-373.

FURTHER READING

Daruna JH. *Introduction to Psychoneuroimmunology.* New York, NY; Academic Press; 2004.

Greeneltch KM, Haudenschild CC, Keegan AD, Shi Y. The Opioid Antagonist Naltrexone blocks acute endotoxic shock by inhibiting tumor necrosis factor-alpha production. *Brain Behav Immun.* 2004;18:476-484.

Matters GL, Harms JF, McGovern C, Fitzpatrick L, Parikh A, Nilo N, Smith JP. Opioid Antagonist Naltrexone Improves Murine Inflammatory Bowel disease. *J Immunotoxicology.* 2008;5:179-187.

Moore E, Wilkinson S. *The Promise of Low Dose Naltrexone Therapy Potential Benefits in Cancer, Autoimmune, Neurological and Infectious Disorders.* Jefferson, NC; McFarland and Co Inc.; 2009.

Zagon IS, Kreiner S, Heslop J, Conway A, Morgan CR, McLaughlin P. Prevention and Delay in Progression of Human Pancreatic Cancer by Stable Overexpression of the Opioid Growth Factor Receptor. *International Journal of Oncology.* 2008;33;317-323.

Zagon IS, Verderame MF, Mclaughlin PJ. The Biology of the Opioid Growth Factor Receptor. *Brain Res Rev.* 2002:38:351-376.

ABOUT THE AUTHOR

Paul Battle, PA-C received his Physiology degree from University of California, Davis. He went on to complete his Physician Assistant training at Emory University School of Medicine in 1981. He is in practice at Boulder Longevity Institute and Barolat Neuroscience in Denver.

Chapter 4
New Treatment Modalities to Improve Immunity and Fight Infections

Eve E. Bralley, Ph.D.; David M. Brady, N.D., D.C., C.C.N., DACBN; Richard S. Lord, Ph.D;, J. Alexander Bralley, Ph.D.

ABSTRACT

The intestinal tract contains 80% of the body's immune system. Gut microbial balance has significant effects on immune status. New molecular techniques using polymerase chain reactions (PCR) allow for fast, accurate identification of gut microbes including anaerobes which were difficult to culture and quantitate using older methods. The recent rise in incidence of MRSA infections is becoming a significant problem. These new molecular techniques allow us to detect the presence of multiple genes conferring drug resistance in bacteria in a stool sample including mecA, the gene that confers resistance to methicillin. sIgA is a mainline defense against infection at mucosal linings. New data will be presented which associates deficiencies of sIgA in the gut with increased incidence of opportunistic microbial and parasitic infection.

Analysis of gut microbial balances, resistance genes and sIgA levels allows for unique treatment strategies to be developed which enhance immune function and fight infection. These strategies use individualized combinations of pre- and probiotics, anti-microbials, and gut-healing nutrients based on the test results of the patient. The aims of this paper are:
1. To learn how new molecular techniques can identify anaerobes and drug resistance genes using a single stool sample.
2. To learn how gut microbial balance, drug resistance genes and sIgA production can affect the immune system.
3. To learn how to effectively interpret laboratory results and design individualized treatment protocols that will enhance immune function and fight infection.

Keywords: PCR, dysbiosis, parasite, commensal immunity, drug resistance genes, anaerobic bacteria, secretory IgA.

INTRODUCTION

The intestinal tract contains 80% of the body's immune system. Gut microbial balance has significant effects on immune status.[1] New molecular techniques using polymerase chain reactions (PCR) allow for fast, accurate identification of gut microbes including anaerobes which were difficult to culture and quantitate using older methods. These new molecular techniques allow us to detect the presence of multiple genes conferring drug resistance in bacteria in a stool sample including mecA, the gene that confers resistance to methicillin.[2,3] Secretory IgA (sIgA) is a mainline defense against infection at mucosal linings.[4,5] New data will be presented which associates deficiencies of sIgA in the gut with increased incidence of parasitic infection.[6]

Analysis of gut microbial balances, parasites, drug resistance genes and sIgA levels allows for unique treatment strategies to be developed which enhance immune function and fight infection.[7] These individualized treatment strategies use combinations of pre- and probiotics, anti-microbials, and gut-healing nutrients based on the test results of the patient. The aims of this paper are:
1. To learn how new molecular techniques can identify anaerobes and drug resistance genes using a single stool sample.
2. To learn how gut microbial balance, drug resistance genes and sIgA production can affect the immune system.
3. To learn how to effectively interpret laboratory results and design individualized treatment protocols that will enhance immune function and fight infection.

THE IMPORTANCE OF MUCOSAL IMMUNITY

The population of the micro biota of the human gastrointestinal (GI) tract is widely diverse and complex, with a high population density. In the colon there are over 10^{11} bacterial cells per gram and over 400 different species. These bacterial cells outnumber host cells by at least a factor of 10.[8] This microbial population has important influences on host physiological, nutritional, and immunological processes. In fact, this biomass should more rightly be considered a rapidly adapting, renewable organ with considerable metabolic activity and significant influence on human health. Consequently, there is renewed and growing interest in identifying the types and activities of these gut microbes.[9]

The normal, healthy balance in micro biota provides colonization resistance to pathogens. Since anaerobes comprise over 95% of these organisms, their analysis is of prime importance. Overgrowth of any one of the more than 400 microbial species in the healthy human gut can produce adverse clinical effects. Excessive colonization of the gut by undesirable microorganisms alters the metabolic or immunologic status of the host.[10,11] When this state leads to disease or dysfunction, it has been termed "dysbiosis" to distinguish it from the correct balance denoted as orthobiosis.[12] Symptoms and conditions thought to be caused or complicated by dysbiosis include inflammatory bowel diseases, irritable bowel syndrome, inflammatory or autoimmune disorders, food allergy/sensitivity, atopic eczema, unexplained fatigue, arthritis, mental/emotional disorders in children and adults, malnutrition, and breast and colon cancer.[13-16]

Anaerobic bacteria are the predominant microorganisms in the human GI tract, outnumbering aerobes by a factor of 10,000 to 1. The most abundant and beneficial or benign anaerobes are *Bifidobacterium, Bacteroides, Fusobacterium, Clostridium, Eubacterium, Peptococcus,* and *Peptostreptococcus. Bifidobacterium* and *Lactobacillus spp.* can comprise up to 25% of the total flora in a healthy adult. A great many other species are present, but in lesser numbers.[17] An imbalance in proportion and numbers of these species can be induced by broad-spectrum antibiotic use. This leads to the dominance of other bacterial species, including *Pseudomonas, Enterobacter, Serratia, Klebsiella, Citrobacter, Proteus, Providencia,* and fungi, especially yeasts such as *Candida.* In health, the upper GI tract is sparsely populated with microorganisms. The gram-positive, facultative forms such as *Streptococcus, Staphylococcus,* and *Lactobacillus* typically survive gastric secretions and bile acids.[18] In the distal ileum concentrations of bacteria increase and the gram-negative bacteria such as *Bacteroides, Bifidobacterium, Fusobacterium,* and *Clostridium* outnumber the gram-positive species. Beyond the ileocecal valve, the bacterial concentration increases steeply to 10^{12} colony-forming units per milliliter of fecal material. By the time they are passed from the body in stools, the large majority of the bacteria are no longer viable.

ACCURATE IDENTIFICATION OF GUT MICROBES
Difficulties in Accurately Assessing Micro Biota Content

Most studies of micro biota in the GI tract have used fecal samples. These do not necessarily represent the populations along the entire GI tract from stomach to rectum. Conditions and species can alter greatly along this tract and generally run from lower to higher population densities. Fecal samples most appropriately represent organisms growing in the colon. In addition, >98% of fecal bacteria will not grow in the presence of oxygen. Therefore, standard fecal culture techniques miss the majority of organisms present.

Polymerase Chain Reaction (PCR)

One of the most important and profound contributions to molecular biology is the advent of the polymerase chain reaction (PCR). PCR, a DNA and RNA-based technology, is a powerful tool which can detect a unique DNA sequence of an infectious agent in any body fluid enabling fast and accurate identification. PCR does not depend on the ability of an organism to grow in culture. Furthermore, PCR is fast, sensitive, and capable of copying a single DNA sequence of a viable or non-viable cell over a billion times within 3-5 hours. In addition, PCR methodology requires only 1-5 cells for detection, whereas a positive culture requires an inoculum equivalent to about 1000 to 5000 cells, making PCR the most sensitive detection method available. (Approximately, 1,000 times more sensitive).[19]

Advantages of PCR amplifications of target microbial DNA for organism detection over traditional culture techniques are many:
- Ability to detect nonviable organisms that are not retrievable by culture based methods.
- Ability to detect and identify organisms that cannot be cultured or are extremely difficult to grow (e.g. anaerobes).
- More rapid detection and identification of organisms that grow slowly (e.g. mycobacterium and fungi).

- Ability to detect previously unknown organism directly in clinical specimens by using broad range DNA primers.
- Ability to quantitate infectious organisms' burden in patient specimens for better clinical responsiveness.

Conventional Versus New Technologies

Conventional bacteriological methods such as microscopy, culture, and identification are used for the analysis and/or quantification of the intestinal microbiota.[20-22] Limitations of conventional methods are their low sensitivities,[23] their inability to detect non-cultivatable bacteria and unknown species, their time-consuming aspects, and their low levels of reproducibility due to the multitude of species to be identified and quantified. In addition, the large differences in growth rates and growth requirements of the different species present in the human gut indicate that quantification by culture is bound to be inaccurate

Another problematic issue with present stool analysis procedures is that of transport time to the laboratory after collection. Culture dependent analysis requires the sample be collected in a nutrient broth to maintain microbial viability. The problem with this protocol is that it allows for continued growth of species during transport and until the sample is actually plated out for culture. Significant changes in the balance of microbes can occur, since some species will more actively grow at the expense of others, and each microbe has specific requirements for viability. DNA analysis eliminates this problem by placing the specimen in formalin vials for transport. The formalin immediately fixes all organisms, capturing the exact balance present at the time of collection.

Preliminary transport studies performed by Scott *et al* show a significant decrease in fecal *Bifidobacter sp.* from collection to 3 days in the nutrient broth mixture (Figure 1). In contrast, *Staphylococcus aureus* had a 5-fold increase in CFUs/gram of fecal matter in one day in the nutrient broth (Figure 2). *Candida sp.* also grew exponentially in the nutrient broth, and peaked on day two (Figure 3). The stool samples fixed in formalin provided consistent readings from collection to day 3. It is possible that due to this issue of transport, Candida infections have been grossly over-reported for decades.

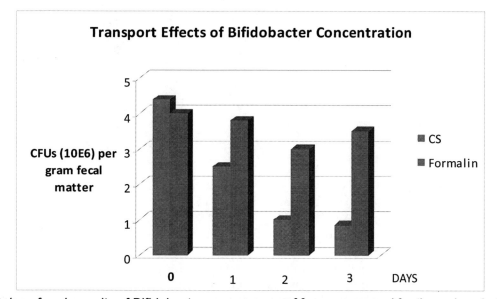

Figure 1: Colony forming units of Bifidobacter sp. per gram of feces measured for three days in fecal matter collected both in culture broth and formalin.

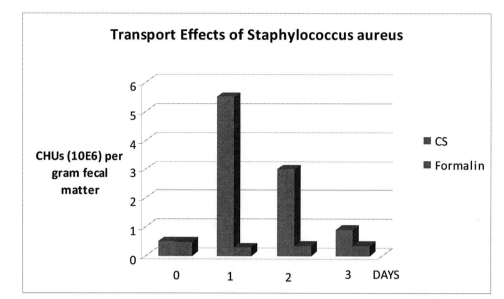

Figure 2: Colony forming units of Staphylococcus aureus per gram of feces measured for three days in fecal matter collected both in culture broth and formalin.

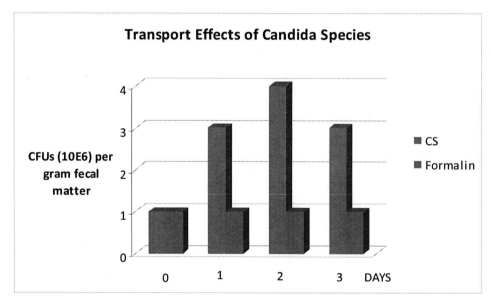

Figure 3: Colony forming units of Candida sp. per gram of feces measured for three days in fecal matter collected both in culture broth and formalin.

PARASITOLOGY

Parasitology is yet another field of microbiology to be greatly improved with genetic molecular technologies. Parasite infections are a major cause of nonviral diarrhea even in developed countries. Classically, parasites have been identified by microscopy and enzyme immunoassays.[24] In recent studies, molecular techniques have proven to be more sensitive and specific than classic laboratory methods.[24-26] Because Giardia cysts are shed sporadically and the number may vary from day to day, laboratories have adopted multiple stool collections to help increase identification rates for all parasite examinations.[26] And, even with the advent of antigen detection systems, there has long been uncertainty in diagnosis when no ova or parasites are found. Due to the nearly 100% sensitivity and specificity of DNA analysis combined with the need for very low amounts of genomic DNA (as low as 2.5 cells per gram),[26] the multiple specimen collections, and technically challenging microscopic identification have

24

been alleviated. With PCR technology, just one fecal sample is all that is needed for 100% sensitivity and specificity in parasitology examinations.

ANTIBIOTIC-RESISTANT GENES

The development of bacterial resistance to antibiotic drugs involves an active change or mutation in the microbial genome, which changes the microbe's metabolic or structural responsiveness to the mechanism of the drugs' action. This genetic change is passed in the population as cells replicate. This genetic material can also be passed on to other strains of bacteria through plasmid sharing. The development of antibiotic resistance is becoming a serious public health issue as overuse of antibiotics continually selects for mutated strains that have developed resistance.

The human intestinal micro biota represents over 400 species. All antibiotic resistance strategies that bacteria develop are encoded in one or more genes. These genes are readily shared among and across species and genera and even among distantly related bacteria. These genes confer resistance to different classes of drugs, and their sequences are known. Therefore, using PCR techniques, they can be readily detected in large populations such as those found in fecal material.

The knowledge of the presence of a drug resistance gene may be quite significant for the clinician when considering treatment of a patient for a pathogen infection. For example, suppose a pathogen is detected in a stool analysis. An analysis of the presence of antibiotic resistance genes is also performed on the sample. Subsequent drug sensitivities are then run on the pathogen and it is found to be sensitive to two antibiotics. But suppose there is also a drug resistant gene present in the sample to one of the drugs (a very possible scenario). It would be imperative, then, that this drug is not used in treating the patient. Otherwise, even though the pathogen is killed the other organisms that have the gene conferring resistance to the drug would thrive relative to other microbes present. This would set up a potentially dangerous situation, where antibiotic resistance is maintained in the population because that gene can be readily spread to other organisms present in the individual as well as the environment.[27,28] Knowledge of the presence of antibiotic-resistant genes in fecal specimens, therefore, represents a significant advance in the treatment of patients and maintenance of health.

SECRETORY IGA

The lymphoid tissue of the intestinal mucosa secretes immunoglobulin A into the lumen of the GI tract as a first line of defense against microbes and antigens. Produced by plasma cells at the basement membrane of the GI tract, two molecules of IgA are connected by protein chains connecting the heavy chains, forming dimeric sIgA that is transported to the luminal surface of the gut. The term sIgA denotes this difference from monomeric IgA measured in serum. Secretory IgA (sIgA) forms immune complexes with pathogens and allergens, which prevents them from binding to and penetrating the intestinal mucosa.[29] A high antigenic load can result in depressed sIgA, even in healthy, asymptomatic individuals. With time, this decrease in resistance can lead to dysbiosis and an increased risk of infection of parasites and allergy.[30,31]

Suppression of sIgA has also been associated with the stress response. The level of sIgA is down-regulated during periods of chronic stress, whereas acute stress induces mobilization and results in a transient increase in sIgA.[32-34] Reduced physical activity and excess body fat in children have also been demonstrated to result in decreased levels of sIgA and increased incidence of upper respiratory infection.[35] Relaxing activities have been demonstrated to increase positive effect and sIgA, while reducing negative effect and sIgA suppression.[36] Perhaps it is summarized best by Alshuler when she states, "*Cortisol suppresses secretory immunoglobulin A (sIgA) in the gastrointestinal tract, which leads to impaired gut antigen sampling. Furthermore, cortisol alters the consistency of the gastrointestinal mucosal barrier. The combined result of these effects is an enhanced immune response to gut-derived antigens and increased translocation of antigenic material to systemic circulation.*"[37] Stress plays an important role in the compromise of the gastrointestinal mucosal immune response and the development of pan-allergy to foods and potentially the development of autoimmune phenomena via antigen-antibody complex cross-reactivity and molecular mimicry. Fecal sIgA evaluation may be beneficial in the overall assessment of the stress response and the management of leaky gut, infection, food allergy, inflammatory arthritis, immunogenic thyroiditis, autoimmunity, and other chronic diseases.[38-48]

25

CASE REPORTS
Case Report 1
Clinical History

A 52-year-old male reported general good health, but was interested in losing weight. Clinician intake information revealed heartburn, gas, diarrhea, oral thrush, and a history of antibiotic use due to chronic diarrhea. Prevacid was used for heartburn relief.

Laboratory Results

A plasma IgG4 test revealed multiple food sensitivities with egg, milk, peanut, and wheat being severe (Figure 4). Stool testing revealed very low levels of the predominant bacteria, *Bacteroides spp.*, *Clostridia spp., and Bifidobacter spp.*, and infection with the opportunistic bacteria *Citrobacter spp.*, *Klebsiella oxytoca, and Salmonella spp.* (Figure 5). No yeast or parasites were identified. The drug-resistance gene, aacA/aphD, was positive indicating antibiotic resistance to the aminoglycoside class of drugs. Total short-chain fatty acids (SCFAs) were low and anti-gliadin antibody was very high. The stool test also revealed signs of maldigestion and malabsorption with elevated fecal triglycerides, vegetable fibers, and long-chain fatty acids (LCFAs) (Figure 6).

IgG Food Antibodies

Methodology: ELISA

Negative	Foods to Avoid		
	Mild **+1 and +2**	**Moderate** **+3 and +4**	**Severe** **+5**
Aspergillus Cantaloupe Corn Crab Lobster Oat Orange Pea, Green Pinto Bean Pork Salmon Shrimp Tomato Walnut	Beef Tuna Chicken Mustard Greens Rice Strawberry Turkey	Almond Cashew Garlic Sunflower Soybean	Egg, Whole Milk Peanut Wheat

Figure 4: IgG4 food antibody measurement in whole blood.

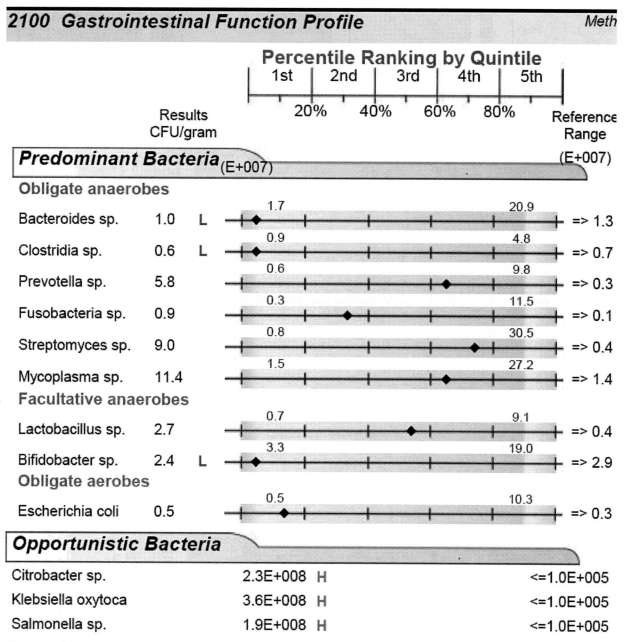

	Results CFU/gram			Reference Range

Predominant Bacteria (E+007)

Obligate anaerobes

Bacteroides sp.	1.0	L	=> 1.3
Clostridia sp.	0.6	L	=> 0.7
Prevotella sp.	5.8		=> 0.3
Fusobacteria sp.	0.9		=> 0.1
Streptomyces sp.	9.0		=> 0.4
Mycoplasma sp.	11.4		=> 1.4

Facultative anaerobes

Lactobacillus sp.	2.7		=> 0.4
Bifidobacter sp.	2.4	L	=> 2.9

Obligate aerobes

Escherichia coli	0.5		=> 0.3

Opportunistic Bacteria

Citrobacter sp.	2.3E+008	H	<=1.0E+005
Klebsiella oxytoca	3.6E+008	H	<=1.0E+005
Salmonella sp.	1.9E+008	H	<=1.0E+005

Figure 5: Measurement of predominant and opportunistic bacteria in feces using molecular techniques including PCR.

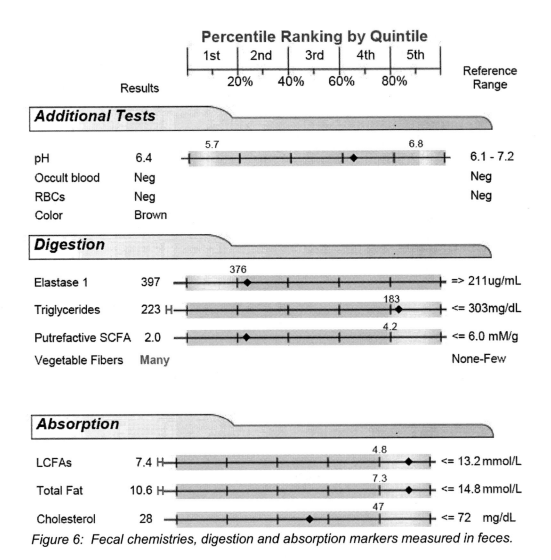

Figure 6: Fecal chemistries, digestion and absorption markers measured in feces.

Treatment

The clinician did not want to treat the opportunistic bacteria with antibiotics due to his history of heavy antibiotic use. Her main focus was healing the gut by removing offending foods, reinoculating with good bacteria, and repairing the intestinal permeability as determined by the multiple IgG food sensitivities. The patient was prescribed a gluten-free diet, high-dose *Bifidobacter spp.* probiotic, a prebiotic formula containing inulin, oligofructose, beta-glucan, and larch arabinogalactan, soluble and insoluble fiber, digestive enzymes, high-dose glutamine powder, and betaine hydrochloride with pepsin. The patient was recommended to discontinue the Prevacid.

Follow-up (3 months)

Bowel movements are becoming more formed and patient has begun to lose weight. Follow-up testing revealed a shift in the predominant bacteria, but still not in balanced proportions. *Citrobacter spp.*, and *Salmonella spp.* are gone. *Klebsiella oxytoca* is still present but the infection has decreased from 2.0 E+008 CFU's to 3.6 E+008 CFU's/gram of stool. Anti-gliadin antibody has decreased, but he still has low total SCFAs, elevated triglycerides, vegetable fibers, and LCFAs. The clinician continued current protocol, but added colostrum and increased the dose of betaine hydrochloride because he still suffered from heartburn.

Follow-up (9 months)

Patient was mentally unprepared to accept how dramatic his improvements in his health and vitality were. He had a 65-pound weight loss, and normal, formed bowel movements 2-3 times per day. He no longer suffers from heartburn, or gas.

Follow-up IgG4 testing showed an improvement from 16 food sensitivities (5 severe) to 3, with egg and milk still severe. Predominant bacteria are relatively balanced with *Bacteroides spp., Clostridia spp., and Bifidobacter spp* in normal range and no opportunistic bacteria present. Digestion and absorption markers have normalized with the exception of vegetable fibers.

Discussion

The patient's heavy use of antibiotics in the past has resulted in dysbiosis. The gut microbial population is important in colonization resistance, and the protection of the epithelial layer of the intestines. In this patient's case, dysbiosis was accompanied with opportunistic bacterial infection and severe intestinal permeability. The use of Prevacid, an acid blocker, only worsened the symptoms by sustaining hypochlorhydria, which directly affects digestion. The clinician's approach of removing gluten, reinoculating the healthy bacteria, and providing nutrient and immune support to the intestinal wall worked to improve the patient's overall health and well-being.

Case Report 2
Clinical History

A 45-year-old female presents with chronic gastrointestinal pain, gas, and bloating. She has been previously diagnosed with and treated for Cryptosporidium and Blastocystis hominis. She has a highly stressful life working full-time and raising three children, one with special needs.

Laboratory Results

A gastrointestinal function profile was run. Most parameters were normal with the exception of the presence of three parasites, and a low total fecal sIgA (Figure 7).

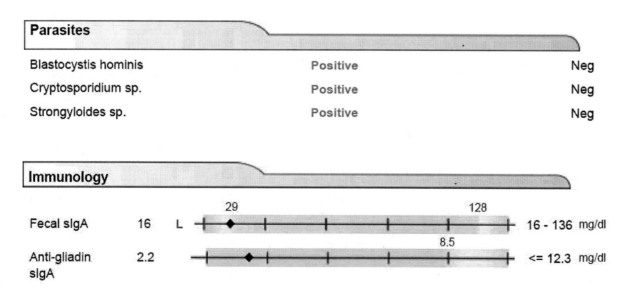

Figure 7. Gastrointestinal function profile.

Often times when fecal sIgA is low, the ability to fight off pathogens is hindered. In this case example the patient has three parasites, and a very low fecal sIgA. Working on increasing sIgA production is paramount to treating the parasite infection. When treating parasites alone, without improving gut mucosal health and sIgA production, the likelihood for re-infection is high.

Treatment

The clinician recommended high dose glutamine powder (10g/day), *Saccharomyces boulardii*, fish oil, multi-vitamin mineral and adrenal support including the calming herbs Rhodiola, and Ashwaganda, Lemon Balm, and Valerian. The clinician also counseled on stress reduction techniques, and mindful eating.

Follow-up (6 months)

The patient reports almost complete relief from symptoms. Her energy level has improved, and is more able to cope with stressful events in her life. Follow-up lab testing revealed an increase in total sIgA, and an absence of parasites.

Discussion

Intestinal function was restored by working on managing stress, supporting adrenal function, and repairing the epithelial layer. Gut immunity was improved, allowing for proper eradication of parasites humans are frequently exposed to.

CONCLUDING REMARKS

The use of new molecular techniques allows for more accurate assessment of gut microbial populations, parasites, drug resistance genes, and secretory IgA levels that can be used to develop unique treatment strategies to improve human health, and patient outcomes.

REFERENCES

1. Macpherson AJ, Harris NL. Interactions between commensal intestinal bacteria and the immune system. *Nat Rev Immunol.* 2004;4:478-485.
2. Mohanasoundaram KM, Lalitha MK. Comparison of phenotypic versus genotypic methods in the detection of methicillin resistance in *Staphylococcus aureus*. *Indian J Med Res.* 2008;127:78-84.
3. Krishnan PU, Miles K, Shetty N. Detection of methicillin and mupirocin resistance in Staphylococcus aureus isolates using conventional and molecular methods: a descriptive study from a burns unit with high prevalence of MRSA. *J Clin Pathol.* 2002;55:745-748.
4. Fagarasan S. Evolution, development, mechanism and function of IgA in the gut. *Curr Opin Immunol.* 2008;20:170-177.
5. Suzuki K, Ha SA, Tsuji M, Fagarasan S. Intestinal IgA synthesis: a primitive form of adaptive immunity that regulates microbial communities in the gut. *Semin Immunol.* 2007;19:127-135.
6. Bungiro RD, Jr., Sun T, Harrison LM, Shoemaker CB, Cappello M. Mucosal antibody responses in experimental hookworm infection. *Parasite Immunol.* 2008;30:293-303.
7. Tlaskalova-Hogenova H, Stepankova R, Hudcovic T, et al. Commensal bacteria (normal microflora), mucosal immunity and chronic inflammatory and autoimmune diseases. *Immunol Lett.* 2004;93:97-108.
8. Rowland IR. Toxicology of the colon: Role of the intestinal microflora. In: Gibson G, MacFarlane G, eds. *Human Colonic Bacteria: Role in Nutrition, Physiology, and Pathology.* Boca Raton, FL: CRC Press; 1995:292.
9. Mackie RI, Sghir A, Gaskins HR. Developmental microbial ecology of the neonatal gastrointestinal tract. *Am J Clin Nutr.* 1999;69:1035S-1045S.
10. Van Eldere J, Robben J, De Pauw G, Merckx R, Eyssen H. Isolation and identification of intestinal steroid-desulfating bacteria from rats and humans. *Appl Environ Microbiol.* 1988;54:2112-2117.
11. Rogers GB, Carroll MP, Serisier DJ, *et al.* Use of 16S rRNA gene profiling by terminal restriction fragment length polymorphism analysis to compare bacterial communities in sputum and mouthwash samples from patients with cystic fibrosis. *J Clin Microbiol.* 2006;44:2601-2604.
12. Galland L, Barrie S. Intestinal dysbiosis and the causes of diseases. *J Advancement Med.* 1993;6:67-82.
13. Braun J, Sieper J. Rheumatologic manifestations of gastrointestinal disorders. *Curr Opin Rheumatol.* 1999;11:68-74.
14. Aydin SZ, Atagunduz P, Temel M, Bicakcigil M, Tasan D, Direskeneli H. Anti-Saccharomyces cerevisiae antibodies (ASCA) in spondyloarthropathies: a reassessment. *Rheumatology (Oxford).* 2008;47:142-144.

15. Scanu AM, Bull TJ, Cannas S, et al. Mycobacterium avium subspecies paratuberculosis infection in cases of irritable bowel syndrome and comparison with Crohn's disease and Johne's disease: common neural and immune pathogenicities. *J Clin Microbiol.* 2007;45:3883-3890.

16. Penders J, Stobberingh EE, van den Brandt PA, Thijs C. The role of the intestinal micro biota in the development of atopic disorders. *Allergy.* 2007;62:1223-1236.

17. Moore WE, Holdeman LV. Human fecal flora: the normal flora of 20 Japanese-Hawaiians. *Appl Microbiol.* 1974;27:961-979.

18. Draser BS, Hill MJ. *Human Intestinal Flora.* New York, NY: Academic Press; 1974.

19. Forbes BA, Sahm DF, Weissfeld AS, Baron EJ. *Bailey & Scott's diagnostic microbiology.* 10th ed. St. Louis, MO: Mosby; 1998.

20. O'Sullivan DJ. Methods of analysis of the intestinal microflora. In: Tannock GW, ed. *Probiotics: a critical review.* Wymondham, UK: Horizon Scientific Press; 1999:23-44.

21. Tannock GW. Analysis of the intestinal microflora: a renaissance. *Antonie Van Leeuwenhoek.* 1999;76:265-278.

22. Finegold SM, Rolfe RD. Susceptibility testing of anaerobic bacteria. *Diagn Microbiol Infect Dis.* 1983;1:33-40.

23. Dutta S, Chatterjee A, Dutta P, et al. Sensitivity and performance characteristics of a direct PCR with stool samples in comparison to conventional techniques for diagnosis of Shigella and enteroinvasive *Escherichia coli* infection in children with acute diarrhoea in Calcutta, India. *J Med Microbiol.* 2001;50:667-674.

24. Verweij JJ, Blange RA, Templeton K, et al. Simultaneous detection of *Entamoeba histolytica, Giardia lamblia,* and *Cryptosporidium parvum* in fecal samples by using multiplex real-time PCR. *J Clin Microbiol.* 2004;42:1220-1223.

25. Morgan UM, Pallant L, Dwyer BW, Forbes DA, Rich G, Thompson RC. Comparison of PCR and microscopy for detection of *Cryptosporidium parvum* in human fecal specimens: clinical trial. *J Clin Microbiol.* 1998;36:995-998.

26. Ghosh S, Debnath A, Sil A, De S, Chattopadhyay DJ, Das P. PCR detection of Giardia lamblia in stool: targeting intergenic spacer region of multicopy rRNA gene. *Mol Cell Probes.* 2000;14:181-189.

27. Bergeron MG, Ouellette M. Preventing antibiotic resistance through rapid genotypic identification of bacteria and of their antibiotic resistance genes in the clinical microbiology laboratory. *J Clin Microbiol.* 1998;36:2169-2172.

28. Martineau F, Picard FJ, Grenier L, Roy PH, Ouellette M, Bergeron MG. Multiplex PCR assays for the detection of clinically relevant antibiotic resistance genes in staphylococci isolated from patients infected after cardiac surgery. The ESPRIT Trial. *J Antimicrob Chemother.* 2000;46:527-534.

29. Brandtzaeg P, Bjerke K, Kett K, *et al.* Production and secretion of immunoglobulins in the gastrointestinal tract. *Ann Allergy.* 1987;59(5 Pt 2):21-39.

30. Schreiber RA, Walker WA. Food allergy: facts and fiction. *Mayo Clin Proc.* 1989;64:1381-1391.

31. Cunningham-Rundles C. Analysis of the gastrointestinal secretory immune barrier in IgA deficiency. *Ann Allergy.* 1986;57:31-35.

32. Hucklebridge F, Clow A, Evans P. The relationship between salivary secretory immunoglobulin A and cortisol: neuroendocrine response to awakening and the diurnal cycle. *Int J Psychophysiol.* 1998;31:69-76.

33. Hucklebridge F, Lambert S, Clow A, Warburton DM, Evans PD, Sherwood N. Modulation of secretory immunoglobulin A in saliva; response to manipulation of mood. *Biol Psychol.* 2000;53:25-35.

34. Kugler J, Reintjes F, Tewes V, Schedlowski M. Competition stress in soccer coaches increases salivary. Immunoglobin A and salivary cortisol concentrations. *J Sports Med Phys Fitness.* 1996;36:117-120.

35. Cieslak TJ, Frost G, Klentrou P. Effects of physical activity, body fat, and salivary cortisol on mucosal immunity in children. *J Appl Physiol.* 2003;95:2315-2320.

36. Kreutz G, Bongard S, Rohrmann S, Hodapp V, Grebe D. Effects of choir singing or listening on secretory immunoglobulin A, cortisol, and emotional state. *J Behav Med.* 2004;2:623-635.

37. Alshuler L. Stress: Thief in the Night. *Int J Integrative Med.* 2001;3.

38. Ansaldi N, Palmas T, Corrias A, *et al.* Autoimmune thyroid disease and celiac disease in children. *J Pediatr Gastroenterol Nutr.* 2003;37:63-66.

39. Gladman D. Gastrointestinal-related arthritis and psoriatic arthritis. *Curr Opin Rheumatol.* 1991;3:575-580.

40. Marker-Hermann E, Schwab P. T-cell studies in the spondyloarthropathies. *Curr Rheumatol Rep.* 2000;2:297-305.
41. Martinez-Gonzalez O, Cantero-Hinojosa J, Paule-Sastre P, Gomez-Magan JC, Salvatierra-Rios D. Intestinal permeability in patients with ankylosing spondylitis and their healthy relatives. *Br J Rheumatol.* 1994;33:644-647.
42. Mielants H. Reflections on the link between intestinal permeability and inflammatory joint disease. *Clin Exp Rheumatol.* 1990;8:523-524.
43. Petru G, Stunzner D, Lind P, Eber O, Mose JR. [Antibodies to Yersinia enterocolitica in immunogenic thyroid diseases]. *Acta Med Austriaca.* 1987;14:11-14.
44. Pishak OV. [The colonization resistance of the mucous membrane of the large intestine in patients with rheumatoid arthritis in a period of exacerbation]. *Mikrobiol Z.* 1999;61:41-47.
45. Stebbings S, Munro K, Simon MA, *et al.* Comparison of the faecal microflora of patients with ankylosing spondylitis and controls using molecular methods of analysis. *Rheumatology (Oxford).* 2002;41:1395-1401.
46. Takuno H, Sakata S, Miura K. Antibodies to *Yersinia enterocolitica* serotype 3 in autoimmune thyroid diseases. *Endocrinol Jpn.* 1990;37:489-500.
47. Tiwana H, Walmsley RS, Wilson C, *et al.* Characterization of the humoral immune response to Klebsiella species in inflammatory bowel disease and ankylosing spondylitis. *Br J Rheumatol.* 1998;37:525-531.
48. Tomer Y, Davies TF. Infection, thyroid disease, and autoimmunity. *Endocr Rev.* 1993;14:107-120.
49. Hoverstad R. The normal microflora and short-chain fatty acids. Paper presented at: Proceedings of the Fifth Bengt E. Gustafsson Symposium; June 1-4, 1988; Stockholm, Sweden.

ABOUT THE AUTHOR

Primary author Dr. Eve Bralley has several years of experience in Integrative and Functional Medicine as a certified clinical nutritionist, educator, and researcher. She completed her Ph.D. in Pharmacology from the University of Georgia, with emphasis in nutraceutical product development. She currently works with Metametrix Clinical Laboratory and is involved in physician consultations, product development, and research.

Chapter 5
New Research on Molecular Mechanisms and Prevention of Alzheimer's Disease

Stanislaw R. Burzynski, M.D., Ph.D.,
Founder & President, Burzynski Clinic (Houston, Texas, USA)

ABSTRACT

Alzheimer's disease (AD) was first described more than a century ago. During the last 25 years, it has been accepted that abnormal proteins forming amyloid-β (Aβ) plaques and tau tangles are responsible for the pathology of the disease. Despite the availability of drugs, which were developed to prevent the formation of these abnormal proteins, minimal progress has been made in the treatment and prevention of AD.

Our research indicates that amyloid precursor protein (APP) is involved not only in the pathology of AD, but also plays an important physiological role in the consolidation of memory. For this reason, therapy for AD should attempt to normalize the mechanism involved in memory processing in addition to a strategy to block formation of pathogenic proteins, and repair damage caused by them. Our study indicates that during the early phase of memory consolidation there is a possibility for formation of the following fragments of APP: spectrin-like, p47-like protein, and peptide recognition tag scotophobin (SP). We propose that the normal function of APP and its homologues is to facilitate memory processing during the initial stage until protein synthesis takes place. Ultimately, the synthesis of new proteins, rather than the formation of APP fragments, decides whether an experience is translated into long-term memory.

Based on the results of research done by our team and experiments conducted by others, we introduced Supplement B, which may correct abnormal mechanisms and improve AD-related decrease of memory. The supplement consists of phenylacetylglutamine (PG), curcumin, and piperine. PG may facilitate the formation of physiological fragments of APP, and decrease Aβ and tau protein-related neurodegeneration. Curcumin decreases generation of Aβ, inflammation, neurodegeneration, oxidative damage, and reduces tau-phosphorylation. The addition of piperine markedly increases absorption and concentration of curcumin and PG in blood.

In conclusion, it is proposed that the physiological function of APP is to facilitate consolidation of memory. The abnormal activity of genes in AD and resulting damage and impairment of brain function can be addressed through the use of supplements containing PG, curcumin, and piperine. These claims need to be supported through further animal research and human clinical trials.

Keywords: Alzheimer's disease, amyloid-β, APP, memory consolidation, curcumin, phenylacetylglutamine.

INTRODUCTION

Alzheimer's disease (AD) was first described more than a century ago. At present, it is the most common neurodegenerative disease, with more than 20 million cases worldwide and approximately 5 million new cases each year.[1,2] During the last 25 years, it has been accepted that abnormal proteins forming amyloid-β (Aβ) plaques and tau tangles are responsible for the pathology of the disease.[1] Despite the availability of drugs, which were developed to prevent the formation of these abnormal proteins, minimal progress has been made in the treatment and prevention of AD.[2]

Our research indicates that amyloid precursor protein (APP) is involved not only in the pathology of AD, but also plays an important physiological role in the consolidation of memory.[3] For this reason, therapy for AD should attempt to normalize the mechanism involved in memory processing in addition to a strategy to block formation of pathogenic proteins, and repair damage caused by them.

This paper will offer a brief history of AD and the molecular mechanisms of AD, and will present the research of our team at Burzynski Clinic (Drs. Elwira Ilkowska-Musial and Stanislaw R. Burzynski) and Accelrys, Inc. (Dr. Anna Tempczyk-Russell). The possibility of using the results of these studies and the formulation of a supplement B to help decrease of memory will also be discussed.

THE HISTORY AND PATHOLOGY OF ALZHEIMER'S DISEASE

In April 1906, in Frankfurt, Germany, a 56-year-old patient named Auguste D died of a disease characterized by progressive memory loss, hallucinations, and neurological symptoms. The patient's physician, Dr. Alois Alzheimer analyzed her brain by using newly developed silver staining methods, which helped him to identify two types of abnormal deposits: neuritic plaques and neurofibrillary tangles.[1] Six months later, Dr Alzheimer presented his findings at the 37th Meeting of the Society of Southwest German Psychiatrists in Tubingen, Germany and described a new disease, named after him by Emil Kraepelin as Alzheimer's disease (Figure 1).

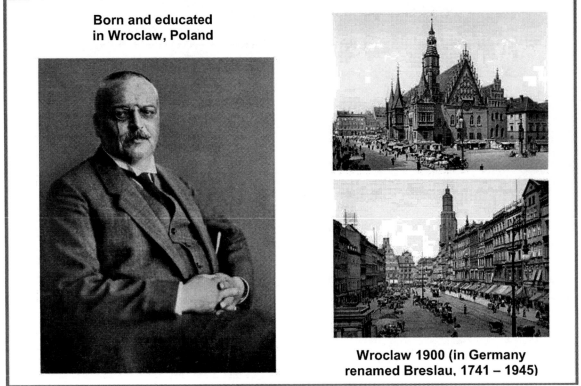

Born and educated in Wroclaw, Poland

Wroclaw 1900 (in Germany renamed Breslau, 1741 – 1945)

Figure 1. Dr Alois Alzheimer

Over the past quarter of a century, after the chemistry of the pathological deposits was explained, two molecules have enjoyed a doubtful fame: 1) Aβ and 2) the microtubule-binding protein tau. Most of the research conducted concentrated on Aβ. In 1984, Glenner and Wong formulated the "amyloid hypothesis".[4] According to this hypothesis, Aβ accumulation results in the formation of neuritic plaques which are responsible for the death of neurons. Current research proves that this hypothesis does not provide sufficient explanation.[5] Synaptic function – synaptic plasticity and long-term potentiation (LTP) – is damaged before detection of Aβ deposits in mouse models of AD.[6] It was found that Aβ is derived from asymmetric cleavage of APP, and both Aβ and APP are normal products of the neurons[7,8] (Figure 2).

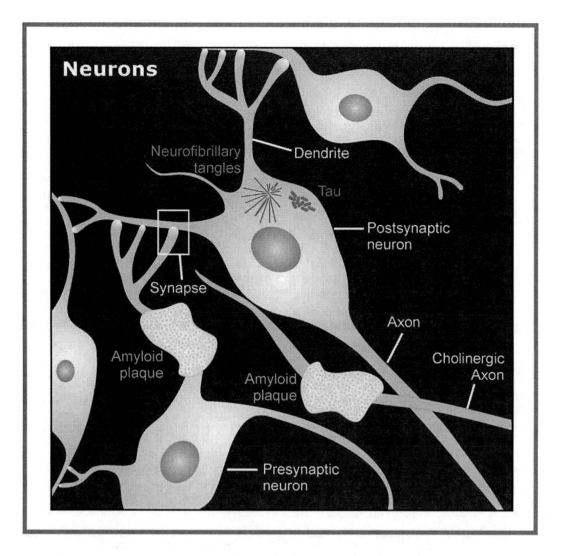

Figure 2. Amyloid Plaques and Neurofibrillary Tangles are Important Pathological Features of Alzheimer's Disease

AMYLOID PRECURSOR PROTEIN

The APP superfamily contains 34 proteins: APP (8 human and 8 rat isoforms) and the amyloid precursor-like proteins APLP1 (3 human and 4 rat isoforms) and APLP2 (3 human and 8 rat isoforms)[9] (Figure 3).

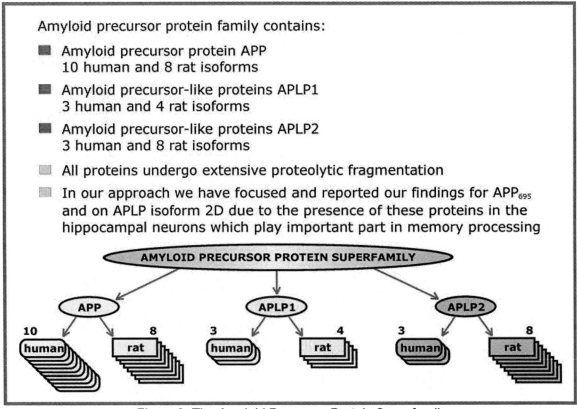

Amyloid precursor protein family contains:

- Amyloid precursor protein APP
  10 human and 8 rat isoforms

- Amyloid precursor-like proteins APLP1
  3 human and 4 rat isoforms

- Amyloid precursor-like proteins APLP2
  3 human and 8 rat isoforms

- All proteins undergo extensive proteolytic fragmentation

- In our approach we have focused and reported our findings for APP$_{695}$ and on APLP isoform 2D due to the presence of these proteins in the hippocampal neurons which play important part in memory processing

Figure 3. The Amyloid Precursor Protein Superfamily

In our approach, we have focused and reported our findings for APP$_{695}$ and APLP isoform 2D due to their evident presence in the hippocampal neurons, which play an important role in memory processing. APP$_{695}$ consists of 695 amino acids and is inserted into the neuronal membrane. Only a small fragment is present inside the neuron, but most of the protein is winding outside the cell as extracellular domain consisting of growth factor like domain (GFLD), copper-binding domain (CuBd), acidic, central APP domain (CAPPD), and a linker which connect to transmembrane and APP intracellular domain (AICD) (Figure 4).

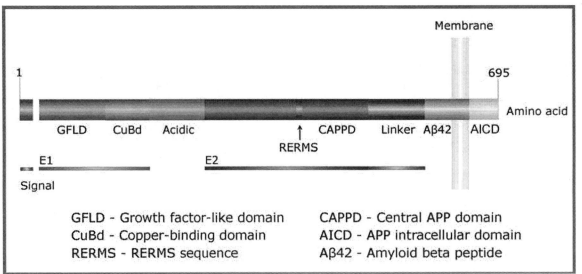

Figure 4. The Domain Structure of Amyloid Precursor Protein

During memory processing, APP is broken down into numerous fragments by a number of proteolytic enzymes; the best known are α-, β-, and γ-secretases.[10] Alpha-secretase activity was found in three enzymes: ADAM9, ADAM10, and ADAM17 (α-disintegrin and metalloproteinase family enzyme).[11] β-secretase was identified as BACE1 (β-site APP-cleaving enzyme 1). The γ-secretase is a complex consisting of presenilin1 and 2 (PS1 and PS2), nicastrin, anterior pharynx-defective, and presenilin enhancer 2.

There are two different pathways for processing APP: physiological non-amyloidogenic pathway and pathological amyloidogenic pathway (Figure 5). In the physiological pathway, APP is cleaved by α- and γ-secretase and Aβ is not formed. However, in the pathological pathway, the cleavage is done by β- and γ-secretase and results in formation of Aβ.

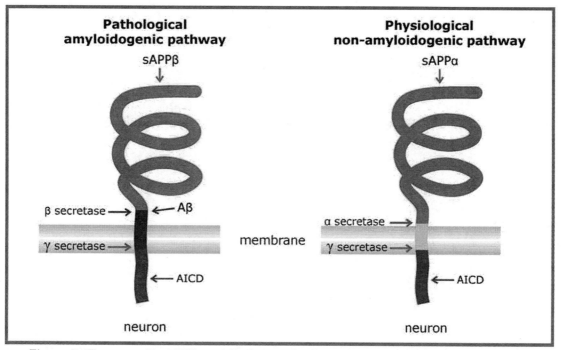

Figure 5. There are Two Different Pathways for Processing Amyloid Precursor Protein

α-secretase activity, which releases soluble APP α (sAPPα) into the extracellular space, occurs very early in the acquisition of memory.[12] Both sAPPα and Aβ are transported inside the neuron through clathrin-coated pits and processed in endosomes, the Golgi system, and the endoplasmic reticulum (Figure 6).[13] The resulting protein fragments are transported to the membrane and can be secreted to the extracellular space. Some Aβ and APP fragments may remain outside the neuron since the beginning. The fate of APP fragments other than Aβ is not well studied.

In addition to forming amyloid plaques, Aβ localizes at synapses and leads to synaptic degeneration.[11] Venkitaramani et al found that small aggregates (oligomers) of Aβ are the most damaging and most disruptive to memory and learning.[5] Whilst Almeida et al[14] and Gregori et al[15] found that Aβ interferes with protein sorting and trafficking and inhibits mitochondria and proteasome and ubiquitin function.

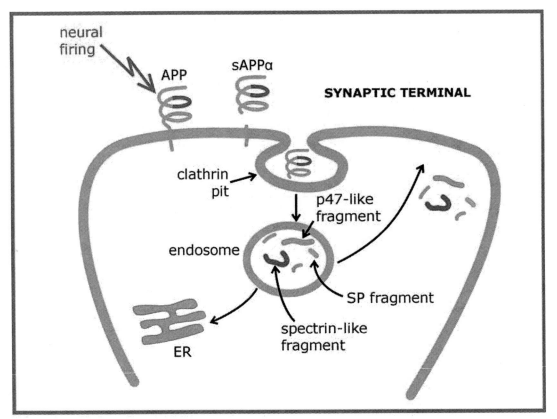

Figure 6. Formation of Amyloid Precursor Protein Fragments During Early Memory Consolidation

THE STAGES OF MEMORY

Memories originate from the connections between neurons at the synapses where the axon of one neuron meets any of the adjacent neuron dendrites.[16] Frequent firing of synapses activates protein synthesis and formation of postsynaptic density. A new postsynaptic terminal is then formed through dendritic spine. Long-term memory is stored in specific neuronal circuits. It is proposed that specific circuits have peptide recognition tags.

Proposed Physiological Role of Amyloid Precursor Protein

Our research indicates the existence of a spectrin-like structure formed by acidic and RERMS-containing domains, the resemblance of the secondary structure of CAPPD fragment to the adaptor protein p47, and the presence of amino acid motifs of peptide tag scotophobin (SP) in CAPPD and the intracellular domains of APP.[3] Fragments of spectrin and p47 play an important part in early memory consolidation, actin polymerization, and maturation and cycling of synaptic vesicles. In addition, SP motifs may form synaptic tags. The following discussion briefly reviews these three mechanisms.

Neural firing, which induces memory, causes a marked increase of actin in dendrites and dendritic spines.[17] Dynamic changes in the actin cytoskeleton are essential for remodeling of dendritic spines.[18] Actin polymerization in dendrites and dendritic spines occurs within the first two minutes of electric stimulation, but is not sufficient for memory consolidation.[19] The initial step involves depolarization, which is followed by an influx of calcium inside the neuron through NMDA receptors.[20] Calcium activates enzymes sensitive to calcium, such as calpain and kinases.[21] Calpain causes the breakdown of spectrin, which is necessary for stabilization of actin filaments.[22] This leads to the formation of a framework on which the neuritic spine assumes the final configuration and becomes the postsynaptic terminal.[19] The actin network binds spectrin, which is responsible for it's attachment to the membrane.[23] Based on the results of our study, spectrin-like fragments of APP may repolymerize with actin and help attach the actin network to the membrane, influencing the shape and chemistry of synapses.

38

A different process takes part in a presynaptic terminal. The primordial presynaptic site is converted into a mature presynaptic active zone within 15-60 minutes.[24] The integral part of this process is maturation and priming of synaptic vesicles. Protein p47 participates in this process and activates the complex that regulates the function of synaptic vesicles (SNARE complex).[25]

Synaptic tags or labels were proposed as the mechanisms to assure synaptic specificity during memory processing.[26] Peptide SP was introduced by Ungar as a synaptic label.[26] It is proposed that SP motifs released during fragmentation of APP and related proteins may form peptide recognition tags.[3]

To summarize, our study indicates the possibility of the formation of spectrin-like fragments of APP, the p47-like protein, and peptide recognition tags, during the early phase of memory consolidation. We propose that the normal function of the APPs and their homologs is to facilitate memory processing during the initial stage until protein synthesis takes place. Ultimately, the synthesis of new proteins, rather than the formation of APP fragments, decides whether an experience is translated into a long-term memory.[27] These claims, however, require confirmation by further studies in biological systems.

SUPPLEMENTS WHICH MAY IMPROVE ALZHEIMER'S DISEASE-RELATED DECREASE OF MEMORY

Based on the results of research done by our team and the experiments conducted by others, we introduced supplement B, which may correct abnormal mechanisms and improve AD-related decrease of memory (Figure 7).[28]

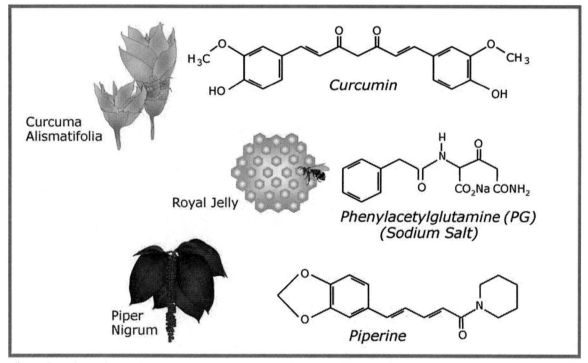

Figure 7. Supplement B Contains Phenylacetylglutamine, Curcumin, and Piperine

The supplement consists of phenylacetylglutamine (PG), curcumin, and piperine. PG may facilitate the formation of physiological fragments of APP through the increased expression of actin 87, neprilysin, and septin. Its antioxidant and anti-inflammatory properties may also reduce the damage caused by Aβ (Figure 8). PG can also decrease tau protein-related neurodegeneration through expression of α-tubulin, and promote tissue repair by increasing signaling through the hedgehog pathway and decreasing signaling by the Notch and Akt pathways (Figure 9). Curcumin decreases the formation of Aβ, inflammation, neurodegeneration, and oxidative damage (Figure 10). It also reduces tau hyperphosphorylation. Animal testing and human clinical trials have confirmed the benefits of curcumin in the treatment of AD. The addition of piperine markedly increases the absorption and concentration of curcumin (up to 20 times) and PG in blood.

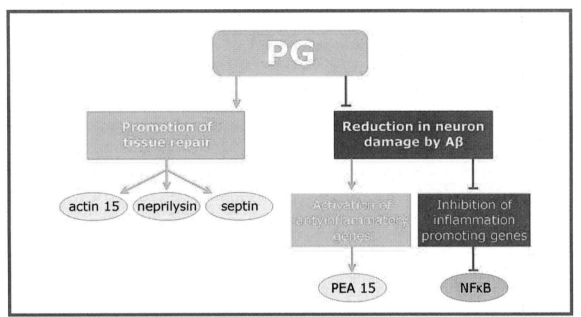

Figure 8. PG Promotes Physiological Activity of Amyloid Precursor Protein and Protects Against Aβ

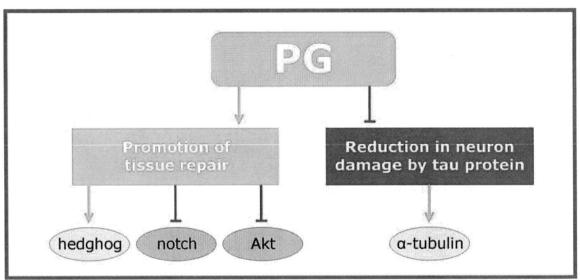

Figure 9. PG Promotes Tissue Repair and Protects Against Tau Protein

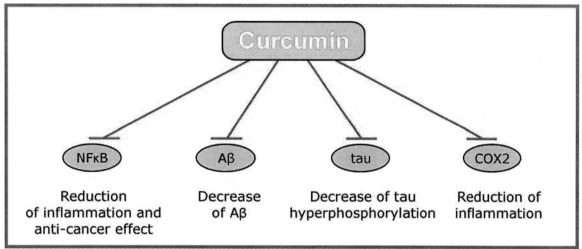

Figure 10. Effect of Curcumin on Genes in Alzheimer's Disease

CONCLUDING REMARKS

It is proposed that the physiological function of APP is to facilitate consolidation of memory. The abnormal activity of genes in AD causes abnormal APP processing and decrease of memory. The pathological activity of these genes may be normalized through the use of supplements containing PG, curcumin, and piperine. However, these claims need to be supported through further animal research and human clinical trials.

REFERENCES

1. Goedert M, Spillantini MG. A century of Alzheimer's disease. *Science* 2006;314:777-781.
2. Roberson ED, Mucke L. 100 years and counting: Prospects for defeating Alzheimer's disease. *Science* 2006;314:781-784.
3. Burzynski SR, Tempczyk-Russell A, Ilkowska-Musial E. Amyloid precursor protein (APP) and related protein fragmentation in consolidation of memory. Presented at Neuroscience 2007, the Society's Annual Meeting; November 3-7, 2007; Sand Diego, California.
4. Glenner GG, Wong CW. Alzheimer's disease and Down's syndrome: sharing of a unique cerebrovascular amyloid fibril protein. *Biochem Biophys Res Commun.* 1984;122:1131-1135.
5. Venkitaramani DV, Chin J, Netzer WJ, Gouras GK, Lesne S, Malinow R, Lombroso PJ. B-amyloid modulation of synaptic transmission and plasticity. *J Neurosci.* 2007;27:11832-11837.
6. Hsia AY, Masliah E, McConlogue L, Yu GQ, Tatsuno G, Hu K, Kholodenko D, Malenka RC, Nicoll RA, Mucke L. Plaque-independent disruption of neural circuits in Alzheimer's disease mouse models. *Proc Natl Acad Sci USA.* 1999;96:3228-3233.
7. Masters CL, Simms G, Weinman NA, Multhaup G, McDonald BL, Beyreuther K. Amyloid plaque core protein in Alzheimer disease and Down syndrome. *Proc Natl Acad Sci USA.* 1985;82:4245-4249.
8. Haass C, Schlossmacher MG, Hung AY, Vigo-Pelfrey C, Mellon A, Ostaszewski BL, Lieberburg I, Koo EH, Schenk D, Teplow DB, Selkoe DJ. Amyloid β-peptide is produced by cultured cells during normal metabolism. *Nature* 1992;359:322-325.
9. LeBlanc AC, Xue R, Gambetti P. Amyloid precursor protein metabolism in primary cell cultures of neurons, astrocytes, and microglia. *J Neurochem.* 1996;66:2300-2310.
10. Reinhard C, Hebert SS, De Strooper B. The amyloid-β precursor protein: integrating structure with biological function. *EMBO J.* 2005;24:3996-4006.
11. LaFerla FM, Green KN, Oddo, S. Intracellular amyloid-β in Alzheimer's disease. *Nat Rev Neurosci.* 2007;8:499-509.
12. Nitsch RM, Slack BE, Wurtman RJ, Growdon JH. Release of Alzheimer amyloid precursor derivatives stimulated by activation of muscarinic acetylcholine receptors. *Science* 1992;258:304-307.
13. Conboy L, Murphy KJ, Regan CM. Amyloid precursor protein expression in the rat hippocampal dentate gyrus modulates during memory consolidation. *J Neurochem.* 2005;95:1677-1688.
14. Almeida CG, Takahashi RH, Gouras GK. β-amyloid accumulation impairs multivesicular body sorting by inhibiting the ubiquitin-proteasome system. *J Neurosci.* 2006;26:4277-4288.

15. Gregori L, Fuchs C, Figueiredo-Pereira ME, Van Nostrand WE, Goldgaber D. Amyloid β-protein inhibits ubiquitin-dependent protein degradation *in vitro*. *J Biol Chem*. 1995;270:19702-19708.
16. Burzynski SR. Genetics of brain aging (II): Genetic mechanisms in encoding and consolidation of memory. In: Klatz R, Goldman R, eds. *Anti-Aging Therapeutics Volume IX*. Chicago, IL: A4M; 2007:79-88.
17. Lin B, Kramar EA, Bi X, Brucher FA, Gall CM, Lynch G. Theta stimulation polymerizes actin in dendritic spines of hippocampus. *J Neurosci*. 2005;25:2062-2069.
18. Segura I, Essmann CL, Weinges S, Acker-Palmer A. Grb4 and GIT1 transduce ephrinB reverse signals modulating spine morphogenesis and synapse formation. *Nat Neurosci*. 2007;10:301-310.
19. Lynch G, Rex CS, Gall CM. LTP consolidation: Substrates, explanatory power, and functional significance. *Neuropharm* 2007;52:12-23.
20. Abraham WC, Williams JM. Properties and mechanisms of LTP maintenance. *Neuroscientist* 2003;9:463-474.
21. Kennedy MB. Signal-processing machines at the postsynaptic density. *Science* 2000;290:750-754.
22. Vanderklish P, Saido TC, Gall C, Arai A, Lynch G. Proteolysis of spectrin by calpain accompanies theta-burst stimulation in cultured hippocampal slices. *Mol Brain Res*. 1995;32:25-35.
23. DeMali KA, Wennerberg K, Burridge K. Integrin signaling to the actin cytoskeleton. *Curr Opin Cell Biol*. 2003;15:572-582.
24. Friedman HV, Bresler T, Garner CC, Ziv NE. Assembly of new individual excitatory synapses: time course and temporal order of synaptic molecule recruitment. *Neuron* 2000;27:57-69.
25. Pye VE, Beuron F, Keetch CA, McKeown C, Robinson CV, Meyer HH, Zhang X, Freemont PS. Structural insights into the p97-Ufd1-Np14 complex. *Proc Natl Acad Sci USA*. 2007;104:467-472.
26. Ungar G. *Molecular mechanisms in learning and memory*. New York: Plenum Press 1970.
27. Costa-Mattioli M. Switching memories ON and OFF. *Science* 2008;322:874-875.
28. Burzynski SR. Genetics of brain aging (I): Gene silencing in neurons. In: Klatz R, Goldman R, eds. *Anti-Aging Therapeutics Volume IX*, Chicago, IL: A4M; 2007:71-78.

ABOUT THE AUTHOR

Dr. Stanislaw Burzynski graduated with honors in 1967. From 1970 to 1977 he was a faculty member at Baylor College of Medicine in Houston. In 1977 he established Burzynski Research Institute. Dr. Burzynski is the discoverer of antineoplastons, and the author of the new theory of aging, and more than 231 patents and 295 publications.

Chapter 6
Modification of the NAD+/NADH Ratio Via Oxaloacetic Acid Supplementation to Mimic Calorie Restriction Metabolic Pathways and Increase Lifespan

Alan B. Cash, B.S., M.S.
Managing Partner, Terra Biological LLC (San Diego, California, USA)

ABSTRACT

Diet supplementation with the human metabolite oxaloacetic acid has been found to provide some of the same benefits as a calorie restricted diet, including: increases in average and maximal lifespan, reduction in fasting glucose levels, fat reduction, and potentially a reduction in cancer incidence. The realized health benefits are due to oxaloacetic acid being able to create an increase in the NAD+/NADH ratio, a key intercellular condition found within the calorie restricted state.

Keywords: calorie restriction mimetic, lifespan, nad+/nadh ratio, diabetes, cancer, oxaloacetic acid

INTRODUCTION

The search for methods to extend human lifespan has spanned all of human history. Within the last 100 years, the most robust method to increase the average and maximal lifespan in laboratory tests with animals has been to enforce a severe diet and restrict calorie consumption by 25% to 40% less than the consumption of the normally fed control group. Mammals such as mice, rats, and dogs have a significantly longer lifespan when they are placed on this highly restricted diet.[1,2] Clinical calorie restriction studies in primates and humans have not yet determined if humans or primates will live longer, due to the longer lifespan of these species. However, examinations of human populations that have undergone reduced calorie consumption, such as on the island of Okinawa, Japan, have shown an increase in average lifespan and in the number of centenarians.[3] Additionally, clinical trials in both primates and humans have shown significant improvements in cardiovascular health (the number one cause of death in humans), and reductions in fasting glucose levels and triglycerides when placed on a calorie restricted diet.[4,5] Primate models showed that calorie restriction provided protection against Type II diabetes.[6]

Calorie restriction, as used herein, is the limitation of total calories derived from carbohydrates, fats, or proteins to a level 25% to 40% below that of control animals fed an unrestricted diet. The life-expanding result of a calorie restricted diet was first observed at Cornell University in 1935 on rats.[7] Since that time, the diet has been shown to increase the lifespan of yeast, worms, flies, spiders, fish, mice, and dogs, a very wide variety of species.[1,2] In addition to the increase in lifespan, there are many health benefits attributed to dietary restriction reported in the literature. These include:

- Decreases in cancer incidence and progression, with up to a 55% decrease in the incidence of cancer (mice, meta-analysis).[8]
- Decreases in neurodegenerative diseases in animal models of Alzheimer's and Parkinson's disease.[9,10]
- Protection against the development of Type II diabetes.[6,11]
- Reduction in cardiovascular risk and, in particular atherosclerosis.[4-6]
- Reduction in inflammatory diseases, such as auto-immune type disease.[12]
- Reduction in body fat.[13]

These are significant benefits; however there are also significant disadvantages to calorie restriction:

- Animals under calorie restriction are lighter in weight than fully fed organisms. This may have severe consequences in territory disputes and mating.
- Puberty occurs later.[14]
- Humans under caloric restriction report being hungry for at least the first 30 days of the process (but after six months, appetite seems to normalize).[15]
- It is a very, very difficult diet to follow.

43

For many years, scientists have struggled to understand how calorie restriction works. Recently, there has been a focus on changes in gene expression changes between calorie restricted animals and the control animals.[16] Calorie restriction increases the activity of genes associated with DNA cellular repair and energy metabolism[17] while decreasing genes associated with creating and storing fat.[16] Rather than preventing aging, "calorie restriction induces a more youthful gene expression profile associated with longer life and health-span".[18]

Calorie Restriction and the NAD+/NADH Ratio

The activation of beneficial genes that can extend health-span and lifespan is a very exciting development in our understanding of the phenomenon, because it allows us to examine methods other than calorie restriction to activate these same genes. One method to activate these genes is to create the same intercellular conditions as calorie restricted cells, preferably without near starvation.[19,20] One consistent intercellular condition within the calorie restricted state is an increase in nicotinamide adenine dinucleotide (NAD+), and a decrease in the reduced version of NAD+, NADH.[21,22] This increase in the NAD+/NADH ratio has been shown to be associated with increases in lifespan. In 2003, it was shown that increases in the NAD+/NADH ratio using genetic engineering increased the lifespan of yeast.[21] Later, in 2007 it was shown that increasing the amount of NAD+ precursors increased lifespan in yeast,[23] that increasing NAD+ in the mitochondria increased cellular survival during genotoxic events,[24] and that increasing the regeneration of NAD+ increased human cell lifespan in vitro.[25] As can be seen, increasing the NAD+/NADH ratio has a strong association with longevity.

We examined different ways to increase the NAD+/NADH ratio in order to see if we could stimulate the genes that result in longer health span and lifespan. Calorie restriction is a proven method to increase the NAD+/NADH ratio, but is very difficult to follow, and is impractical for the general population. Prolonged exercise also increases the NAD+/NADH ratio due to gluconeogenesis. As an alternate method of increasing the NAD+/NADH ratio, we examined the use of human metabolic molecules to decrease NADH and increase NAD+.

USING OXALOACETIC ACID SUPPLEMENTATION TO MODIFY THE NAD+/NADH RATIO

Oxaloacetate is a Krebs cycle intermediate metabolite and is central to energy metabolism. Mutations that cause a lack of oxaloacetate result in a bleak prognosis for the patient, with mental retardation followed by death, typically within early childhood.[26] Excess amounts of oxaloacetate, such as from a nutritional supplement, are readily absorbed in the stomach and are measured in the bloodstream within one hour.[27] Within the cytosol of the cell, oxaloacetate can engage in several reactions, but a highly favorable reaction is the conversion of oxaloacetate into malate via the enzyme malate dehydrogenase (Gibbs Free Energy difference of -29.7). During this conversion into malate (another Krebs cycle intermediate), NADH is converted to NAD+. This both lowers the NADH level and increases the NAD+ level, leading to a significant change in the NAD+/NADH ratio.

The increase in cellular NAD+/NADH levels typically occurs in the cytoplasm, but has also been measured inside the mitochondria. Micro-molar concentrations of oxaloacetate increase the NAD+ level in the mitochondria by 50%, and due to the concurrent reduction in NADH, have been measured in vitro to increase the NAD+/NADH ratio within the mitochondria by 900%.[28] The increase in the NAD+/NADH ratio in the mitochondria occurred within minutes. Vitamin C appears to assist in the transfer of oxaloacetate across the inner mitochondrial membrane.[28] Increasing NAD+ levels in the mitochondria have been directly shown to increase cellular lifespan,[24] although the increase in overall lifespan could also be due to delivery of a potent antioxidant[29-32] directly into the mitochondria. Oxaloacetate has been shown to be protective of brain mitochondrial DNA when exposed to toxins.[33] The protective effect of oxaloacetate on mitochondrial DNA may be a factor in decreasing aging, as premature mitochondrial damage greatly resembles aging in mice models.[34-37].

Testing Oxaloacetic Acid as a Calorie Restriction Mimetic

To test our hypothesis that oxaloacetate can mimic the intercellular NAD+/NADH ratio conditions of the calorie restricted state, and thereby mimic the positive health effects of calorie restriction without the necessary reduction in caloric intake, we tested oxaloacetic acid supplementation on worms (*Caenorhabditis elegans*), Fruit Flies (*Drosophila melanogaster*), C57BL/6 Mice (*Mus musculus*), and humans. In the short-lived species of worms, fruit flies, and mice, we saw an increase in lifespan ranging from 20 to 25%, similar to what would be seen in calorie restricted animals (See Figure 1). Our largest data base is with the short-lived *C. elegans* worm, which showed a 20% increase in mean lifespan (p << 0.001) and a 13% in maximal lifespan (p < 0.005) as opposed to similar control worms. The lifespan increase in humans has not been proven, however, due to the necessary length of the test.

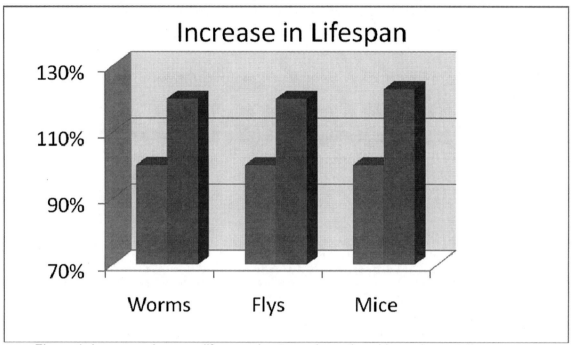

Figure 1. Increases in mean lifespan due to oxaloacetic acid supplementation.

In mice, we performed gene expression analysis on liver tissue of the mice supplemented with oxaloacetic acid and compared it to both calorie restricted mice and normally fed control mice. The calorie restricted mice showed 1,763 changes in gene expression as compared to the normally fed mice. In contrast, the oxaloacetic acid supplemented mice only showed gene expression changes in 765 mice. Many of these gene expression changes may be outliers due to the methodology of the experiment. However, 363 of the genes that changed in expression levels were common to both the calorie restricted mice and the oxaloacetic acid supplemented mice. Many of these common genes regulate DNA repair, transcription, glucose metabolism, and fat production and storage. Of the 363 common genes that changed expression levels, 98% of them exhibited similar directional expression. For example, the *FOXO3a* gene, which is involved in glucose homeostasis and starvation response,[38] was up-regulated in expression in both the calorie restricted animals and the oxaloacetic acid supplemented animals. Genes controlling fatty acid biosynthesis and cholesterol biosynthesis were down-regulated in both the calorie restricted animals and in the oxaloacetic acid supplemented animals. These included the *ACAA1, CNBP, FASN, IDI1, NDUFAB1, PCX*, and *SC5D* genes. Up-regulating the *FOXO3a* gene will lead to improvements in glucose system functioning, whereas down-regulation of the genes that create and store fat leads to reduced overall weight in the animals, as the supplemented animals have less fat.

Similar to calorie restricted humans, oxaloacetate has been shown to be an effective agent for reducing glucose levels. A clinical trial by Yoshikawa shows that 100 to 1,000 mg of the sodium salt of oxaloacetic acid is effective in lowering the blood and urine glucose levels of diabetic patients. Yoshikawa initially investigated oxaloacetic acid for diabetes treatment after identifying the compound as the active ingredient extracted from the Asian mountain shrub *Euonymus alata* (Winged Euonymus or Burning Bush),[27] a traditional herb used for hundreds of years and still in use today to treat diabetes in Asian countries.[39,40] In the clinical trial, fasting glucose levels were brought to normal levels in the majority of diabetic patients without any noted side effects. In animal studies, Yoshikawa showed that sodium oxaloacetate increased the uptake of glucose by tissues 300% in diabetic animals, and 180% in normal animals.[27] In patients with normal glucose levels, fasting glucose is dropped only a small amount, but the amplitude of the changes in fasting glucose levels is dropped by greater than 50%, indicating improved glucose regulation, as would be expected based on the gene response. A more recent study in 2003 study showed that oxaloacetate inhibits zinc-mediated pancreatic islet cell death and diabetes in animal models.[41]

Mimicking Calorie Restriction as a Method to Support Glucose Metabolism – A Case Study

Here we report a case study on a 73 year old Hungarian woman, weight of 89 kg, with a history of difficult to treat type 2 diabetes. The trial was a "grass-roots" look at glucose levels performed by the patient with a glucose test strip meter under normal living conditions. The unsolicited data was supplied to us as the developer of the nutritional supplement product. Unfortunately, no other measurements were taken by the patient other than blood glucose levels, but the number of readings taken by the patient is impressive, and does show statistically significant results.

At the start of the study, the woman was on the following medications:

- Diaprel MR/ (80 mg) 2 per day – extended release Gliclazide (80 mg), a once per day diabetic drug.
- Pentoxyl-EP (400 mg) 1 per day – contains pentoxifylline, used for intermittent claudication (a symptom complex characterized by leg pain and weakness brought on by walking, with the disappearance of the symptoms following a brief rest).
- Merckformin (1000 mg) 1 per day - (Metformin, Glucophage) – used for type 2 diabetes.
- Glycerine sol (0.5 dl) after dinner.
- Avandamet 1 per day – a combination of metformin and rosiglitazone used for the treatment of type 2 diabetes.

The woman's fasting glucose levels fluctuated between 8 and 11 mmol/L, her glucose levels rose as high as12 mmol/L after a meal.

In addition to her current medicines, the patient self-started 200 mg/day benaGene (1 capsule), an over-the-counter nutritional supplement composed of 100 mg 3-carboxy-3-oxopropanoic acid (oxaloacetic acid) and 100 mg ascorbic acid (Vitamin C). During the study the patient increased the use of benaGene to 400 mg/day (two capsules), and then 600 mg/day (3 capsules).

By the end of the 70-day study the patient's fasting glucose levels had dropped to a range between 7 and 8 mmol/L, and glucose levels after a meal remained more consistent in the 7 to 8.5 mmol/L range – levels not achievable with the three prescription medications the patient was consuming. Using linear trend analysis, the patient's fasting glucose levels dropped 23% from the start of the test to the end of the test. Her glucose levels after a meal dropped 34.5%, indicating a major improvement in glucose management and glucose tolerance. Comparison of the various glucose levels in the first half of the trial versus the second half of the trail yields a p value of < 0.001, indicating a very significant difference between the first half and second half of the trial. The reduction in glucose levels occurred despite a reduction in the amount of Mercformin used – from 1000 mg/day to 850 mg/day during the study. The patient also stopped using Pentoxyl-EP and glycerol by the end of the study. The data from this case study is graphed in Figure 2.

Improvement in this patents glucose levels and glucose tolerance with the bioidentical human metabolic compound oxaloacetic acid, an over-the-counter dietary supplement, is a low-risk option that has been shown to successfully support proper glucose functioning.

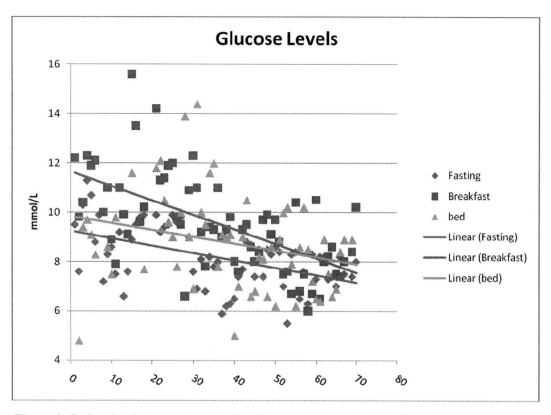

Figure 2. Daily blood glucose levels of a 73-year old female diabetic patient taken under fasting conditions, after breakfast and prior to bed.

Using Oxaloacetic Acid to Mimic Calorie Restriction and Reduce Body Fat

While genes are fixed, the manner in which genes are expressed changes constantly in response to the environment and food consumed.[42,43] Drastically cutting calories over an eight week period (such as during calorie restriction) has been shown to decrease the expression of the genes associated with the production and storage of fat.[16] In a similar fashion, oxaloacetic acid supplementation down-regulates genes that include the *ACAA1*, *FASN*, *NDUFAB1*, and *PCX* genes, which are associated with fatty acid biosynthesis, along with *CNBP*, *IDI1* and *SC5D*, which are associated with cholesterol biosynthesis (mouse data). Reducing the gene expression leads to less fat production and storage. This may allow dieters a genomic method to better maintain their weight after a diet, by slowing down the pathways that create and store fat.

Mimicking Calorie Restriction as a Method to Reduce Cancer Incidence

Calorie restriction is one of the most effective means to delay the onset of cancer,[8,44-46] and has provided a mechanism to treat cancer.[47,48] In addition, fasting prior to chemotherapy treatment has been shown to increase the effectiveness of the chemotherapy, allowing better survival rates (in mice), by allowing the toxins to better target cancer cells and reduce the side effects on normal cells.[49] Unfortunately, calorie restriction is difficult to perform over a lifetime, and may present a "quality of life" challenge to those with existing cancer. Certain compounds can "mimic" many of the physiological effects seen in the calorie restricted state, without the reduction in calories.[20,50] These calorie restriction "mimetics", which include the natural compound resveratrol and the diabetes drug metformin, have also been shown to reduce cancer incidence and growth.[51-53]

Oxaloacetic acid supplementation has been shown to eliminate the ability of some cancer cell types to reproduce, while not affecting normal tissues. A 20 uM level of oxaloacetate in contact with human A549 lung cancer *tissue in vitro* resulted in differential massive debris within the cancer tissue, but

47

not within normal tissue. The massive debris resulted in the inability of the cancer tissue to reproduce, even if the cancer tissue was moved away from the oxaloacetate solution for a period of six weeks.[54]

Calorie restriction and calorie restriction mimetics change the expression of genes that regulate the body.[55] The tie between genes expressed under calorie restriction that increase lifespan and decrease cancer proliferation may have been first hypothesized by Anisimov.[56] Further to that hypothesis, it was shown that increased activation of the longevity gene *FOXO3* encoded a protein to prevent cancer and predict a better outcome for breast cancer patients.[57] More recently, it was shown that *FOXO3* is needed to induce apoptosis (programmed cell death) in gastric cancer cells.[58] Pinkston *et al* documented that genes that increase the lifespan of *C. elegans* (worms) also inhibit tumor growth.[59] Arden reviews the *FOXO* genes for potential new therapeutic targets for a broad spectrum of cancers. Her review indicated that *FOXO1* is a tumor suppressor gene. She also reports that "*FOXO3* can override IkB stimulation of cell cycle progression, proliferation, and tumorigenesis in mice, further supporting *FOXO3* as a candidate tumor suppressor gene."[60] A further review by Reagan-Shaw *et al* also indicates *FOXO* transcription factors as targets for cancer management.[61]

Our research with gene chip technology in mice shows that oxaloacetate supplementation increases the expression of the *FOXO1* and *FOXO3* genes by approximately 40% and 70%, respectively, which is similar to the increases in gene expression seen in calorie restriction. Thus, in addition to the role of oxaloacetate in creating inter-cellular "junk" in cancer cells as noted by Farah (2007), oxaloacetate may also provide a potential gene expression-based support for reducing cancer incidence.

Reported Side Effects of Oxaloacetic Acid Supplementation

Oxaloacetic Acid supplementation has been commercially available as an over-the-counter nutritional supplement in Canada and Europe for approximately three years. During that time, there have been surprising side effects noted by the consumers. These include:

- Improvements in sleep
- Reduction in constipation
- Immediate relief from altitude sickness
- Reduction in sugar cravings
- Reduction in hunger pains during voluntary fasting
- Increased "feeling of peace"

The mechanisms behind these side effects are not understood at this time.

CONCLUDING REMARKS

While increases in human lifespan have not been proven with the supplement oxaloacetic acid due to the normal length of the human lifespan, short lived species such as worms, flies, and mice that have had oxaloacetic acid supplementation have been documented to live approximately 20% longer than control animals, similar to that seen in calorie restricted animals.

Oxaloacetic acid has been shown in humans to support and improve glucose system functioning, similar to that seen in calorie restricted volunteers. The genomic pathways that create and store fat are down-regulated with oxaloacetic acid supplementation (mice data).

Using human metabolites to mimic the intercellular conditions of the calorie restricted metabolic state and thereby achieve the health benefits of calorie restriction (without the necessary reduction in calories) may be an important improvement to the human condition.

REFERENCES

1. Koubova J, Guarente L. How does calorie restriction work? *Genes Dev.* 2003;17:313-321.
2. Lawler DF, Larson BT, Ballam JM, *et al.* Diet restriction and ageing in the dog: major observations over two decades. *Br J Nutr.* 2008;99:793-805.
3. Willcox BJ, Willcox DC, Todoriki H, *et al.* Caloric restriction, the traditional Okinawan diet, and healthy aging: the diet of the world's longest-lived people and its potential impact on morbidity and life span. *Ann N Y Acad Sci.* 2007;1114:434-455.
4. Holloszy JO, Fontana L. Caloric restriction in humans. *Exp Gerontol.* 2007;42:709-712.

5. Fontana L, Meyer TE, Klein S, Holloszy JO. Long-term calorie restriction is highly effective in reducing the risk for atherosclerosis in humans. *Proc Natl Acad Sci U S A.* 2004;101:6659-6663.
6. Lane MA, Ingram DK, Roth GS. Calorie restriction in nonhuman primates: effects on diabetes and cardiovascular disease risk. *Toxicol Sci.* 1999;52:41-48.
7. McCay CM CM, Maynard LA. The effect of retarded growth upon the length of the life span and upon the ultimate body size. *Journal of Nutrition.* 1935;10:63-79.
8. Dirx MJ, Zeegers MP, Dagnelie PC, van den Bogaard T, van den Brandt PA. Energy restriction and the risk of spontaneous mammary tumors in mice: a meta-analysis. *Int J Cancer.* 2003;106:766-770.
9. Qin W, Zhao W, Ho L, *et al.* Regulation of forkhead transcription factor FoxO3a contributes to calorie restriction-induced prevention of Alzheimer's disease-type amyloid neuropathology and spatial memory deterioration. *Ann N Y Acad Sci.* 2008;1147:335-347.
10. Love R. Calorie restriction may be neuroprotective in AD and PD. *Lancet Neurol.* 2005;4:84.
11. Lane MA, Tilmont EM, De Angelis H, *et al.* Short-term calorie restriction improves disease-related markers in older male rhesus monkeys *(Macaca mulatta). Mech Ageing Dev.* 2000;112:185-196.
12. Gugliucci A, Kotani K, Taing J, *et al.* Short-Term Low Calorie Diet Intervention Reduces Serum Advanced Glycation End Products in Healthy Overweight or Obese Adults. *Ann Nutr Metab.* 2009;54:197-201.
13. Nicklas BJ, Wang X, You T, et al. Effect of exercise intensity on abdominal fat loss during calorie restriction in overweight and obese postmenopausal women: a randomized, controlled trial. *Am J Clin Nutr.* 2009;89:1043-1052.
14. Van der Spuy ZM. Nutrition and reproduction. *Clin Obstet Gynaecol.* 1985;12:579-604.
15. Anton SD, Han H, York E, Martin CK, Ravussin E, Williamson DA. Effect of calorie restriction on subjective ratings of appetite. *J Hum Nutr Diet.* 2009;22:141-147.
16. Dhahbi JM, Mote PL, Wingo J, Tillman JB, Walford RL, Spindler SR. Calories and aging alter gene expression for gluconeogenic, glycolytic, and nitrogen-metabolizing enzymes. *Am J Physiol.* 1999;277:E352-360.
17. Castelein N, Hoogewijs D, De Vreese A, Braeckman BP, Vanfleteren JR. Dietary restriction by growth in axenic medium induces discrete changes in the transcriptional output of genes involved in energy metabolism in Caenorhabditis elegans. *Biotechnol J.* 2008;3:803-812.
18. Cao SX, Dhahbi JM, Mote PL, Spindler SR. Genomic profiling of short- and long-term caloric restriction effects in the liver of aging mice. *Proc Natl Acad Sci U S A.* 2001;98:10630-10635.
19. Lane MA, Ingram DK, Roth GS. The serious search for an anti-aging pill. *Sci Am.* 2002;287:36-41.
20. Ingram DK, Zhu M, Mamczarz J, *et al.* Calorie restriction mimetics: an emerging research field. *Aging Cell.* 2006;5:97-108.
21. Lin SJ, Ford E, Haigis M, Liszt G, Guarente L. Calorie restriction extends yeast life span by lowering the level of NADH. *Genes Dev.* 2004;18:12-16.
22. Easlon E, Tsang F, Skinner C, Wang C, Lin SJ. The malate-aspartate NADH shuttle components are novel metabolic longevity regulators required for calorie restriction-mediated life span extension in yeast. *Genes Dev.* 2008;22:931-944.
23. Belenky P, Racette FG, Bogan KL, McClure JM, Smith JS, Brenner C. Nicotinamide riboside promotes Sir2 silencing and extends lifespan via Nrk and Urh1/Pnp1/Meu1 pathways to NAD+. *Cell* 2007;129:473-484.
24. Yang H, Yang T, Baur JA, *et al.* Nutrient-sensitive mitochondrial NAD+ levels dictate cell survival. *Cell* 2007;130:1095-1107.
25. van der Veer E, Ho C, O'Neil C, *et al.* Extension of human cell lifespan by nicotinamide phosphoribosyltransferase. *J Biol Chem.* 2007;282:10841-10845.
26. Ahmad A, Kahler SG, Kishnani PS, *et al.* Treatment of pyruvate carboxylase deficiency with high doses of citrate and aspartate. *Am J Med Genet.* 1999;87:331-338.
27. Yoshikawa K. Studies on the anti-diabetic effect of sodium oxaloacetate. *Tohoku J Exp Med.* 1968;96:127-141.
28. Haslam JM, Krebs HA. The permeability of mitochondria to oxaloacetate and malate. *Biochem J.* 1968;107:659-667.
29. Desagher S, Glowinski J, Premont J. Pyruvate protects neurons against hydrogen peroxide-induced toxicity. *J Neurosci.* 1997;17:9060-9067.

30. Puntel RL, Nogueira CW, Rocha JB. Krebs cycle intermediates modulate thiobarbituric acid reactive species (TBARS) production in rat brain in vitro. *Neurochem Res.* 2005;30:225-235.
31. Puntel RL, Roos DH, Grotto D, Garcia SC, Nogueira CW, Rocha JB. Antioxidant properties of Krebs cycle intermediates against malonate pro-oxidant activity in vitro: a comparative study using the colorimetric method and HPLC analysis to determine malondialdehyde in rat brain homogenates. *Life Sci.* 2007;81:51-62.
32. Berry EV, Toms NJ. Pyruvate and oxaloacetate limit zinc-induced oxidative HT-22 neuronal cell injury. *Neurotoxicology* 2006;27:1043-1051.
33. Yamamoto HA, Mohanan PV. Effect of alpha-ketoglutarate and oxaloacetate on brain mitochondrial DNA damage and seizures induced by kainic acid in mice. *Toxicol Lett.* 2003;143:115-122.
34. Wei YH, Lee HC. Oxidative stress, mitochondrial DNA mutation, and impairment of antioxidant enzymes in aging. *Exp Biol Med (Maywood).* 2002;227:671-682.
35. Navarro CL, Cau P, Levy N. Molecular bases of progeroid syndromes. *Hum Mol Genet.* 2006;15 Spec No 2:R151-161.
36. McKiernan SH, Tuen VC, Baldwin K, Wanagat J, Djamali A, Aiken JM. Adult-onset calorie restriction delays the accumulation of mitochondrial enzyme abnormalities in aging rat kidney tubular epithelial cells. *Am J Physiol Renal Physiol.* 2007;292:F1751-1760.
37. Alexeyev MF, Ledoux SP, Wilson GL. Mitochondrial DNA and aging. *Clin Sci (Lond).* 2004;107:355-364.
38. Huang H, Tindall DJ. Dynamic FoxO transcription factors. *J Cell Sci.* 2007;120:2479-24787.
39. Fang XK, Gao Y, Yang HY, *et al.* Alleviating effects of active fraction of Euonymus alatus abundant in flavonoids on diabetic mice. *Am J Chin Med.* 2008;36:125-140.
40. Park SH, Ko SK, Chung SH. *Euonymus alatus* prevents the hyperglycemia and hyperlipidemia induced by high-fat diet in ICR mice. *J Ethnopharmacol.* 2005;102:326-335.
41. Chang I, Cho N, Koh JY, Lee MS. Pyruvate inhibits zinc-mediated pancreatic islet cell death and diabetes. *Diabetologia* 2003;46:1220-1227.
42. Mead M. Nutrigenomics: The Genome-Food Interface. *Environ Health Perspect.* 2007;115:A582-A589.
43. Brown L, van der Ouderaa F. Nutritional genomics: food industry applications from farm to fork. *Br J Nutr.* 2007;97:1027-1-35.
44. Hursting SD, Lavigne JA, Berrigan D, Perkins SN, Barrett JC. Calorie restriction, aging, and cancer prevention: mechanisms of action and applicability to humans. *Annu Rev Med.* 2003;54:131-152.
45. Mai V, Colbert LH, Berrigan D, et al. Calorie restriction and diet composition modulate spontaneous intestinal tumorigenesis in Apc(Min) mice through different mechanisms. *Cancer Res.* 2003;63:1752-1755.
46. Firestein R, Blander G, Michan S, *et al.* The SIRT1 deacetylase suppresses intestinal tumorigenesis and colon cancer growth. *PLoS ONE.* 2008;3:e2020.
47. Seyfried TN, Kiebish M, Mukherjee P, Marsh J. Targeting energy metabolism in brain cancer with calorically restricted ketogenic diets. *Epilepsia* 2008;49 Suppl 8:114-116.
48. Zhou W, Mukherjee P, Kiebish MA, Markis WT, Mantis JG, Seyfried TN. The calorically restricted ketogenic diet, an effective alternative therapy for malignant brain cancer. *Nutr Metab (Lond).* 2007;4:5.
49. Raffaghello L, Lee C, Safdie FM, *et al.* Starvation-dependent differential stress resistance protects normal but not cancer cells against high-dose chemotherapy. *Proc Natl Acad Sci U S A.* 2008;105:8215-8220.
50. Contestabile A. Benefits of caloric restriction on brain aging and related pathological States: understanding mechanisms to devise novel therapies. *Curr Med Chem.* 2009;16:350-361.
51. Harikumar KB, Aggarwal BB. Resveratrol: a multitargeted agent for age-associated chronic diseases. *Cell Cycle.* 2008;7:1020-1035.
52. Wang W, Guan KL. AMP-activated protein kinase and cancer. *Acta Physiol (Oxf).* 2009;196:55-63.
53. Cazzaniga M, Bonanni B, Guerrieri-Gonzaga A, Decensi A. Is it time to test metformin in breast cancer clinical trials? *Cancer Epidemiol Biomarkers Prev.* 2009;18:701-705.
54. Farah IO. Differential modulation of intracellular energetics in A549 and MRC-5 cells. *Biomed Sci, Instrum* 2007;43:110-115.

55. Dhahbi JM, Mote PL, Fahy GM, Spindler SR. Identification of potential caloric restriction mimetics by microarray profiling. *Physiol Genomics.* 2005;23:343-350.
56. Anisimov VN. Insulin/IGF-1 signaling pathway driving aging and cancer as a target for pharmacological intervention. *Exp Gerontol.* 2003;38:1041-1049.
57. Hu MC, Lee DF, Xia W, *et al*. IkappaB kinase promotes tumorigenesis through inhibition of forkhead FOXO3a. *Cell* 2004;117:225-237.
58. Yamamura Y, Lee WL, Inoue K, Ida H, Ito Y. RUNX3 cooperates with FoxO3a to induce apoptosis in gastric cancer cells. *J Biol Chem.* 2006;281:5267-5276.
59. Pinkston JM, Garigan D, Hansen M, Kenyon C. Mutations that increase the life span of *C. elegans* inhibit tumor growth. *Science* 2006;313:971-975.
60. Arden KC. Multiple roles of FOXO transcription factors in mammalian cells point to multiple roles in cancer. *Exp Gerontol.* 2006;41:709-717.
61. Reagan-Shaw S, Ahmad N. The role of Forkhead-box Class O (FoxO) transcription factors in cancer: a target for the management of cancer. *Toxicol Appl Pharmacol.* 2007;224:360-368.

CONFLICT OF INTEREST

Alan Cash is an officer in a commercial venture involving calorie restriction mimetics, including the sale of oxaloacetic acid supplemented with vitamin C as "benaGene™".

ABOUT THE AUTHOR

Alan Cash is a physicist focused on the metabolic energy pathways of calorie restriction and methods to reproduce the effects of calorie restriction with small molecules rather than extreme diets. Collaborations include the US National Institute on Aging's "Interventions Testing Program" which investigates treatments with the potential to extend lifespan and delay disease.

Chapter 7
Public Health Decline in the Nineteenth Century and Its Subsequent Decline in the Twentieth and Twenty-First Centuries[†]

Paul Clayton
Visiting Fellow, School of Life Sciences, Oxford Brookes University (United Kingdom)
Judith Rowbotham
Department of History & Law, Nottingham Trent University (United Kingdom)
[†] This chapter is an extended re-working of three papers published in the *Journal of the Royal Society of Medicine*[1-3]

ABSTRACT

Analysis of the mid-Victorian period in the UK reveals that life expectancy at age 5 was as good as or better than exists today, and the incidence of degenerative disease was 10% of ours. Their levels of physical activity and hence calorific intakes were approximately twice ours. They had relatively little access to alcohol and tobacco; and due to their correspondingly high intake of fruits, wholegrains, oily fish, and vegetables, they consumed levels of micro- and phyto-nutrients at approximately ten times the levels considered normal today. This paper relates the nutritional status of the mid-Victorians to their freedom from degenerative disease; and extrapolates recommendations for the cost-effective improvement of public health today.

Keywords: Public health, dietary shift, degenerative disease, Victorian

INTRODUCTION

The mid-Victorian period is usually defined as the years between 1850 and 1870 but in nutritional terms it is a slightly longer period, lasting until around 1880. During these 30 years a generation grew up with probably the best standards of health ever enjoyed by a modern state. The British population had risen significantly and had become increasingly urbanised, but the great public health movement had not yet been established and Britain's towns and cities were still notoriously unhealthy environments. Despite this, Britain and its world-dominating empire were supported by a workforce, an army, and a navy comprised of individuals who were healthier, fitter, and stronger than we are today. They were almost entirely free of the degenerative diseases which maim and kill so many of us, and although it is commonly stated that this is because they all died young, the reverse is true; public records reveal that they lived as long – or longer – than we do in the 21st century.

These findings are remarkable, as this brief period of great good health predates not only the public health movement but also the great 20th century medical advances in surgery, infection control, and drugs. They are also in marked contrast to popular views about Victorian squalor and disease, views that have long obscured the realities of life and death during that 'period of equipoise'.

Recent research indicates that the mid-Victorians' good health was entirely due to their superior diet. This period was, nutritionally speaking, an island in time; one that was created and subsequently squandered by economic and political forces. This begs a series of questions. How did this brief nutritional 'golden age' come about? How was it lost? And could we recreate it?

One key contributory factor was what used to be called the Agricultural Revolution; a series of developments in agricultural practice that massively improved crop and livestock yields. This slow green revolution started in the late seventeenth century, gradually accelerated until the mid-19th century, and underpinned both modern urbanisation and the associated Industrial Revolution. Arguably the most critical agricultural development was a more complex system of crop rotation, which greatly improved both arable output and animal husbandry. In the 1730's a new breed of innovative land-owner (epitomized by Marquis 'Turnip' Townshend) introduced new systems of crop rotation from Sweden and The Netherlands, and new crops like the swede. The new crop rotation systems avoided the need to let land lie fallow one year in three, and instead used a four or five year cycle in which turnips and clover were used as two of the crops because of their ability to replenish the soil. These new systems created immense gains in food productivity. Between 1705 and 1765 English wheat exports increased ten-fold, while the increased availability of animal feed meant that most livestock no longer had to be slaughtered at the onset of winter and that fresh (instead of salted) meat became cheaper and more widely available throughout the year.

Population shifts also played a key contributory role. The bulk of the population had always lived on the land but by 1850, as revealed by the 1851 census, more Britons were living and working in towns than in the countryside. The agricultural improvements of the previous 150 years meant that agriculture produced far more than before, but used far fewer people to achieve this. As a result, people moved to towns to find work: Britain was the first modern consumer society and there was real demand for workers in an increasing number of urban industries. Traditionally, urban life expectancy was significantly lower than rural life expectancy, but from the mid-Victorian period on this difference disappears.

Victorian society was very different to traditional society. It was a class society as we understand it today rather than the older, more deferential model, and this created enormous social tensions. For the very poor, towns remained deeply unpleasant places to live, and it can be argued that for many, the social structure of towns even got worse. As more of the working classes moved into towns, more of the middle classes moved out to create the beginnings of suburbia. The great Victorian commentator Thomas Carlyle claimed that in cities, little tied one human being to another except for the 'Cash Nexus', where employer and employee met in an uncomfortable wage and profit-driven relationship, as Mrs Gaskell revealed in books like *North and South*.

In many ways, however, urban socio-economic conditions were getting better. Trades unions and philanthropists were slowly but surely improving urban working conditions and wages throughout the last half of the century. The threats of political instability which had seemed most threatening in towns up to the late 1840s were largely dispersed during the mid-Victorian era, as a result of changes in the political and legal systems. For example, the Great Reform Act of 1832 was followed by the 1867 Reform Act, which meant that most male urban heads of households were now able to vote. In 1845 the notorious Corn Laws were finally repealed.

One of the most important results of the political changes was that the interests of the landed classes were no longer protected. Traditionally, parliament had always sought to protect the income of farmers and landowners, and after the end of the Napoleonic Wars, this stance had seen the introduction of the highly unpopular Corn Laws from 1815. These kept the price of grain at a level that ensured agricultural prosperity, but they had a disastrous effect on the price of food. This particularly affected the new urban, industrial workforce, which was heavily dependent on bread as a staple food. The Corn Laws kept the price of bread artificially high, even during economic depressions such as the 1840s, a decade which became notorious as the 'Hungry 40's'.

The post-Great Reform Act parliament, however, was susceptible to pressure from groups such as the Anti-Corn Law League led by Richard Cobden and Joseph Bright. When the situation was exacerbated by the Irish Great Potato Famine, Prime Minister Sir Robert Peel, the grandson of a mill-owner, forced through the repeal of the Corn Laws. From that time on farming interests were under pressure to produce cheap food because it had become clear that the prosperity of the country depended on industrial rather than on agricultural output. As the Great Exhibition of 1851 underlined, Britain had become the Workshop of the World.

Improved agricultural output and a political climate dedicated to ensuring cheap food lead to a dramatic increase in the production of affordable foodstuffs; but it was the development of the railway network that actually brought the fruits of the agricultural and political changes into the towns and cities, and made them available to the mid-Victorian working classes.

The start of the modern railway age is usually marked by the opening of the Stockton & Darlington line in 1825. From the late 1830s on, progress was impressively rapid. Important long-distance lines came first, followed by smaller local lines criss-crossing the country. The London and Birmingham line opened in 1838, part of Brunel's London to Bristol route the same year, and the London and Southampton line in 1840. By the mid century the key lines were already laid. The railway system grew exponentially, reaching 2500 miles by 1845, and continued to expand, carrying goods as well as passengers. Thanks to trains, producers were now supplying the urban markets with more, fresher and cheaper food than was previously possible. This boosted urban demand for fresh foodstuffs, and pushed up agricultural output still further. A survey of food availability in the 1860s, through sources such as Henry Mayhew's survey of the London poor, shows very substantial quantities of affordable vegetables and fruits now pouring into the urban markets.

This fortunate combination of factors produced a sea change in the nation, and in the nation's health. By 1850 Britain's increasing domestic productivity and foreign power had created a national mood of confidence and optimism which affected all levels of society. Driven by better nutrition, far more than the new schemes of clean air and water, which only began to have an effect from the 1870s and onwards, adult life expectancy increased from the 1850s until by 1875 it matched or surpassed our own.[4] The health and vitality of the British population during this period was reflected in the workforces and armed forces that powered the transformation of the urban landscape at home, and drove the great expansion of the British Empire abroad.

Unfortunately, negative changes that would undermine these nutritional gains were already taking shape. Thanks to her dominant global position, and developments in shipping technology, Britain had created a global market drawing in the products of colonial and US agriculture, to provide ever-cheaper food for the growing urban masses. From 1875 onwards, and especially after 1885, rising imports of cheap food basics were increasingly affecting the food chain at home. Imported North American wheat and new milling techniques reduced the prices of white flour and bread. Tinned meat arrived from the Argentine, Australia, and New Zealand, which was cheaper than either home-produced or refrigerated fresh meat also arriving from these sources. Canned fruit and condensed milk became widely available.

This expansion in the range of foods was advertised by most contemporaries, and by subsequent historians, as representing a significant 'improvement' in the working class diet. The reality was very different. These changes undoubtedly increased the variety and quantity of the working class diet, but its quality deteriorated markedly. The imported canned meats were fatty and usually 'corned' or salted. Cheaper sugar promoted a huge increase in sugar consumption in confectionery, now mass-produced for the first time, and in the new processed foods such as sugar-laden condensed milk, and canned fruits bathed in heavy syrup. The increased sugar consumption caused such damage to the nation's teeth that by 1900 it was commonly noted that people could no longer chew tough foods and were unable to eat many vegetables, fruits, and nuts.[5] For all these reasons the late-Victorian diet actually damaged the health of the nation, and the health of the working classes in particular.

The decline was astonishingly rapid. The mid-Victorian navvies, who as seasonal workers were towards the bottom end of the economic scale, could routinely shovel up to 20 tons of earth per day from below their feet to above their heads.[6] This was an enormous physical effort that required great strength, stamina, and robust good health. Within two generations, however, male health nationally had deteriorated to such an extent that in 1900, 5 out of 10 young men volunteering for the second Boer War had to be rejected because they were so undernourished. They were not starved, but had been consuming the wrong foods.[7,8] This reality is underlined by considering army recruitment earlier. The recruiting sergeants had reported no such problems during previous high profile campaigns such as the Asante War (1873-4) and Zulu War (1877-8).

The fall in nutritional standards between 1880 and 1900 was so marked that the generations were visibly and progressively shrinking. In 1883, the infantry were forced to lower the minimum height for recruits from 5ft 6inches to 5ft 3 inches. This was because most new recruits were now coming from an urban background instead of the traditional rural background (the 1881 census showed that over three-quarters of the population now lived in towns and cities). Factors such as a lack of sunlight in urban slums (which led to rickets due to Vitamin D deficiency) had already reduced the height of young male volunteers. Lack of sunlight, however, could not have been the sole critical factor in the next height reduction, a mere 18 years later. By this time, clean air legislation had markedly improved urban sunlight levels; but unfortunately, the supposed 'improvements' in dietary intake resulting from imported foods had had time to take effect on the 16-18 year old cohort. It might be expected that the infantry would be able to raise the minimum height requirement back to 5ft.6inches. Instead, they were forced to reduce it still further, to a mere 5ft. British officers, who were from the middle and upper classes and not yet exposed to more than the occasional treats of canned produce, were far better fed in terms of their intake of fresh foods and were now on average a full head taller than their malnourished and sickly men.

In 1904, and as a direct result of the Boer disaster, the government set up the Committee on Physical Deterioration. Its report, emphasising the need to provide school meals for working class children, reinforced the idea that the urban working classes were not only malnourished at the start of the twentieth century but also (in an unjustified leap of the imagination, reinforced by folk memories of the 'Hungry 40's) that they had been so since the start of nineteenth century industrial urbanisation.[5,9] This profound error of thought was incorporated into subsequent models of public health, and is distorting and damaging healthcare to this day.

The crude average figures often used to depict the brevity of Victorian lives mislead because they include infant mortality, which was tragically high. If we strip out peri-natal mortality, however, and look at the life expectancy of those who survived the first 5 years, a very different picture emerges. Victorian contemporary sources reveal that life expectancy for adults in the mid-Victorian period was almost exactly what it is today. At 65, men could expect another ten years of life; and women another eight (the lower figure for women reflects the high danger of death in childbirth, mainly from causes unrelated to malnutrition).[4,10,11] This compares surprisingly favourably with today's figures: life expectancy at birth (reflecting our improved standards of neo-natal care) averages

75.9 years (men) and 81.3 years (women); though recent work has suggested that for working class men and women this is lower, at around 72 for men and 76 for women.[12]

If we accept the working class figures, which are probably more directly comparable with the Victorian data, women have gained three years of life expectancy since the mid-Victorian period while men have actually fallen back by 3 years. The decline in male life expectancy implicates several causal factors; including the introduction of industrialised cigarette production in 1883, a sustained fall in the relative cost of alcohol and a severe decline in nutritional standards, as outlined below. The improvement in female life expectancy can be partly linked to family planning developments but also to other factors promoting women's health such as improvements in dress. Until widespread accessible family planning facilities arrived after the First World War, women's health could be substantially undermined by up to 30 years of successive pregnancies and births.[13-15] These figures suggest that if twentieth century women had not also experienced the negative impacts of tobacco consumption becoming respectable, along with an increased alcohol intake and worsening nutrition as they began to consume the imported delicacies originally preserved mainly for the men, (all those things which had cost their men folk 3 years), they would have gained 6 years.

Given that modern pharmaceutical, surgical, anaesthetic, scanning, and other diagnostic technologies were self-evidently unavailable to the mid-Victorians, their high life expectancy is very striking, and can only have been due to their health-promoting lifestyle. But the implications of this new understanding of the mid-Victorian period are rather more profound. It shows that medical advances allied to the pharmaceutical industry's output have done little more than change the manner of our dying. The Victorians died rapidly of infection and / or trauma, whereas we die slowly of degenerative disease. It reveals that with the exception of family planning, the vast edifice of twentieth century healthcare has not enabled us to live longer but has in the main merely supplied methods of suppressing the symptoms of degenerative diseases which have emerged due to our failure to maintain mid-Victorian nutritional standards.[16] Above all, it refutes the Panglossian optimism of the contemporary anti-aging movement whose protagonists use 1900 – a nadir in health and life expectancy trends – as their starting point to promote the idea of endlessly increasing lifespan. These are the equivalent of the get-rich-quick share pushers who insisted, during the dot.com boom, that we had at last escaped the constraints of normal economics. Some believed their own message of eternal growth; others used it to sell junk bonds they knew were worthless. The parallels with today's vitamin pill market are obvious, but this also echoes the way in which Big Pharma trumpets the arrival of each new miracle drug.

In short, the majority of even the poorest mid-Victorians lived well, despite all their disadvantages and what we would now consider discomforts. Those that survived the perils of childbirth and infancy lived as long as we do, and were healthier while they were alive. Their prolonged good health was due to their high levels of physical activity, and as a consequence, how and what they ate. We could learn a good deal from them.

HOW THE MID-VICTORIANS WORKED

Due to the high levels of physical activity routinely undertaken by the Victorian working classes, calorific requirements ranged between 150% and 200% of today's historically low values. Almost all work involved moderate to heavy physical labour, and often included that involved in getting to work. Seasonal and other low-paid workers often had to walk up to 6 miles per day.[17] While some Victorian working class women worked from home (seamstressing for instance) more went out to work in shops, factories and workshops, necessitating long days on their feet, plus the additional burden of housework.[17,18] Many single women were domestics, either live-in servants or daily workers. This was particularly physically demanding, as very few households had male servants, so women did all the heavy household work from scrubbing floors to heaving coals upstairs. Men worked on average 9-10 hours / day, for 5.5 to 6 days a week, giving a range from 50 to 60 hours of physical activity per week.[18] Factoring in the walk to and from work increases the range of total hours of work-related physical activity up to 55 to 70 hours per week. Women's expenditure of effort was similarly large.[18] Married women had also domestic chores in their own homes after work, and in addition, their daily dress up to the 1890s at least (when the development of the tailor-made costume reduced both corseting and the weight of numerous layers of fabric) involved real physical effort just in moving around. Male leisure activities such as gardening and informal football also involved substantial physical effort.

Using average figures for work-related calorie consumption, men required between 280 (walking) and 440 calories (heavy yard work) per hour; with women requiring between 260 and 350 calories per hour. This gives calorific expenditure ranges during the working week of between 3000 to 4500 calories / day (men) and 2750 to 3500 (women).

Total calorific requirements were likely to have been even higher during the winter months; with less insulated and less warmed homes, working class Victorians used more calories to keep warm than we do. The same held true for workplaces, unless the work (certain factory operations, blacksmithing, etc) heated the environment to unhealthy levels. At the top end of the physical activity range were the 'navigators', the labourers who built (largely without machinery) the roads and railways that enabled the expansion of the British economy. These men were expending 5000 calories or more per day.

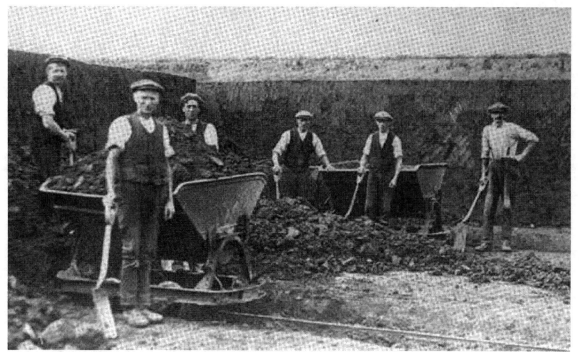

Figure 1. 'Moulders' at the Murston brickfields. The 'moulders' shaped clay into bricks, each man making close on 1000 every hour for an 8½ hour day and a 58 hour week. One brickie is on record as having made 986,091 bricks between April and September.

In short, the mid-Victorians ate twice as much as we do, but due to their high levels of physical activity remained slim; overweight and obesity were relatively rare, and (unless associated with ill-health) were generally identified as phenomena associated with the numerically smaller middle and upper-middle class. But it is not just the amount of food the mid-Victorians consumed that is so unfamiliar; the composition of their diet was also very different from our own.

WHAT THE MID-VICTORIANS ATE
Vegetables, Green and Root
Onions were amongst the cheapest vegetables, widely available all year around at a cost so negligible that few housewives budgeted what cost them around a halfpenny (even cheaper if bruised) for a bunch containing at least a dozen. They might become slightly more expensive in the late spring, when leeks could be substituted.[19] Watercress was another cheap staple in the working class diet, available at a halfpenny for four bunches in the period April to February.[19] The Jerusalem artichoke was consumed from September through to March, often home-grown as it was one of the easiest vegetables to grow in urban allotments.[20] Carrots and turnips were inexpensive staples, especially during the winter months. Cabbage was also cheap and readily available, along with broccoli. Fresh peas were available and affordable from June to July, with beans from July to September.[19]

Fruit

Apples were the cheapest and most commonly available urban fruits from August through to May; with cherries taking over in the May-July period, followed by gooseberries in June up to August, then plums and greengages in July through to September.[19] Dried fruits and candied peel were always cheaply available, and used to sweeten desserts such as bread puddings and for cakes and mincemeat. They were also consumed as an afternoon snack, particularly by children, according to Victorian cookery books[20, 21] and many other sources from Dickens to Mayhew. All fruits and vegetables were organically grown, and therefore had higher levels of phytonutrients than the intensively grown crops we eat today.[22]

Legumes and Nuts

Dried legumes were available all year round and widely used (e.g., pease pudding). The chestnut was the most commonly consumed nut and one of the most commonly eaten street snacks in the chestnut season, running from September through to January. Filberts or hazelnuts were available from October through to May; walnuts were another regularly bought seasonal nut. Imported almonds and Brazil nuts were more expensive, but widely consumed around Christmas as a 'treat'. Coconuts were also imported, often given as presents or won at fairs; commonly grated for use in cakes and desserts.[19]

Fish and Seafoods

The herring was one of the most important fish in the Victorian urban diet; fresh in the autumn, winter, and spring; dried and salted (red herring) or pickled/soused all year round. Red herrings were a staple of the working class diet throughout the year because they were easily cooked (e.g., Idylls of the Poor). Other favourites were cheap and easily obtainable varieties with better keeping qualities than the more vulnerable white fish, including sprats, eels, and shellfish (oysters, mussels, cockles, whelks). Of the white fish consumed, cod, haddock, and John Dory were preferred. Typically, and unlike today, the whole fish was consumed including heads and roes.[19] Fish was available from Monday evening to Friday evening; with broken and day old fish or eels and shoreline shellfish available on Saturdays, as fishermen did not go out over the weekends.[23]

Meats

Consumption of meat was considered a mark of a good diet and its complete absence was rare: consuming only limited amounts was a poverty diet.[23] Joints of meat were, for the poor, likely to be an occasional treat. Yet only those with the least secure incomes and most limited housing, and so without either the cooking facilities or the funds, would be unlikely to have a weekly Sunday joint; even they might achieve that three or four times a year, cooked in a local cookhouse or bakery oven. Otherwise, meat on the bone (shin or cheek), stewed or fried, was the most economical form of meat, generally eked out with offal meats including brains, heart, sweetbreads, liver, kidneys, and 'pluck', (the lungs and intestines of sheep). Pork was the most commonly consumed meat. All meats were from free-range animals.

Eggs and Dairy Products

Many East End [of London] households kept hens in their backyards, and Robert's study of Lancashire suggests similar patterns.[14] Keeping a couple of hens could produce up to a dozen eggs per household per week. There were fears about adulteration of milk (frequently watered-down). Butter did not feature largely in the working-class diet. Dripping was a preferred substitute in the days before cheap margarine. Hard cheeses, as opposed to soft cheeses, were favoured by the working classes as a regular part of their diet, partly because even when the heel of the cheese was too hard to eat, the ends could be toasted.

Alcohol

Beer was the most commonly consumed form of alcohol, but with an alcohol content significantly lower than today's beers. Careful reading of contemporary sources including cookery and domestic economy books suggest that the alcohol percent of beer consumed in the home was probably only 1% to 2%; often less as it was watered down, especially for consumption by women and children.[21,24,25] In pubs, the alcohol content of beer was more regulated and generally higher, ranging from 2% to 3%. These are still weak beers, compared to today's average of around 5%. Spirits were more intermittently consumed by men and rarely by women: respectability and gin did not go together.[26] Working class men and women seldom drank wine, except for port or sherry. A third or more of households were temperate or teetotal, partly due to the sustained efforts of the anti-alcohol movement.[27,28]

Tobacco

Pipe smoking was widespread but intermittent amongst working class males, and a cigar or cheroot might be smoked on special occasions. Snuff had largely fallen out of favour, as had chewing tobacco. The big expansion in mass tobacco consumption by the working classes did not take place until after 1883, when industrial cigarette production was introduced.[29] It was not until the twentieth century that women of all classes became major consumers of tobacco, under the pressure of heavy advertising.

Adulterants

Some adulterants commonly used in Victorian foods were well-known to be toxic even then: lead chromate in mustard, mercury and arsenic compounds as colorants in confectionery, and picrotoxin in beer all undoubtedly contributed to ill health. In contrast, modern nutritional biochemistry reveals that some of the other common 'adulterants' have potentially significant health benefits. The hawthorne used to extend tea, for example, contained vaso- and cardio-protective flavonoids.[31-35] The coriander in beer may have had some anthelmintic activity,[36] and the watering down of beer and spirits was – from a health perspective – a generally good thing!

Dietary Summary

Mid-Victorian working class men and women consumed between 50% and 100% more calories than we do, but because they were so much more physically active than we are today, overweight and obesity hardly existed at the working class level. The working class diet was rich in seasonal vegetables and fruits; with consumption of fruits and vegetables amounting to 8 to 10 portions per day. This far exceeds the current national average of around 3 portions, and the government-recommended 5-a-day. The mid-Victorian diet also contained significantly more nuts, legumes, whole grains and omega three fatty acids than the modern diet. Much meat consumed was offal, which has a higher micronutrient density than the skeletal muscle we largely eat today.[37] Prior to the introduction of margarine in the late Victorian period, dietary intakes of trans fats were very low. There were very few processed foods and therefore little hidden salt, other than in bread. Recipes suggest that significantly less salt was then added to meals. At the table, salt was not usually sprinkled on a serving but piled at the side of the plate, allowing consumers to regulate consumption in a more controlled way. The mid-Victorian diet had a lower calorific density and a higher nutrient density than ours. It had a higher content of fibre (including fermentable fibre), and a lower sodium / potassium ratio. In short, the mid-Victorians ate a diet that was not only considerably better than our own, but also far in advance of current government recommendations. It more closely resembles the Mediterranean diet, proven in many studies to promote health and longevity; or even the 'Paleolithic diet' recommended by some nutritionists.[38]

In terms of alcohol consumption, the comparisons with today are also revealing. Many contemporary reports suggest that around a fifth of Victorian working class men might, when employed, spend up to a fifth of their income on beer.[39] Assuming an average urban income ranging from £1 to £4 per week, and given mid-century pub prices of 3d to 8d per pint for beer, the reported expenditure would account for around 16 pints to 20 per week maximum, or between 3 and four pints per night. As Victorian beer generally had an alcohol content ranging between 1 and 3.5%,[40] this is equivalent to one and a half to two pints of beer per day in contemporary terms. Seen in this light, the huge Victorian concerns about drunkenness in the Victorian working classes appear to be more a reflection of respectable morality than a real public health issue.[41] Cost implications ensured that for most, the Victorian 'alcohol problem' was certainly less significant than it is in our time, when the frequency of public drunkenness and levels of injury and illness have become a serious public health concern.[42] Finally, mid-Victorian tobacco consumption was very much lower than today.

These new findings reveal that, contrary to received wisdom, the mid-Victorians ate a healthier diet than we do today. This had dramatic effects on their health and life expectancy.

HOW THE MID-VICTORIANS DIED

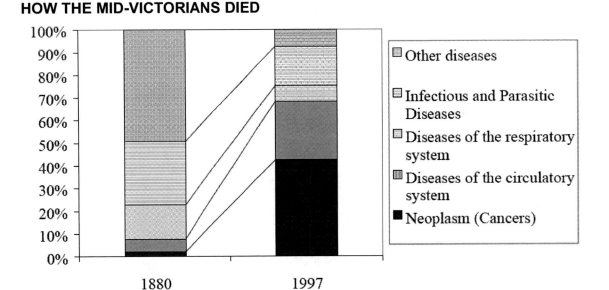

*Figure 2. Causes of Death in England and Wales: 1880 and 1997.
Reprinted from Charlton 2004, 2, 9.*

The overall pattern of Victorian causes of death broadly resembles that found in developing countries today, with infection, trauma, and infant / mother mortality in the pole positions, and non-communicable degenerative disease being relatively insignificant.

Common causes of death[43,44] included:

1. Infection including TB and other lung infections such as pneumonia; epidemics (scarlet fever, smallpox, influenza, typhoid, cholera, etc), with spread often linked to poor sanitation: and the sexually transmitted diseases.
2. Accidents/trauma linked to work place and domestic conditions. Death from burns was an important cause of death among women, due largely to a combination of open hearth cooking, fashions in dress, and the use of highly flammable fabrics.
3. Infant / mother mortality.[44] This was generally due to infection, although maternal haemorrhage was another significant causative factor.
4. Heart failure. This was generally due to damage to the heart valves caused by rheumatic fever, and was not a degenerative disease. Angina pectoris does not appear in the registrar general's records as a cause of death until 1857 – and then as a disease of old age – although the diagnosis and its causes were recognised.[45-48]

Uncommon causes of death included:

1. Coronary artery disease (see above)
2. Paralytic fits (strokes, see *Webster's Dictionary*). Stroke was mainly associated with the middle and upper classes who ate a diet in which animal derived foods had a more significant role, and who consumed as a result rather less fruits and vegetables. Strokes were generally non-fatal, at least the first time; although mortality rates increased with each subsequent stroke.[43]
3. Cancers were relatively rare.[43] While the Victorians did not possess sophisticated diagnostic or screening technology, they were as able to diagnose late stage cancer as we are today; but this was an uncommon finding. In that period, cancer carried none of the stigma that it has recently acquired, and was diagnosed without bias. For example, in 1869 the Physician to Charing Cross Hospital describes lung cancer as '… one of the rarer forms of a rare disease. You may probably pass the rest of your students life without seeing another example of it.'[49]

Not only were cancers very uncommon compared to today, they appear to have differed in other key respects. James Paget (of Paget's Disease) built a large practice on the strength of diagnosing breast cancer, which he did by sight and palpation – that is at Stages 3 and 4. In this group he describes a life expectancy of 4 years after diagnosis, extending to eight or more with surgery.[50] The corresponding figures today are stage 3: 50% survival at 10 years if given surgery, chemo- and radio-therapy, and stage 4: overall survival about 15 months. These figures suggest that breast cancer during the Victorian period was significantly less rapidly progressive than is the case today, probably due to the Victorians' significantly higher intakes of a range of micro- and phyto-nutrients which slow cancer growth.

In summary, although the mid-Victorians lived as long as we do, they were relatively immune to the chronic degenerative diseases that are the most important causes of ill health and death today.

WHAT DID THE VICTORIANS EVER DO FOR US?

The implications of the mid-Victorian story are far-reaching, because, unlike the paleolithic scenario, details of the mid-Victorian lifestyle and its impact on public health are extensively documented. Thus, the mid-Victorian experience clearly shows us that:

1. Degenerative diseases are not caused by old age (the 'wear and tear' hypothesis); but are driven, in the main, by chronic malnutrition. Our low energy lifestyles leave us depleted in anabolic and anti-catabolic co-factors; and this imbalance is compounded by excessive intakes of inflammatory compounds. The current epidemic of degenerative disease is caused by the widespread problem of multiple micro- and phyto-nutrient depletion (Type B malnutrition.)
2. With the exception of family planning and antibiotics, the vast edifice of twentieth century healthcare has generated little more than tools to suppress symptoms of the degenerative diseases which have emerged due to our failure to maintain mid-Victorian nutritional standards.
3. The only way to combat the adverse effects of Type B malnutrition, and to prevent and / or cure degenerative disease, is to enhance the nutrient density of the modern diet.

THE CASE FOR SUPPLEMENTS

Our levels of physical activity and therefore our food intakes are at an historic low. To make matters worse, when compared to the mid-Victorian diet, the modern diet is rich in processed foods. It has a higher sodium/potassium ratio, and contains far less fruit, vegetables, wholegrains, and omega 3 fatty acids. It is lower in fibre and phytonutrients, in proportional and absolute terms; and, because of our high intakes of potato products, breakfast cereals, confectionery, and refined baked goods, may have a higher glycemic load. Given all this, it follows that we are inevitably more likely to suffer from dysnutrition (multiple micro- and phytonutrient depletion) than our mid-Victorian ancestors.

This is supported by survey findings on both sides of the Atlantic; the USDA's 1994 to 1996 Continuing Survey of Food Intakes by Individuals,[51,52] and the National Diet & Nutrition Surveys[53] both show that many individuals today are unable to obtain RNI values of a variety of vitamins and minerals. Malnutrition in the UK is now reckoned to contribute to illness-related costs in excess of £7.3 billion per annum.[54] Since it would be unacceptable and impractical to recreate the mid-Victorian working class 4000 calorie/day diet, this constitutes a persuasive argument for a more widespread use of food fortification and/or properly designed food supplements. Most supplements on the market are incredibly badly designed. They are assembled by companies that do not understand the real nutritional issues that confront us today, and sell us pills containing irrational combinations and doses that can do more harm than good.

To insist, as orthodox nutritionists and dieticians do, that only whole fruit and vegetables contain the magical, health-promoting ingredients represents little more than the last gasp of the discredited and anti-scientific theory of vitalism *("Vitalism – the insistence that there is some big, mysterious extra ingredient in all living things – turns out to have been not a deep insight but a failure of imagination."* – Daniel Dennett.) Even the stately FSA concedes that fruit juices count towards your 5-a-day, as do freeze-dried powdered extracts of fruits and vegetables. As our knowledge of phytochemistry and phytopharmacology increases, it has become perfectly acceptable to use rational combinations of the key plant constituents in pill or capsule form.

These arguments are developed in *Pharmageddon*,[56] a medical textbook which illustrates how micro- and phyto-nutrients can be specifically combined in order to prevent and treat the chronic degenerative diseases that characterise and dominate the 20th and 21st centuries; and how they

61

could be integrated into our food chain in order to reduce the contemporary and excessively high risks of the degenerative diseases to the far lower mid-Victorian levels.

CONCLUDING REMARKS

In light of the huge body of evidence linking diet to health, many researchers are now studying the dietary intakes of different groups of people and attempting to tease out such esoteric factors as, for example, just how much omega 3 fish oil is necessary to reduce the risk of Alzheimer's; or how what dose of flavonoids should be consumed to reduce the risk of stomach cancer.

Most of this research is patently a waste of time. Current generations are, from an historical point of view, anomalous. Our historically low levels of physical activity and consequently food intakes mean that even those groups consuming the highest levels of berry fruits, green leaf vegetables, or oily fish, are still well below optimal (mid-Victorian) levels of consumption.

For example, eminent scientists working with dietary elements thought to reduce the risk of cancer have commented that although 'pharmacological levels' of compounds such as flavonoids or salicylates have strong anti-cancer properties *in vitro*, there is little evidence that dietary (or 'physiological') levels of intake have any protective effects in humans.

In contrast the mid-Victorians, with their far greater intakes of fruits and vegetables, which were organic and in many cases contained significantly higher concentrations of phytonutrients than our intensively grown crops do[57,62] were consuming 'pharmacological' levels of these valuable and protective compounds. This would explain why they were so effectively protected against cancer, and heart disease, and all the other degenerative, non-communicable disorders. And it would also explain why, with our very low 'physiological' intakes, we are so terribly prone to these largely avoidable diseases.

We believe also that the on-going search for disease susceptibility genes is ahistoric and therefore largely misinformed. The mid-Victorian gene pool was not significantly different to our own, yet their incidence of degenerative disease was approximately 90% less.[4] In the high-nutrient mid-Victorian environment, the vast majority of the population was protected; and the combination of high levels of physical activity and an excellent diet enhanced the expression of a coordinated array of health-promoting genes.[63,64] As the nutrient tide has receded, increasing numbers of genetic polymorphisms have become exposed,[65] thus making current genome-wide association studies (GWAS) largely redundant. If we take this argument to an extreme, and progress to a diet totally devoid of micronutrients, all polymorphisms become disease-associated. It follows that the pharmaceutical industry's attempts to develop genomically derived and individualized treatments such as RNA interference and ISPC are unlikely to impact on public health. The steel vessel of Public Health is rent open, and the drug companies are selling us high-priced pots of caulk.

Do not, therefore, look to the drug companies to provide remedies for the appalling state of our health; or to our politicians who seem unable, in many cases, to see far beyond the brims of their parliamentary troughs. Look, instead, to the food and beverage industries, and to a lesser extent the supplement companies, who may well step up to the plate with better designed foods and nutritional programmes once the currently profoundly counter-productive regulatory system has been re-drafted.

REFERENCES

1. Clayton P, Rowbotham J. An unsuitable and degraded diet? Part 1: Public health lessons from the mid-Victorian working class diet. *J Roy Soc Med.* 2008;101:282-289.
2. Clayton P, Rowbotham J. An unsuitable and degraded diet? Part 2. Realities of the mid-Victorian diet. *J Roy Soc Med.* 2008;101:350-357.
3. Clayton P, Rowbotham J. An unsuitable and degraded diet? Part 3. Victorian consumption patterns and their health benefits. *J Roy Soc Med.* 2008;101:454-462.
4. Charlton J, Murphy M, eds. *The Health of Adult Britain 1841-1994.* London, UK: National Statistics; 2004.
5. Burnett J, Oddy D, eds. *The Origins and Development of Food Policies in Europe.* London, UK: Leicester University Press; 1994.
6. Coleman T. *The Railway Navvies.* London, UK: Pelican; 1968.
7. Rowntree BS. *Poverty, a Study of Town Life London: Centennial Edition.* London UK: Policy Press; 2001.
8. Garrow J. Starvation in hospital [Editorial]. *British Medical Journal.* 1994;308:934.
9. Colquhoun A, Lyon P, Alexander E. Feeding minds and bodies: the Edwardian context of school meals. *J Nutrit Health Sci.* 2001;31:117-125.
10. McKeown T. *The Modern Rise of Population.* London, UK: Edward Arnold; 1976.

11. McNay K, Humphries J, Klasen S. Death and Gender in Victorian England and Wales: Comparisons with Contemporary Developing Countries. Cambridge, UK: Cambridge Working Papers in Economics, University of Cambridge; 1998.
12. Joyce M. The Right to Live: health, democracy and inequality. Available at : http://www.iwca.info/cgi-bin/iwcacte.pl? Accessed August, 2006.
13. Harris B. Gender, health and welfare in England and Wales since industrialisation. *Research in Economic History.* 2008;26:157-204.
14. Roberts E. *A Woman's Place.* Oxford, UK: Blackwell; 1984.
15. Ross E. *Love and Toil Motherhood in Outcast London 1870-1918.* London, UK: Oxford University Press; 2002.
16. Colgrove J. The McKeown Thesis: A Historical Controversy and Its Enduring Influence. *Am J Public Health.* 2002;92:725-729.
17. Steadman Jones G. *Outcast London. A study in the relationship between classes in Victorian Society.* London, UK: Penguin; 1984.
18. 8th Report of the Medical Officer of the Privy Council, 1865, Parliamentary Papers, XXXIII, 1866.
19. Mayhew H. *London Labour and the London Poor.* London, UK; 1861-1862.
20. Kirton J. *Buy Your Own Cherries.* Norwich, UK: Jarrold & Sons; 1862.
21. *Plain Cookery Recipes.* London, UK: Nelson; 1875.
22. Halvorsen BL, Holte K, Myhrstad MC, et al. A systematic screening of total antioxidants in dietary plants. *J Nutr.* 2002;132:461-471.
23. Walton JK. Fish and Chips and the British Working Class, 1870-1940. Leicester, UK: Leicester University Press; 1992.
24. Wigglesworth E. *The Brewers and Licensed Victuallers Guide.* Leeds, UK: Green & Co; 1849.
25. Newsholme A, Scott M. *Domestic Economy.* London, UK: Swann Sonnenschein; 1892.
26. Wood H. Danesbury House. Edinburgh, UK: Scottish Temperance League; 1860:112-156.
27. Harrison B. *Drink and the Victorians: The Temperance Question in England, 1815-1872.* 2nd ed. Edinburgh, UK: Keele University Press; 1994.
28. Berridge V. *Current and future alcohol policy: the relevance of history.* History and Policy Papers. Available at http://www.historyandpolicy.org/archive/policy-paper-38.html Accessed February, 2006.
29. Hilton M. *Smoking in British popular culture 1800-2000.* Manchester, UK; Manchester University Press: 2000.
30. Brixius K, Willms S, Napp A, Tossios P, Ladage D, Bloch W, Mehlhorn U, Schwinger RH. Crataegus special extract WS 1442 induces an endothelium-dependent, NO-mediated vasorelaxation via eNOS-phosphorylation at serine 1177. *Cardiovasc Drugs Ther.* 2006;20:177-184.
31. Asgary S, Naderi GH, Sadeghi M, Kelishadi R, Amiri M. Antihypertensive effect of Iranian Crataegus curvisepala Lind.: a randomized, double-blind study. *Drug Exp Clin Res.* 2004;30:221-225.
32. Kim SH, Kang KW, Kim KW, Kim ND. Procyanidins in crataegus extract evoke endothelium-dependent vasorelaxation in rat aorta. *Life Sci.* 2000;67:121-131.
33. Veveris M, Koch E, Chatterjee SS. Crataegus special extract WS 1442 improves cardiac function and reduces infarct size in a rat model of prolonged coronary ischemia and reperfusion. *Life Sci.* 2004;74:1945-1955.
34. Walker AF, Marakis G, Simpson E, Hope JL, Robinson PA, Hassanein M, Simpson HC. Hypotensive effects of hawthorn for patients with diabetes taking prescription drugs: a randomised controlled trial. *Br J Gen Pract.* 2006;56:437-443.
35. Xie ML, Mao CP, Gu ZL, Chen KJ, Zhou WX, Guo CY. Effects of xiaoyu tablet on endothelin-1, nitric oxide, and apoptotic cells of atherosclerotic vessel wall in rabbits. *Acta Pharmacol Sin.* 2002;23:597-600.
36. Eguale T, Tilahun G, Debella A, Feleke A, Makonnen E. *In vitro* and *in vivo* anthelmintic activity of crude extracts of *Coriandrum sativum* against *Haemonchus contortus*. *J Ethnopharmacol.* 2007;110:428-433.
37. McCance RA, Widdowson EM. *The Composition of Foods.* 6th ed. London, UK: Food Standards Agency; 2006.
38. O'Keefe JH Jr, Cordain L. Cardiovascular disease resulting from a diet and lifestyle at odds with our Paleolithic genome: how to become a 21st-century hunter-gatherer. *Mayo Clin Proc.* 2004;79:101-108.

39. Harrison B. *Drink and the Victorians: The Temperance Question in England, 1815-1872.* 2nd ed. Edinburgh, UK: Keele University Press; 1994.

40. Berridge V. *Current and future alcohol policy: the relevance of history.* History and Policy Papers. Available at http://www.historyandpolicy.org/archive/policy-paper-38.html Accessed February, 2006.

41. Swift R. Behaving Badly: Irish Migrants and Crime in the Victorian City. In: Rowbotham J, Stevenson K, eds. *Criminal Conversations: Victorian Crimes, Social Panic and Moral Outrage.* Columbus, OH: Ohio University Press; 2005.

42. Williams R. The pervading influence of alcoholic liver disease in hepatology. *Alcohol Alcohol.* 2008;43:393-397.

43. Smith EB. *The People's Health.* London, UK: Croom Helm; 1979.

44. Woods R. *The Demography of Victorian England and Wales.* Cambridge, UK: Cambridge University Press; 2000.

45. Burns A. *Observations on some of the most frequent and important diseases of the heart; on aneurism of the thoracic aorta; on preternatural pulsation in the epigastric region; and on the unusual origin and distribution of some of the large arteries of the human body.* Edinburgh, UK: Bryce; 1809.

46. Heberden W. Some Account of a Disorder of the Breast. Presented to the Royal College of Physicians, London, 1768. Published in: *Medical Transactions.* London, UK: Royal College of Physicians; 177: 59-67.

47. Morgagni GB. *De sedibus et causis morborum per anatomen indagatis libri quinque.* Vol 1. Venice, Italy: 1761. [Italian].

48. Virchow R. *Die Cellularepathologie in ihrer begrundung auf physiologische and pathologische Gewebelehre.* Berlin, Germany: Hischwald; 1858. [German].

49. Hyde Salter H. *Lancet.* July 3rd, 1869.

50. Paget J. On the average duration of life in patients with scirrhous cancer of the breast. *Lancet* 1856;1:62-63.

51. USDA2: US Department of Agriculture, Agricultural Research Service. *Food and Nutrient Intakes by Individuals in the United States, by Sex and Age, 1994–96. Nationwide Food Surveys Report No. 96-2.* Washington, DC: US Department of Agriculture, Agricultural Research Service; 1998.

52. USDA1: US Department of Agriculture, Agricultural Research Service. *Food Survey Research Group: The Continuing Survey of Food Intakes by Individuals and the Diet and Health Knowledge Survey, 1994–96.* CD-Rom data.

53. Gregory J *et al.* National Diet and Nutrition Surveys. London, UK: HMSO.

54. Elia M, Stratton R, Russell C, Green C, Pan F. *The cost of disease-related malnutrition in the UK: considerations for the use of oral nutritional supplements (ONS) in adults.* BAPEN New Health Economic Report; 2005.

55. Bardia A, Tleyjeh IM, Cerhan JR, Sood AK, Limburg PJ, Erwin PJ, Montori VM. Efficacy of antioxidant supplementation in reducing primary cancer incidence and mortality: systematic review and meta-analysis. *Mayo Clin Proc.* 2008;83:23-34.

56. Clayton P. *Pharmageddon: The Limits of Pharmaceutical Medicine – and What Lies Beyond.* London, UK: Royal Society of Medicine Press: 2009.

57. Carbonaro M, Mattera M, Nicoli S, Bergamo P, Cappelloni M, Modulation of antioxidant compounds in organic vs conventional fruit (peach, *Prunus persica L.*, and pear, *Pyrus communis L.*) *J Agr Food Chem.* 2002;50:5458-5462.

58. Dani C, Oliboni LS, Vanderlinde R, Bonatto D, Salvador M, Henriques JA. Phenolic content and antioxidant activities of white and purple juices manufactured with organically- or conventionally-produced grapes. *Food Chem Toxicol.* 2007;45:2574-2580.

59. Pérez-López AJ, López-Nicolas JM, Núñez-Delicado E, Del Amor FM, Carbonell-Barrachina AA. Effects of agricultural practices on color, carotenoids composition, and minerals contents of sweet peppers, cv. Almuden. *J Agric Food Chem.* 2007;55:8158-8164.

60. Gill C. 2008. Personal communication.

61. Lester GE, Manthey JA, Buslig BS. Organic vs conventionally grown Rio Red whole grapefruit and juice: comparison of production inputs, market quality, consumer acceptance, and human health-bioactive compounds. *J Agric Food Chem.* 2007;55:4474-4480.

62. Halvorsen BL, Holte K, Myhrstad MC, *et al.* A systematic screening of total antioxidants in dietary plants. *J Nutr.* 2002;132:461-471.

63. Ornish D, Magbanua MJ, Weidner G, *et al.* Changes in prostate gene expression in men undergoing an intensive nutrition and lifestyle intervention. *Proc Natl Acad Sci U S A.* 2008;105:8369-8374.
64. Traka M, Gaspar AV, Melchini A, et al. Broccoli Consumption Interacts with GSTM1 to Perturb Oncogenic Signalling Pathways in the Prostate. PLoS ONE. 2008;3:e2568. doi:10.1371/journal.pone.0002568.
65. Ames BN, Elson-Schwab I, Silver EA. High-dose vitamin therapy stimulates variant enzymes with decreased coenzyme binding affinity (increased K(m)): relevance to genetic disease and polymorphisms. *Am J Clin Nutr.* 2002;75:616-658.

ABOUT THE AUTHOR

Primary author Dr. Paul Clayton graduated Summa cum Laude at Edinburgh University, and subsequently did a PhD in medical pharmacology at the MRS Brain Metabolism Unit, Edinburgh. He then served as a senior advisor to Committee on Safety of Medicines. For last 30 years PC has specialised in the pharmacology of food and food derivates. He consults to Coca Cola, Proctor & Gamble, Arla Foods, Danisco, HFL and many other companies in the food and beverage sector. He is the author of Health Defence, the first textbook of pharmaconutrition (now going to 3rd edition), and PharmacoNutrition (to be published by the Royal Society of Medicine Press in Spring of '09). PC is currently developing clinical trials of pharmaconutritional interventions in Hungary, where he is Scientific Director of the new Szent-Gyorgyi Institute.

PERMISSION STATEMENT

Chapter 8
Adrenal Dysfunction: An Evidence-Based Review of the Causes and Consequences of Hypocortisolism

Lena D. Edwards, M.D.
Owner and President, Balance Health & Wellness Center (Lexington, KY USA);
Andrew H. Heyman, M.D., MHSA
Adjunct Assistant Professor, University of Michigan (Ann Arbor, MI USA)

INTRODUCTION

The role of the adrenal glands in the stress response and the importance of proper adrenal gland function in health maintenance have long been described.[1,2] Extensive medical literature exists confirming the adverse consequences of chronic stress on normal human physiology. Yet many patients who seek medical treatment for their symptoms of chronic stress are often dismissed or misdiagnosed. Treatment is then often misdirected at symptom relief rather than on correction of the true underlying pathophysiological processes. Despite our extensive understanding of chronic stress and its effects on the hypothalamic-pituitary-adrenal (HPA) axis, disagreement and speculation about the existence of adrenal fatigue or hypoadrenia as a distinct clinical entity persists. Although the literature is not as abundant, the presence of primary adrenally-mediated hypocortisolism has been cited.[3-5]

Integrity of the HPA axis is essential for maintaining homeostasis. Exposures to any stressors results in the stimulation of the "stress system" thereby inducing a myriad of adaptive hormonal responses designed to re-establish disrupted homeostasis and to promote survival of the organism. These adaptive reactions include such changes as a reduction in appetite and increases in thermogenesis, arousal, analgesia, blood pressure, heart rate, and attention. These "fight or flight" responses are intended to be short lived as the organism either survives or succumbs to the stressor(s). Once an organism has been chronically subjected to the stress system response, initial physiological adaptive mechanisms paradoxically lead to demise of the organism via abnormal adrenal hormone production, aberration of diurnal patterns of adrenal hormone release, and ultimately overt reductions in adrenal gland hormone productions.

The neuroendocrine system, of which the adrenals are an integral component, is complex and directly affects the aging process via the intricate interplay of numerous hormones and organ systems. Despite the increase in life expectancy of our population, many patients are not enjoying optimal health and often succumb to premature death from numerous comorbidities. The development of disease and premature death is profoundly influenced by exposure to chronic stressors, and there are extensive studies outlining the relationship between chronic stress, aging, and hormonal deficiencies including menopause, andropause, somatopause, adrenopause, and thyropause. Early identification and treatment of the physiologic consequences of chronic stress may lead to a reduction in patient morbidity and mortality.[6-9]

Many clinical syndromes including 'burnout', fibromyalgia (FMS), chronic pain, chronic fatigue syndrome (CFS), Post-traumatic Stress Disorder (PTSD), chronic pelvic pain, and asthma have been shown to be associated with hypocortisolism and HPA axis dysfunction.[3,5,10] Yet our medical training has not emphasized investigation of these endocrinological aberrations as causative in patients with these and other conditions. Rather, traditional medical practices promote identification and treatment of the extremes of the adrenal gland dysfunction spectrum, namely Addison's disease and Cushing's disease. Baschetti astutely describes how CFS, as one example, shares 43 clinical features with Addison's disease. He goes on further to suggest that with such "impressive clinical overlap", clinicians should assess cortisol production in patients with chronic fatigue even if the classical signs and symptoms of Addison's disease are lacking.[11]

ADRENAL DYSFUNCTION
Adrenal Anatomy and Hormones
The adrenal glands lie directly above the kidneys and are divided into two distinct areas. The outer adrenal cortex accounts for 80 to 90 percent of the gland volume while the inner adrenal medulla comprises the remainder. The adrenal cortex is comprised of three layers, the zona glomerulosa, the zona fasiculata, and the zona reticularis. The zona glomerulosa produces mineralocorticoids. Glucocorticoids are produced the zona fasiculata, and to a lesser extent the zona reticularis. The adrenal androgens are produced by the zona reticularis. The inner portion of the gland, the adrenal medulla, is the site of catecholamine production. The rate limiting step of steroid hormone production is the conversion of cholesterol to pregnenolone, which requires adequate amounts of properly functioning cytochrome P450 enzymes. The function and potency of the adrenal hormones is largely dictated by their structural configuration, the presence of serum carrier proteins, and the evolution of receptors to which the hormones must bind to exert their effects.[12,13] It is in part through effects on these mechanisms that chronic stress induces both absolute and "relative" adrenal hormone deficiencies.

Cortisol is the major glucocorticoid secreted by the adrenal cortex and is often referred to as the "stress hormone" since it is essential in the stress response ("fight or flight") system. It is released via hypothalamic corticotropin-releasing hormone (CRH) stimulation of pituitary adrenocorticotropic hormone (ACTH), both of which are released during periods of stress. The primary role of cortisol is to restore homeostasis after short periods of physiological stress. In high concentrations, cortisol has potent metabolic effects as a catabolic hormone in all organs and tissues except the liver. Under its influence, gluconeogenesis, glycogenolysis, and lipolysis increase. Other systemic effects of elevated glucocorticoids include increased gastric acid secretion, decreased collagen production, reduced diuresis, reduced bone formation, and hippocampal neuronal damage. Cortisol elevation also impairs thyroid hormone production and function, and causes numerous aberrations in immune system regulation and function.[7,8,12-15]

Proposed Mechanisms Underlying the Evolution of Hypocortisolism
Although many of the deleterious effects of chronic stress have been attributed to elevations in cortisol, ample evidence also implicates hypocortisolism in disease development. There is much speculation as to how hypocortisolism evolves after periods of prolonged stress. Reduced availability of cortisol may be due not only to primary depletion of the adrenal glands but also to secondary mechanisms involving reductions in biosynthesis of hormones at different levels of the HPA axis. Since integrity of HPA axis function and predictable patterns of diurnal cortisol release are essential for maintaining homeostasis during periods of stress, much of the available research on stress induced diseases and hypocortisolism has focused on disturbances in these mechanisms.[3,5,10,16,17]

An increase in hypothalamic release of CRF with subsequent adaptive down-regulation of CRF receptors at the level of the pituitary gland has also been proposed. Although this has been demonstrated in animal studies, replication of such a process in human subjects has been difficult but may be indirectly implied.[3] Yehuda *et al* and others have suggested that an increase in the sensitivity of the HPA axis to hypercortisolism induced negative feedback may be the cause, however further study is needed to fully elucidate these mechanisms.[18,19] Hellhammer and Wade have postulated a developmental model whereby hypocortisolism via a hypoactive HPA axis may develop after prolonged periods of chronic stress. This consequence evolves after an initial period of HPA axis hyperactivity and hypercortisolism. They speculate hypocortisolism may occur as a type of maladaptive "over compensation" of the self preservation mechanisms designed to protect the metabolic machinery from the effects of persistent cortisol elevation.[19]

Heim and colleagues have reviewed studies on the effects of chronic stress on the adrenal glands and have concluded, "There is a considerable body of evidence of reduced adrenal gland activity and reactivity in human subjects living under conditions of chronic stress."[3] Their conclusion is congruent with some of the authors' review of the literature and clinical experiences. Some have proposed the term "adrenal fatigue" to describe such a relative state of adrenal insufficiency. Indeed, findings of low basal cortisol levels, elevation in ACTH levels, and reduction in cortisol responses to ACTH and CRH stimulation have been demonstrated in patients with syndromes including FMS, CFS, PTSD, and chronic pelvic pain.[3,10,22-24] Moreover, chronic stress can result in reduced adrenocortical activity without development of overt diseases as some human studies have shown.[16] Chronic stress-induced reduction in basal adrenal activity may account for many of the early signs and symptoms of adrenal insufficiency.[10,11,16,25] Additionally, there is significant overlap between the symptoms of hypocortisolism and the signs and symptoms of adrenal insufficiency in critically ill patients. Such patients have been showed to have impaired adrenal gland release of cortisol either through direct adrenal injury, adrenal gland unresponsiveness, and lack of substrate for cortisol production.[26-28]

Another mechanism through which adrenally mediated hypocortisolism may develop is via a reduction in adrenal gland volume. Certainly, this notion is plausible since some human studies have demonstrated adrenal hypertrophy during periods of acute stress.[29] Unfortunately, studies demonstrating primary adrenally mediated hypocortisolism are not found in the literature in abundance. One study by Scott and colleagues did find this to be the case in CFS patients. In their study, Scott *et al* found CFS patients to have suboptimal adrenal cortisol production in response to stimulation testing which was felt to be secondary to reduction in adrenal gland size as evidenced by computed tomography.[4]

Metabolic Consequences of Hypocortisolism

An essential physiological consequence of hypocortisolism is an increase in the inflammatory response and immune system activation. This increase in inflammatory signaling is due in part to loss of counterregulation by normal glucocorticoid activity. Consequently, the upregulation of numerous inflammatory pathways increases susceptibility to the development of autoimmune diseases, inflammation, neoplasias, chronic pain, atopy, allergies, and asthma.[3,6,10,16,30,31] Studies have found elevated levels of pro-inflammatory cytokines in patients with stress related disorders including PTSD, CFS, and FMS.[32-35] Breast cancer patients demonstrate significant post-treatment exhaustion and have been shown to have significantly altered HPA axis activity in combination with elevated interleukin (IL)-6 levels, flattened cortisol curves, increased mortality, and metastases. Furthermore, the more flattened the cortisol curve the worse the prognosis and the earlier the mortality.[36,37] Other studies have found elevations in IL-1β, natural killer cells, antinuclear auto-antibodies, thyroid antibodies, and prostaglandins in patients with PTSD, in patients with intrusive traumatic memories, in sexually abused girls, and in patients with CFS, FMS, and chronic pelvic pain respectively.[3,32-34]

Hypocortisolism also indirectly allows an in increase in catecholamine activity since cortisol normally suppresses catecholamine release. As a result, there is an increase in sympathetic nervous system activity. Increased levels of catecholamines have been observed in patients with both PTSD and FMS.[16,17,35]

Although clearly maladaptive, the physiologic changes induced by hypocortisolism and HPA axis hypoactivity may actually be protective and may have evolved to ensure survival of the organism. McEwen was the first to describe the concepts of allostasis and allostatic load and described them as the unchecked negative cumulative effects of chronic stress on normal physiological function. He outlines four conditions that lead to an increase in allostatic load: 1) repeated assaults from multiple stressors (increasing risk for hypertension, myocardial infarction and atherosclerosis); 2) lack of adaptation; 3) prolonged response due to delayed shutdown (associated with depression, hippocampal atrophy, osteoporosis, insulin resistance); and 4) inadequate cortisol response (leading to loss of counterregulation of cytokines IL-6, tumor necrosis factor (TNF), increased auto-immune and inflammatory conditions, atherosclerosis, FMS, and persistent fatigue. [36]

Studies have shown increased mortality in patients with high allostatic loads and decreased allostatic loads in hypocortisolemic patients. Extrapolating from these findings, Fries *et al* postulate that, "Hypocortisolism is a protective response dampening chronic HPA axis activity and thereby reducing the damaging effects of the glucocorticoid response to daily hassles at the expense of symptoms such as high stress sensitivity, pain, and fatigue.[10] Further supporting their proposal that hypocortisolism is actually a protective response, Fries and colleagues have observed comparable groups of pregnant women and found those with lower morning cortisol levels had higher daily stress compared to their counterparts experiencing normal or low daily stress loads. The authors speculate that the hypocortisolism may be a counter-regulatory protective mechanism designed to protect placental corticotrophin-releasing factor (CRF) from maternal cortisol.[10]

Raison and Miller also portend that enhanced stimulation of the immune system may be protective. In individuals suffering from recurrent or ongoing infectious assaults, reduced glucocorticoid signaling impairs the normally adaptive inhibitory mechanisms thereby promoting the body's ability to mount adequate retaliatory defenses.[17] Other authors have coined term "sickness response" to describe the anorexia, fatigue, anhedonia, hyperesthesia, and concentration difficulties often accompanying the body's response to infection. In his 1988 paper, Hart wrote that the sickness response results from the body's adaptive attempts to ration and prioritize its defenses to better eliminate the pathogen. Many symptoms of the sickness response mimic those of stress related bodily disorders, and an association between hypocortisolism induced FMS and the sickness response has been observed.[3,10,17,21] The notion that hypocortisolism is actually protective is intriguing and further investigation will likely find this to be the case.

CONCLUDING REMARKS

The clinical implications of HPA axis dysfunction and aberrations in the normal diurnal pattern of cortisol release have been well recognized in the medical literature. Although hypercortisolism has long been thought to mediate many stress induced metabolic derangements, research continues to emerge highlighting the role of hypocortisolism in physiologic comprise and disease development. Because of the extensive nature of this topic as well as the overabundance of supporting medical literature, this paper serves as an initial introduction to and a general overview of the topic of hypocortisolism. Although numerous theories exist attempting to define the cascade of events leading to stress induced hypocortisolism, the mechanisms through which it evolves have not been fully elucidated. It is conceivable that when a hypermetabolic adrenal gland is subjected to persistent stress, the transition from hyper- to hypocortisolism may occur as a result of primary adrenal dysfunction. It is by this mechanism we propose adrenal dysfunction, and what some term 'adrenal fatigue' may evolve.

Clinicians are rigorously trained to identify and treat the extremes of adrenal dysfunction (Addison's disease and Cushing's disease). Instruction on the early of adrenal dysfunction but who do not yet manifest the extremes of disease remains lacking. A higher degree of clinical awareness about the clinical presentations of HPA axis dysfunction and hypocortisolism is essential to properly diagnose and treat patients who present with this 'subclinical' systemic process.

We hope this paper provides readers with a better understanding of the complexity of the stress system response, its effects on the HPA axis, and the clinical consequences of adrenal gland dysregulation. We also suggest adrenal fatigue, or 'burn out' of the adrenal gland consequent to chronic stress, represents only one form of primary hypocortisolism and clinicians should be cautious not to be short sighted in their understanding and treatment of the complexity of HPA axis dysfunction and the role it also plays in the development of hypocortisolism.

REFERENCES

1. Cannon WB. Stresses and strains of homeostasis. *Am J Med Sci*. 1935;189:1-4.
2. Tattersall RB. Hypoadrenia or "A Bit of Addison's Disease". *Medical History*. 1999;43:450-467.
3. Heim C, Ehlert U, Hellhammer DH. The potential role of hypocortisolism in the pathophysiology of stress-related bodily disorders. *Psychoneuroendocrinology.* 2000;25:1-35.
4. Scott LV, Teh J, Reznek R, Martin A, Sohaib A, Dinan TG. Small adrenal glands in chronic fatigue syndrome: a preliminary computer tomography study. *Psychoneuroendocrinology*. 1999;24:759-768.
5. Tintera JW. The hypoadrenocortical state and its management. *New York State Journal of Medicine*. 1955;55:1869-1876.
6. Seeman TE, Singer BH, Rowe JW, Horwitz RI, McEwen BS. Price of adaptation-allostatic load and its health consequences. MacArthur studies of successful aging. *Arch Intern Med*. 1997;157:2259-2268.
7. Chrousos GP. Organization and integration of the endocrine system. *Sleep Med Clin*. 2007; 2:125-145.
8. Tsigos C, Chrousos GP. Hypothalamic-pituitary-adrenal axis, neuroendocrine factors and stress. *Psychosom Res*. 2002;53:865-871.
9. Epel ES. Psychological and metabolic stress: A recipe for accelerated cellular aging? *Hormones*. 2009;8:7-22.
10. Fries E, Hesse J, Hellhammer J, Hellhammer DH. A new view on hypocortisolism. *Psychoneuroendocrinology*. 2005;30:1010-1016.

11. Baschetti R. Chronic fatigue. *CMAJ.* 2006;175:386.

12. Nussey S, Whitehead S. *Endocrinology: An Integrated Approach.* Oxford, UK: BIOS Scientific Publishers Ltd; 2001.

13. Blakemore C, Jennet S. *The Oxford Companion to the Body.* New York, NY: Oxford University Press; 2001.

14. McAuley MM, Kenny RA, Kirkwood TT, Wilkinson DD, Jones JJ, Miller VM. A mathematical model of aging-related and cortisol induced hippocampal dysfunction. *BMC Neurosci.* 2009;10:26.

15. Besedovsky HO, Del Rey A, Sorkin E. Integration of activated immune cell products in immune endocrine feedback circuits. In: Oppenheim JJ, Jacobs DM, eds. *Leukocytes and Host Defense Feedback Volume 5.* New York, NY: Oppenheim; 1984: 200.

16. Gunnar MR, Vazquez DM. Low cortisol and flattening of expected daytime rhythm: potential indices of risk in human development. *Dev Psychopathol.* 2001;13:515-538.

17. Raison CL, Miller AH. When not enough is too much: the role of insufficient glucocorticoid signaling in the pathophysiology of stress-related disorders. *Am J Psychiatry.* 2003;160:1554-1565.

18. Yehuda R, Teicher MH, Trestman RL, Leven good RA, Siever LJ. Cortisol regulation in posttraumatic stress disorder and major depression: a chronobiological analysis. *Biol Psychiatry.* 1996;40:79-88.

19. Yehuda R. Sensitization of the hypothalamic-pituitary-adrenal axis in posttraumatic stress disorder. *Ann NY Acad Sci.* 1997;821:57-75.

20. Hellhammer J, Schlotz W, Stone AA, Pirke KM, Hellhammer D. Allostatic load, perceived stress, and health: A prospective study in two age groups. *Ann NY Acad Sci.* 2004;1032:8-13.

21. Hellhammer DH, Wade S. Endocrine correlates of stress vulnerability. *Psychother. Psychosom.* 1993;60:8-17.

22. Heim C, Ehlert U, Hanker JP, Hellhammer DH. Abuse-related posttraumatic stress disorder and alterations of the hypothalamic-pituitary-adrenal axis in women with chronic pelvic pain. *Psychosom Med.* 1998;60:309-318.

23. Cleare AJ, Miell J, Heap E, Sookdeo S, Young L, Malhi GS, O'Keane V. Hypothalamic-pituitary-adrenal axis dysfunction in chronic fatigue syndrome, and the effects of low-dose hydrocortisone therapy. *J Clin Endocrinol Metab.* 2001;86:3545-3554.

24. Heim C, Ehlert U, Hanker JP, Hellhammer DH. Abuse-related posttraumatic stress disorder and alterations of the hypothalamic-pituitary-adrenal axis in women with chronic pelvic pain. *Psychosom Med.* 1998;60:309-318.

25. Baschetti R. Chronic fatigue syndrome, exercise, cortisol and lymphadenopathy. *J Intern Med.* 2005;258:291-292.

26. Chang SS, Liaw SJ, Bullard MJ, Chiu TF, Chen JC, Liao HC. Adrenal insufficiency in critically ill emergency department patients: a Taiwan preliminary study. *Acad Emerg Med.* 2001;8:761-764.

27. Rivers EP, Blake HC, Dereczyk B, Ressler JA, Talos EL, Patel R, Smithline HA, Rady MY, Wortsman J. Adrenal Dysfunction in Hemodynamically Unstable Patients in the Emergency Department. *Academic Emergency Medicine.* 1999;6:626-630.

28. Marik PE, Pastores SM, Annane D, Meduri GU, Sprung CL, Arlt W, et al. Recommendations for the diagnosis and management of corticosteroid insufficiency in critically ill adult patients: Consensus statements from an international task force by the American College of Critical Care Medicine. *Crit Care Med.* 2008;36:1937-1949.

29. Hart BL. Biological basis of the behavior of sick animals. *Neurosci Behavior Rev.* 1988;60:309-318.

30. McEwen B. Protective and damaging effects of stress mediators. *N Engl J Med.* 1998;338:171-179.

31. Patarca-Montero R, Antoni M, Fletcher MA, Klimas NG. Cytokine and other immunologic markers in chronic fatigue syndrome and their relation to neuropsychological factors. *Appl Neuropsychol.* 2001;8:51-64.

32. Torpy DJ, Papanicolaou DA, Lotsikas AJ, Wilder RL, Chrousos GP, Pillemer SR. Responses of the sympathetic nervous system and the hypothalamic-pituitary-adrenal axis to interleukin-6: a pilot study in fibromyalgia. *Arthritis Rheum.* 2000;43:872-880.

33. Spivak B, Shohat B, Mester R, Avraham S, Gil-Ad I, Bleich A, Valevski A, Weizman A. Elevated levels of serum interleukin-1β in combat-related posttraumatic stress disorder. *Biol Psychiatry.* 1997;42:345-348.

34. DeBellis MD. Antinuclear antibodies and thyroid function in sexually abused girls. *J Trauma Stress.* 1996;9:369-378.

35. Liberzon I, Abelson JL, Flagel SB, Raz J, Young EA. Neuroendocrine and psychophysiologic responses in PTSD: a symptom provocation study. *Neuropsychopharmacology*. 1999;21:40-50.
36. Bower JE, Ganz PA, Aziz N, Olmstead R, Irwin MR, Cole SW. Inflammatory responses to psychological stress in fatigued breast cancer survivors: relationship to glucocorticoids. *Brain, Behavior, and Immunity*. €2007;21:251-258.
37. Sephton S, Sapolsky R, Kraemer H, Spiegel D. Diurnal cortisol rhythm as a predictor of breast cancer survival. *J Natl Cancer Inst*. 2000;92:994-1000.

ABOUT THE AUTHORS

Dr. Lena Edwards is the president and owner of Balance Health & Wellness Center in Lexington, KY. She is a Board Certified Internist and Board Certified and Fellowship Trained in Anti-Aging/Functional/Regenerative Medicine with over ten years of clinical experience. In addition to running her solo medical practice full-time, she is also the medical director of Seasons Salon and Spa and the health and wellness columnist for Business Lexington, a prominent local business publication. She is also actively involved in teaching, writing, and speaking on topics relating to anti-aging, health, and wellness. Her special interests are bio-identical hormone replacement and adrenal gland dysfunction.

Dr. Andrew Heyman is a nationally recognized expert in natural medicine, involved in the field of Integrative and Anti-Aging Medicine for over two decades with extensive experience in nutrition, vitamins, herbology, Chinese medicine, manual therapies and more. He serves as faculty in the Department of Family Medicine at the University of Michigan, where he received his medical degree. Dr. Heyman also holds a Masters in Health Services Administration from the University of Michigan School of Public Health and was the first administrator for the University of Michigan Complementary and Alternative Medicine Research Center where he was responsible for administering a $7 million NIH grant to research alternative therapies for cardiovascular diseases. Dr. Heyman currently has several leadership positions in the field of Anti-Aging Medicine. He is the national clinical chair of the Consortium of Academic Health Centers for Integrative Medicine, a collaboration of 50 North American universities (including Harvard, Stanford, Duke, Columbia, Yale and more) that all maintain a strong interest in the combination of conventional with natural therapies. Dr. Heyman remains clinically active as well, which includes providing medical acupuncture at the University of Michigan, in addition to teaching medical students and residents about natural therapies. He also directs a medical spa and several private practices in Michigan and Virginia. He has consulted to physicians, health systems and public health professionals seeking to develop wellness, lifestyle and nutrition programs.

Chapter 9
An Integrative Approach to Treating Prostate Cancer
Isaac Eliaz, M.D., M.S., L.Ac.
Founder & Medical Director, Amitabha Medical Clinic and Healing Center (Sebastopol, CA USA)

ABSTRACT
This paper will outline an integrative approach to treating prostate cancer, with the emphasis being on maximum diagnosis and minimum intervention.

Keywords: prostate cancer, integrative, modified citrus pectin, MCP

INTRODUCTION
In order to understand the unique benefits of an integrative approach to treating prostate cancer (PCa), one must first become familiar with the concept of holistic, integrative medicine as a practice. This is an approach to healthcare that draws upon various healing traditions and modalities in order to create a synergistic movement towards health and away from disease.

Conventional treatments, particularly in oncology, focus on attacking and destroying the disease. While this approach has its merits, strictly disease-focused treatments neglect to support the patient's health and vitality. The goal of integrative medicine, on the other hand, is to support health and vitality while at the same time reducing disease (see Figure 1). Naturally, this would also be the goal of any effective integrative PCa treatment.

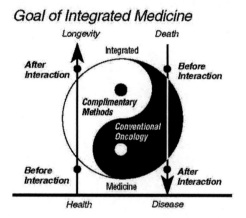

Figure 1. Wellness is represented by two vertical axes/arrows.
The health axis points up with increasing health representing increasing longevity. In contrast as one travels up the disease axis one gets closer to death. A hypothetical patient presenting with a weakened vitality and an aggressive cancer would show up on the axes at the points labeled "before interaction." The goal of integrative medicine is to use a combination of conventional and complimentary methods to increase health and decrease the disease resulting in the patient ending up at the points "after the interaction."

PCa is a heterogeneous disease ranging from a physiological, "non-malignant" process to a disease that can kill you in months. Therefore, the basic principles in the treatment of PCa are maximum diagnosis and minimum intervention. So what does this mean on a practical level?

THE FIRST STEP: EVALUATION

The first step in evaluating a person newly diagnosed with PCa is to create a broad and extensive baseline – one that focuses on both the health and the disease aspects. Unfortunately, however, many evaluations – even those performed by the leading institutions in this country –lack much of the basic information critical to designing intelligent treatment protocols.

Understanding the Patient

In order for a person to get back to optimal health, they first need to know where on the health and disease axis they are. This requires a thorough evaluation. As a doctor, that means listening to the patient in order to get a feel for his health status. How well is he taking care of himself? Does he exercise, walk, maintain a healthy diet, and use stress reduction methods? How quickly will he respond to a health concern or health opportunity? For example, a man notices a change in urinary frequency – does he call his doctor the same day, or does he wait six months before reporting it?

Another factor to evaluate is the willingness of the patient to address his own condition. Does he have enough flexibility to make the necessary changes in his life – and to follow through with them? This information is absolutely critical to making assessments as well as my recommendations.

A physician can think that a particular patient needs to walk one hour a day, alter their diet, take six different supplements, change their job, etc. But making the above recommendations without considering if the person is able (or willing) to follow them would be an example of doctor-driven medicine. In patient-driven medicine, which is the calling card of any good integrative doctor, the reality of the patient's situation will always determine the plan.

Gathering Essential Data

The initial evaluation always has a number of components, which when combined will give the clinician a better ability to assess the health and disease status of the person. These include:

1. Detailed history and intake.
2. Thorough physical exam.
3. Additional diagnostic methods, such as pulse diagnosis.
4. Laboratory work – prostate specific antigen (PSA), hormonal profile, prostate cancer gene 3 (PCA3) test, etc.)
5. Imaging – ultrasound, MRI, bone scan.
6. Biopsies, if needed.

Since it is not possible to cover all of these components in detail in this paper, the focus will remain on the four main issues: blood tests, urine tests, imaging, and biopsies.

Important Blood Tests
Prostate Specific Antigen (PSA)

It is important to measure both the total and free levels of PSA, as well as to track the magnitude of changes and the speed at which the patient's PSA is increasing. Much could be said about PSA evaluation, but for now, simply remember these key points:

- Low PSA doesn't necessarily mean a slow-growing disease.
- Rate of change is very important.
- PSA can actually have seasonal variations.
- It is essential to evaluate the PSA in relationship to the size of the prostate. For example, a PSA of 4.5 with a prostate of 30ml is more worrisome than a PSA of 7.5 with a prostate of 110ml (very large). That is because a normal prostate secretes PSA at an average rate of 0.07ng/ml. For the 30ml patient, this natural production accounts for 2.1 out of the total score of 4.5 – only half. For the 7.5 patient, however, it accounts for all of the PSA.
- Prostatitis is quite non-specific, and will also elevate the PSA. So, elevated PSA with urinary symptoms (a common complaint in cases of prostatitis) is less worrisome than the same PSA without any complaints.

Prostatic Acid Phosphatase (PAP)

This test was used regularly before PSA gained popularity, and still plays an important role in the initial evaluation. The finding of a PAP elevation signifies that there is a higher risk that the PCa is outside the prostate and that the cancer is a more aggressive type. This is an essential component of initial "staging" of PCa. This information can be used to guide selections for further diagnostic tests, and ultimately, to guide recommendations for an integrative treatment plan.

Hormonal profile

The hormone profile is very important. For example, a patient with PCa who has a high testosterone level will respond better to treatment compared to a patient with the same disease, but lower testosterone levels. The following basic lab tests are critical for all PCa patients:

- Total Estrogens: As men age, testosterone is increasingly converted to estrogens. This tendency is compounded by exposure to environmental toxins, xenoestrogens, and toxic heavy metals. The clinician will often see an increase in total estrogens and estrogen to testosterone ratio, and a decrease in 2-hydroxy estrogen to 16-hydroxy estrogen to ratio. These hormonal changes are major factors in the pathogenesis of PCa and contribute greatly to the increased incidence of PCa. It is in restoring this critical hormonal balance that complementary and integrative medicine has come to play a leading role in the prevention of PCa.
- Estradiol
- Estrone sulfate
- Testosterone (both total and free)
- Progesterone
- DHEA-S
- Dihydrotestosterone (DHT)
- Prolactin: Higher levels (including high-normals) are associated with a worse prognosis.
- Carcinoembyronic antigen (CEA): The cancer tends to be more aggressive when this colon cancer marker is elevated.
- Insulin-like growth Factor -1 (IGF-1): When elevated, this also indicates a more aggressive disease. However, this marker has proved to be of limited clinical value, possibly due to laboratory detection issues.
- Thyroid function: Thyroid function is also important as it can indicate the speed of the individual's metabolism. In cancerous conditions, the body will often attempt to slow down the thyroid in an attempt to slow down the disease. As such, the problem is not really in the thyroid – it is simply an adaptive response of the body. For that reason, exercise caution when considering thyroid support in a patient with cancer. From the perspective of health and disease, if the disease is moving faster than the health aspect, speeding up that aspect is not a good idea. If, on the other hand, the patient is winning their fight, speeding up can allow for more healing to be accomplished in a shorter period of time.

Inflammatory and Viscosity Markers

- HbA1c: This is a marker for glucose metabolism. Altered blood sugar regulation is a risk factor for cancer and a stimulus to cancer cell proliferation. Blood sugar dysregulation is part of metabolic syndrome which promotes inflammation.
- Fibrinogen: This is an indicator of blood viscosity or thickness, and signifies a decrease in the fluidity of movement of blood and therefore oxygen and nutrients to cells. Congestion, poor nutrient delivery, and lowered oxygen availability to cells promotes abnormal cell development. Cancer cells also use fibrin in the bloodstream to conceal their presence. Cancer predisposes a patient to increased viscosity and thus an increased risk of blood clots and pulmonary embolism which can be life threatening.
- Lipoprotein(a) [Lp(a)]: This is one of the factors measured in a thorough lipid metabolism evaluation and is an indication of viscosity.

- Cardio or ultrasensitive C-reactive protein (CRP): This is an important general marker for inflammation which is one of the primary drivers of abnormal cell proliferation.

Important Urine Tests
Prostate Cancer Gene 3 (PCA3) Test

The PCA3 test is a gene-based test carried out on a urine sample. PCA3 is highly specific to PCa – and therefore, in contrast to PSA, it is not increased by common conditions such as benign prostatic enlargement (BPH) or inflammation of the prostate (prostatitis).

There are four scenarios in which PCA3 could help in making better decisions in diagnosing and treating PCa. Using this test, a doctor can determine:

1. Which men with ≥ 1 negative biopsy have a high probability of a positive repeat biopsy.
2. Which men with an elevated PSA level (between 2.5 and 10 ng/mL) or a low PSA level but a suspicious digital rectal examination DRE have a high probability of a positive first biopsy.
3. Which men with PCa have a high probability of significant PCa.
4. Which men with PCa have a high probability of disease progression on watchful waiting.

The PCA3 test has yet to be cleared or approved by the US Food and Drug Administration (FDA). However, this test is available and is being used by some of the most progressive physicians working with PCa patients today.

Imaging

A good baseline requires good imaging. Unfortunately, an ultrasound taken in the average urologist's office is unacceptable. Some reliable state-of-the-art imaging techniques include:

- Color Doppler flow ultrasound: This is an excellent and cost-effective imaging method. The limitation is that at the present time very few doctors know how to do it well. For those lucky enough to be in the Bay Area, however, The University of California, San Francisco (UCSF) is one of the best imagers in the country.
- Endorectal MRI with spectroscopy: This is an advance in imaging where two modalities are used and compared. It is used to help determine the probability of organ confined disease, or to see if the cancer has spread to seminal vesicles or regional lymph nodes.
- Bone scan: This is a scan that may be ordered for initial staging of PCa if aggressive disease is suspected from the biopsy report.

Biopsy

Biopsies are the gold standard for confirmation of PCa. So why even write about them? Well, it is clear that biopsies are over-performed. When are they really needed? The basic question one should ask when it comes to biopsies is: Will the biopsy make a difference in the treatment plan? Certain patients with localized disease are adamant about following their imaging and staying on watchful waiting – and for them, repeat biopsies will make no difference whatsoever. However, the disadvantage of this approach is that the aggressiveness of the cancer may increase over time and biopsy provides a way of monitoring for these changes. Following blood markers and non-invasive imaging techniques closely can often provide enough information to see if there is an expansion of the disease. These decisions are ultimately the patient's choice after weighing carefully the pros and cons.

Biopsies provide important information on the grade of the disease, the Gleason score, and how extensively the disease has spread on the local level. Knowing the level of aggressiveness of the cancer and whether it is localized or has extended beyond the prostate gland itself are crucial pieces of information for formulating an effective integrative treatment strategy. However, biopsies have the following disadvantages:

- Side effects, including long-term pain, possible infections, and disturbance in urination.
- Spread of disease. Although there are no good studies to confirm this point, we do know that for patients with negative RT-PCR (meaning, no PCa cells are detected systemically), half will turn positive after radical prostatectomy. Logically speaking, multiple injuries to the tissue (in this case, caused by 6 to 18 biopsies) will increase

inflammation and angiogenesis, both of which are major contributors toward metastasis.

- False negative is another concern. False negatives can range from 20 to 40 percent, depending on how many biopsies are done, what imaging techniques are used, and who is doing them.

If a PCa patient can get good imaging routinely, his PSA is low, and his disease is clearly localized to a small part of the prostate, follow-up without biopsy is a viable choice – one that will likely become more popular over time. PCA3 can also prevent unnecessary biopsies, as mentioned before. But of course, making this decision is easier if you have all the laboratory data and know how to interpret it.

If a patient is undergoing biopsies, supplementation with modified citrus pectin (MCP) – at a dosage of 15 g/day for a week before biopsies, and for the three to four weeks after – is critical. This protocol can reduce the chance of cancer spreading due to the procedure.

TREATMENT
Conventional Treatments
Conventional treatment paths will vary depending on the patient's situation, but options include localized treatments, androgen deprivation therapy, cyrotherapy, and high intensity focused ultrasound (HIFU).

Localized Treatments
- External radiation (3D conformal) therapy: This has been improved as intensity modulated radiation therapy (IMRT), where the intensity can be modified based on the location – delivering more radiation to the tumor, and less to the surrounding tissue.
- Seed implants: This is another form of radiation in which radioactive seeds are implanted into the prostate gland, in order to concentrate the activity while reducing damage to surrounding tissue.
- Radical Prostatectomy or prostate removal: This should be a last resort, as it tends to result in a high number of undesirable effects – including erectile dysfunction and urinary incontinence. However, advancements in surgical procedures may soon change that.

Androgen Deprivation Therapy
Combined hormonal therapy (or the use of more than one hormone-modulating drug) can yield positive results when used appropriately over a long period of time. However, monotherapy – the use of a single agent (such as Casodex) without suppression of testosterone – offers the best quality of life. This method is preferable in cases of less aggressive disease, where the quality of life and sexual function are a major consideration

Cryotherapy
This technique freezes the abnormal tissue. Side effects are also an issue for long-term quality of life. The skill of the practitioner is often a crucial element in the outcome. In adition, preparatory interventions which shrink the prostate gland prior to surgery will improve the changes of a successful outcome.

High Intensity Focused Ultrasound (HIFU)
This technique uses sound waves to increase the temperature of the tissue to kill the prostate cells. This method is currently in clinical trials in the US but has been used successfully in other parts of the world on thousands of men. Urologists in the US who have been trained to do HIFU take American patients out of the country for the procedure. This procedure seems to have the lowest side effect profile.

Complementary Treatments

Any beneficial integrative program for PCa will always begin with dietary modification. These are some of the most critical changes a patient can make, and they can have a very big impact on prostate health in the long term.

Key Dietary Modifications

The first dietary modification should be the elimination of red meats. Meat contains high amounts of arachidonic acid, and some by-products of arachidonic acid have promoted PCa in animals. In addition, well-done and cured meats (such as bacon, salami, and ham) can also promote PCa, so consumption of these meats should be limited as well.

Omega-3-rich fish has been shown to be beneficial for PCa patients. With that said, PCa patients should be wary of fish that are also high in mercury (such as swordfish and tuna).

Finally, several servings of cruciferous vegetables (cabbage, Brussels sprouts, broccoli, and cauliflower) a day can help to fight PCa and reduce risk of the disease. In test tube and animal studies, these foods have been shown to have potent anticancer activity – likely due to several of their active compounds, including indole-3-carbinol, 5 glucaric acid (calcium D-glucarate), and sulforaphane. But the protective effects of cruciferous vegetables are also thought to be due to their high concentration of the carotenoids lutein and zeaxanthin, as well as their stimulatory effects on the breakdown of environmental carcinogens associated with prostate PCa.

Whatever their primary mode of action may be, the value of "eating your vegetables" has been borne out in a number of clinical studies. Research has indicated as much as a 41 percent decreased risk of PCa among men eating three or more servings of cruciferous vegetables per week, as compared with those eating less than one serving per week.

Critical Supplements

Conventional approaches to PCa focus on attacking and destroying it with procedures such as seed implant, radical prostatectomy, radiation therapy, cryotherapy, or hormonal therapy. These approaches are not always successful at eradicating the disease and are often associated with side effects that severely impact quality of life. In addition, these approaches do not support the overall health and vitality of the patient.

The goal of integrative medicine, on the other hand, is to support a person's health and vitality while at the same time reducing the disease. Conventional treatments can be complemented by nutrients to boost the immune system, modulate hormones, usher the toxins out of the body, and much more. In some cases, nutrients have shown promise in preventing and controlling PCa.

Studies have shown that combining nutrients that have different mechanisms of action in effective amounts allows the cancer to be attacked from all sides at once. In addition to their anticancer properties, many nutrients have specific health-promoting properties. These nutrients can be categorized according to their beneficial principles:

- Anti-tumor
- Prevention of cancer metastasis
- Detoxification and liver support
- Hormonal modulation
- Anti-microbial
- Anti-inflammatory
- Antioxidant
- Anti-angiogenesis
- Immune enhancement

By selecting nutrients that have multiple mechanisms of action we create a program which simultaneously impacts the cancer cells from a number of angles as well as supporting the patient's immune response, thus creating an additive beneficial effect.

Modified Citrus Pectin (MCP)

One such nutrient with multiple beneficial properties is modified citrus pectin (MCP). For this reason, it is one of the foundational supplements for treatment of PCa at Amitabha Clinic. Research both in vitro and in vivo has elucidated several mechanisms of action that give MCP powerful anticancer effects. Clinical evidence has shown that a specific modified citrus pectin product – administered in dosages of 5 g three times daily following prostatectomy, radiation, or cryosurgery – can increase the time of PSA doubling in men with PCa, thus slowing disease progression. Additionally, in vitro studies on MCP's effect on a PCA3 human PCa cell line plated on a human endothelial cell monolayer showed a significant 80.7 percent cytotoxicity.

Earlier research at Wayne State University demonstrated that MCP, when given orally, had an inhibitory effect on carbohydrate-mediated tumor growth, angiogenesis, and metastasis in vivo, and showed a dose-dependent inhibition of tumor angiogenesis on breast and colon cancer cell cultures using human umbilical vein endothelial cells in vitro.

Recent advances have introduced a new, more potent form of this compound, which has since demonstrated even more compelling results among a group of late-stage cancer patients. In late 2007, researchers at Albert-Ludwigs University in Freiburg, Germany enrolled 49 patients, each with advanced state solid tumors of varying types – colon cancer, PCa, breast cancer, kidney cancer, lung cancer, cervical cancer, liver cancer, and pancreatic cancer, among others. Each patient had completed conventional treatments, including surgery, chemotherapy, and radiation without success. Nearly 90 percent of the cancers had metastasized. During the trial, patients were administered 5 g of MCP orally, three times a day. They would later be evaluated for clinical benefit – including pain reduction, improved physical functioning, increased appetite and sleep, and reduced fatigue. At just eight weeks, the results were already overwhelmingly positive, with 20.7 percent of the patients showing an overall clinical benefit response and stabilization of disease. By the conclusion of the study, response rates continued to improve, with a majority of the patients showing improved quality of life and pain reduction. And perhaps most remarkably, one patient with metastasized PCa demonstrated a 50 percent decrease in PSA levels at 16-weeks, accompanied by a significant increase in clinical benefit.

More recent research, performed at Columbia University and just accepted for publication, points to the potential mechanism of this action. Laboratory results indicate that MCP can inhibit cell proliferation and apoptosis in PCa cell lines (including androgen-dependent and androgen-independent cells), induce apoptosis by the cleavage of caspase-3, and inhibit cell proliferation by reducing MAP kinase signaling.

In the initial interview of a PCa patient, an evaluation of potential toxicities and exposures should be performed, through careful history taking and laboratory testing. Heavy metals, in conjunction with the abundant presence of environmental toxins and xenoestrogens, constitute a dangerous insult to the body through DNA damage, hormonal modulation, immune suppression, oxidative stress, and hyper-inflammation. Since they are of particular concern in PCa, addressing toxicity is a fundamental part of an effective approach to treatment.

The chelation properties of MCP have been confirmed in several clinical trials – showing that in healthy individuals, this natural compound can safely and gently increase the urinary excretion of toxic metals such as mercury, cadmium, arsenic and lead. These results have been paired with significant improvement in various clinical symptoms, suggesting that MCP's ability to remove heavy metals and environmental toxins on an ongoing basis may be of great benefit to cancer patients.

A published five-case study report describes a significant toxic burden in a patient with unusually aggressive PCa. This 59-year old with a PCa diagnosis and a suspected history of metal toxicity had a confirmed highly elevated lead level using urine collection post EDTA challenge. He began a combined treatment regimen using hormonal therapy, intravenous and oral nutrient treatments including MCP combined with alginates at 3 capsules twice daily on an empty stomach. At three months, his lead level decreased 49 percent, his PSA dropped from 102 to <0.1, and we have seen a resolution of his bone metastasis. This represents a remarkable success for a patient with aggressive disease. By using this safe, oral chelation supplement, this patient's lead burden was reduced significantly, with a corresponding enhancement in his response to an integrative treatment approach.

It must be noted, however, that the preparation used in the above research (PectaSol) is the only form of MCP that has been validated in human clinical trials. This is important, as not all MCP products are the same – and no other product on the market matches the chemical specifications of PectaSol. If the molecular weight of the MCP is too high, it cannot be absorbed into the bloodstream. If it is too low, or doesn't have the right structure, it won't effectively block all the galectin sites, which is one of MCP's modes of action in inhibiting metastasis. To achieve comparable results to any of these clinical studies, the same preparation should be used, in appropriate doses according to the patient's needs (Table 1).

Table 1. The Use of Modified Citrus Pectin

MCP Application	Use (Take on an empty stomach)
Active Cancer	15 g/day (5 g TID)
Biopsy	15 g/day (5 g TID) Take one week before procedure and two weeks after.
Heavy Metal Chelation	High body burden levels: 15 g/day (5 g TID) Lower levels: 15 g/day for 5 days a month, 5 g/day the rest of the month
Cancer Prevention	5 g/day ongoing

Medicinal Mushrooms

Another cornerstone nutrient in integrative PCa protocols is the use of combined medicinal mushrooms. Medicinal mushrooms have been well researched for their anti-tumor and immune-stimulating effects, and are absolutely essential for the maintenance of vitality. They are important for maintaining long-term health and are even more critical for individuals who have cancer.

For patients who are new to using mushrooms, beginning with a "priming" dose for one to two months is recommended. This dose should be two or three times the maintenance level. After this, the patient can continue taking the normal maintenance dose, which is typically the suggested dose.

It is important for a patient to supplement with medicinal mushrooms on a long-term basis, as some of their benefits require an extended time of consumption. Ideally, a patient should supplement with many different mushrooms in order to obtain optimal protection. In the case of cancer, for example, beneficial mushrooms include Coriolus, Cordyceps, Reishi, Polyporus, Maitake, Agaricus, Shiitake, Hericium, Auricularis, Poria, and Tremella. At Amitabha Clinic, we use a unique formula consisting of six varieties of medicinal mushrooms, all grown on cancer fighting immune enhancing herbs.

Combining Selected Nutrients

There are a number of other nutrients that have extensive research demonstrating value in an integrative approach to treating PCa. We select and modify each patient's program over time in conjunction with their use of conventional therapy approaches. There are a number of products on the market that combine compounds that greatly enhance compliance. Prior to a surgical intervention the goal is to shrink the prostate, lower tumor volume, reduce inflammation, and protect tissue integrity.

To this end, the clinician may select from several possible nutrient groups. Hormonal modulators, such as the indole-3-carbinol (I3C) metabolite diindolylmethane (DIM), a phytochemical found in cruciferous vegetables, have been shown to induce growth inhibition, apoptosis, and antiangiogenic activity in multiple cancer cell lines and tumors.

Mineral supplements such as zinc have shown no observable toxicity and inhibit the growth of lung and PCa cells grown in xenograft mice models models. Similarly, the herbal saw palmetto with its liposterolic component has been shown to significantly reduce the concentration of 5alpha-dihydrotestosterone (DHT) in the prostate and result in a significant increase in apoptosis and significant decrease in pathological tumor grade and frank tumor incidence.

The use of anti-inflammatories such as quercetin and curcumin should also be incorporated into individual integrative programs. Quercetin has an antioxidant and anti-inflammatory activity and prevents cancer. It inhibits the growth of certain malignant cells in vitro, as well as histamine and most cyclin-dependent kinases, and also displays unique anticancer properties. Curcumin, the major active constituent of the dietary spice turmeric, also has potential for the prevention and therapy of cancer. Preclinical data have shown that curcumin can both inhibit the formation of tumors in animal models of carcinogenesis and act on a variety of molecular targets involved in cancer development.

Prospective and retrospective epidemiological studies indicating an inverse relationship between lycopene intake and PCa risk have similarly been supported by in vitro and in vivo experiments. These studies show that oral lycopene is bioavailable, accumulates in prostate tissue, and is localized to the nucleus of prostate epithelial cells. In addition to antioxidant activity, in vitro experiments indicate other mechanisms of chemoprevention by lycopene including induction of apoptosis and antiproliferation in cancer cells, anti-metastatic activity, and the upregulation of the antioxidant response element leading to the synthesis of cytoprotective enzymes.

Another example in the selective use of supplements in an integrative approach is the use of Vitamin D-3. Because of its mechanism as a differentiating agent, I avoid using it during radiation. Baseline 25(OH) vitamin D levels should be obtained and monitored during vitamin D therapy.

Table 2 shows supplement dosages and mechanisms of action which you may find useful in guiding your selection of different combinations. Of course, one of the many strengths of nutritional and herbal therapies is the ability to combine nutrients that have similar properties to get a stronger, synergistic effect. Using nutritional blends that are formulated to encompass many different therapeutic aspects is one way to do this. These blends often use lower amounts of individual ingredients and work synergistically to produce a stronger effect than the recommended larger dose of a single ingredient, as listed in the table below.

New cell culture research delineates the role of this type of poly-botanical blend in PCa cell proliferation. A recently-completed study – performed in collaboration with Columbia University Medical Center and pending publication – determined that a 33-ingredient formula can induce G2/M cell cycle arrest and apoptosis in both androgen-dependent (AD) and androgen-independent (AI) PCa cell lines at very low concentrations. Moreover, this formula was shown to inhibit AKT and MAPK signal pathways, suggesting its suppression of PCa progression in both AD, and more importantly AI PCa, for which there is currently no curative therapy

This synergistic blend of nutrients, in combination with MCP, forms a basic protocol. From this foundation, you may include additional medicinal mushrooms and nutrients (or more of specific herbs or nutrients) as warranted by the patient's health and disease status.

Table 2. Selected Valuable Nutrients for Treating Prostate Cancer

Nutrient or Herb	General Use (Total amounts per day)	Highlighted Properties
Modified Citrus Pectin (MCP)	15 g/day on an empty stomach (1-2 hours from other supplements)	Anti-tumor Prevents metastasis Anti-angiogenic Toxic metal chelation
Medicinal mushrooms	4-12 g/day	Immune enhancement Detoxification/liver support
Curcumin (turmeric root extract 95% curcuminiods)	1,500-4,500 mg/day	Cytotoxic/anti-tumor Hormonal modulation Detoxification/liver support
Chinese herbs	varies	Cytotoxic/anti-tumor Multiple properties
Saw Palmetto berry extract Pygeum bark extract	100-600mg/day	Cytotoxic/ anti-tumor Hormonal Modulation Anti-inflammatory
Lycopene	10-30 mg/day	Cytotoxic/ anti-tumor Antioxidant
Artemisinin	200-1,200 mg/day	Cytotoxic/anti-tumor, use carefully- can weaken digestion
Selenium	200 mcg-3,600 mcg/day (depending on length of application)	Cytotoxic/anti-tumor Antioxidant
Thymic protein A	As directed	Immune enhancement
Stinging nettles root	150-400 mg extract a day	Immune enhancement
Soy isoflavones.	100- 1,000 mg/day,	Anti-angiogenic, bone protection, prevents metastasis
DIM (Diindolymethane)	50-300 mg a day	Hormonal modulation
Garlic	Varies	Anti-microbial
Cayenne	Varies	Anti-inflammatory
Green tea extract	50-500 mg/day	Antioxidant Hormonal modulation
Vitamin D-3	1,000 IU- 6,000 IU/day Monitor kidney function with high doses	Promotes cell differentiation
Zinc	30-50 mg/day	Antioxidant Hormonal modulation
Vitamin E	400-1,200 IU/day	Antioxidant
Vitamin C	1,000-6,000 mg/day	Antioxidant Other multiple functions
Qurecetin	250-2,000 mg/day	Antioxidant Anti-inflammatory Reduces drug resistance
Conjugated linoleic acid (CLA)	3,000 mg/day	Cytotoxic Promotes cell differentiation
Resveratrol from red grape extract (*Vitus vinifera*) or *Polygonum cuspidatum* root extract)	20-200 mg/day	Antioxidant
Broccoli extract 22:1 (*Brassica oleracea*)	50-200 mg/day	Antioxidant Anti-inflammatory
Alpha lipoic acid	100-400 mg/day	Antioxidant
Pomegranate	100-500 mg/day	Antioxidant Anti-inflammatory

CONCLUDING REMARKS

Studies continue to attempt to elucidate the complex issues surrounding which populations of men may benefit from the various interventions available – with age, PSA, Gleason score, co-morbidities, and quality of life issues all factoring into the equation. One thing, however, is clear: The use of natural, safe compounds – with no side effects, and which improve not only prostate health but the health and balance of many organs and systems – will be of benefit to every patient.

This type of integrative, holistic approach to protocol design – which is focused on the patient and honors the basic principles of health and disease – may delay the need for invasive approaches in some men, augment a watchful waiting approach for others, and reduce side effects for those choosing to undergo conventional treatments.

FURTHER READING

Awad AB, Fink CS. Phytosterols as anticancer dietary components: evidence and mechanism of action. *J Nutr.* 2000;130:2127-2130.

Awad AB, Fink CS, Williams H, Kim U. In vitro and in vivo (SCID mice) effects of phytosterols on the growth and dissemination of human prostate cancer PC-3 cells. *Eur J Cancer Prev.* 2001;10:507-513.

Awad AB, Gan Y, Fink CS. Effect of beta-sitosterol, a plant sterol, on growth, protein phosphatase 2A, and phospholipase D in LNCaP cells. *Nutr Cancer.* 2000;36:74-78.

Baldus SE, Zirbes TK, Weingarten M, Fromm S, Glossmann J, Hanisch FG, *et al.* Increased galectin-3 expression in gastric cancer: correlations with histopathological subtypes, galactosylated antigens and tumor cell proliferation. *Tumour Biol.* 2000;21:258-266.

Boileau TW, Liao Z, Kim S, Lemeshow S, Erdman JW Jr, Clinton SK. Prostate carcinogenesis in N-methyl-N-nitrosourea (NMU)-testosterone-treated rats fed tomato powder, lycopene, or energy-restricted diets. J Natl Cancer Inst. 2003;95:1578-1586.

Bresalier RS, Mazurek N, Sternberg LR, Byrd JC, Yunker CK, Nangia-Makker P, Raz A. Metastasis of human colon cancer is altered by modifying expression of the beta-galactoside-binding protein galectin 3. *Gastroenterology.* 1998;115:287-296.

Bresalier RS, Yan PS, Byrd JC, Lotan R, Raz A. Expression of the endogenous galactose-binding protein galectin-3 correlates with the malignant potential of tumors in the central nervous system. *Cancer.* 1997;80:776-787.

Chen HH, Zhou HJ, Fang X. Inhibition of human cancer cell line growth and human umbilical vein endothelial cell angiogenesis by artemisinin derivatives in vitro. *Pharmacol Res.* 2003;48:231-236.

Cohen JH, Kristal AR, Stanford JL. Fruit and vegetable intakes and prostate cancer risk. *J Natl Cancer Inst.* 2000;92:61-68.

Deeb D, Xu YX, Jiang H, Gao X, Janakiraman N, Chapman RA, Gautam SC. Curcumin (diferuloyl-Methane) enhances tumor necrosis factor-related apoptosis-inducing ligand-induced apoptosis in LNCaP prostate cancer cells. *Mol Cancer Ther.* 2003;2:95-103.

Deliliers GL, Servida F, Fracchiolla NS, Ricci C, Borsotti C, Colombo G, Soligo D. Effect of inositol hexaphosphate (IP(6)) on human normal and leukaemic haematopoietic cells. *Br J Haematol.* 2002;117:577-587.

Dong Y, Zhang H, Hawthorn L, Ganther HE, Ip C. Delineation of the molecular basis for selenium-induced growth arrest in human prostate cancer cells by oligonucleotide array. *Cancer Res.* 2003;63:52-59.

Duffield-Lillico AJ, Dalkin BL, Reid ME, Turnbull BW, Slate EH, Jacobs ET, Marshall JR, Clark LC; Nutritional Prevention of Cancer Study Group. Selenium supplementation, baseline plasma selenium status and incidence of prostate cancer: an analysis of the complete treatment period of the Nutritional Prevention of Cancer Trial. *BJU Int.* 2003;91:608-612.

Eliaz I, Rode D. The effect of modified citrus pectin on the urinary excretion of toxic elements. Presented at: Fifth Annual Conference of Environmental Health Scientists: Nutritional Toxicology and Metabolomics; 2003; University of California, Davis.

Eliaz I, Hotchkiss AT, Fishman ML, Rode D. The effect of modified citrus pectin on urinary excretion of toxic elements. *Phytother Res.* 2006;20:859-864.

Eliaz I, Weil E, Wilk B. Integrative medicine and the role of modified citrus pectin/alginates in heavy metal chelation and detoxification – five case reports. *Forsch Komplement Med* (2006). 2007;14:358-364.

Finkelstein MP, Aynehchi S, Samadi AA, Drinis S, Choudhury MS, Tazaki H, Konno S. Chemosensitization of carmustine with maitake beta-glucan on androgen-independent prostatic cancer cells: involvement of glyoxalase I. *J Altern Complement Med.* 2002;8:573-580.

Frydoonfar HR, McGrath DR, Spigelman AD. The effect of indole-3-carbinol and sulforaphane on a prostate cancer cell line. *ANZ J Surg.* 2003;73:154-156.

Fullerton SA, Samadi AA, Tortorelis DG, Choudhury MS, Mallouh C, Tazaki H, Konno S. Induction of apoptosis in human prostatic cancer cells with beta-glucan (Maitake mushroom polysaccharide). *Mol Urol.* 2000;4:7-13.

Ghosh J, Myers C Jr. Arachidonic acid metabolism and cancer of the prostate. *Nutrition.* 1998;14:48-57.

Guess B, Jennrich R, Johnson H, Redheffer R, Scholz M. Using splines to detect changes in PSA doubling times. *Prostate.* 2003;54:88-94.

Guess B, Scholz M, *et al.* Modified citrus pectin (MCP) increases the prostate specific antigen doubling time in men with prostate cancer: a phase II clinical trial. Presented at: Science of Whole Person Healing Conference; 2003; Washington, DC.

Guzey, M., S. Kitada, et al. Apoptosis induction by 1alpha,25-dihydroxyvitamin D3 in prostate cancer. *Mol Cancer Ther.* 2002;1(9): 667-77.

Haese A, Van Poppel H, Marberger M, Mulders P, Abbou C, Boccon-Gibod L, Stenzl A, Huland H, De La Taille A, Schalken J. The value of the PCA3 assay in guiding decision which men with a negative prostate biopsy need immediate repeat biopsy: preliminary European data. *Eur Urol Suppl.* 2007;6:48.

Hsu DK, Dowling CA, Jeng KC, Chen JT, Yang RY, Liu FT. Galectin-3 expression is induced in cirrhotic liver and hepatocellular carcinoma. *Int J Cancer.* 1999;81:519-526.

Jenkins DJ, Kendall CW, D'Costa MA, Jackson CJ, Vidgen E, Singer W, *et al.* Soy consumption and phytoestrogens: effect on serum prostate specific antigen when blood lipids and oxidized low-density lipoprotein are reduced in hyperlipidemic men. *J Urol.* 2003;169:507-511.

Kelly WK, Scher HI, Mazumdar M, Vlamis V, Schwartz M, Fossa SD. Prostate-specific antigen as a measure of disease outcome in metastatic hormone-refractory prostate cancer. *J Clin Oncol.* 1993;11:607-615.

Kim L, Rao AV, Rao LG. Effect of lycopene on prostate LNCaP cancer cells in culture. *J Med Food.* 2002;5:181-187.

Kristal AR, Lampe JW. Brassica vegetables and prostate cancer risk: a review of the epidemiological evidence. *Nutr Cancer.* 2002;42:1-9.

Kucuk O, Sarkar FH, Sakr W, Djuric Z, Pollak MN, Khachik F, *et al.* Phase II randomized clinical trial of lycopene supplementation before radical prostatectomy. *Cancer Epidemiol Biomarkers Prev.* 2001;10:861-868.

Kune GA. Eating fish protects against some cancers: epidemiological and experimental evidence for a hypothesis. *J Nutr Med.* 1990;1:139-44.

Lai H, Singh NP. Selective cancer cell cytotoxicity from exposure to dihydroartemisinin and holotransferrin. *Cancer Lett.* 1995;91:41-46.

Lee MM, Gomez SL, Chang JS, Wey M, Wang RT, Hsing AW. Soy and isoflavone consumption in relation to prostate cancer risk in China. *Cancer Epidemiol Biomarkers Prev.* 2003;12:665-668.

Lee WR, Hanks GE, Hanlon A. Increasing prostate-specific antigen profile following definitive radiation therapy for localized prostate cancer: clinical observations. *J Clin Oncol.* 1997;15:230-238.

Leitzmann MF, Stampfer MJ, Wu K, Colditz GA, Willett WC, Giovannucci EL. Zinc supplement use and risk of prostate cancer. *J Natl Cancer Inst.* 2003;95:1004-1007.

Marks LS, Fradet Y, Deras IL, Blase A, Mathis J, Aubin SM, *et al.* PCAA3 Molecular Urine Assay for prostate cancer in men undergoing repeat biopsy. *Urology.* 2007;69:532-535.

Liu WK, Xu SX, Che CT. Anti-proliferative effect of ginseng saponins on human prostate cancer cell line. *Life Sci.* 2000;67:1297-1306.

Miyazaki J, Hokari R, Kato S, Tsuzuki Y, Kawaguchi A, Nagao S, Itoh K, Miura S. Increased expression of galectin-3 in primary gastric cancer and the metastatic lymph nodes. *Oncol Rep.* 2002;9:1307-1312.

Moon BK, Lee YJ, Battle P, Jessup JM, Raz A, Kim HR. Galectin-3 protects human breast carcinoma cells against nitric oxide-induced apoptosis: implication of galectin-3 function during metastasis. *Am J Pathol.* 2001;159:1055-1060.

Moore JC, Lai H, Li JR, Ren RL, McDougall JA, Singh NP, Chou CK. Oral administration of dihydroartemisinin and ferrous sulfate retarded implanted fibrosarcoma growth in the rat. *Cancer Lett.* 1995;98:83-87.

Nachshon-Kedmi M, Yannai S, Haj A, Fares FA. Indole-3-carbinol and 3,3'-diindolylmethane induce apoptosis in human prostate cancer cells. *Food Chem Toxicol.* 2003;41:745-752.

Nakamura M, Inufusa H, Adachi T, Aga M, Kurimoto M, Nakatani Y, *et al.* Involvement of galectin-3 expression in colorectal cancer progression and metastasis. *Int J Oncol.* 1999;15(1): 143-8.

Nangia-Makker P, Hogan V, Honjo Y, Baccarini S, Tait L, Bresalier R, Raz A. Inhibition of human cancer cell growth and metastasis in nude mice by oral intake of modified citrus pectin. *J Natl Cancer Inst.* 2002;94:1854-1862.

Nangia-Makker P, Honjo Y, Sarvis R, Akahani S, Hogan V, Pienta KJ, Raz A.Galectin-3 induces endothelial cell morphogenesis and angiogenesis. *Am J Pathol.* 2000;156:899-909.

Norrish AE, Ferguson LR, Knize MG, Felton JS, Sharpe SJ, Jackson RT. Heterocyclic amine content of cooked meat and risk of prostate cancer. *J Natl Cancer Inst* 1999;91:2038-2044.

Palombo JD, Ganguly A, Bistrian BR, Menard MP. The antiproliferative effects of biologically active isomers of conjugated linoleic acid on human colorectal and prostatic cancer cells. *Cancer Lett.* 2002;177:163-172.

Pienta KJ, Naik H, Akhtar A, Yamazaki K, Replogle TS, Lehr J, Donat TL, Tait L, Hogan V, Raz A. Inhibition of spontaneous metastasis in a rat prostate cancer model by oral administration of modified citrus pectin. *J Natl Cancer Inst.*1995;87:348-353.

Platt D, Raz A. Modulation of the lung colonization of B16-F1 melanoma cells by citrus pectin. *J Natl Cancer Inst.*1992;84:438-442.

Rose DP, Connolley JM. Omega-3 fatty acids as cancer chemopreventive agents. *Pharmacol Ther.* 1999;83:217-244.

Santa María Margalef A, Paciucci Barzanti R, Reventós Puigjaner J, Morote Robles J, Thomson Okatsu TM. Antimitogenic effect of Pygeum africanum extracts on human prostatic cancer cell lines and explants from benign prostatic hyperplasia. *Arch Esp Urol.* 2003;56:369-378. [Spanish].

Sartor CI, Strawderman MH, Lin XH, Kish KE, McLaughlin PW, Sandler HM. Rate of PSA rise predicts metastatic versus local recurrence after definitive radiotherapy. *Int J Radiat Oncol Biol Phys.* 1997;38:941-947.

Saxe GA, Hébert JR, Carmody JF, Kabat-Zinn J, Rosenzweig PH, Jarzobski D, Reed GW, Blute RD. Can diet in conjunction with stress reduction affect the rate of increase in prostate specific antigen after biochemical recurrence of prostate cancer? *J Urol.* 2001;166:2202-2207.

Schuurman AG, van den Brandt PA, Dorant E, Goldohm RA. Animal products, calcium and protein and prostate cancer risk in the Netherlands Cohort Study. *Br J Cancer.* 1999;80:1107-1113.

Sharma G, Singh RP, Agarwal R. Growth inhibitory and apoptotic effects of inositol hexaphosphate in transgenic adenocarcinoma of mouse prostate (TRAMP-C1) cells. *Int J Oncol.* 2003;23:1413-1418.

Singh NP, Lai H. Selective toxicity of dihydroartemisinin and holotransferrin toward human breast cancer cells. *Life Sci.* 2001;70:49-56.

Singh RP, Agarwal C, Agarwal R. Inositol hexaphosphate inhibits growth, and induces G1 arrest and apoptotic death of prostate carcinoma DU145 cells: modulation of CDKI-CDK-cyclin and pRb-related protein-E2F complexes. *Carcinogenesis.* 2003;24:555-563.

Sliva D, Sedlak M, Slivova V, Valachovicova T, Lloyd FP Jr, Ho NW. Biologic activity of spores and dried powder from Ganoderma lucidum for the inhibition of highly invasive human Breast and prostate cancer cells. *J Altern Complement Med.* 2003;9:491-497.

Strum S, Scholz M, *et al.* Modified citrus pectin slows PSA doubling time: a pilot clinical trial. Presented at: International Conference on Diet and Prevention of Cancer; 1999; Tampere, Finland.

Weiss T, McCulloch M, *et al.* Modified citrus pectin induces cytotoxicity of prostate cancer cells in co-cultures with human endothelial monolayers. Presented at: International Conference on Diet and Prevention of Cancer; 1999; Tampere, Finland.

Yan J, Katz A. PectaSol-C® Modified Citrus Pectin Induces Apoptosis and Inhibition of Proliferation in Human and Mouse Androgen Dependent and Independent Prostate Cancer Cells. Integr Cancer Ther. 2010; In Press.

Yu L, Blackburn GL, Zhou JR. Genistein and daidzein downregulate prostate androgen-regulated transcript-1 (PART-1) gene expression induced by dihydrotestosterone in human prostate LNCaP cancer cells. *J Nutr.* 2003;133:389-392.

Zhou JR, Yu L, Zhong Y, Blackburn GL. Soy phytochemicals and tea bioactive components synergistically inhibit androgen-sensitive human prostate tumors in mice. *J Nutr.* 2003;133:516-521.

Zhou JR, Yu L, Zhong Y, Nassr RL, Franke AA, Gaston SM, Blackburn GL. Inhibition of orthotopic growth and metastasis of androgen-sensitive human prostate tumors in mice by bioactive soybean components. *Prostate.* 2002;53:143-153.

ABOUT THE AUTHOR

Dr Isaac Eliaz is an internationally renowned lecturer, author, researcher, product formulator, and integrative clinical practitioner. As a physician who also holds a Masters Degree in Chinese Medicine, Dr. Eliaz has the combination of in-depth training to truly integrate the wisdom of traditional medical approaches with Western or conventional medicine. He is the founder of both EcoNugenics, Inc. and Amitabha Medical Clinic and Healing Center in Sebastopol, California, where he specializes in the integrative treatment of cancer, cardiovascular disease, and other chronic illnesses through the thoughtful application of both Western medicine and complementary and alternative approaches.

Chapter 10
Toxic Heavy Metals as Causative Agents of Chronic Illnesses and Cancer:
Clinically Proven Treatments and Detoxification Modalities

Rita Ellithorpe, M.D.
Founder, Tustin Longevity Center (Tustin, California USA)

ABSTRACT

Increasing accumulations of low levels of multiple heavy metals in our environment are a legacy of our industrialized society. There is compelling evidence to suggest that toxic heavy metals (e.g. arsenic, cadmium, mercury, lead, aluminum, and nickel) are associated with diseases of aging, such as cancer and cardiovascular disease. The eminent health risks of toxins must be addressed, and health care professionals need to be aware of effective detoxification and treatment protocols to enhance patient care. One of the underlying mechanisms of heavy metal toxicity is oxidative damage, in particular, free radical oxidation of cell membranes. Recent published research and clinical experience have identified several approaches to combat the assaults of heavy metal toxins and counter their harmful effects. One such approach is the integration of specialized heavy metal diagnostics and treatment with calcium disodium ($CaNa_2$) EDTA chelation suppositories for reduction of long-term toxicity, lipid replacement therapy (LRT) for cellular membrane fortification, and specific anti-oxidants that address cellular/tissue damage along with lifestyle changes. Recent clinical research in aged men of treatment with chelation suppositories along with supportive therapies demonstrated a significant ($P<0.05$) reduction in a variety of symptoms of prostate conditions, improved cardiovascular blood markers, and excretion of multiple heavy metals. The detoxification and removal of heavy metal toxins along with supplemental repair of damaged cellular membranes and enhancement of mitochondrial function are paramount considerations for medical practitioners and may lead to beneficial advances in the field of anti-aging medicine. The aims of this paper are to:
1. Promote awareness of the ubiquitous nature of heavy metal toxicity and the impact it has on the health of the world's population.
2. Emphasize the importance of the diagnosis and detection of heavy metals in the blood, urine, and feces.
3. Introduce various integrative approaches of metal detoxification and cellular repair.

INTRODUCTION

Increasing accumulations of low levels of multiple heavy metals in our environment are a legacy of our industrialized society. The air we breathe, the food we eat, and the water we drink are contaminated with heavy metals. There is compelling evidence to suggest that toxic heavy metals (e.g. arsenic, cadmium, mercury, lead, aluminum, and nickel) are associated with diseases of aging, such as cancer and cardiovascular disease. Cancer is now the number cause of death in adults and in children aged 1-15, yet the impact of toxins is still not being taken seriously by mainstream medicine.

Toxins are everywhere. They invade our bodies and cause devastating disease. Heavy metals (and other toxins) exert their deleterious effects by damaging cell membranes, promoting the production of free radicals, and causing oxidative stress. Figure 1 shows a cell membrane. The image on the left is that of a healthy membrane, while that on the right is of a membrane that has been damaged by oxidative stress. The phospholipids that make up the lipid bilayer of the cell membrane are very susceptible to oxidation by the free radicals generated by heavy metals and other toxins. Figure 2 illustrates the devastating effect that free radicals have on cells.

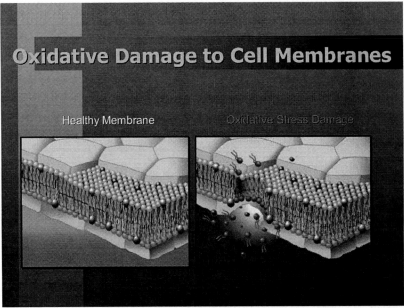

Figure 1. Heavy Metals Cause Oxidative Damage to Cell Membranes

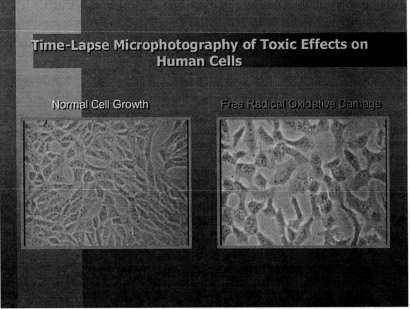

Figure 2. Heavy Metal Induced Oxidative Damage on Human Cells

The most significant toxic heavy metals are lead, cadmium, mercury, aluminum, nickel, and arsenic, however no heavy metal is safe – all damage cell membranes. The problem with heavy metals is that they are stored in the body, thus meaning that continual exposure to low levels ultimately leads to high levels. Furthermore, exposure to multiple heavy metals compounds the danger. Most research studies in the effects of heavy metal exposure and accumulation are conducted on isolated metals (typically lead or mercury) alone. However, if you test your patients you will find that many of them have multiple heavy metals stored within their body. This is a global problem. Many foreign countries do not have environmental protection laws, and pollution from industrial processes such as smelting is being carried by the jet stream and contaminating our environment. The Environmental Protection Agency (EPA), the Food and Drug Administration (FDA), the Centers for Disease Control (CDC), and state health departments are all monitoring our exposure to these cell-damaging agents, and it is time that we all began to take preventive measures against chronic low level metal toxicity.

The official stance on lead is that blood levels of <30 mcg/dL carry no risk. The results of a study by Lustberg and Silbergeld (Fig. 3) show that this is clearly not the case.[1] This study used follow-up data from the Second National Health and Nutrition Examination Survey (NHANES II) to evaluate the association between lead exposure and mortality in the United States. Results showed that individuals with baseline blood lead levels of 20 to 29 mcg/dL had 46% increased all-cause mortality, 39% increased circulatory [cardiovascular] mortality, and 68% increased cancer mortality compared with those with blood lead levels of less than 10 mcg/dL. The authors of this study concluded: "Individuals with blood lead levels of 20 to 29 mcg/dL in 1976 to 1980 (15% of the US population at that time) experienced significantly increased all-cause, circulatory, and cancer mortality from 1976 through 1992. Thus, we strongly encourage efforts to reduce lead exposure for occupationally exposed workers and the 1.7 million Americans with blood lead levels of at least 20 mcg/dL."

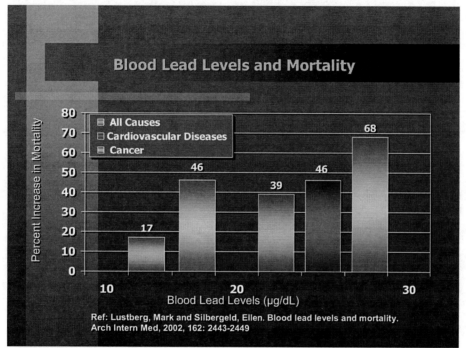

Figure 3. The Relationship between Blood Levels and Mortality

My own research on 251 of my patients revealed that the blood of every single patient tested contained heavy metals. However, what was more frightening was the discovery that 22% of blood samples contained significantly elevated levels of heavy metals and 17% contained potentially toxic levels of heavy metals (Fig. 4). In addition, 39% of samples contained significantly elevated levels of multiple metals – not one, not two, but three or four or five. So, from these two studies we can deduce that blood lead levels of <30 mcg/dL are far from harmless, and that it is very likely that we all have heavy metals in our blood.

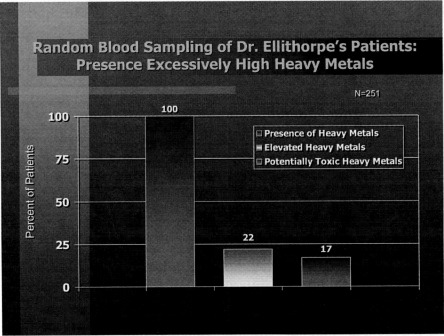

Figure 4. Personal Study of Presence of Heavy Metals in Blood Samples

HEAVY METALS, CHRONIC ILLNESS, AND CANCER
Aluminum

Aluminum is everywhere. Sources of aluminum include:

- Aluminum cookware
- Aluminum foil
- Antacids
- Antiperspirant
- Baking powder (containing aluminum)
- Buffered aspirin
- Canned acidic foods
- Food additives
- Lipstick
- Medications and drugs (anti-diarrheal agents, hemorrhoid medications, vaginal douches)
- Processed cheese
- "Softened water"
- Tap water

Aluminum is associated with a number of health conditions, including: respiratory problems (coughing, asthma), bone disease, skeletal problems, skin rashes, neurological development problems in children, and Alzheimer's disease. The relationship between aluminum and Alzheimer's disease is well established. Several studies have linked elevated aluminum concentrations in drinking water to an increased risk of Alzheimer's disease. While a case-control study by Rondeau *et al* found an association between Alzheimer's disease and lifetime exposure to aluminum in antiperspirants and antacids.[2] Results of this study revealed that the more antiperispirant and/or aluminum antacids that was used, the more likely the person would develop Alzheimer's disease, With the increased risk being as high as 300% in high users.

Arsenic

Like aluminum, arsenic is abundant in our modern environment. Sources of arsenic include:

- Air pollution
- Antibiotics given to commercial livestock
- Certain marine plants
- Chemical processing
- Coal fired power plants
- Defoliants
- Drinking water
- Drying agents for cotton
- Herbicides
- Insecticides
- Meat (from commercially raised poultry and cattle)
- Metal ore smelting
- Pesticides
- Seafood (fish, mussels, oysters)
- Specialty glass
- Wood preservatives

Arsenic is classified as a class I human carcinogen. Inorganic arsenic is now known to increase the risk of cancers of the lung, skin, bladder, liver, kidney, and prostate. At last, the EPA has proposed to reduce the exposure limit from 50 parts per billion to 5 parts per billion. Cancer is just one of the health problems associated with arsenic, others include: sore throats, lung irritation, nausea and vomiting, low red and white blood cell count, abnormal heart rhythm, damage to blood vessels, sensation of pins and needles, darkening of skin, and the appearance of small corns and warts.

The vast majority of my patients have a low white blood cell count. When I started practicing medicine 30 years ago, a white blood cell count of 6.0-7.0 $x10^3/mm^3$ was the norm. Now, I am regularly seeing patients with white blood cell counts of 4.1, 3.5, and 2.5 $x10^3/mm^3$. In fact, one patient, a 19-year-old male, had a white blood cell count of just 1.9 $x10^3/mm^3$. He was placed on a detoxification and cell repair program, and within four to six months his white blood cell had risen to a far healthier 6.7 x $10^3/mm^3$.

Cadmium

Sources of cadmium include:

- Air pollution
- Art supplies
- Bone meal
- Cigarette smoke
- Food (coffee, fruits, grains, and vegetables grown in cadmium-laden soil
- Meat (kidneys, liver, poultry)
- Freshwater fish
- Fungicides
- Highway dusts
- Incinerators
- Mining
- Nickel-cadmium batteries – a highly significant source of cadmium
- Oxide dusts
- Paints
- Phosphate fertilizers
- Power plants
- Seafood (crab, flounder, mussels, oysters, scallops)
- Sewage sludge
- "Softened" water

- Smelting plants
- Welding fumes

Health conditions associated with cadmium include: vomiting, diarrhea, kidney disease, fragile bones, and prostate cancer.

Mercury

Sources of mercury include:
- Air pollution
- Batteries
- Cosmetics
- Dental amalgams
- Diuretics (mercurial)
- Electrical devices and relays
- Explosives
- Foods (grains)
- Fungicides
- Fluorescent lights
- Freshwater fish (especially large bass, pike, and trout
- Insecticides
- Mining
- Paints
- Pesticides
- Petroleum products
- Saltwater fish (especially large halibut, shrimp, snapper, swordfish, and shellfish)
- Tap water

Mercury vapor is the most toxic form of mercury. If you have mercury amalgam dental fillings, every time you eat or drink something hot you are outgassing mercury into your body. Mercury accumulates in the brain and kidneys. It is able to transfer across the placental membrane, and thus into the developing fetus.

Lead

Lead is well known for its toxic effects upon the body. Sources of lead include:
- Air pollution
- Ammunition (shot and bullets)
- Bathtubs (cast iron, porcelain, steel)
- Batteries
- Canned foods
- Ceramics
- Chemical fertilizers
- Cosmetics
- Dolomite
- Dust
- Foods grown around industrial areas
- Gasoline
- Hair dyes and rinses
- Leaded glass
- Newsprint and colored advertisements
- Paints
- Pesticides
- Pewter
- Pottery

- Rubber toys
- Soft coal
- Soil
- Solder
- Tap water
- Tobacco smoke
- Vinyl "mini-binds"

In the 1990's there was a big movement to remove lead from paints and gas. However, as petrochemicals burn better if you add metal to them, the gas companies switched lead for nickel – another toxic heavy metal.

Lead affects the central nervous system, the kidneys, and the reproductive system. It also causes anemia, memory problems, decreased reaction time, and weakness in the fingers, wrists, and ankles. Last, but most certainly not least, it is also carcinogenic. Children are far more susceptible to the toxic effects of lead. Symptoms and signs of lead toxicity in children include: anemia, severe stomachache, muscle weakness, brain damage, a stunting of mental and physical growth, learning difficulties, and behavioral problems.

Nickel

Nickel is present in many day-to-day items, yet it is a toxic heavy metal. Sources of nickel include:
- Appliances
- Buttons
- Ceramics
- Cocoa
- Cold-wave hair permanents
- Cooking utensils
- Cosmetics
- Coins
- Dental Materials
- Food (chocolate, hydrogenated oils, nuts, and food grown near industrial areas)
- Hair spray
- Industrial waste
- Jewelry
- Medical implants
- Metal refineries
- Metal tools
- Nickel-cadmium batteries
- Orthodontic appliances
- Shampoo
- Solid-waste incinerators
- Stainless steel kitchen utensils
- Tap water
- Tobacco and tobacco smoke
- Water faucets and pipes
- Zippers

Numerous health problems are associated with nickel, including: apathy, blue-colored lips, contact dermatitis, diarrhea, dizziness, fever, headache, gingivitis, insomnia, nausea, rapid heart rate, skin rashes, shortness of breath, stomatitis, and vomiting. It is also a known carcinogen.

DIAGNOSIS AND TREATMENT

Laboratory Diagnosis of Heavy Metal Toxicity

There are several different ways of determining the presence of heavy metals within the body. Hair analysis is one option. For this, you simply snip of a small piece of the patient's hair and send it off to a laboratory. The reading you get from hair analysis is a delayed reading, so it is temporal in terms of exposure time. Heavy metal levels in hair do correlate with tissue levels. However, it is important to note that hair products may interfere with testing. I do not use hair analysis anymore because other methods, such as urine testing, are more clinically useful.

Urine testing is very useful as it assesses retention. What this means is that lets you see how a patient responds to a challenge. Urine testing is especially good for assessing chronic low level exposure. Testing is performed pre and post provocation. A number of provocation agents are available. Ethylenediaminetetraacetic acid (EDTA) is probably the most well known provocation agent. EDTA is FDA approved and is classified as generally regarded as safe (GRAS). It chelates everything. Other agents include 2,3-dimercapto-1-propanesulfonic acid (DMPS) and dimercaptosuccinic acid (DMSA), however I prefer to use EDTA. To carry out a urinary challenge, I give the patient 1500 mg of EDTA intravenously, collect their urine for six hours, and then I send it off to the laboratory. Figure 5 is an example of a typical report. The majority of reports I receive show very elevated levels of lead and mercury.

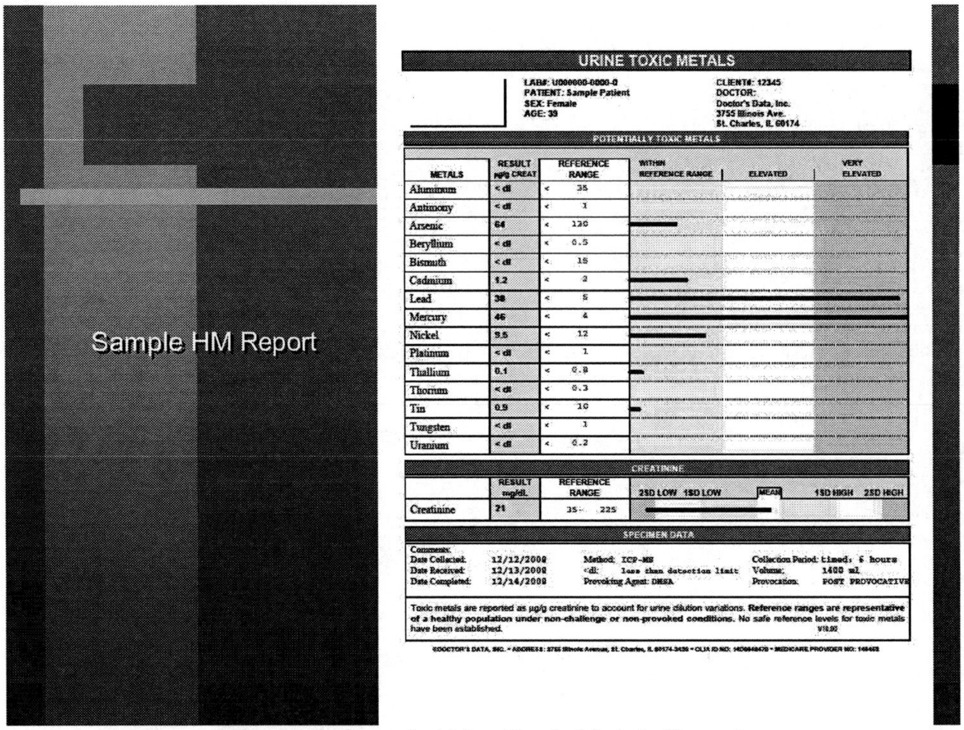

URINE TOXIC METALS

LAB#: U000000-0000-0
PATIENT: Sample Patient
SEX: Female
AGE: 39

CLIENT#: 12345
DOCTOR:
Doctor's Data, Inc.
3755 Illinois Ave.
St. Charles, IL 60174

POTENTIALLY TOXIC METALS

METALS	RESULT µg/g CREAT	REFERENCE RANGE	WITHIN REFERENCE RANGE	ELEVATED	VERY ELEVATED
Aluminum	< dl	< 35			
Antimony	< dl	< 1			
Arsenic	64	< 130			
Beryllium	< dl	< 0.5			
Bismuth	< dl	< 15			
Cadmium	1.2	< 2			
Lead	38	< 5			
Mercury	46	< 4			
Nickel	9.5	< 12			
Platinum	< dl	< 1			
Thallium	0.1	< 0.8			
Thorium	< dl	< 0.3			
Tin	0.9	< 10			
Tungsten	< dl	< 1			
Uranium	< dl	< 0.2			

CREATININE

	RESULT mg/dL	REFERENCE RANGE	2SD LOW	1SD LOW	MEAN	1SD HIGH	2SD HIGH
Creatinine	21	35– 225					

SPECIMEN DATA

Comments:
Date Collected: 12/12/2008 Method: ICP-MS Collection Period: timed: 6 hours
Date Received: 12/13/2008 <dl: less than detection limit Volume: 1400 ml
Date Completed: 12/14/2008 Provoking Agent: DMSA Provocation: POST PROVOCATIVE

Toxic metals are reported as µg/g creatinine to account for urine dilution variations. Reference ranges are representative of a healthy population under non-challenge or non-provoked conditions. No safe reference levels for toxic metals have been established.

Figure 5. Sample Urine Toxic Metals Report

Another method of assessing heavy metals is red blood cell mineral analysis. This type of analysis enables you to determine intracellular levels of minerals (which includes heavy metals). It is useful for assessing recent exposure, while also letting you know if a patient has adequate levels of beneficial minerals, for example calcium. Red blood cell mineral analysis should be performed regularly in patients following a detoxification program.

The final method of assessing heavy metal levels is fecal metal testing. The primary route of elimination of heavy metals is via the feces. This type of testing is useful for assessing dietary and environmental exposure to heavy metals, however it should not replace pre and post provocation testing of urinary heavy metals.

Clinically Proven Treatments and Detoxification Modalities

The aims of treatment are to remove toxins, repair damaged cells, and revitalize health. EDTA is an essential part of a heavy metal detoxification program. In the past, EDTA tended to be given intravenously. However, intravenous chelation was never popular with patients as it is expensive, time consuming (it takes 3-6 hours), and invasive. The good news is that we now have at our disposal a much cheaper and far less time consuming way of using EDTA – in suppository format. EDTA suppositories can be used in combination with intravenous, oral, and transdermal EDTA, or as a stand-alone therapy.

We conducted pharmacokinetic studies to compare the bioavailability of EDTA in the suppositories with that of intravenously delivered EDTA. Unsurprisingly, the bioavailability of intravenous EDTA was 100%. In comparison, the bioavailability of the EDTA in the suppositories was 36%. However, we also found that the tissue penetration of the EDTA in the suppositories was nearly 4-times that of the intravenous EDTA. Furthermore, the intravenously delivered EDTA was detectable in the blood for just 1.5 hours, whereas the rectally delivered EDTA was detectable in the blood for more than 8 hours. So, the rectal suppository has better tissue penetration and is longer acting than intravenous EDTA.

Figure 6 illustrates the effect of treatment on a 9-year-old boy who lived near a lead battery plant. Heavy metal analysis was carried out on this child, and the results showed that his urine contained surprisingly little lead. However, we treated him with a 1000 mg EDTA suppository and the next day his urine contained 325.6 mcg of lead. EDTA is very effective at chelating lead.

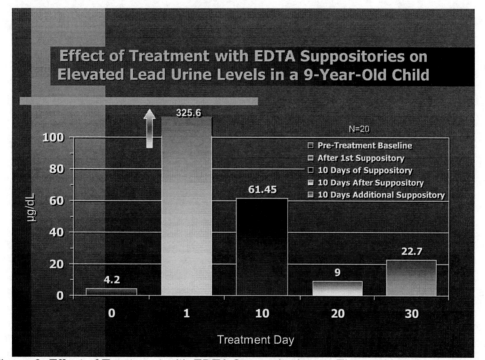

Figure 6. Effect of Treatment with EDTA Suppositories on Elevated Lead Urine Levels in a 9-Year-Old Child

We also conducted a study on the effect of treatment with EDTA suppositories in men with chronic prostate problems. For this study the participants were scored for urinary symptoms, pain symptoms, and quality of life (QOL) both before and after treatment. As can be seen in Figure 7, the results showed that urinary symptoms, pain symptoms, and quality of life all improved significantly after treatment with EDTA suppositories.

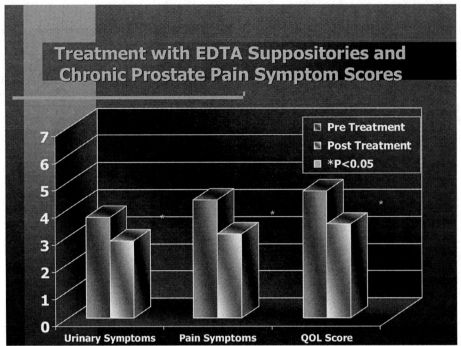

Figure 7. Treatment with EDTA Suppositories and Chronic Prostate Pain Symptom Scores

Case Studies
Case Study 1
FK was a 42-year-old female. She suffered from fibromyalgia and chronic fatigue, and was hypothyroid. Testing revealed elevated levels of several heavy metals, especially arsenic (Ar). She was treated with EDTA suppositories, and within just four months her arsenic, lead (Pb), mercury (Hg), and nickel (Ni) levels were significantly lower – her arsenic level had fall from 220 mcg to just 4.5 mcg! Furthermore, she was feeling much better, her energy levels had improved, she was in less pain, and she was able to increase her daily activity levels.

Case Study 2
KM was a 55-year-old female. She suffered from chronic lower back pain and fatigue, and was hypothyroid. Testing revealed that her mercury level was 30 mcg. Following treatment with EDTA suppositories it fell to 2.6 mcg. A year later, she was full of energy and her back pain was stable.

Case Study 3
MO was a 52-year-old male. He suffered from chronic anxiety and panic attacks, hypertension, and lower back pain. This man was an electrician, and so his risk of exposure to heavy metals was high. He also ate a lot of fish. Not too surprisingly, testing revealed that he had elevated levels of mercury and lead. Treatment was begun and his mercury and lead levels dropped. However because of his occupation and his love of fish they kept on creeping up again, but we did manage to get them under control. At follow-up two years later his anxiety was greatly improved, his blood pressure had dropped, and his lower back pain had improved.

CONCLUDING REMARKS
Over the last 8 years or so I have treated more than 3000 patients with more than 300,000 doses of EDTA suppositories. The beauty of this treatment is that is a non-invasive, quick, easy, inexpensive, safe, FDA-approved, and clinically proven method of reducing heavy metal burden. However, prescribing EDTA suppositories is not the only thing to consider. Emphasis should also be placed on cell membrane repair, the importance of a healthy diet, and reducing the risk of heavy metal exposure. Many patients report similar benefits after following such a program, these benefits include: improved mental clarity,

increased energy, increased endurance, reduced blood pressure, enhanced cardiovascular performance, improved libido, improved erectile dysfunction, improvement in prostate conditions, and improved overall quality of life.

REFERENCES

1. Lustberg M, Silbergeld E. Blood lead levels and mortality. *Arch Intern Med*. 2002;162:2443-2449.
2. Rondeau V, Commenges D, Jacqmin-Gadda H, Dartigues JF. Relation between aluminum concentrations in drinking water and Alzheimer's disease: an 8-year follow-up study. *Am J Epidemiol*. 2000;152:59-66.

ABOUT THE AUTHOR

Dr. Rita Ellithorpe is the founder and medical director of Tustin Longevity Center. She received her medical degree in 1982 from The Chicago Medical School/University of Health Science in North Chicago, IL. From there she completed her internship in family practice at Womack Army Hospital, Fort Bragg, NC in 1983. At Fort Knox, KY, she served as an emergency room staff physician, general medical officer and flight surgeon as Chief of the Aviation Clinic from 1983-1990.

Dr. Ellithorpe participated in cancer investigations with Dr. Stanislaw Bruzynski at his research institute in Houston, Texas and was later published as a co-author in literature describing his unique therapy. A staff physician and Director of Women's Studies at Whitaker Wellness Medical Clinic in Newport Beach, CA, she went on to help in the development of natural medicinal therapies at Great Smokies Medical Center in Asheville, North Carolina. Dr. Ellithorpe holds a second doctorate in integrative medicine focusing on health at the cellular level. Dr. Ellithorpe is a graduate and guest faculty member of Capitol University of Integrative Medicine, Washington, D.C.

Chapter 11

Using Customized Age Reducing Exercise (CARE) for Longevity and Active Prevention of Brain Degenerative Diseases and Other Disorders

Erik Flowers, M.A.
Director, C.A.R.E. Fit Center (Los Angeles, CA USA)

ABSTRACT

Customized Age Reducing Exercise (CARE) is an integrated program of cognitive exercise that retrains the brain and body systems to create a neurogenetic response. Developmental benefits of CARE include: heightened reflexes, improved balance, greater strength and self-confidence, sharper auditory perception, more developed somatosensory system, and improved visual cognition. CARE can help mitigate or reverse brain degenerative diseases, senior falling, concussive disorders, essential tremors, anxiety/mood swings, depression, lack of focus, and short-term memory loss. CARE can be of benefit to many people, including: mobile/immobile people aged 40; athletes, former athletes with a history of concussions, and professional bodybuilders; people with dementia/Alzheimer's disease, Parkinson's disease, Huntington's disease, post traumatic stress disorder (PTSD), attention deficit hyperactivity disorder (ADHD), HIV+, depression, mood disorders, and addictions. The aims of this paper are to introduce CARE, to stress the urgent need for a practical exercise solution that promotes longevity and preventative self-care, and to discuss why retraining areas of strength, balance and reflexes help adults aged 40+ and special populations.

Keywords: anti-aging exercise, senior exercise, preventative care, health and fitness, exercises for brain degenerative disease, longevity

INTRODUCTION

Customized Age Reducing Exercise (CARE) is an integrated program of cognitive exercise that retrains the brain and body systems to create a neurogenetic response. Developmental benefits of CARE include: heightened reflexes, improved balance, greater strength and self-confidence, sharper auditory perception, more developed somatosensory system, and improved visual cognition. CARE can help mitigate or reverse brain degenerative diseases, senior falling, concussive disorders, essential tremors, anxiety/mood swings, depression, lack of focus, and short-term memory loss. CARE can be of benefit to many people, including: mobile/immobile people aged 40; athletes, former athletes with a history of concussions, and professional bodybuilders; people with dementia/Alzheimer's disease, Parkinson's disease, Huntington's disease, post traumatic stress disorder (PTSD), attention deficit hyperactivity disorder (ADHD), HIV+, depression, mood disorders, and addictions. The aims of this paper are to introduce CARE, to stress the urgent need for a practical exercise solution that promotes longevity and preventative self-care, and to discuss why retraining areas of strength, balance and reflexes help adults aged 40+ and special populations.

CUSTOMIZED AGE REDUCING EXERCISE

The concept of CARE was developed over 30-years while working with people aged 40+ in equipped, ill-equipped and unequipped environments. CARE is an accessible, affordable, integrated, multi-sensory, program of simultaneous cognitive exercise and physical movements that retrains the brain and body systems to create a neurogenetic response.

Multiple systems contribute to our ability to balance in standing and moving environments. The sensory (i.e., vision, somatosensory, and vestibular) systems provide us with information about the surrounding environment. The motor system uses the information from the sensory system to produce coordinated postural muscle activity to help us keep our balance.

CARE is about safely rebuilding strength, balance, and reflexes for people aged 40 and over 40 and special populations. Although this is a supplemental exercise program it does not replace recommended cardiovascular or strength training.

Why We Should CARE?

The National Institute on Aging declares that regular exercise and physical activity "can reduce the risk of developing some disease and disabilities that develop as people grow older."[1] Whilst the Fisher Center for Alzheimer's Research Foundation says: "Regular exercise during your middle years may lower your risk of developing Alzheimer's disease [and Dementia] in old age."

CARE video documentation and personal testimonials show positive results for: agile adults 40+, populations with dementia, HIV, depression, essential tremors, addiction recovery, less mobile seniors, professional athletes, and bodybuilders. CARE can also be of benefit to people with: attention deficit disorder (ADD), ADHD, PTSD, multiple sclerosis (MS), and other brain degenerative disorders.

CARE addresses the brain and the body's need for engagement, vigilance, and resilience. Developmental benefits of CARE include: greater strength, improved balance, heightened reflexes, sharper auditory perception, a more developed somatosensory system, improved visual cognition, and added self-esteem – all of which help to regenerate brain function. CARE takes just ten minutes a day.

If, personally, professionally, and as a nation, we are CARE-less and don't cogitate, mobilize, and correct our imbalances we will get sicker. In 2009, the US spent twice as much per capita on health care as European countries, but we are twice as sick with chronic disease. In the US, 95% of the health care dollar is spent on treatment and just 5% is spent on prevention.

Who Should CARE?

A Baby Boomer (a person born1946-1964) turns 50 every eight seconds. Boomers have gone back to social exercise environments. They thought they could do it themselves, purchasing home equipment from major department stores – basically buying all the equipment they could jam into living rooms, garages, basements, even bedrooms. Almost all of that equipment ended up at the thrift store. Eventually, Baby Boomers realized they needed help and realized a social setting was more conducive to positive results, thus they have gradually migrated back to gyms and fitness centers.

After age 40 we lose 5% brain volume per year, 10% muscle mass per year, and 10% cardiovascular volume per year – if we don't CARE. In 2009, Dementia affected 35 million people worldwide. That number is expected to double in the next 20-years. In the US, the average treatment cost of after-fall hip surgery is $20,000. Baby Boomers are the key to our nation's future health care costs.

The three basics of living an active CARE-ing lifestyle as you age are:

- Move, move, and move (add 2-4 years);
- Find a challenging hobby or activity (add 2 years)
- Don't be a loner (add 3-5 years).

How CARE Works

CARE emphasizes prevention not protection. The difference is: "Protective" you put up a rickety fence and hope a strong wind doesn't blow it down; "Preventative" you build a solid wall, fortify it, armor it, and guard it. CARE exercises spark new neuropathways by alerting the reticular activating system, which puts the brain and body at a heightened sense of awareness, pumping adrenaline to the processing centers of the brain which sends messages to "recognize," "move," and most importantly "look out" for yourself and that when you react you do not hurt someone. That is the essence of CARE-ing.

Rikli and Jones correctly state that group or individualized exercise programs designed to improve functional mobility should be based on as much information as possible to maximize program effectiveness and participant safety.[3] This is why CARE uses a 10-point assessment system, including three standardized tests measuring strength, balance, and flexibility.

CARE Assessments

- Goals:
  - Personal goals: Before any assessments are administered, the client will likely have a personal perception of what can be improved. For example: The CARE trainer asks, "What would you like to get out of this training?" The client may answer, "I would like to improve my balance."
  - Trainer goals: After the assessments, the CARE trainer may have a greater perception of what exercises could benefit the client. For example: The client has difficulty rising from a

chair. The trainer can then prescribe an exercise plan that would emphasize balance and strength.

- Purpose: Help the client become stronger, more mobile, and improve their reflexes in order to help prevent falls, stop shaky hands, aid circulation, etc; to improve their lifestyle and mitigate aging issues.
- Postural charting (including gate).
- Auditory: Auditory perception is the second slowest reacting sensory system. Does the client use a hearing aid? Test: The trainer can test functional hearing by standing 5-10 feet from the client and instructing the client to first close their eyes. The trainer then claps three times. The client must duplicate the pattern (or indicate that they heard with an affirmative nod.) Auditory perception is checked by instructing the client to first close their eyes. The trainer says any short word (for example, "cake" or "stop") and asks the client to repeat what they heard.
- Vision: Visual perception is the slowest reacting sensory system. Does the client wear glasses? And, if so, for what purpose? The trainer asks the client if they have a valid driver's license. The DMV administers an eye test and also measures decision-making skills and reflexes with their required driving test. The trainer also has the client reach for various objects at various distances, heights, and angles. This tests their somatosensory inputs for controlling balance. The fastest reacting sensory system is the somatosensory system.
- Psy-Phy (pronounced "Sci-Fi"): The trainer asks the client about their aches and pains. These physiological and psychological symptoms can additionally help the trainer understand what the client's body is communicating. Interpreting the language of the body can help in healing.
- Mini Mental-State Exam (MMSE): This brief test goes a long way to demonstrate client orientation, short-term memory, concentration, language abilities, and motor skills.
- 10-Q Checklist/Physical Problems Affecting Memory: 1) HIV or syphilis; 2) anemia; 3) thyroid (forgetfulness, weight gain, depression, dry skin, coldness, joint/muscle ache, fatigue); 4) liver/kidney (GGT scan/liver enzyme + alcohol abuse); 5) diabetes; 6) heart issues (EKG; supplement with omega 3-6-9); 7) mini-strokes; 8) carotid artery blockage (MRI); 9) insomnia (polysomnogram PSO); 10) nutrition (dietician).
- CARE assessment: This is comprised of 20 questions that provides medical, sociological, physiological, genealogical, psychological and therapeutic information, and can stand alone as a comprehensive evaluation tool. A "yes" to 3 of the 20 questions indicates the client requires CARE. 1) Are you over 45-years of age? 2) Have you had mini strokes? 3) Are you taking steroidal medication for any reason? 4) Do you sit a lot? 5) Do you have lower back problems? 6) Is your blood pressure 140/90 mmHg or higher, or have been told your blood pressure is too high? 7) Are you 15 or more pounds overweight? 8) Is your cholesterol level 240mg/dL or higher? 9) Do you have an abnormal heartbeat? 10) Is it true you do not have a regular exercise program? 11) Do you smoke? 12) Does your family have a history of heart disease? 13) Does your family have a history of strokes before 60-years-old? 14) Do you live alone? 15) Do you have diabetes or take medication to control your blood sugar? 16) Do you take medication for depression or excessive mood shifts? 17) Is it true you have never played catch? 18) Do you seem to be forgetting things more and more? 19) Do you eat fast food two or more times a week? 20) Is it true that you are on hormone replacement therapy?
- General fitness: The following fitness tests were developed by Rikli and Jones:[3]
  - Strength: 1) Chair stand (measures lower body muscular strength for walking, getting out of a chair, tub or car, prevent falls); 2) Arm curl (measures upper body strength for lifting, carrying, holding).
  - Flexibility: Back scratch test (shoulder flexibility for getting dressed, combing hair, reaching, and posture).
  - Mobility: 8-foot-up-and-go measures balance for overall mobility.

Why is 40 The Un-Magic Number?

Theoretically, 40 is not the benchmark age. More realistically, the stop-gap number is 45. By 40 we have done our best to create a comfortable lifestyle. Ironically, it is around that age many of us begin to "lose it." Not only do we have more medical issues due to 15-20 unneeded pounds, but we've also CARE-lessly created personal family problems and our savings likely need a stimulus package. At 40 we've lost our momentum. But we deny it for about five years. But there is good news: We have as many neurons in our brain as there are stars in the sky. And: It is possible to teach old dogs new tricks.

In his bestselling book *Spark: The Revolutionary New Science of Exercise and the Brain*, John Ratey quotes the noted neuroscientist William Greenough, who says: "Exercise optimizes your mind-set to improve alertness, attention and motivation; it prepares and encourages nerve cells to bind together which allows for new information; and, it spurs the development of new nerve cells in the brain's processing centers." Ratey then goes on to ask Greenough what he believes is the optimal exercise plan. Greenough answers: "Nobody's done that research yet. Maybe in the next five years we'll know a lot more."[4]

CARE fills the void of exercise knowledge now. CARE is not exclusively a fall prevention program, nor exclusively a brain-buster program. CARE comes before the fall. CARE can be done at home, in assisted living facilities, senior residences, hospitals and medical centers, at medical offices, and be implemented into city recreation programs.

There are over 100 specific exercises and moves used with CARE clients. The CARE program is prescribed for 10-minutes a day, 6-days a week, for 6-weeks, with weekly visits by a CARE trainer. The CARE client contract states: "After six weeks, it is highly recommended that the client maintain the program by requesting an extension, or periodic exercise updates. The client agrees to share at least one exercise with a family member or friend."

REFERENCES

1. Exercise & Physical Activity: Your Everyday Guide from the National Institute on Aging. National Institute on Aging. Available at: http://www.nia.nih.gov/HealthInformation/Publications /ExerciseGuide/ Accessed March 22, 2010.
2. To Ward off Alzheimer's, Exercise. Fisher Center for Alzheimer's Research Foundation. Available at: http://www.alzinfo.org/newsarticle/templates/archivenewstemplate.asp?articleid=127&zoneid=9 Accessed March 22, 2010.
3. Rikli RE, Jones JC. Senior Test Manual, Human Kinetics. 2007.
4. Ratey J, Hagerman E. Spark: The Revolutionary New Science of Exercise and the Brain. Little Brown & Co; 2008.

ABOUT THE AUTHOR

Erik Flowers has been an exercise specialist for more than 30-years. He developed Customized Age Reducing Exercise (CARE) at his gym, Body Builders Gym, Los Angeles. He has trained staff at Alzheimer's centers, presented at wellness workshops, conducted exercise seminars at addiction recovery facilities, and personally trains agile 40+ and less mobile seniors.

Chapter 12
Traumatic Brain Injury – Hormonal Dysfunction Syndrome: "The Stealth Syndrome"

Mark L. Gordon, M.D., FAAFP
Clinical Professor, USC Keck School of Medicine (Los Angeles, CA USA);
Medical Director, Millennium Health Centers, Inc. and TBI-MedLegal (Encino, CA USA)

ABSTRACT

Until recently we have accepted the progressive and often premature loss of hormones as being a genetically predisposing process that we will all experience. It has also been considered as that natural sequence of events triggering the aging process. But there is nothing natural about a process that can be precipitated prematurely by external forces which can take from us our youth and ability to endure the challenges inherent in maintaining a long, productive, quality of life.

Traumatic brain injury (TBI) can be a condition that causes premature aging. It can result from a number of insults to both the exterior and interior aspects of the brain's encasement – the skull. Exteriorly, blunt force trauma caused by an object, an explosion, a shock wave, as well as by G-forces induced by an amusement park ride, can cause TBI. Whilst internal causes of TBI include anoxia, hemorrhagic bleeding, subarachnoid hemorrhage, x-rays, and toxins found in our air, water, and food, as well as numerous medications that can drastically influence hormonal homeostasis.

Regardless of the causation, the affect can be the production of a group of chemicals called caspases. These chemicals lead to a progressive dysfunction between the hypothalamus and pituitary gland with subsequent loss of hormonal regulation and production through a process called apoptosis. In effect, the wiring between these two areas is damaged or destroyed, interrupting hormonal communication.

It has been documented that the deficiencies of growth hormone (GH), testosterone, estrogen, progesterone, thyroid, and cortisol (singularly and in combination), are responsible for the majority of psychological, physiological, and physical symptoms that are characteristic of post-concussion syndrome (PCS), post-traumatic stress syndrome (PTSS), and post traumatic brain injury (PTBI).

Symptoms frequently precede the detection of the underlying hormone deficiencies, that is, if they are even looked at. In one clinical study, 56% of the group had one or more hormonal deficiencies within 3-months of the neurotrauma.[1]

Radiologic assessment of the intracranial impact of TBI has become a science unto itself with the newer technologies helping to better define damaged areas of the brain. A number of contemporary radiologic studies have statistically documented common areas of the brain that fall first victim to TBI. It was not surprising to see that the hippocampus was a commonly damaged area, as we know that many patients with TBI suffer from memory related deficits.

Early laboratory assessment of the patient with TBI can monitor and document the sometime sudden if not progressive decrease in hormones. Then the logical challenge becomes treatment based upon replacement or supplementation of the insufficient or deficient hormone(s).

Traditionally, treatment has been with psychotropic drugs and psychotherapy, with poor quality of life outcome. This has been nothing more than treating the superficial symptoms and not the underlying cause and that is the "Stealth Syndrome".

This paper will consider the incidence, clinical course, diagnosis, and treatment of post TBI hormonal dysfunction syndrome – pTBI-HDS.

Keywords: traumatic brain injury, TBI, post TBI hormonal dysfunction syndrome, pTBI-HDS

INTRODUCTION AND OVERVIEW

Until recently we have accepted the progressive and often premature loss of hormones as being a genetically predisposing process that we will all experience. It has also been considered as that natural sequence of events triggering the aging process. But there is nothing natural about a process that can be precipitated prematurely by external forces which can take from us our youth and ability to endure the challenges inherent in maintaining a long, productive, quality of life.

Traumatic brain injury (TBI) can be a condition that causes premature aging. It can result from a number of insults to both the exterior and interior aspects of the brain's encasement – the skull. Exteriorly, blunt force trauma caused by an object, an explosion, a shock wave, as well as by G-forces induced by an amusement park ride, can cause TBI. Whilst internal causes of TBI include anoxia, hemorrhagic bleeding, subarachnoid hemorrhage, x-rays, and toxins found in our air, water, and food, as well as numerous medications that can drastically influence hormonal homeostasis.

Regardless of the causation, the affect can be the production of a group of chemicals called caspases. These chemicals lead to a progressive dysfunction between the hypothalamus and pituitary gland with subsequent loss of hormonal regulation and production through a process called apoptosis. In effect, the wiring between these two areas is damaged or destroyed, interrupting hormonal communication.

It has been documented that the deficiencies of growth hormone (GH), testosterone, estrogen, progesterone, thyroid, and cortisol (singularly and in combination), are responsible for the majority of psychological, physiological, and physical symptoms that are characteristic of post-concussion syndrome (PCS), post-traumatic stress syndrome (PTSS), and post traumatic brain injury (PTBI).

Symptoms frequently precede the detection of the underlying hormone deficiencies, that is, if they are even looked at. In one clinical study, 56% of the group had one or more hormonal deficiencies within 3-months of the neurotrauma.[1]

Radiologic assessment of the intracranial impact of TBI has become a science unto itself with the newer technologies helping to better define damaged areas of the brain. A number of contemporary radiologic studies have statistically documented common areas of the brain that fall first victim to TBI. It was not surprising to see that the hippocampus was a commonly damaged area, as we know that many patients with TBI suffer from memory related deficits.

Early laboratory assessment of the patient with TBI can monitor and document the sometime sudden if not progressive decrease in hormones. Then the logical challenge becomes treatment based upon replacement or supplementation of the insufficient or deficient hormone(s).

Traditionally, treatment has been with psychotropic drugs and psychotherapy, with poor quality of life outcome. This has been nothing more than treating the superficial symptoms and not the underlying cause and that is the "Stealth Syndrome".

This paper will consider the incidence, clinical course, diagnosis, and treatment of post TBI hormonal dysfunction syndrome – pTBI-HDS.

TRAUMATIC BRAIN INJURY – HORMONAL DYSFUNCTION SYNDROME
A Change in Concepts Based Upon Science

In the beginning of the anti-aging revolution, physicians (interventional endocrinologists) accepted the onset and progression of hormone deficiencies as being a part of the natural aging process. This was loosely taken to be around the 4th decade of life when males start to loose testosterone and females begin the downward spiral leading to menopause due to estrogen, progesterone, and testosterone deficiencies. During this progression there are three variable but significant adverse changes in one's psychological, physiological, and physical wellbeing that seems to correlate greater with pituitary hormone deficiencies than with one's age.

Although the relationship between neurotrauma and hormonal deficiencies has been in the medical literature for decades, its place in clinical medicine has been obscured until recently. Nonetheless, there is still academic resistance challenging the criteria that we use to define someone with a hormonal deficiency as well as the optimal treatment.

Incidence

pTBI-HDS is typically associated with severe head traumas with a Glasgow Coma Score (lowest 3 and highest 15) of less than 7 or 8 with loss of consciousness and coma. Survivors of such head trauma often suffer from impairment of cognition, language, and mood, as well as physical functioning. However, more recent research by Kelly *et al* suggest that relatively mild head trauma can be enough to cause a TBI with development of hormone regulatory dysfunction.[2] Motor vehicle accidents and sports, such as boxing, martial arts, wresting, football, are common causes of TBI. As are slip and falls, blunt trauma, and shaken trauma. Even seemingly innocuous rides at amusement parks can be violent enough to cause jarring of the stock of the pituitary that can predispose us to TBI.

An estimated 1.9 million Americans sustain a TBI each year with approximately 52,000 of those people dying from their injuries on the spot. Anywhere between 300,000 and 380,000 end up in an emergency room or are hospitalized for observation. The remaining individuals "shake it off" and go home unaware of the smoldering process that continues as they sleep. Of those that survive, many will go on to develop progressive hormonal deficiencies (accelerated by subsequent TBI), which leads to pTBI-HDS. This "Stealth Syndrome" is frequently subtle, frequently unaddressed, and frequently under-diagnosed. The leading causes of TBI are:

- Falls (28%)
- Motor vehicle-traffic crashes (20%)
- Struck by/against events (19%)
- Assaults (11%)
- Other causes (22%)[3]

Veterans and Traumatic Brain Injury

Neurologists affiliated with the U.S. military now estimate that up to 30% of troops who have been on active duty for 4-months or longer (in both Iraq and Afghanistan) are at risk of some form of disabling neurological damage. This is partly based on the knowledge that closed head injuries far outnumber the penetrative head injuries on which official statistics are based. So, while official figures put the number of U.S. troop casualties in Iraq and Afghanistan at 22,600 (as of November 2006), there may be up to 150,000 already suffering from TBI.

These same neurologists are among those who have highlighted the Bush administration's neglect of its injured troops. They emphasize the need for prompt diagnosis and evaluation of troops who have sustained TBI, as well as improved methods for screening returning troops for brain damage and better monitoring of injured troops' progress during treatment and rehabilitation. The Veterans Affairs and Armed Services Committee set aside $3.75 million for the creation of a computer-based system for the measurement of cognitive functions in troops before and after deployment to war zones. The pre-deployment testing was started this past year at Fort Collins, Kentucky. Congress recently authorized $450 million from the Iraq spending bill for research into TBI.

Symptomatology

Whether the trauma is mild, moderate, or severe it still can cause the brain's ability to regulate important life maintaining hormones to fail. The loss of these hormones increases the risk of heart attack, stroke, emotional instability, depression, anxiety, mood swings, memory loss, fatigue, confusion, amnesia, poor cognition, learning disabilities, decreased communication skills, poor healing, frequent infections, poor fracture healing, poor skin quality, increased body fat, decreased muscle strength and size, infertility, and loss of sex drive.

Neuroradiology

Radiologic evidence for identification of specific neuroimaging findings indicative of TBI has been advanced with use of the 1.5- and 3.0-Tesla high-field MRI. Orrison *et al* assessed 100 unselected consecutive examinations of professional unarmed combatants to determine the extent of identifiable TBI findings. The percentage of positive findings and the localization of lesions were quantified using the checklist that included the MRI findings previously reported in the medical literature. Seventy-six percent of the unarmed combatants had at least one finding that may be associated with TBI: 59% hippocampal atrophy, 43% cavum septum pellucidum, 32% dilated perivascular spaces, 29% diffuse axonal injury,

24% cerebral atrophy, 19% increased lateral ventricular size, 14% pituitary gland atrophy, 5% arachnoid cysts, and 2% had contusions.[4] The improved resolution and increased signal-to-noise ratio on 1.5- and 3.0-Tesla high-field MRI systems defines the range of pathological variations that may occur in professional unarmed combatants. Additionally, the use of a systematic checklist approach insures evaluation for all possible TBI-related abnormalities. This knowledge can be used to anticipate the regions of potential brain pathology for radiologists and emergency medicine physicians, and provides important information for evaluating unarmed combatants relative to their safety and long-term neurocognitive outcome.

Clinical Course

There are three phases to post TBI hormonal deficiency syndrome: acute, recovery, and the chronic phase. Aimaretti *et al* found GH deficiency and secondary hypogonadism were the most common acquired pituitary defects induced by TBI in the transition phase (pediatric to adolescent). The results of this study suggest that it is extremely important to give all prepubescent children who have sustained a head injury a total hormone assessment, because that head injury may cause pTBI-HDS, which could cause a whole range of problems, including short stature, personality changes, functional disability, and problems with language skills and school skills.[5] The most recent literature suggests that hormone levels should be determined immediately after the injury and then again a few weeks later.

Schneider *et al* studied the prevalence of anterior pituitary insufficiency at 3 and 12-months after TBI. Results showed that 56% of TBI patients had anterior pituitary insufficiency at 3-months and 36% at 12-months.[1] Leal-Cerro *et al* conducted a similar study investigating the prevalence of TBI-mediated hypopituitarism in patients who had sustained a severe TBI within the last five years. Results showed that 17% had gonadotrophin deficiency, 6.4% had adrenocortiocotrophic (ACTH) deficiency, 5.8% had thyroid stimulating hormone (TSH) deficiency, and 1.7% developed diabetes insipidus. Overall, 24.7% of participants developed some type of pituitary hormone deficiency.[6]

Kelly *et al* found that chronic GH deficiency developed in 18% of patients with complicated mild, moderate, or severe TBI, and was associated with depression and diminished quality of life.[7] Whilst Powner *et al* found that chronic hormonal deficiencies occur in 30-40% of patients after TBI, with 10-15% of patients having more than one deficiency.[8] Like Kelly, Powner documented 15-20% of TBI patients go on to develop GH deficiency. Results of the study by Powner *et al* also showed that 15% of TBI patients developed gonadal hormone deficiencies and 10-30% developed hypothyroidism. The researchers found that chronic adrenal failure was widespread amongst TBI patients and that nearly a third had elevated prolactin levels.[8]

Koponen *et al* conducted a 30-year follow-up study on patients who had suffered TBI to determine the occurrence of psychiatric disorders. Their results showed that 48.3% of study participants had had an axis I disorder that began after TBI. The most common disorders after TBI were: major depression (26.7%), alcohol abuse or dependence (11.7%), panic disorder (8.3%), specific phobia (8.3%), and psychotic disorders. Nearly a quarter (23.3%) developed at least one personality disorder. These findings led the researchers to conclude: "The results suggest that TBI may cause decades-lasting vulnerability to psychiatric illness in some individuals. TBI seems to make patients particularly susceptible to depressive episodes, delusional disorder, and personality disturbances. The high rate of psychiatric disorders found in this study emphasizes the importance of psychiatric follow-up after traumatic brain injury."[9]

Assessing Neurotrauma-Related Hormonal Dysfunction

In order to optimally treat pTBI-HDS those hormones that are insufficient or deficient need to be identified. Important points to remember when you suspect that a patient may have sustained a potential neurotrauma are:

- It is vital not to use the intensity of the trauma to predict the onset of post TBI hormonal dysfunction syndrome – even the most subtle of injures can precipitate TBI.
- It is vital that you perform comprehensive hormonal testing immediately after the precipitating event to establish a baseline (insulin-like growth factor-1, TSH, luteinizing hormone, follicle stimulating hormone, prolactin, cortisol, etc).
- Do not use age as a predictor. Even in a 45-year-old patient it is vital to inquire about any historical head trauma – even head trauma that occurred in their childhood.

- Although GH cannot be used at present for the treatment of TBI, it can still be used to treat adult GH deficiency syndrome (AGHDS). However, being aware of the etiology of such a deficiency is extremely important because you may need to adopt a totally different approach to a patient's treatment.
- Consider early hormonal supplementation to minimize the psychological, physiological, and physical sequelae.
- Hormonal assessments can be done at three-month intervals from the date of injury, or more frequently based upon treatment.
- A comprehensive cognitive, laboratory, radiological, and confrontational examination of the TBI patient is being developed by the Millennium and will be available at www.tbimedlegal.com.

CONCLUDING REMARKS

There are already 4.7 million people walking around with the residual affects of TBI. On top of this number there are an additional 300,000 - 380,000 more individuals who have sustained a significant TBI. At the present time, treatment has been based upon therapies that only mask the underlying condition of hormonal deficiencies and do nothing to correct them.

In order to address the 300,000 plus returning veterans with TBI, the government has set up a center at Fort Collins Kentucky under Dr. Twillie, who puts the soldiers through a battery of tests to measure different cognitive functions. Visual tests show how fast and accurately a soldier can recognize letters, a driving simulator gives soldiers the feeling of driving under different environmental conditions and a Nintendo Wii game system, with its motion-sensitive controller, helps with coordination skills. Once a soldier's individual deficiencies are identified, therapy can be designed to help retrain the brain to overcome those problems, Twillie said.

In a review of the available government protocols, there was no document found that discussed* the association of TBI with hormonal deficiencies in light of the overwhelming medical literature that addresses the underlying and stealth condition of pTBI-HDS.

For that reason, the Millennium Health Centers, Inc. though it's new division of "TBIMedLegal", has set up a free to veterans program of hormonal assessment. Once veterans have been documented as being deficient they can return to their physician for treatment. If you are interested in participating with this patriotic program please visit www.tbimedlegal.com and sign in under "physicians sign-in".

REFERENCES

1. Schneider HJ, Schneider M, Saller B, Petersenn S, Uhr M, Husemann B, von Rosen F, Stalla GK. Prevalence of anterior pituitary insufficiency 3 and 12 months after traumatic brain injury. *Eur J Endocrinol.* 2006;154:259-265.
2. Kelly JP. Traumatic brain injury and concussion in sports. *JAMA.* 1999;282:989-991.
3. Langlois JA, Rutland-Brown W, Thomas KE. Traumatic brain injury in the United States: emergency department visits, hospitalizations, and deaths. Atlanta (GA): Centers for Disease Control and Prevention, National Center for Injury Prevention and Control; 2006.
4. Orrison WW, Hanson EH, Alamo T, Watson D, Sharma M, Perkins TG, Tandy RD. Traumatic brain injury: a review and high-field MRI findings in 100 unarmed combatants using a literature-based checklist approach. *J Neurotrauma.* 2009;26:689-701.
5. Aimaretti G, Ambrosio MR, Di Somma C, Gasperi M, Cannavò S, Scaroni C, De Marinis L, Baldelli R, Bona G, Giordano G, Ghigo E. Hypopituitarism induced by traumatic brain injury in the transition phase. *J Endocrinol Invest.* 2005 Dec;28(11):984-989.
6. Leal-Cerro A, Flores JM, Rincon M, Murillo F, Pujol M, Garcia-Pesquera F, Dieguez C, Casanueva FF. Prevalence of hypopituitarism and growth hormone deficiency in adults long-term after severe traumatic brain injury. *Clin Endocrinol (Oxf).* 2005;62:525-532.
7. Kelly DF, McArthur DL, Levin H, Swimmer S, Dusick JR, Cohan P, Wang C, Swerdloff R. Neurobehavioral and quality of life changes associated with growth hormone insufficiency after complicated mild, moderate, or severe traumatic brain injury. *J Neurotrauma.* 2006;23:928-942.
8. Powner DJ, Boccalandro C, Alp MS, Vollmer DG. Endocrine failure after traumatic brain injury in adults. *Neurocrit Care.* 2006;5:61-70.

9. Koponen S, Taiminen T, Portin R, Himanen L, Isoniemi H, Heinonen H, Hinkka S, Tenovuo O. Axis I and II psychiatric disorders after traumatic brain injury: a 30-year follow-up study. *Am J Psychiatry*. 2002;159:1315-1321.

ABOUT THE AUTHOR

Originally residency trained and board certified in family medicine (1984), Dr. Mark L. Gordon continued his medical education in clinical orthopedics (1990), cosmetic dermatology (1993), and sports medicine (1995) prior to culminating in interventional endocrinology (1997) – a term which he coined in 2003. Dr. Gordon has been a strong advocate of the promotion of preventive medicine through the correction of underlying hormonal deficiencies. He was instrumental in opening up the recognition of traumatic brain injury as a cause of hormonal deficiency in the hallmarked presentation on ESPN's Outside the Lines (2007). His book, *The Clinical Application of Interventional Medicine* (2008), is recognized by his peers as a dissertation on the standards of care and assessment for anti-aging medicine. His academic standards and medical knowledge have been recognized by UCLA and USC, where he holds the position of Clinical Professor (1998). As medical director of CBS Studios (2001), he has been used for projects at HBO, CBS, ESPN, CNN, FOX, and a number of international programs. Dr. Gordon is owner and medical director of Millennium Health Centers -- Medicine for the 21st century, in Encino California. Most recently (5/2009), Dr. Gordon was the expert on the first litigated case of TBI causing a subsequent myocardial infarction.

Chapter 13
Metabolic Syndrome: Syndrome X, Y, Z … ?

Stephen Holt, M.D., LLD (Hon.) ChB., PhD, DNM, FRCP (C) MRCP (UK), FACP,
FACG, FACN, FACAM, KSG
Distinguished Professor of Medicine (Emerite),
New York Department of Integrative Medicine at NYCPM (New York, NY USA)

Reproduced, with permission, in part from the *Townsend Letter.*

ABSTRACT

Metabolic syndrome, or "syndrome X," as it is often called, is the variable combination of obesity, hypercholesterolemia and hypertension, linked by an underlying resistance to insulin. This condition is often associated with excess insulin secretion. The syndrome was first described by Reaven in 1998, but its principal component of obesity was not initially emphasized. Retrospective data from the National Health Nutritional Survey for the period 1988 to 1994 implied that 47-million Americans had metabolic syndrome. Today, it is estimated that 1 in every 4 adults in the United States (approximately 70-million individuals) has metabolic syndrome. The fact that metabolic syndrome is so common and that it is associated with serious negative health outcomes, qualifies it as the number-1 public health problem facing several Western societies.

Although the metabolic syndrome is identified as a major cause of cardiovascular disease, it is less apparent that it increases deaths and disabilities from all causes, and underlies numerous diseases, including: female reproductive disorders (polycystic ovary syndrome (PCOS)), non-alcoholic fatty-liver disease, non-alcoholic steatohepatitis, gestational diabetes mellitus, significant changes in body eicosanoid status, inflammatory disease, poor cognitive function, Alzheimer's disease and certain cancers.

The aim of this paper is to show how a multifaceted approach, which includes lifestyle changes and nutritional interventions, can help to both prevent and treat metabolic syndrome.

INTRODUCTION

Metabolic syndrome, or "syndrome X," as it is often called, is the variable combination of obesity, hypercholesterolemia and hypertension, linked by an underlying resistance to insulin. This condition is often associated with excess insulin secretion. The syndrome was first described by Reaven in 1998,[1] but its principal component of obesity was not initially emphasized. Retrospective data from the National Health Nutritional Survey for the period 1988 to 1994 implied that 47-million Americans had metabolic syndrome.[2] Today, it is estimated that 1 in every 4 adults in the United States (approximately 70-million individuals) has metabolic syndrome. The fact that metabolic syndrome is so common and that it is associated with serious negative health outcomes, qualifies it as the number-1 public health problem facing several Western societies.

Although the metabolic syndrome is identified as a major cause of cardiovascular disease, it is less apparent that it increases deaths and disabilities from all causes, and underlies numerous diseases, including: female reproductive disorders (polycystic ovary syndrome (PCOS)), non-alcoholic fatty-liver disease, non-alcoholic steatohepatitis, gestational diabetes mellitus, significant changes in body eicosanoid status, inflammatory disease, poor cognitive function, Alzheimer's disease and certain cancers.[3]

RETHINKING THE MANAGEMENT OF METABOLIC SYNDROME

Excessive dietary intake of refined sugar, lack of exercise, poorly defined genetic tendencies, environmental toxins, and adverse lifestyles contribute variably to the pathogenesis of the metabolic syndrome.[3] Current pharmaceutical and surgical approaches to management of the syndrome have many obvious disadvantages and limitations. It has been suggested by Federal Government researchers that focused treatments of the individual components of the syndrome (hypercholesterolemia, obesity, and hypertension) are unlikely to provide a better outcome than "integrated" management strategies.[2] This suggestion is consistent with dietary attempts to restrict refined carbohydrate intake, and it helps to explain the short-term success of some low carbohydrate diets for weight control.[3] The notion of "integrative" management strategies as first line options for metabolic syndrome opens the door for "alternative" management with dietary supplements.

First-Line Management Options for Metabolic Syndrome

Metabolic syndrome has variable clinical manifestations, which I have attempted to incorporate in a new, unifying concept of disease.[3] This concept extends far beyond the existing definition of syndrome X as obesity, hypertension, and hypercholesterolemia, linked by underlying insulin resistance.[3] In order to take account of this unifying concept, I have coined the term syndrome X, Y and Z...to incorporate the many other diseases that are linked to insulin resistance (Figure 1).

Effective prevention and treatment of metabolic syndrome involves a multifaceted approach directed at all of its cardinal components.[3] Current allopathic treatments (drugs) for syndrome X have been too specifically focused on the individual components of metabolic syndrome (e.g. anti-hypertensive therapy, cholesterol-lowering drugs, etc.) While pharmaceutical interventions should be applied where necessary, they most often form a "back-up plan" for its management. In contrast, the natural techniques of lifestyle modification, and nutritional or nutraceutical interventions (or both), may provide versatile and potent first-line options for the management of syndrome X.[3]

In many cases, treating obesity must involve the management of syndrome X, but syndrome X may occur infrequently in an individual of normal body weight and not all overweight people have syndrome X (Table 1). Failing to diagnose or manage syndrome X in the obese individual is negligent medical practice (Table 1). There is no doubt that syndrome X is both under-diagnosed and under-treated in both conventional and alternative medical practices.

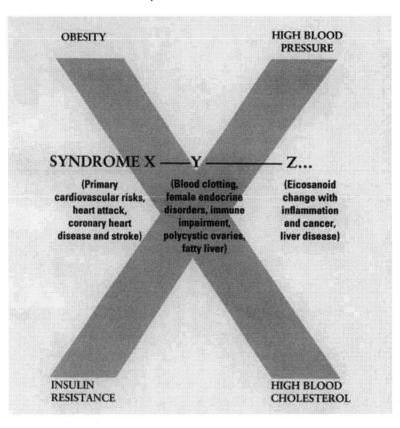

Figure 1: The concept of syndrome X, Y and Z..., which includes the constellation of the four hallmark components of syndrome X (metabolic syndrome) (large X in the figure), to which are added other diseases, accounting for the Y and Z...component. The terms syndrome X, Y and Z... are designed to emphasize the wide range of disabilities associated with the metabolic syndrome.

Nutritional Factors for Syndrome X
Clear Benefits of Dietary Fiber i Syndrome X

Many types of soluble fiber may benefit individuals with syndrome X, through their effects on appetite or satiety regulation, body weight, and blood cholesterol levels.[3] Evolution of research into soluble components of dietary fiber has led to the discovery of fractions of oat soluble fiber (beta-glucans) that have been shown to effectively lower blood cholesterol, reduce postprandial blood glucose, induce satiety, and suppress appetite.[4-7] Although the glucocolloids that contain these beta-glucan fractions of oat fiber have physicochemical properties that modulate upper gastrointestinal motility by delaying gastric emptying,[8] or by retarding or impeding the absorption of specific (macronutrients such as glucose and fats), they also have intrinsic metabolic effects (IMEF).

These IMEF occur, in part, as a consequence of the prebiotic actions of fiber and fermentation of soluble fiber in the colon to yield short-chain fatty acids, including propionic, acetoacetic, and butyric acids. Of these, propionic acid can enter the portal circulation of the liver, and may interfere with cholesterol synthesis by blocking the activity of hydroxymethyl-glutaryl coenzyme A (HMG CoA) reductase, a key enzyme in the synthetic pathway of cholesterol.[3,6] Other types of soluble fiber are of value in blunting postprandial blood glucose responses, e.g. soy fiber, pectin, and guar gum.[9,10]

Table 1. Syndrome X nutritional factors are composed of nutrients, botanicals, herbs and extracts that are of potential value in the nutritional management of metabolic syndrome X, associated with obesity. Some listed substances may provide nutritional support for diets used in the management of diabetes mellitus. (Adapted from Holt et al[10])

FACTOR	THERAPEUTIC EFFECTS
Soluble fiber e.g. oat beta glucan	Soluble fiber reduces post-prandial blood glucose, reduces blood cholesterol, improves glucose tolerance, regulates bowel function, primes the immune system, probably by a prebiotic effect. In addition, soluble fiber promotes satiety and it has other intrinsic metabolic effects. Plays a pivotal role in nutritional management of syndrome X and weight control, especially in children.
Soy Protein (25 g/day)	Soy protein reduces blood cholesterol and its isoflavone content may reduce platelet "stickiness" and exert valuable antioxidant functions. Value of vegetable protein rotation in diets. Soy has many other health benefits and it is an ideal dietary substrate for use in diabetes mellitus and syndrome X. Soy is not toxic.
Omega 3 fatty acids (EPA)	Omega 3 fatty acids are best taken in fish oil concentrates, high in EPA, presented in enteric coated capsules for greater compliance and bioavailability. Plant precursors of omega 3 fatty acids (e.g. flaxseed oils, walnut oils, macadamia etc. are not reliable sources of active fatty acids). Fish oil sensitizes insulin by acting on PPAR receptors and it has multiple health benefits including: cardiovascular benefits, anti-inflammatory actions etc.
Chromium	Several studies imply that chromium in various forms may assist in blood cholesterol reduction, weight control and they may sensitize the actions of insulin.
Alpha lipoic acid	A powerful anti-oxidant which plays a specific role in combat against advanced glycation end-products (AGES), with possible reduction in tissue complications in states of dysglycemia. Has a specific insulin sensitizing role, but should not be given by parenteral administration.
Vanadium	An insulin sensitizer of variable value.
Antioxidants	Including but not limited to anthocyanadins, ellagic acid, turmeric, bioflavonoids, direct or indirect anti-oxidant vitamins or minerals e.g. Vitamin E, C, A, selenium, zinc etc. Anti-oxidants are often misused and mis-formulated. Anti-oxidants should be given with REDOX balance to access all body tissues, hydrophilic and lipophillic properties. Single high dose antioxidants are best avoided, especially by unopposed intravenous administration.
Starch blockers and fat blockers	White kidney bean extract, soluble fiber, chitin of variable value.
Cinnamon	An insulin mimetic.
Maitake	Weak insulin sensitizing effect with both whole mushroom powder and fractions. <u>Not</u> a stand-alone weight control or syndrome X nutritional factor.
Green coffee bean extract	Polyphenols e.g. chlorogenic acid assists in correction of dysglycemia, with specific effects on hepatic glucose synthesis.
Green tea	Very potent antioxidant with widespread health benefits, including effects on glucose metabolism. Distinguished content of catechins, especially EGCG.
Hoodia gordoni	Proposed as a non-stimulant appetite suppressant due to its content of steroidal glycosides.

The glycemic index (GI) and the glycemic load of food are relevant to the dietary guidelines or nutritional support that may counteract exaggerated glycemic responses in syndrome X.[3,8] In simple terms, the GI is a way of describing the ability of different foods to cause a post-prandial rise in blood sugar. Foods laden with simple sugars can be expected to cause a rapid rise in blood glucose to high levels which, in turn, triggers insulin secretion from the pancreas. Such foods have a high GI.[3,8,10]

A major component of the GI is related to altered rates of sugar absorption, at least after acute sugar intake.[8] Upward swings in blood glucose are determined to a significant degree by rapid rates of transfer of glucose to its site of maximal absorption in the small bowel, which is a function of the rate of gastric emptying.[3,8,10] Speedy absorption of sugar pushes blood glucose levels to high ranges (a high glycemic response). In simple terms, repeated, rapid, roller coaster swings in post-prandial blood glucose tend to "flog the pancreatic islet cell mass to death".[3,10] The concept of GI or load becomes more complex with mixed diets.[3]

Essential Fatty Acids and Metabolic Syndrome

The influence of eicosanoids on glucose and insulin homeostasis has been partially defined,[11] however the effects of insulin resistance (or lack) on eicosanoid pathways is less clear.[3,10] Many individuals with syndrome X have a dietary status where eicosanoid pathways are driven towards the production of prothrombotic and pro-inflammatory prostaglandins.[3,11,12] This may occur, in part, as a consequence of common dietary deficiencies of certain essential fatty acids (omega-3 fatty acids) or alteration in the ratio of omega-6 and omega-3 essential fatty acid dietary intake. This shift towards "deviant" prostaglandins is aggravated by insulin resistance, ketoacidosis, and the diabetic diathesis.[11-13]

There is evidence that eicosanoid production can be altered by insulin lack or excess and hyperglycemia. Animal studies show increases in circulating metabolites of prostaglandin E2 (PGE2) production after the experimental induction of diabetes with streptozotocin.[12] This rise in PGE2 metabolites is also found in diabetic humans.[13] Thus, both the circumstances that contribute to the development of insulin resistance and syndrome X can be expected to contribute to changes in the body eicosanoid status that have a detrimental effect on health.

This metabolic change in eicosanoid status is manifested mainly by a quantitative difference in the types of eicosanoid (prostaglandins) produced. "Active" omega-3 fatty acids (eicosapentaenoic acid (EPA) and docosahexaenoic acid (DHA)) found in fish oil supplements, can assist in correcting "deviant" pathways of eicosanoid production. The dosage of fish oil required to induce a therapeutic effect in this context is higher than the dosages that are typically used in clinical practice (greater than 2g/day).

Enteric coated fish oil capsules are preferred for clinical use because they can provide up to 3-times the bioavailability of active omega-3 fatty acids compared with regular fish oil capsules or liquids.[3,10] Powerful arguments can be made to reject the use of "regular" fish oil capsules because compliance is poor with dosages in excess of 2g/day, which may be required for a "therapeutic effect".

Fish oil liquids are obsolete for use in professional practice because of their variable absorption, poor compliance, and tendency to spontaneously decompose and form damaging lipid peroxides. Furthermore, it is known that among eicosanoid precursors, EPA can enhance insulin sensitivity, presumably through effects on peroxisome proliferator-activated receptor alpha (PPAR-α) receptors, which regulate the actions of insulin.[3] Natural clinicians must finally appreciate that omega-3 fatty acid precursors found in vegetable oils (e.g. flax, walnut, macadamia, etc.) are not reliable ways of achieving the desired influence of active omega-3 fatty acids. Omega-3 precursor conversion rates to EPA may be as little as 2% conversion of the total precursor dose in a 24-hour period.

Diets intended to combat syndrome X should contain liberal amounts of omega-3, and where appropriate, omega-6 fatty acids, in the correct balance with one another, together with a strictly controlled intake of refined carbohydrates, a restricted salt intake, an increased intake of fiber intake, and an increased proportion of vegetable sources of protein.[3,9,10] Refined carbohydrate-controlled diets require facilitation to make them more effective in the long-term (by attempts to overcome insulin resistance). This usually equates to the effective management of the constellation of problems found within syndrome X (cholesterol, blood pressure, and insulin resistance). Table 1 presents a number of dietary components and supplements[3,10] that can help in preventing and managing metabolic syndrome.

Obesitis – More Than a Novel Concept!

Obesity and excess body fat are both inflammatory conditions. Inflammation is a key factor in the pathophysiology of syndrome X.[14,15] Not only does obesity raise the level of pro-inflammatory messenger molecules in the body, it precipitates or contributes to several disorders of inflammation, including cardiovascular disease, cancer, arthritis, Alzheimer's disease, liver disease, and asthma.[14] This inflammatory disease "link" with obesity further explains the undesirable effects of insulin resistance,[3] and introduces the novel term "obesitis".

The hallmarks of syndrome X and many cases of pre-type 1, or early type 2 diabetes mellitus often involve the presence of insulin resistance.[3,16] Insulin acts by specific receptor binding, which precipitates many intracellular events.[16] Current evidence suggests that insulin resistance is determined partially by chemical mediators that are released from immune competent cells or fat cells.[16,18] For example, elevated levels of the inflammatory cytokine, tumor necrosis factor-alpha (TNF-α) are associated with overnutrition, and reduction of TNF-α activity is associated with weight loss and improvements in insulin resistance.[18] Many factors that link inflammation and tissue damage have come from recent studies of non-alcoholic fatty liver disease, which is a common component of syndrome X.[19] I believe that syndrome X is a major cause of "cryptogenic" cirrhosis.[3]

While the underlying biochemical basis of the relationships between obesity or syndrome X and inflammatory disease remains underexplored,[20] these circumstances permit me to coin the term "obesitis" and propose that anti-inflammatory approaches should not be overlooked as an important part of obesity management.[3,10]

Up to one third of blood levels of the inflammatory cytokine, interleukin (IL)-6, may emanate from adipose tissue and weight loss is often associated with reduction in blood markers of inflammation e.g. C-reactive protein (CRP) and IL-18.[18,20] Popular healthcare authors have attempted to link inflammation with many common diseases, but their interpretation of this important association is limited or naïve because only changes in eicosanoid status are emphasized (e.g. The Zone).[21] While correcting eicosanoid precursor pathways with omega-3 fatty acids is an important anti-inflammatory and insulin sensitizing maneuver, it is not the whole story.[3,10,14,16]

Recent studies have confirmed the anti-inflammatory actions of certain substances that are found in fat tissue.[18,20] These substances have been referred to as adipocytokines, and include leptin, adiponectin, and visfatin.[22,23] Adiponectin is manufactured by fat cells and blood levels of this protein are reduced in states of obesity, insulin resistance, type 2 diabetes mellitus, and atheroma.[22,23] Adiponectin exhibits potent anti-inflammatory effects by suppressing TNF-α synthesis and promoting the availability of anti-inflammatory cytokines, e.g. IL-10 or IL-1-receptor antagonist.[15,24] The plot thickens in "obesitis" where imbalances of pro-inflammatory and anti-inflammatory cytokines exist. These issues are closely linked to immune dysfunction that is common in obesity, syndrome X, and type II diabetes mellitus.[3] The natural clinician can reverse these circumstances, at least partially, with holistic natural interventions.

Table 2. Elements of Syndrome X and Nutritional Factors that May Counteract Them

Insulin resistance – Chromium polynicotinate, vanadium, maitake, green tea polyphenols, mixed berry antioxidants, and alpha lipoic acid may assist insulin function. Beta-glucan fractions of oat soluble fiber may lower blood glucose levels after sugar intake. Green coffee bean extracts alter hepatic glucose metabolism. Cinnamon is an insulin mimetic.
Abnormal blood lipids – Antioxidants and chromium with biotin may exert favorable effects on blood cholesterol. Oat beta-glucan may reduce blood levels of low-density lipoprotein (LDL) cholesterol and triglycerides, and may variably increase high-density lipoprotein (HDL) cholesterol.
Obesity – Starch-blockers may inhibit sugar absorption. Oat beta-glucan may produce a sensation of satiety when taken before meals, and thereby assist in controlling calorie intake. Delayed appetite suppressant effects of fiber occur and smoothing out blood glucose responses may help to stop "sugar craving."
Hypertension – Variable but small reductions in blood pressure result from weight control and lifestyle changes, e.g. exercise, avoidance of substance abuse (alcohol, caffeine, and smoking). Soluble fiber may have modest independent blood pressure-lowering effects.
Oxidative stress and advanced glycation end products – May be reduced by bioflavonoids, ellagic acid, anthocyanidins, alpha lipoic acid, and other antioxidants.
Homocysteine – Vitamins B6, B12, and folic acid may reduce blood homocysteine levels. Homocysteine and hyperuricemia must not be overlooked in syndrome X. Beware of hyperuricemia.

The final common pathway of tissue damage in obesity or syndrome X often involves oxidative damage due to the generation of free radicals, perhaps exacerbated by a reduction in antioxidant defenses in the body.[15,18] Of course, the progression of the complications of obesity and diabetes mellitus is related to oxidative tissue stress, with the development of advanced glycation end products (AGES).[3] Therefore, the treatment of obesity-related disease seems quite incomplete without supporting antioxidant body functions in the clinical management of the obese or overweight person (Tables 1 and 2), especially in the presence of co-existing syndrome X.

Circadian Biorhythms, Sleep, Obesity, and Syndrome X

Sleep deprivation, overweight status, and syndrome X appear to be inextricably linked in many people. The mechanisms of this association are not fully understood. Reduction in sleep duration in healthy young men is associated with major changes in levels of hormones (ghrelin and leptin) that increase hunger and appetite, thereby promoting weight gain.[25] An established association between short sleep duration and obesity has led to the proposition that more sleep is necessary to prevent obesity.[25-28] Sometimes, restoring sleep patterns alone can promote weight loss.[26,28]

Chronic lack of sleep increases an individual's susceptibility to syndrome X. Furthermore, "forced" sleep deprivation in healthy young adults appears to be diabetogenic, as evidenced by detectible alterations of glucose metabolism.[25,27] The diabetogenic effects of sleep deprivation may be hormonally mediated.[25] Sleeplessness has been associated with decreases in the normal nocturnal surge of thyrotropin or growth hormone (GH) and increases in corticosteroid secretion.[26,27] These hormonal changes are often present in the elderly, reinforcing the notion of a potential causal relationship among sleeplessness and/or obesity and premature aging.[25-28]

The relationship between obesity and insomnia may be linked to the excitability of brain cells, most notably the stress-responsive hypocretin/orexin cells in the hypothalamus.[29] Daily stresses may act on the hypothalamus, resulting in sustained stimulation of hypocretin/orexin cells, which could precipitate insomnia and overeating. One may now postulate the link between obesity and other conditions such as fasting, periodic hypoglycemia, and perimenopause, which are all "stressors" that could serve to excite hypothalamic neurons.[29]

The restoration of sleep patterns of optimum quality and duration can be expected to improve the management of obesity, but stress management appears to be a very important additional factor in obesity management, because of its beneficial effect on sleep patterns and body metabolism that favors weight control.[25-28] It has been suggested that weight gain around the menopause is due to hormonal changes. I reject this hypothesis and propose that this perimenopausal weight gain is more likely to be due to sleep deprivation, which often accompanies the transition of menopause. Failure to restore sleep biorhythms in the menopausal female thwarts all attempts to control unpleasant transitional symptomatology.

Inducing sleep by the use of certain hypnotic drugs has to be seriously questioned in the management of the overweight individual, and it may be quite undesirable in certain circumstances.[30] For reasons that remain unclear, drugs such as Ambien® (zolpidem) may cause weight gain, binge eating, and bizarre behavior.[30] Clearly, natural ways to healthy sleep are preferred over pharmaceutical interventions. Comprehensive plans to engage in positive lifestyle change, together with the use of synergistic dietary supplements are attractive first-line management options for common sleep disorders.[28] Sleeping naturally has been described in programs that involve lifestyle change and the use of nutritional support for sleep with dietary supplements.[28] Sleep is a major area for intervention with natural healthcare.

Implications for Effective Management of Obesity (A Summary)

Integrative medicine can offer the optimal pathway to the management of an overweight status and/or syndrome X, if the modern science of allopathic medicine is complemented or/replaced by holistic care (Table 3.). Many people can shed a few pounds of bodyweight in the short tem, but sustained weight control involves many management principles, other than diet, drugs or supplements alone.[31]

The last thing that is required in the new millennium is another diet promise for weight loss. That said, carbohydrate restriction in the short-term can result in apparently safe and effective, accelerated weight loss.[31] However, long-term restriction of carbohydrate intake is probably neither safe nor effective and compliance is a problem.[31] Low carbohydrate diets result often in rebound weight gain, largely

114

because of lack of compliance, and the documented failure of carbohydrate restriction alone to overcome insulin resistance (syndrome X).[31]

Table 3. A Holistic Management Plan for Obesity

A Holistic Weight Management Program for Natural Clinicians	
FACTORS TO ADDRESS	**ACTIONS**
Mutual acceptance of weight status, required commitments and targets for weight and health management	Weight assessment BMI measurement Fat distribution Definition of realistic weight loss targets with health focus. Avoid unrealistic weight loss expectations.
Identify and exclude specific secondary causes of obesity	Congenital disorder, thyroid disease, Cushing's syndrome, psychiatric disease, drugs, surgery, metabolism and insulin resistance syndrome, syndrome X, etc.
Is metabolic syndrome X present?	The overweight person with syndrome X has increased risk of many diseases (syndrome X, Y, Z…) Failure to address insulin resistance syndrome in the presence of obesity is incomplete medical management.
Diet	Tailored to specific weight control targets and objectives. Short-term accelerated weight loss with low carbohydrate approach, Long-term maintenance with balanced diet includes: restricted simple sugar, trans-fatty acids and saturated fats; moderate protein intake (1g/Kg) with vegetable protein inclusion; moderate salt intake. Planning required for special circumstances of liver disease, diabetes mellitus, hypertension and, again, beware of syndrome X.
"Obesitis"	All factors that may suppress inflammation are worthy interventions. The common pathway of inflammation often involves oxidative stress. Various nutraceuticals may suppress inflammation and/or independently or simultaneously sensitize the actions of insulin, e.g. alpha-lipoic acid, hydrophilic and lipophilic antioxidants, and the versatility and power of EPA, given in enteric coated capsules for compliance and bioavailability.
Correct Biorhythm	Reductions in sleep duration and quality promote weight gain, abnormal glucose metabolism, and insulin resistance. Without healthy sleep, weight loss cannot be sustained and eating disorders emerge, especially nocturnal "fridge-raiding"
Behavior Modification	Many approaches, but altered attitudes to food and removal of positive reinforcements to overeating. Frequent social gluttony
Exercise	Movement is an absolute prerequisite for weight control. Energy into the body must be balance by energy expenditure. Aerobic exercise must be matched to physical fitness levels. Panacea benefits from exercise are apparent.
Adjunctive Approach	Dietary supplements for weight control are often associated with illegal treatment claims for obesity and many have a poor scientific basis for their use. Stimulant weight loss supplements should be avoided in the mature, obese person. Reductions in net calorie intake are the goal, but modern nutraceutical technology has combined appetite suppression with attempts to alter metabolic changes associated with obesity e.g. dysglycemia and insulin resistance syndrome, the hallmark of syndrome X. Drugs used in weight control have onerous side effects. *Hoodia gordonii* shows promise for non-stimulant appetite suppression and it can be combined with natural substances that alter dysglycemia e.g. green tea and chlorogenic acid (found in green coffee bean) etc.
Surgical Intervention?	A variety of approaches are possible, e.g. gastric banding. Surgery for obesity results in a circumstance of forced malnutrition. The clinical course and natural history of the post-obesity surgery patient has not been evaluated in the long-term. The nutritional status of the post-surgical obese individual is often mismanaged. A big question mark exists with obesity surgery in children and teenagers. Careful selection required for surgery, but holistic care of these patients must occur to decrease post-surgical morbidity and mortality. Surgery is "the last ditch".

115

Without positive lifestyle change there cannot be a health benefit from any weight control program. I have great reservations about the increasing use of surgery for weight control, even though recent studies imply that laparoscopic gastric-banding techniques are reported to be more effective than diet and lifestyle interventions for weight control.[32] However, improvements in some components of syndrome X and obesity are to be expected as a consequence of certain surgical procedures; and short-term quality of life measures may improve.[32]

Some recent comparative studies of obesity surgery[32] have involved patients who would not normally receive surgery for obesity. However, obesity surgery comes with complications and its outcome is often related to the existing health of the patient and the skill of the surgeon. There may be at tendency to overestimate the value and safety of bariatric surgery and its use in teenagers poses worrisome issues because of the lack of long-term follow up studies. It is not known exactly when the risk-benefit ratio of surgery is most favorable. Non-invasive management obesity must always be perceived as the first-line option.[3] Surgery has been proposed as able to reverse several components of syndrome X, but the presence of syndrome X, *per se*, cannot be considered an indication for surgery.

Drugs for weight control are often undesirable interventions because of side effect profiles.[30] Nutritional approaches are often safe and they are assumed to be cost effective when used in an appropriate manner.[28,31,33] Unfortunately, dietary supplements used for weight control are purveyed often with weak evidence of efficacy.[33] Natural substances that reduce appetite by stimulant mechanisms may compound cardiovascular risks in the obese individual who may already have hypertension and cardiovascular risk factors (syndrome X). The removal of ephedra (ma huang) as a dietary supplement for weight control was appropriate because of the misuse of this otherwise useful dietary supplement.[33] Indeed, the U.S. Federal Trade Commission has taken a strong position that dietary supplements cannot carry a weight loss claim which is regarded as a "drug claim".

Recent studies with putative, non-stimulant appetite suppressants such as *Hoodia gordonii* and *Caralluma fimbriata* extract are very promising because controlled intake of calories is the key initiative in weight control.[33,34]

CONCLUDING REMARKS

Changes in lifestyle, and nutritional interventions with condition-specific dietary supplements,[10] may have more to offer for the prevention and treatment of syndrome X or obesity than do existing allopathic management strategies(Table 3).[3,10] Combating the specific components of syndrome X has become one of the most important public health initiatives in Western Society.[3,10] This initiative continues to be often ignored. In particular, the increasingly global initiative for achievement of a healthy body weight must be comprehensive in its tactics.[3,10] Weight control diets require modification and facilitation with revised dietary guidelines and the help of lifestyle changes used with key dietary supplements or functional foods.[3,10,31,33]

REFERENCES

1. Reaven GM. Banting Lecture 1988. Role of insulin resistance in human diabetes. *Diabetes* 1988;37:1595-1607.
2. Ford ES, Giles WH, Dietz W. The prevalence of metabolic syndrome in the US population. *JAMA* 2002;297:356-359.
3. Holt S. *Combat Syndrome X, Y and Z...* Newark, NJ: Wellness Publishing; 2002.
4. Braaten JT, Wood PJ, Scott FW, *et al*. Oat beta-glucan reduces blood cholesterol concentration in hypercholesterolemic subjects. *Eur J Clin Nutr.* 1994;48:465-474.
5. Inglett GE. The United States of America as represented by the Secretary of (Washington, DC), assignee. *Soluble hydrocolloid food additives and method of making.* US Patent 6 060 519. August 7, 1998.
6. Glore SR, Van Treeck D, Knehans AW. Guild M. Soluble fiber and serum lipids. A literature review. *J Am Diet Assoc.* 1994;94:425-436.
7. Hallfrisch J, Schofield DJ, Behall KM. Diets containing soluble oat extracts improve glucose and insulin responses of moderately hypercholesterolemic men and women. *Am J Clin Nutr.* 1995;61:379-82.
8. Holt S, Heading CR, Carter D, *et al*. Effect of gel fiber on gastric emptying and absorption of glucose and paracetamol in humans. *Lancet* 1979;1:636-639.

116

9.   Holt S. *The Soy Revolutio*n. New York, NY: Dell Publishing, Inc.; 1999.
10. Holt S, Wright JV, Taylor TV. *Syndrome X Nutritional Factors*. Newark, NJ: Wellness Publishing; 2003.
11. Robertson RP. Eicosanoids as pluripotential modulators of pancreatic islet function. *Diabetes* 1988;37:367.
12. Axelrod L, Levine T. Plasma prostaglandin levels in rats with diabetes mellitus and diabetic ketoacidosis. *Diabetes* 1982;31:994.
13. McRae JR, Day RP, Metz SA, *et al*. Prostaglandin E2 metabolite levels during diabetic ketoacidosis. *Diabetes* 1985;34:761
14. Handelsman Y. Guest Editorial. *Metabolic Syndrome and Related Disorders*. 2005;3:281-283.
15. Matsuzawa Y, Funahashi T, Nakamura T. Molecular mechanism of Metabolic Syndrome X: contribution of adipocytokines adipocyte-derived bioactive substances. *Ann NY Acad Sci*. 1999;892:146-154.
16. Bloomgarden ZT. Concepts of insulin resistance. *Metabolic Syndrome and Related Disorders*. 2005;3:284-293.
17. Pirola L, Johnston AM, Van Obberghen E. Modulation of insulin action. *Diabetologia*. 2004;47:170-184.
18. Wellen KE, Hotamisligil GS. Inflammation, stress, and diabetes. *J Clin Invest*. 2005;115:1111-1119.
19. Bloomgarden ZT. Non-alcoholic fatty liver disease and malignancy as complications of insulin resistance. *Metabolic Syndrome and Related Disorders*. 2005;3:316-327.
20. Grimble RF. Inflammatory status and insulin resistance. *Curr Opin Clin Nutr Metab Care*. 2002;5:551-559.
21. Sears B. *The Anti-Inflammation Zone*. Regan Books; 2005.
22. Bloomgarden ZT. Cardiovascular complications of insulin resistance. *Metabolic Syndrome and Related Disorders*. 2005;3:305-315.
23. Fonseca VA, Bratcher C, Thethi T. Pharmacological treatment of the insulin resistance syndrome in people without diabetes. *Metabolic Syndrome and Related Disorders*. 2005;3:332-338.
24. Angulo P. Nonalcoholic fatty liver disease. *N Engl J Med*. 2002;346:1221-1231.
25. Spiegel K, Tasali E, Penev P, Van Cauter E. Sleep curtailment in healthy young men is associated with decreased leptin levels, elevated ghrelin levels, and increased hunger and appetite. *Ann Intern Med*. 2004;141:846-850.
26. Taheri S. The link between short sleep duration and obesity: we should recommend more sleep to prevent obesity? *Arch Dis Child*. 2006;91:881-884.
27. Kohatsu ND, Tsai R, Young T, VanGilder LF, Burmeister, Stromquist AM, Merchant JA. Sleep Duration and Body Mass Index in a Rural Population. *Archives of Internal Medicine*. 2006;166:1701-1705.
28. Holt S. *Sleep Naturally*. Little Falls, NJ: Wellness Publishing Inc.; 2003.
29. Horvath TL, Bing Gao, X. Input organization and plasticity of hypocretin neurons: Possible clues to obesity's association with insomnia. *Cell Metabolism*. 205;1:279-286.
30. Barrett J, Underwood A. Perchance to...Eat? *Newsweek*. 2006;March 27:54.
31. Holt S. *Enhancing Low Carb Diets*. Wellness Publishing; 2004.
32. O'Brien PE, Dixon JB, Laurie C, *et al*. Treatment of mild to moderate obesity with laparoscopic adjustable gastric banding or an intensive medical program: a randomized trial. *Ann Intern Med*. 2006;144:625-633.
33. Holt S. *Supreme Properties of Hoodia Gordonii*. Wellness Publishing; 2005.
34. Rajendran, R, Rajendran, K. *Caralluma extract products and processes for making the same*. US Patent 7 390 516. June 24, 2008.

ABOUT THE AUTHOR

Dr. Stephen Holt is Distinguished Professor of Medicine (Emerite), Scientific Advisor, Natural Clinician LLC is a best selling author, award winning medical teacher, researcher and clinician. He has published several hundred articles in peer review medical literature and he is the author of more than 20 books.

Chapter 14
Calorie Restriction Mimetics: Natural Therapeutics

Stephen Holt, M.D., LLD (Hon.) ChB., PhD, DNM, FRCP (C) MRCP (UK), FACP,
FACG, FACN, FACAM, KSG
Distinguished Professor of Medicine (Emerite),
New York Department of Integrative Medicine at NYCPM (New York, NY USA)

Reproduced, with permission, in part from the Townsend Letter.

ABSTRACT

A quest of modern medical practice is to promote longevity (long life in good health). Anti-aging medicine is oversubscribed with "band-aid" approaches in the relentless pursuit of the "fountain of youth". The only intervention that has been shown to extend average and maximal lifespan in a wide variety of living organisms is the restriction of calorie intake.

It appears that the application of calorie restriction of the order of 30-50% below average free-feeding calorie intake may induce an inhibitory effect on many aspects of aging, including aging processes in non-human primates and most probably humans.

As experimental studies over the past two decades started to define the beneficial biochemical and physiological effects of calorie restriction, scientists started to propose that there were a variety of substances (drugs and natural compounds) that could mimic these desirable effects on body structures and functions. In the late 1990s, scientists started to propose the notion that there were calorie restriction mimetics that have anti-aging properties as a consequence of their ability to induce biological changes that occurred as a consequence of direct reductions of overall calorie intake.

The aim of this paper is to examine the biological effects of calorie restriction and to introduce the concept of calorie restriction mimetics.

INTRODUCTION

A quest of modern medical practice is to promote longevity (long life in good health). Anti-aging medicine is oversubscribed with "band-aid" approaches in the relentless pursuit of the "fountain of youth". The only intervention that has been shown to extend average and maximal lifespan in a wide variety of living organisms is the restriction of calorie intake.[1-5] While genetic manipulations could enhance lifespan, modern science has a long way to go before this futuristic intervention can be applied.

There are thousands of articles that focus on the ability of significant reductions in calorie intake and their effects on enhancing lifespan and reducing the incidence and prevalence of age-related diseases.[1-8] It appears that the application of calorie restriction of the order of 30-50% below average free-feeding calorie intake may induce an inhibitory effect on many aspects of aging, including aging processes in non-human primates and most probably humans.[1-8] Much research has been performed on calorie restriction in rodents, but it appears that biological responses to calorie restriction are quite similar in primates[5] and other species.

Despite isolated arguments to the contrary, it seems that calorie restriction is an effective longevity promoting strategy for humans, but the widespread application of the degree of dietary restriction required to retard aging creates compliance problems of an insurmountable magnitude. It is a monumental task to change the eating habits of a nation, but the North American continent has a recalcitrant problem with "food-portion-size distortion," resulting in excessive calorie intake. This issue is a pivotal component of the obesity epidemic in North America, and elsewhere.

There are many proponents of the use of food restriction strategies for anti-aging, with targets of food intake at about 40% of an average calorie intake of 2,000 calories per day, or thereabouts. The first observations of the lifespan enhancing ability of calorie restriction were made more than 70-years ago.[9] These observations lay somewhat dormant in the medical literature until the 1950s when the pioneer of modern calorie restriction interventions, Professor Roy Walford started to popularize his concepts of the 120-year diet.[10] In brief, Walford discussed the advantage of the "high/low diet," where he suggested a combination of "under-nutrition without malnutrition."

The proposals of Professor Walford involved the careful application of a calorie restricted diet that was "nutrient dense" with the provision of vital and essential nutritional cofactors, most notably vitamins and minerals with phytonutrients.[10] Interests in calorie restriction have accelerated to a point where this approach has generated great interest as a research focus for the US National Institute of Aging. Recent research has expanded beyond laboratory animals to human interventions using dietary calorie restriction or substances that can mimic the biological changes that are seen in the presence of significant reductions of daily calorie intake (so-called "calorie restriction mimetics"). Conservative scientists sometimes demand to see more research into the human effects of calorie restriction as an anti-aging strategy, but it seems prudent to accept this intervention as a valid, reliable, and safe approach to enhancing lifespan.[1-10]

As experimental studies over the past two decades started to define the beneficial biochemical and physiological effects of calorie restriction, scientists started to propose that there were a variety of substances (drugs and natural compounds) that could mimic these desirable effects on body structures and functions. In the late 1990s, scientists started to propose the notion that there were calorie restriction mimetics that have anti-aging properties as a consequence of their ability to induce biological changes that occurred as a consequence of direct reductions of overall calorie intake.[9] Many experiments involving reduction of total calorie intake (up to a level of 70% less than the *ad libitum* dietary intake in animals) show that calorie restriction improves a number of biomarkers of aging, with overt evidence of improved general health.[2-11]

The use of calorie restriction mimetics, in isolation of significant dietary calorie reduction, has the naïve appeal to some of providing an "easy option" for longevity promotion, but it seems quite reasonable to conclude that the combined use of calorie restriction mimetics with tolerable reductions of overall calorie intake would act in a highly synergistic manner. This approach seems to be deeply rooted in good scientific agreement, derived from almost eight decades of research.[1-10]

While one may acknowledge the call for more research on the use of calorie restriction as a longevity promoter in humans, the benefits of this intervention appear to be well documented and highly credible. A key health initiative that has been repeatedly promoted for the U.S. nation is an overall restriction of calorie intake, in what have been somewhat futile attempts to reverse the obesity epidemic.[12]

CALORIE RESTRICTION AND CALORIE RESTRICTION MIMETICS
Biological Effects of Calorie Restriction

A simple understanding of the biochemical and physiological effects of calorie restriction explains why this intervention can extend average lifespan (defined as the average number of years that an organism is expected to live).[9,10] There is a major and added bonus to the intervention – calorie restriction induces the prolongation of maximum lifespan (defined as the greatest number of years that a living organism can survive).[9,10]

It is efficient to classify several areas of the biological outcome of calorie restriction. These areas include, but may not be limited to, the following: alteration of the expression and actions of many key enzyme systems that control body metabolism and protein synthesis, reduction of the accumulation and removal of damaged protein, modulation of normal processes of cell death (apoptosis), modification of the actions of chaperone molecules, secondary reduction in protein/sugar cross-linking (glycosylation), variable reversal of dysglycemia, reduction of chronic inflammation and inflammatory markers, hormetic effects, inhibition of glycolysis with insulin sensitizing actions and specific influences on genes that alter cell repair or death (e.g. Sir2 gene or the human homologous SIRT1 gene).[1-10,13-16]

Individuals who interpret the data in Table 1 with some degree of skepticism should recognize that essentially all species of animals, that have had their responses to calorie restriction studied, have shown overall parallel biochemical or physiological outcomes.[5] In addition, scientists and physicians who are focused on anti-aging medicine have developed a consensus opinion that the effects noted in animals are often present in non-human primates and humans.[5,9]

The support for calorie restriction interventions in longevity medicine is bolstered by results from human experiments that involved eight scientists who followed a calorie restriction protocol for almost two years.[5] In this study, the human volunteers exhibited similar physiological changes that were observed in primates who had been subjected to similar levels of calorie restriction.[5] These are truly exciting observations which are quite compatible with information from population studies or epidemiological findings of the health benefits that result generally from the retention of a normal or low-weight range as a consequence of calorie restriction or moderation.[12]

Table 1. The biophysiological and clinical outcomes that have been described in many experiments that have utilized calorie restriction, or in some cases, calorie restriction mimetics.[1-10,13-16]

- Favorable effects on cardiovascular structure and function, with reductions in heart rate, blood pressure, LDL cholesterol, and triglycerides.
- Improvements in insulin sensitivity and overall normalization of blood glucose levels.
- Increase in protein synthesis and the elimination of abnormal proteins from the body. Enhanced action of chaperone molecules, which contribute to the synthesis and maintenance of essential proteins, with the benefit of enhanced elimination of damaged proteins.
- Modulation of the process of "orderly cell death" (apoptosis) with improvement in the repair and maintenance of integrity of DNA. Secondary benefits on transcription.
- Reduction of oxidative stress to tissues by diminution of free radical generation in a quantitative and qualitative manner.
- Reduction in body temperature.
- Reduction in body fat mass, including visceral adiposity, with concomitant increase in muscle mass.
- Beneficial effects on hormonal secretions that tend to fall with age, e.g. DHEA and growth hormone.
- Improvements in brain function, including memory, cognition, and perhaps mood.
- Spontaneous enhancement of an ability to engage in physical activity.
- Stimulation of growth factors, e.g. brain-derived neurotrophic factor (BDNF).
- Weight loss.

Calorie Restriction Mimetics

A calorie restriction mimetic can be defined as a pharmaceutical or chemical compound or natural agent which has the ability to reproduce one or more principal biological effects of calorie restriction.[9] There are many putative calorie restriction mimetic compounds that have variable effects on body structures and functions (Table 2).[1-9] It appears that these agents can be administered to humans or animals to induce substantially similar biochemical or physiological changes that have been documented to occur when significant dietary restriction of calories has been undertaken. One may assume that there may be great inter-individual and intra-individual variation in the human response to a calorie restriction mimetic. For example, some of these mimetics may have primary effects on genetic controls of aging, whereas others may have more specific effects on glucose metabolism. In other words, the biochemical versatility of calorie restriction mimetics is quite variable.

It seems obvious that there is a highly complex cascade of biological events that occurs with calorie restriction, which matches, in part, the even more complicated cascade of events that determines aging. I have repeatedly reminded myself and other practitioners of integrative medicine that the power of synergy is a pivotal component of natural therapeutics.[17] While many practitioners of biointegrative medicine have rejected, in part, the flawed concept of the single drug receptor actions in therapeutics, it continues to surprise me that many physicians or healthcare givers are using single supplement or natural product interventions. For example, resveratrol has been heralded as a key anti-aging supplement and its effects are likely to be significantly enhanced by the synergistic action of other calorie restriction mimetics.

Against this background, I have undertaken a review of putative calorie restriction mimetics that have good scientific agreement for their use in longevity promotion. Of course, efficacy is important in attempts to mimic the biological actions of calorie restriction, but safety is a key issue. Table 2 provides an incomplete list of calorie restriction mimetics, but it focuses upon those that appear to be evidence-based with credible scientific support for their biological effects in animals or humans.[1-10,13-19] Analysis of these putative calorie restriction mimetics permits the rational and logical synergistic formulation of a dietary supplement that can be expected to provide nutritional support for the modification of body structures and functions that change favorably with calorie restriction.

Table 2. Putative calorie restriction mimetics. Prescription drugs are excluded, along with biological substances involved in biotechnology research.

AGENT	COMMENT
Metformin	Increased insulin sensitivity, reduction of glucogenesis, inhibition of excessive glucose absorption, enhanced glycolysis by increasing gene expression that encodes for glucokinase and liver-specific pyruvate kinase. Modulation of stress responses, with the activation of AMPK.
Resveratrol*	A polyphenol that stimulates Sir2 gene, promotes DNA structure and function, resulting in reduced or modulated apoptosis. Proven anticancer benefits with beneficial cardiovascular effects, including potent antioxidant activity. Effects on apoptosis are complex, operating through mechanisms of hormesis, dependent on the ratio of resveratrol to other related molecules that alter "pro and anti-apoptotic" factors. These latter effects are dependent on receptor targets and other modulating factors.
Carnosine*	A combination of amino acids, which inhibits cross-linking of proteins and formation of AGEs, enhances glutamate action in the brain, stimulating nitric oxide with improvement in brain function and memory. A classic anti-aging factor that increases average lifespan, but not maximum lifespan in rodents. Arguably a calorie restriction mimetic, but it has important potential synergistic actions in the natural therapeutics of anti-aging.
Avocado*	Concentrated dosages of mannoheptulose from avocado improve insulin sensitivity and blood glucose levels, with thermogenic effects on fat deposits in muscle. Enhances lifespan in mice.
Gymnema*	Alkaloids (gymnemosides) have glucose regulating effects.
2-deoxyglucose	Increases insulin sensitivity, reduces blood glucose, but toxic in high dosages; and not recommended for routine use because of narrow window of safety versus therapeutic effect.
Aminoguanidine	Reduces abnormal protein accumulation, prevents glycosylation and reduces AGEs
Hydroxycitrate	May reduce calorie intake? Largely withdrawn because of liver toxicity.
Adiponectin	A role in fat metabolism, perhaps mediating the effects of calorie restriction.
Thiazolidinediones	Insulin sensitizing drugs, variable and onerous side effects.
Iodoacetate	Prevention against toxic metabolites of glucose.
Modulators of NPY	Calorie restriction stimulates the production of the neuropeptide NPY, which stimulates normal eating and increases in body weight.
Exandin	An example of a glucagon-like-peptide (GLP) which counteracts the effects of glucagon, reduces plasma glucose and suppresses food intake, involved in insulin release.
PYY3-36	A peptide (gut hormone) that inhibits food intake by actions on the hypothalamus, with secondary effects on glucose metabolism.
Leptin	Stimulates fat metabolism and reduces body weight. Involved in the hormonal responses that occur with calorie restriction. May be a principal mediator of the clinical effects of calorie restriction.
Alpha Lipoic Acid*	Valuable antioxidant with insulin sensitizing actions.
Cinnamon*	Methylhydroxychalones are insulin mimetics.
Acetyl-L-Carnitine*	Arguably a calorie restriction mimetic, *per se*. Antioxidant with neuroprotective and energizing effects. Facilitates mitochondrial function.
Mixed Antioxidants*	The value of antioxidant protection in anti-aging medicine is well established. The synergistic use of lipophilic and hydrophilic antioxidants provide important synergistic, pro-longevity interventions. While arguably classified as calorie restriction mimetics, grape seed extracts with mixed polyphenols, green tea polyphenols, ellagic acid and maritime pine bark are antioxidants with specific anticancer and beneficial cardiovascular effects. Cancer and cardiovascular disease are the two major causes of premature death.
Oxaloacetate	Specific effects on the Krebs Cycle. Currently not an approved dietary supplement ingredient.
	* Denotes good scientific agreement to use as nutritional support for body structures and functions that are modified with calorie restriction, excluding those with an uncertain safety profile.

Synergistic Calorie Restriction Mimetics: A Novel Anti-Aging Strategy

It would be misleading to think that there is a magic anti-aging pill. I have written and lectured extensively on nutritional factors for anti-aging, but my recommendations for nutritional interventions are qualified consistently by advice on positive lifestyle and the use of multiple interventions that can act as longevity promoters in a cooperative and amplified manner.[1] This short article skims the surface of knowledge on calorie restriction mimetics. These substances constitute one of the most important emerging fields of anti-aging therapeutics in the next decade.

Longevity is unquestionably the legacy of a positive and healthy lifestyle and anti-aging medicine must be defined within the context of advanced preventive medicine. Elegant arguments have prevailed where the prevention or reduction in prevalence of premature causes of death and disability may not have as significant an impact on average and maximum lifespan as has been hitherto supposed. However, there is no doubt that the prevention of fatal illness and the promotion of wellbeing are key initiatives for all practicing physicians.

While the pages of alternative medicine journals are filled with promises of isolated hormonal interventions, dietary supplements, and other options to promote longevity, the idea of calorie restriction remains an important and highly effective approach to anti-aging. Obesity is rapidly becoming the number one preventable cause of premature death and disability and for no other reason (apart from the obvious) dietary calorie restrictions seem to be a very important initiative for many societies that engage in excessive nutrition.[12] It seems strange that we are talking about the health benefits of "under-nutrition" when many billions of people are living with malnutrition. Classic scholars of biointegrative medicine in the Victorian era subscribed to the importance of the theories of "deprivation and excess," in terms of disease promotion. Perhaps we have overlooked these early foundations of medicine?

It is with optimism that I propose the combined use of several dietary supplements that can have additive calorie restriction mimetic effects, to be used with appropriate lifestyle guidance. I am not optimistic that the active restriction of calorie intake in the diet is an achievable intervention for industrialized society, but I believe that the use of natural substances that can reproduce the documented benefits of calorie restriction is a major advance in the anti-aging field.

In summary, my recommendations would include the synergistic use of formulations of dietary supplements that would include key ingredients such as carnosine, resveratrol, gymnema alkaloids, alpha lipoic acid, cinnamon, and avocado, with the added benefits of grape seed extracts, ellagic acid, and pine bark polyphenols. It would be highly advisable to have longitudinal studies that can assess the benefits of calorie restriction mimetics, but it may take many years before, what now seems obvious, becomes apparent in "hard-nosed," scientific language. It appears to be increasingly clear that calorie restriction mimetic compounds have intrinsic health giving benefits in addition to any potential benefits that they may have as a consequence of their ability to mimic the biochemical and physiological effects of the dietary restriction of calories.

I wish to stress the important work of Walford[10] who did not minimize the importance of the avoidance of malnutrition by sustaining the quality and quantity of vitamin, mineral, protein, carbohydrate and lipid intake, while overall calorie intake is reduced. Against this background, I highly recommend that individuals take multivitamin products that have phytochemical and mineral cofactors while they attempt to reduce their calorie intake. Modern practitioners of integrative medicine have switched increasingly to complex vitamin sources that have phytonutrient and mineral co-factors.[20]

We are reminded often that modern processed food is robbed often of vital nutrients and diminishing the intake of the average American diet may lead inevitably to at least occult malnutrition.[20] Experts on the value of exercise continue to promote the anti-aging benefits of physical activity.[21] Recent studies show the beneficial biochemical consequences of endurance exercises which enhance metabolic enzyme activity, improve mitochondrial function, and alter the expression of sirtuins.[21] In addition, exercise promotes insulin sensitivity, assists in the prevention of type 2 diabetes, and reduces gluconeogenesis.[21] Thus, exercise can be considered to have calorie restriction mimetic effects.

There is a frenetic interest among drug manufacturers for the development of calorie restriction mimetics, with their customary oversight of "natural calorie restriction mimetics" that have been already defined and found to be safe in the human food chain. We have entered an age of evidence-based natural therapeutics where we must start to correct the underlying complex pathophysiology of aging with holistic medical interventions.[1-23]

REFERENCES

1. Holt S. Specific anti-aging factors for natural clinicians. *Townsend Letter.* 2008;July:90-96.
2. Roth GS, Ingram DK, Lane M. Calorie restriction in primates: will it work and how will we know? *J Am Ger Soc.* 1999;47:896-903.
3. Spindler ST. Calorie restriction enhances the expression of key metabolic enzymes associated with protein renewal during aging. *Ann NY Acad Sci.* 2001;928:296-304.
4. Lee CK, Klopp RG, Weindruch R. Gene expression of aging and its retardation by calorie restriction. *Science* 1999;285:1390-1393.
5. Walford R, Harris SB, Gunion MW. The calorically-restricted, low fat nutrient-rich diet in Biosphere-2 significantly lowers blood glucose, total leukocyte count, cholesterol and blood pressure in humans. *Proc Natl Acad Sci USA.* 1992;89:11533-11537.
6. Cao SX, Dhahbi JM, Mote PL. Genomic profiling of short- and long-term calorie restriction effects in the liver of aging mice. *Proc Natl Acad Sci USA.* 2001;98:10630-10635.
7. Cusi K, De Fronzo RA. Metformin: a review of its metabolic effects. *Diabetes Rev.* 1998;6:89-131.
8. Dhahbi JM, Mote PL, Wingo J, *et al.* Calories and aging alter gene expression for gluconeogenic, glycolytic and nitrogen metabolising enzymes. *Am J Physiol.* 1999;277:E352-360.
9. Kyriazis M. *Anti Aging Medicines.* London, UK: Watkins Publishing; 2005.
10. Walford RL. *The 120 Year Diet: How To Double Your Vital Years.* New York, NY: Simon & Schuster; 1986.
11. Roth GS, Ingram D, Lane MA. Caloric restriction in primates and relevance to humans. *Ann NY Acad Sci.* 2001;928:305-315.
12. Holt S. *Combat Syndrome X, Y and Z.* Little Falls, NJ: Wellness Publishing; 2003.
13. Ingram DK, Anson RM, de Cabo R, *et al.* Development of calorie restriction mimetics as a prolongevity strategy. *Ann N Y Acad Sci.* 2004;1019:412-423.
14. Lane MA, Mattison J, Ingram DK, Roth GS. Calorie restriction and aging in primates: relevance to humans and possible CR mimetics. *Microsc Res Tech.* 2002;59:335-338.
15. Hursting SD, Lavigne JA, Berrigan D, Perkins SN, Barret JC. Calorie restriction, aging and cancer prevention: mechanisms of action and applicability to humans. Ann Rev Med. 2003;54:131-152.
16. Wood JG, Rogina B, Lavu S, *et al.* Sirtuin Activators mimic calorie restriction and delay aging in metazoans. Nature 2004;430:686-689.
17. Holt S. *A Primer of Natural Therapeutics, a Certification Course for Dietary Supplement Counselors.* Little Falls, NJ: Holt Institute of Medicine Press; 2008.
18. Quideau S. Plant "polyphenolic" small molecules can induce a calorie restriction-mimetic lifespan extension by activating sirtuins. *ChemBioChem.* 2004;5:427-430.
19. Dhahbi JM, Mote PL, Fahy G, Spindler S. Identification of potential caloric restriction mimetics by microarray profiling. *Physio Genomics.* 2005;23:343-350.
20. Holt S. Natural therapeutics: observations on multivitamins. *Townsend Letter.* 2009; Feb/Mar.
21. Evans W, Rosenberg IH. *Biomarkers: The 10 Determinants of Aging You Can Control.* New York, NY: Simon & Schuster; 1991.
22. Klatz R. *The Official Anti-Aging Revolution.* Laguna Beach, CA: Basic Health Publications; 2007.
23. Weindruch R, Keenan KP, Carney JM, *et al.* Caloric restriction mimetics. *J Geron.* 2001;56:20-33.

ABOUT THE AUTHOR

Dr. Stephen Holt is Distinguished Professor of Medicine (Emerite), Scientific Advisor, Natural Clinician LLC is a best selling author, award winning medical teacher, researcher and clinician. He has published several hundred articles in peer review medical literature and he is the author of more than 20 books.

Chapter 15
Stem Cell Support:
The Nutraceutical Induction of Adult Stem Cell Recruitment (IASCR)

Stephen Holt, M.D., LLD (Hon.) ChB., PhD, DNM, FRCP (C) MRCP (UK), FACP, FACG, FACN, FACAM, KSG
Distinguished Professor of Medicine (Emerite),
New York Department of Integrative Medicine at NYCPM (New York, NY USA)

Reproduced, with permission, in part from the Townsend Letter.

ABSTRACT
Many different types of stem cells are being used in research and clinical practice throughout the world. Examples of these stem cells include, human embryonic stem cells (ESC), human cord blood or placental stem cells, adult stem cells (ASC), and even animal stem cells (live cell therapy). While there are clear and obvious advantages of the use of ESC as a consequence of their totipotent nature, the use of such cells in general therapeutics presents insurmountable ethical and moral problems. Although the use of human umbilical stem cells tends to overcome ethical problems, work in this field poses special technical challenges. These circumstances have led to major interest in the use of ASC. In ASC procedures, stem cells are harvested, grown, manipulated, and reintroduced. The overall objective of ASC treatments is to implant ASC, which are often coaxed down a pathway of differentiation toward a specific adult somatic cell type in order to replace diseased or ailing tissues.

Innovative scientists have been working on the potential use of mobilized in-situ ASC, as a non-invasive form of stem cell treatment. This is the process of induction of ASC recruitment (IASCR). A decade of research has led to current proposals that endogenous or in situ ASC (most notably bone marrow stem cells) can be mobilized from their niches in the body, with the result that they may migrate to various organs and engage in tissue repair or regeneration. The objective of this article is to highlight the combinations of nutrients, botanicals, or herbals that can play a role in the mobilization of ASC and their antioxidant protection during their migration.

INTRODUCTION
Many different types of stem cells are being used in research and clinical practice throughout the world.[1] Examples of these stem cells include, human embryonic stem cells (ESC), human cord blood or placental stem cells, adult stem cells (ASC), and even animal stem cells (live cell therapy). While there are clear and obvious advantages of the use of ESC as a consequence of their totipotent nature, the use of such cells in general therapeutics presents insurmountable ethical and moral problems.[2,3] Although the use of human umbilical stem cells tends to overcome ethical problems, work in this field poses special technical challenges.[1] These circumstances have led to major interest in the use of ASC. In ASC procedures, stem cells are harvested, grown, manipulated, and reintroduced.[1] The overall objective of ASC treatments is to implant ASC, which are often coaxed down a pathway of differentiation toward a specific adult somatic cell type in order to replace diseased or ailing tissues.

ASC are pluripotent and have different degrees of versatility in their ability to engraft and replace damaged tissues. While some ASC appear limited in their ability to differentiate into different cell types, many recent studies show that such cells (especially stromal bone marrow or adipose tissue-derived) may have great versatility, in some circumstances.[1,4-22] Elegant biotechnology research is being undertaken to transform harvested ASC into highly-specialized "functional" cell types for the potential treatment of disorders such as Parkinson's disease.[1]

There has been a great deal of high quality research in the application of ASC treatments, particularly in the field of human bone marrow transplantation. However, there have been reports of poorly performed ASC treatment in off shore locations, which are alleged to be poorly equipped or devoid of important ancillary services to make ASC treatments safe and effective. Recent revisions to US laws that govern stem cell treatments (Obama legislation) have produced widespread interest in the development of stem cell treatment facilities, especially in centers of healthcare excellence. While stem

125

cell therapies are advancing in a meteoric manner, all current "classic" stem cell treatments provide a series of disadvantages or limitations.[1]

Innovative scientists have been working on the potential use of mobilized in-situ ASC, as a non-invasive form of stem cell treatment.[23,24] This is the process of induction of ASC recruitment (IASCR).[25] A decade of research has led to current proposals that endogenous or in situ ASC (most notably bone marrow stem cells) can be mobilized from their niches in the body, with the result that they may migrate to various organs and engage in tissue repair or regeneration.[23-25] While somewhat futuristic, I have proposed that there may be several means whereby endogenous ASC could be released and promoted to differentiate into desired cell types to treat specific organ damage.[25] This proposal is supported by major advances in the characterization compounds that can induce stem cell differentiation to specific cell types in vitro.[1]

The proposed, non-invasive technology of IASCR has obvious advantages over the processes of harvesting and reintroduction of ASC. These processes form part of current complex treatment programs.[1] A body of evidence has emerged that several pharmaceuticals or natural substances are capable of mobilizing ASC from human bone marrow deposits, but some uncertainty surrounds the ability of mobilized ASC to home into damaged tissue and undertake a process of recruitment that will produce the desired treatment outcome of tissue repair or regeneration. However, diseased or damaged tissues provide complex signals to attract regenerative stem cells and the body has a built in homing system that it utilizes when ASC are part of an "internal repair kit".[1,23-25] The development of IASCR represents a new horizon in stem cell treatments that could make stem cell therapies more portable and cost effective.[25]

The objective of this article is to highlight the combinations of nutrients, botanicals, or herbals that can play a role in the mobilization of ASC and their antioxidant protection during their migration. Earlier work is very important in the current proposals and this research must be acknowledged and applauded.[23,24] I have called the process described in this article IASCR, with the "R" making a certain assumption of ASC Recruitment, justified or otherwise. With further research, the "R" may stand for regeneration or repair of diseased or ailing tissues.

INDUCTION OF ADULT STEM CELL RECRUITMENT
Adult Stem Cells at Work

ASC are ubiquitous in the body and they live in "niches" in many organs.[1] Most research has been performed with ASC of bone marrow origin, where stem cells are encouraged to proliferate to support the presence of blood components, often following marrow ablation. It has been stated that the very presence of ASC in adults poses questions concerning the exact definition of a stem cell.[1] While scientists have no problem in discussing the potential of several stem or progenitor cells to form new cell types or engage in tissue renewal, the concept of "stemness" emerges.[1] In brief, "stemness" is the ability of a stem cell to produce different cell types and their ability to engage in self renewal.[1]

There is a large body of clinical and scientific literature that demonstrates the pluripotent potential of bone marrow ASC.[4-22] Bone marrow ASC have been harvested and reinjected into patients, following varying degrees of laboratory manipulation, in order to treat the consequences of degenerative disease. Variable success is apparent in some anecdotal reports on the Internet. The results of many of these studies are reported in animal experiments in great detail, but many human experiences remain quite anecdotal in their descriptions of clinical outcome.[25] Bone marrow ASC are engaged in the long-term replenishment of all blood elements, but they are composed of a group of non-hematopoietic ASC (stromal cells), which are precursors of bone, cartilage, and skeletal tissues.[24,25] This limited view of ASC has been overturned by many observations of the ability of these ASC to form a much wider range of specific cell types that may play a pivotal role in tissue healing and cellular replacement or regeneration.[4-22] In simple terms, ASC in a variety of niches in the body could migrate and translocate to a site of tissue damage where they may undergo cellular differentiation that improves organ structure and function.[1,4-22]

In their classic article in *Medical Hypothesis*, Jensen and Drapeau[23] describe a hypothesis to support some of the components of what I have termed IASCR. In brief, these scientists highlight the importance of the ability of ASC to target and grow at locations of tissue damage and the ability for this migration to occur after induced mobilization of ASC, most notably from bone marrow. There are other steps to be applied to the concept of IASCR, which may include the use of agents to protect stem cells or

126

improve their functionality and enhance their ability to differentiate into the desired types of adult somatic cells.[25]

Many authors confirm the pluripotent properties and ability of ASC to migrate within the body.[1,4-25] Such studies include the ability of bone marrow ASC to become functional myocytes, hepatocytes, osteocytes, and cells of the central nervous system.[4-24] Available scientific information permits a clear conclusion that ASC have an ability to migrate from their tissues sites of origin and undergo cellular differentiation that results in a variable degree of repair of many different tissues.[1]

The laboratory identification of ASC involves a check for the presence of three characteristics that are hallmarks of "stemness".[1] Firstly, the cells must be able to renew themselves. Secondly, the cells must have the ability to differentiate into specific cell types and, thirdly, the cells must be transplantable with functional engraftment.[1] A characteristic of all stem cells is the presence of telomerase, an important marker found in cancer cells.[1] The presence of telomerase has led to proposals that many types of malignancies originate in stem cells, as a consequence of disorganized cell division.

The residual argument that promoting ASC activity in humans could lead to the development of cancer is not supported by current scientific knowledge or experimentation. At present, it appears to be a reasonable and safe proposal that ASC may be mobilized in the human body without significant adverse effects.[25] The use of ASC technology has been perceived as widely acceptable in medical practice, because it rests on the relative safety and effectiveness of human bone marrow transplantation,[1] but regulatory issues concerning the use of ASC therapy in the US remain to be defined with clarity.

Mobilizing Adult Stem Cells

Several drugs, biological agents, and nutritional factors exert effects on the mobilization and disposition of otherwise quiescent adult stem cells (Table 1).[23-25] A number of nutritional co-factors exert effects on supporting the differentiation of stem cells (e.g. hematopoietic bone marrow stem cells require vitamin D, B12, folic acid, and iron for maturation). Recent studies imply that single or combination formulations of natural substances may promote the mobilization of stem cells.[23-25] Such natural agents include, but may not be limited to: carnosine, blueberries (and other anthocyanidins-containing botanicals), green tea derivatives, and components of algae (fucoidans and pigments).[23-25]

Table 1. Factors that mobilize Adult Stem Cells (ASC) or provide nutritional support (e.g. antioxidant protection) for stem or progenitor cells.

- **DRUGS** (or isolated biologicals in clinical use or trials): IL-1, IL-3, IL-6, stem cell factor(s), erythropoietin, granulocyte-colony stimulating factor (G-CSF), etc.

- **NUTRACEUTICALS**: oleic acid, linolenic acid, blueberry, blue-green algae (AFA), green tea, fucoidan, and vitamin D3. Putative releasers or antioxidant protection may occur with fucoxanthin, beetroot, spirulina, spinach, Ashwagandha, grape seed extract. Cofactors: vitamin B12, folate, etc.

In conventional medical practice, a number of drugs have been utilized to stimulate bone marrow stem cell activity (e.g. granulocyte-macrophage colony-stimulating factor (GM-CSF) or erythropoietin).[26,27] In addition, various combinations of cytokines can facilitate the growth of stem cells in vitro (e.g. IL-1, IL-3, IL-6, erythropoietin, and stem cell factors). In vitro comparisons of specific synergistic formulae of putative stem cell supporting nutrients with the actions of the drug GM-CSF imply that such combinations of nutrients may, in some circumstances, increase bone marrow stem cell proliferation to a degree greater than the drug GM-CSF.[24] Whether or not mobilized ASC can be recruited in a consistent manner and result in engraftment to replace diseased or ailing tissues requires further investigation; and this subject has attracted legal controversies with regulatory authorities or "bounty hunters" who impact the sale of dietary supplements.[28,29]

There have been many anecdotal reports of benefit following the use of nutritional agents to support ASC structure and function, but these reports are largely in testimonial format, often displayed on the internet in multilevel marketing information. However, it is recognized that ASC are often "tissue-specific" in their homing characteristics.[1,17,19,22-24] Moreover, diseased or degenerating cells produce a variety of chemical messengers (e.g. cytokines) or have alterations of cell surface receptors that may attract reparative adult stem cells.[1,17,19] A key, but sometimes overlooked, factor in all ASC technology is to protect the utilized stem cells (in-situ or exogenous allograft administration) from oxidative stress by the use of REDOX balanced antioxidants. Such antioxidants may be present in several nutritional factors that promote stem cell structure and function,[25] for example fucoxanthin in fucoidan-containing brown algae.[30]

Key Contemporary Research

Several scientists have presented experimental or clinical information on the use of specific nutrients or botanicals for the mobilization of ASC.[23-25] There has been considerable examination and controversy concerning the use of *Aphanizomenon-flos aquae* (AFA or blue-green Algae) for use as an enhancer of stem cell mobilization.[28,29] In February 2003, a California court ruled that many statements used in the marketing of a branded form of blue-green algae were deceptive.[28,29] The court ruled that the use of this ingredient was associated with a series of advertising claims that were untrue, unfounded, or likely to mislead, to variable degrees.[28,29] However, more recent research would seem to imply that there is a scientific basis for the use of blue-green algae (AFA) in the nutritional support of stem cell mobilization.[31]

In well conducted experiments, preparations of AFA containing a novel cyanobacterial ligand for human L-selectin was shown to have an important role in stem cell biology.[31] An extract of AFA, enriched with this novel ligand for human L-selectin was studied in laboratory and human experiments.[31] L-selectin is an example of a cell adhesion molecule that plays a role in the retention and mobilization of bone marrow stem cells into the systemic circulation. In brief, scientists showed that oral administration of this extract of AFA contained an L-selectin blocker which promotes the release of stem cells from the bone marrow by interfering with the functions of CXCR4 chemokine receptors that are specific for stromal derived factor-1 (SDF-1).[31]

Any compound that interferes with CXCR4 or SDF-1 will promote stem cell mobilization. These experiments involving the administration of the AFA extract resulted in a 25% increase in the number of circulating stem cells at 1-hour post administration, compared with placebo.[31] Stem cells were measured in blood samples by defining the presence of the CD34+ cell.[31] These results were found to be reproducible in humans. The scientists commented that the mobilization of stem cells with an L-selectin blocker appears to be of a lower magnitude and greater transience of effects than can be achieved by the administration of G-CSF.[31] In separate experiments, scientists have proposed that an enhanced level of circulating CD34+ stem cells is a reasonable indicator of good health.[31]

Several nutrients appear to have an effect on mobilizing bone marrow ASC or stromal cells. For example, vitamin D and 1, 25 dihydroxyvitamin D3 are modulators of several immune functions, including an ability to stimulate the production of progenitor cells.[32] In addition, oleic and linoleic acids have been shown to promote the proliferation of intestinal stem cells and hematopoietic precursor cells, respectively.[33,34] Combinations of these simple nutrients form a significant component of any product used for stem cell support; and they are likely to act in a safe and synergistic manner with specific ASC-mobilizers, such as AFA.[25] The power of synergy in the use of combinations of nutrients and botanicals has been highlighted in recent studies by Bickford *et al.*[24]

In one important in vitro study, Bickford *et al* examined the ability of certain natural substances (nutraceuticals) to work together in a synergistic manner to promote the proliferation of human ASC.[24] In these studies, the scientists directed their attention to hematopoietic (bone marrow) stem cells, with the knowledge that these types of ASC are those that are used routinely in the relatively common practice of human bone marrow transplantation. These studies show that certain nutrients or botanical extracts were able to stimulate bone marrow cell proliferation in a dose-dependent manner.

The experiments by Bickford *et al* were performed using a positive control substance which is known to stimulate bone marrow stem cell activity. The positive control substance used in these experiments was GM-CSF,[26] a substance that is often prescribed by cancer therapists in a routine manner to counteract side effects of toxic drugs that are used in cancer treatments.[26] Chemotherapeutic drugs often result in bone marrow damage and suppression of immune function.

By using GM-CSF as a control, the scientists were able to make laboratory assessments of the ability of various combinations of nutraceuticals (nutrients or botanicals) to induce positive effects on the stimulation and mobilization of bone marrow stem cells.[24] The positive control, using GM-CSF, resulted in an anticipated stimulation of bone marrow cell production by a factor of about 46%.[24] While this ability to stimulate bone marrow cell proliferation was more substantial than the use of any single nutrient or natural substance under investigation, the combined use of natural substances (nutraceuticals) resulted in a greater increase in bone marrow cell proliferation than was observed with GM-CSF.[24] In other words, in these experiments, combinations of nutrients and botanicals (natural agents) worked better than the control drug (GM-CSF).[24]

It is relevant to note that several nutraceuticals that promote ASC production have the additional benefit of antioxidant actions, which may assist in preventing damaged or circulating ASC from oxidative stress (free radical generation).[25] Oxidative stress can attack the viability and impair the potentially beneficial functions of "stimulated" or "mobilized" adult stem cells.[25]

It is quite valuable to examine in detail just how powerful the synergistic effects of nutrient and botanical combinations actually are on bone marrow cell proliferation. Bickford *et al* showed that a combination of blueberry and green tea extracts increased specific types of bone marrow cell proliferation by a factor of up to 70%; and a simple combination of blueberry extract with vitamin D3 caused an increase of about 62%. When blueberry extract was combined with carnosine, an 83% increase in proliferation of bone marrow cells was observed.[24]

The experiments of Bickford *et al* were further extended to the study of various natural substances (nutraceuticals) on the stimulation of stem cells in the bone marrow.[24] ASC can be identified and segregated by identification of surface antigens (laboratory markers). A good example of the presence of such surface antigens is the identification of CD133+ or CD34+ antigen-receptor expressions. In the experiments, the drug GM-CSF increased CD34+ and CD133+ (early stem cells) by a factor of about 48%, but a combination of the natural substances carnosine, blueberry extract, green tea extract, and vitamin D3 increased the markers of early stem cells by 68%.[24] It is gratifying to see how synergistic combinations of natural substances (with no significant adverse effects) can sometimes outperform expensive prescription drugs, such as GM-CSF.

The use of seaweed in stimulating stem cell production has been ascribed to the ability of complex carbohydrates (fucoidans), contained with seaweed, to promote ASC release from bone marrow stores into the peripheral blood or general circulation.[36-39] Fucoidans bind with fibroblast growth factors and promote angiogenesis (new blood vessel growth), however they also have immuno-modulating, anti-inflammatory properties.[36-39] Angiogenesis (promotion of the growth of new blood vessels) has been highlighted as an important process in human stem cell engraftment.[1]

Chris D. Meletis, ND has drawn attention to the stem cell enhancement potential of fucoidan found in marine algae.[36] This polysaccharide compound, found in abundance in Wakame seaweed, has been shown to exert influence on the mobilization of endothelial progenitor cells, associated with the incorporation of such cells into ischemic tissue. It would appear that fucoidan acts through the modulation of the activity of SDF-1.[36-39] In addition, it appears that fucoidan has pro-angiogenic activity which is very important in the process of repair of tissue damage.[36-39] The benefits of fucoidan appear to be particularly important in general tissue repair processes and cardiovascular health.[36]

In brief, it appears that there is a group of miscellaneous botanicals that may have value in induction of ASC mobilization or recruitment. Examples of these botanical agents include: green tea polyphenols,[40] blueberries,[41] other anthocyanidins and vegetables including spirulina, spinach, grape seed extract, and Ashwagandha.[25] There are many potential mechanisms, whereby these botanicals can exert benefit in IASCR. For example, green tea polyphenols have anti-aging, angiogenic, anti-cancer, and cell protective benefits. Blueberries, spinach, and strawberries contain compounds that modulate cell-signaling cascades and have regenerative effects on certain cell populations[42]. Other botanicals that have been mentioned will provide, at least, antioxidant and variable cell regulatory potential.[25]

While it is recognized that ASC are often "tissue specific," they may be somewhat limited by an ability to replace specific cell types that are damaged. However, ASC retain a degree of pluripotency (multipotent) that permits them to differentiate (form a special adult cell identity) into somatic cell types that are present in different organ tissues. Clearly, further investigations of the ability of nutraceuticals to support ASC proliferation and mobilization are required.[25]

Summarizing the Concept of Induction of Adult Stem Cell Recruitment

There are several unresolved issues in the proposals that I make concerning IASCR (Table 2). While it seems clear that ASC release and migration occurs following the use of several nutraceuticals, the question of deployment of mobilized ASC to organs has not been evaluated. Diseased or ailing tissues are known to produce many chemo-attractants for circulating stem cells.[17-19] Intrinsic in the progress of IASCR following stem cell mobilization, is a plausible proposal that homing of progenitor or ASC will occur in a reproducible manner. Questions arise concerning the engagement and recruitment of ASC at target sites. This process must be followed ideally by desired proliferation and engraftment. These matters remain to be clarified.

Table 2. How to Utilize the IASCR[25]

- Mobilize ASC from bone marrow and other niche locations .
- Increase circulation of ASC with semi-continuous, safe stimuli. (Herbs, botanicals and nutrients are preferred to drug approaches – they cost less, and are associated with fewer side effects.
- Protect ASC from oxidative damage.
- Encourage homing to desired target organ (?)
- In-vivo assistance in the differentiation of ASC to replace cell types of the diseased organ has to be developed (the "human petri-dish" approach).
- A body of research demonstrates that human bone marrow ASC are able to "home in" on diseased organs and differentiate into many cell types.

Within the concepts of IASCR rests the possible applications of some substances that can assist in promoting the in vitro differentiation of mobilized stem cells towards desired cell types, in order to regenerate specific disease organs. Many physical or chemical manipulations are applied in the laboratory to transform (manipulate) harvested stem cells, in order that they may be stimulated to differentiate along certain cell lineages. Perhaps these "petri-dish" manipulations of stem cells can be applied in an overall process of IASCR, making the circumstances somewhat like a "human petri-dish" of stem cell differentiation? These matters are quite speculative at present, but it is known that the simple application of key nutrients can have major effects on pathways of differentiation taken by cultured stem cells in vitro.[1]

Formulations for Stem Cell Support

In order to use nutraceutical induction of ASC mobilization or recruitment (IASCR), one must propose a rational basis for this novel procedure.[25] The nutraceuticals that have been shown to have mobilization and protection potential for ASC have potential health benefits that extend beyond the IASCR,[25] such as their antioxidant potential and cell regulatory potentials. Although much further research is required to validate my proposals for the routine use of IASCR, cumulative evidence to date reinforces this promising novel approach for disease management and, perhaps, the promotion of longevity.[25]

In this overview, the power of synergy among nutrients, herbals and botanicals in the facilitation and mobilization of ASC and their potential recruitment by damaged or ailing tissues have become apparent. It seems prudent to conclude that the use of a single stem cell mobilizing factors alone, e.g. AFA, is not likely to be as effective as synergistic combinations of nutraceuticals. These circumstances make several proposals on single or limited combinations of nutrients with botanicals somewhat obsolete. Cumulative scientific studies appear to support the use of more complex synergistic nutraceutical formulations, with greater potential functionality. These proposals supersede several existing patents on stem cell mobilization. Table 3 proposes a complex nutraceutical formulation that can be used in the support of stem cells.

Table 3. One of several proposals for complex synergistic formulations to induce ASC mobilization and antioxidant protection, with ancillary functionality.

- Fatty acids: linolenic and oleic acid
- Antioxidant protectors including anthocyanidins (blueberry and beet root), spirulina, green tea polyphenols, OPC, and fucoxanthin
- Key nutrient support with vitamin D3 for cell proliferation and nutritional support of bone marrow function with vitamin B12 and folate.
- Specific evidence-based stem cell releasers, e.g. AFA, blueberry, vitamin D3, and fucoidan.

CONCLUDING REMARKS

More than a decade of research exists in the use of natural compounds to assist in the mobilization or recruitment of endogenous ASC. I propose the concept of IASCR with the use of nutritional support for stem cell function.[25] This approach appears feasible and readily applicable without any significant risks of adverse effects. This non-invasive area of stem cell technologies appears quite attractive, given the lack of portability and the limitations of current stem cell procedures that require a combination of advanced clinical skills and sophisticated laboratory support.

REFERENCES

1. Scott CR, *Stem Cell Now: A Brief Introduction to the Coming Medical Revolution.* New York, NY: First Plume Printing, Penguin Group; 2006.
2. Mattei JF. The ethical question of the embryo. *Bull Acad Natl Med.* 2000;184:1227-1235.
3. Parker SM. Bringing the 'gospel of life' to American jurisprudence: a religious, ethical, and philosophical critique of federal funding for embryonic stem cell research. *J Contemp Health Law Policy.* 2001;17:771–808.
4. Ferrari G, Cusella-De-Angelis G, Coletta M, *et al.* Muscle regeneration by bone marrow-derived myogenic progenitors. *Science* 1998;279:1528-1530.
5. Orlic D, Kajstura J, Chimenti S, *et al.* Bone marrow cells regenerate infracted myocardium. *Nature* 2001;410:701-705.
6. Kocher AA, Schuster MD, Szabolcs MJ, *et al.* Neovascularization of ischemic myocardium by human bone-marrow-derived angioblasts prevents cardiomyocyte apoptosis, reduces remodeling, and improves cardiac function. *Nat Med.* 2001;7:430-436.
7. Carmeliet P, Luttun A. The emerging role of the bone marrow-derived stem cells in (therapeutic) angiogenesis. *Thromb Haemost.* 2001;86:289-297.
8. Petersen BE, Bowen WC, Patrene KD, et al. Bone marrow as a potential source of hepatic oval cells. *Science* 1999;284:1168-1170.
9. Lagasse E, Connors H, Al-Dhalimy M, et al. Purified hematopoietic stem cells can differentiate into hepatocytes in vivo. *Nat Med.* 2000;6:1229-1234.
10. Pereira R.F, O'Hara MD, Laptev AV, *et al.* Marrow stromal cells as a source of progenitor cells for non-hematopoietic tissues in transgenic mice with a phenotype of osteogenesis imperfecta. *Proc Natl Acad Sci USA.*1998;95:1142-1147.
11. Azizi SA, Stokes D, Augelli BJ, DiGirolamo C, Prockop DJ. Engraftment and migration of human bone marrow stromal cells implanted in the brains of albino rats similarities to astrocyte grafts. *Proc Natl Acad Sci USA.* 1998;95:3908-3913.
12. Prockop DJ, Azizi SA, Colter D, Digirolamo C, Kopen G, Phinney DG. Potential use of stem cells from bone marrow to repair the extracellular matrix and the central nervous system. *Biochem Soc Trans.* 2000;28:341-345.
13. Kopen GC, Prockop DJ, Phinney DG. Marrow stromal cells migrate throughout forebrain and cerebellum, and they differentiate into astrocytes after injection into neonatal mouse brains. *Proc Natl Acad Sci USA.* 1999;96:10711-10716.
14. Polli EE. Transplanting bone-marrow stem cells in the central nervous system. *Haematologica* 2000;85:1009-1010.

15. Mezey E, Chandross KJ, Harta G, Maki RA, McKercher SR. Turning blood into brain: cells bearing neuronal antigens generated in vivo from bone marrow. *Science* 2000;290:1779-1782.

16. Brazelton TR, Rossi FM, Keshet GI, Blau HM. From marrow to brain: expression of neuronal phenotypes in adult mice. *Science* 2000;290:1775-1779.

17. Eglitis MA, Mezey E. Hematopoietic cells differentiate into both microglia and macroglia in the brains of adult mice. *Proc Natl Acad Sci USA.* 1997;94;4080-4085.

18. Lu D, Li Y, Wang L, Chen J, Mahmood A, Chopp M. Intraarterial administration of marrow stromal cells in a rat model of traumatic brain injury. *J Neurotrauma.* 2001;18:813-819.

19. Korbling M, Kutz RL, Khanna A, Ruifrok AC, Rondon G, Albitar M, Chamblin RE, Estrov Z. Hepatocytes and epithelial cells of donor origin in recipients of peripheral blood stem cells. *N Engl J Med.* 2002;346:738-746.

20. Ogawa M. Differentiation and proliferation of hematopoietic stem cells. Blood 1993;81:2844-2853.

21. Socolovsky M, Constantinescu SN, Bergelson S, Sirotkin A, Lodish HF. Cytokines in hematopoiesis: specificity and redundancy in receptor function. *Adv Protein Chem.* 1998;52:141-198.

22. Henschler R, Brugger W, Luft T, Frey T, Mertelsmann R, Kanz L. Maintenance of transplantation potential in ex vivo expanded CD34(+)-selected human peripheral blood progenitor cells. *Blood* 1994;84:2898-2903.

23. Jensen GS, Drapeau C. The use of in situ bone marrow stem cells for the treatment of various degenerative diseases. *Medical Hypotheses.* 2002;59:422-428.

24. Bickford PC, Tan J, Shytle RD, Sanberg CD, El-Badri N, Sanberg PR. Nutraceuticals synergistically promote proliferation of human stem cells. *Stem Cell Dev.* 2006;15:118-123.

25. Holt S. Proceedings at Stem Cell Summit, American Academy of Anti Aging Medicine, September 11, 2009

26. Demetri GD, Griffin JD. Granulocyte colonystimulating factor and its receptor. *Blood* 1991;78:2791-2808.

27. Adamson JW, Eschbach JW. Treatment of the anemia of chronic renal failure with recombinant human erythropoietin. *Annu Rev Med.* 1990;41:349-360.

28. Moran JP. Decision. Teachers for Truth in Advertising v Cell Tech Products, Inc. Superior Court of California for the County of Tulare, Case No. 19777, Feb 20, 2003.

29. Complaint for untrue or misleading advertising (Bus. And Prof. Code Section 17500) and commission of unlawful, unfair and fraudulent business acts and practices (Bus. and Prof. Code Section 17200). Teachers for Truth in Advertising v Cell Tech Products, Inc. Superior Court of California for the County of Tulare, Case No. 19777, Oct 23, 2001.

30. Holt S. Fucose complexes, fucoxanthin fucoid and fat storage. *Townsend Letter.* 2008;June;87-92.

31. Comprehensive marketing and scientific data produced by StemTech Health Sciences Inc., in support of the sales of StemEnhance™, www.stemtechhealth.com and affiliated publications.

32. Mathieu C, Van EE, Decallonne B, Guilietti A, Gysemans V, Bouillon R, Overbergh L. Vitamin D and 1,25-dihydroxyvitamin D3 as modulators in the immune system. *J Steroid Biochem Mol Biol.* 2004;89-90:449-452.

33. Hisha H, Kohdera U, Hirayama M, et al. Treatment of Shwachman syndrome by Japanese herbal medicine (Juzen-taiho-to): stimulatory effects of its fatty acids on hemopoiesis in patients. *Stem Cells.* 2002;20:311-319.

34. Hisha H, Yamada H, Sakurai MH, et al. Isolation and identification of hematopoietic stem cell-stimulating substances from Kampo (Japanese herbal) medicine, Juzentaiho-to. *Blood* 1997;90:1022-1030.

35. Holehouse EL, Liu ML, Aponte GW. Oleic acid distribution in small intestinal epithelial cells expressing intestinal-fatty acid binding protein. *Biochim Biophys Acta.* 1998;1390:52-64.

36. Meletis CD. Stem cell enhancement: fucoidans novel role in tissue repair and heart health. Available at http://www.vrp.com/articles.aspx?ProdID=art2254&zTYPE=2 Accessed November 6, 2009.

37. Boisson-Vidal C, Zemani F, Caligiuri G, Galy-Fauroux I, Colliec-Jouault S, Helley D, Fischer AM. Neoangiogenesis induced by progenitor endothelial cells: effect of fucoidan from marine algae. *Cardiovasc Hematol Agents Med Chem.* 2007;5:67-77.

38. Sweeney EA, Lortat-Jacob H, Priestley GV, Nakamoto B, Papayannopoulou T. Sulfated polysaccharides increase plasma levels of SDF-1 in monkeys and mice: involvement in mobilization of stem/progenitor cells. Blood. 2002;99:44-51.

39. Zemani F, Benisvy D, Galy-Fauroux I, Lokajczyk A, Colliec-Jouault S, Uzan G, Fischer AM, Boisson-Vidal C, Low-molecular-weight fucoidan enhances the proangiogenic phenotype of endothelial progenitor cells. *Biochem Pharmacol.* 2005;70:1167-1175.
40. Song DU, Jung YD, Chay KO, Chung MA, Lee LH, Yang SY, Shin BA, Ahn BW. Effect of drinking green tea on age-associated accumulation of Maillard-type fluorescence and carbonyl groups in rat aortic and skin collagen. *Arch Biochem Biophys.* 2002;397:424-429.
41. Bomser J, Madhavi DL, Singletary K and Smith MA, In vitro anticancer activity of fruit extracts from Vaccinium species. *Planta Med.* 1996;62:212-216.
42. Joseph JA, Shukitt-Hale B, Denisova NA, Bielinski D, Martin A, McEwen JJ, Bickford PC. Reversals of agerelated declines in neuronal signal transduction, cognitive, and motor behavioral deficits with blueberry, spinach, or strawberry dietary supplementation. *J Neurosci.* 1999;19:8114-8121.

ABOUT THE AUTHOR

Dr. Stephen Holt is Distinguished Professor of Medicine (Emerite), Scientific Advisor, Natural Clinician LLC is a best selling author, award winning medical teacher, researcher and clinician. He has published several hundred articles in peer review medical literature and he is the author of more than 20 books.

Chapter 16
Biology and Genetics of Aging

Michael Klentze, M.D., Ph.D.
International Medical Director, Vitallife Corporation Ltd. (Bangkok, Thailand)

ABSTRACT

Aging, like many other biological processes, is subject to regulation by genes that control pathways that have been conserved during evolution in order to keep the balance between apoptosis and growth. Genetic differences partly explain why long-lived people cluster in families. Studies comparing life expectancy in twins and other family members have found that up to 25% of the variation in human lifespan is heritable. The remaining 75% is due to environmental exposures, accidents and injuries, and chance. Very long life, to beyond ages 90 or 100-years, appears to have an even stronger genetic basis. Conversely, several clinical syndromes of "accelerated aging" and death at an early age (the progeroid syndromes) have a known genetic basis. What would be the characteristics of longevity genes in humans? Such genes would function in several important ways. They might slow the rate of age-related senescent changes in cells and tissues, improve the effectiveness of repair mechanisms, and increase resistance to environmental stresses like infection and injury. Longevity genes should also affect a wide spectrum of debilitating age-related conditions. These requirements are consistent with the observation that the elderly children of centenarians have much less diabetes and ischemic heart disease, and better self-rated health, than do age-matched controls. This suggests that they have inherited a longevity gene – or more likely a set of genes – from their long-lived parent that protects against these infirmities.

This paper will discuss our current understanding of the biology and genetics of aging and longevity.

INTRODUCTION

Aging, like many other biological processes, is subject to regulation by genes that control pathways that have been conserved during evolution in order to keep the balance between apoptosis and growth. Genetic differences partly explain why long-lived people cluster in families. Studies comparing life expectancy in twins and other family members have found that up to 25% of the variation in human lifespan is heritable. The remaining 75% is due to environmental exposures, accidents and injuries, and chance. Very long life, to beyond ages 90 or 100-years, appears to have an even stronger genetic basis. Conversely, several clinical syndromes of "accelerated aging" and death at an early age (the progeroid syndromes) have a known genetic basis. What would be the characteristics of longevity genes in humans? Such genes would function in several important ways. They might slow the rate of age-related senescent changes in cells and tissues, improve the effectiveness of repair mechanisms, and increase resistance to environmental stresses like infection and injury. Longevity genes should also affect a wide spectrum of debilitating age-related conditions. These requirements are consistent with the observation that the elderly children of centenarians have much less diabetes and ischemic heart disease, and better self-rated health, than do age-matched controls. This suggests that they have inherited a longevity gene – or more likely a set of genes – from their long-lived parent that protects against these infirmities.

This paper will discuss our current understanding of the biology and genetics of aging and longevity.

BIOLOGY AND GENETICS OF AGING

There are some very important pathways that have been found to be involved in aging and longevity. Among them the insulin/insulin-like growth factor (IGF)-1 pathway, the mammalian target of rapamycin (mTOR) pathway, and the p53 pathways are mostly conserved pathways that impact upon longevity and aging-related diseases such as cancer. We know that most of all cancers arise in the last quarter of lifespan with the frequency increasing exponentially with time. Older people show accumulated mutations in critical genes, especially in the p53 gene, and hypermethylation of genes critical to cell survival in individual cells over a lifetime. Given the crucial role of the p53 gene in apoptosis and tumour prevention, a decline in p53 activity at older ages and an increased hypermethylation in cells of animals could contribute to the observed increases in tumorigenesis and provides a profound understanding between cancer and aging. In addition, we see an accumulation of DNA mutations over lifetime, the increased expression of risk genes, and a decreased expression of genes involved in detoxification. Demethylation of risk genes, hypermethylation of protective genes, and accumulation of mutations in protective genes is a common event in aging. The recent sequencing and annotation of the human genome has raised the possibility of finding genetic alleles (gene variants) that are associated with complex phenotypes (traits) like longevity. One common way that alleles develop is through mutations in a single nucleic acid in a DNA molecule, due to a deletion, insertion, or substitution (e.g. from adenosine to thymine). These are known as single nucleotide polymorphisms, abbreviated as SNPs and pronounced "snips." Since SNPs are the most common type of genetic variation, they are presumed to underlie many of the biological changes in gene activity that affects traits of medical interest. Some SNPs are located in exons, the regions of a gene's DNA that are transcribed into RNA and then translated into proteins. Exonic SNPs – unless they do not result in amino acid changes (because of redundancy in the genetic code) – almost certainly affect protein structure or function. However, even SNPs located in non-coding regions of DNA may be capable of altering phenotype, for example by affecting the likelihood that an exon will be transcribed. There are also "epigenetic" changes that affect transcription but which do not involve changes at the nucleotide level, such as changes in chromatin conformation and packing, and DNA methylation.

Telomere Theory of aging

One possible cause of aging is the shortening of the telomeres, which results in a loss of DNA bases. As the cell divides over and over, these telomeres become shorter and shorter. Telomeres are actually loop-like structures which are associated with an assortment of proteins, the most notable of which are the telomeric repeat-binding factors (TRFs). TRF1 regulates telomere length, assisting the telomerase enzyme, while TRF2 models the telomere into the T-loop structure. The loss of TRF2 from telomeres directly signals apoptosis. Germ cells and tumour cells express the enzyme telomerase, which lengthens the telomeres by adding new processed DNA bases into the loop structure.

Werner's Syndrome

Werner's syndrome (WS), or adult progeria, is a rare inherited disease. Patients are born with normal length telomeres, but they shorten faster then those of non-Werner patients, thus causing accelerated aging. WS is associated with the early onset of many age-related diseases and most closely represents accelerated aging of any of the segmental progerias. The majority of people who have WS are Japanese (attributed to inbreeding). WS is due to a defect or deletion of a single gene, the WRN gene, which results in defects in telomeres and DNA repair. The WRN gene is a member of the helicase family that causes DNA to unwind, a requirement for most forms of DNA repair. Defective WRN protein results in a reduction of p53-mediated apoptotic signaling.

Hutchinson-Gilford Progeria Syndrome

Children with Hutchinson-Gilford progeria syndrome (HGPS), or childhood progeria, are born with short telomeres. Childhood progeria occurs once per 4-8 million births. The disease is caused by a deletion mutation in the gene for lamin A, a filament protein in the nuclear matrix and nuclear lamina that is required for DNA replication and nuclear organization. The point mutation results in the production of a prelamin A that cannot be converted to lamin A because it is missing 50 amino acids. At age 5 the telomeres of a HGPS child are about as long as those of a very elderly person.

In Down's syndrome the telomeres of the immune system cells shorten at an abnormally high rate. Down's syndrome victims are very vulnerable to infection, due to the rapid shortening of the telomeres of their leukocytes (white blood cells). The incidence of diabetes is 5-10 times greater for Down's syndrome victims than for age-matched controls. Nonetheless, Down's syndrome victims show no accelerated vulnerability for breast and prostate cancer, high blood pressure, osteoporosis, or cataracts.

Oxidative Stress, the Insulin-Like Growth Factor-1 Receptor, and Longevity

The rate of aging and lifespan varies greatly among species, and therefore must be under genetic control. Recently, mutations in several genes have been found to markedly increase lifespan (sometimes up to 6-fold) in nematode worms (C. elegans), fruit flies (Drosophila), and mice, apparently by slowing the aging process. There are good reasons to believe that understanding these "longevity genes" will be useful in studying human aging and lifespan. Most biologic pathways, and the genes that control them, have been conserved through evolution and there is no reason to suppose that those which regulate aging and longevity would be an exception. Indeed, several metabolic pathways that affect aging and longevity in one species of animal (e.g. fruit flies) also do so in other species (e.g. nematodes and mice). There are human homologues, with apparently similar functions, to many if not all of the genes in these pathways, although we do not yet whether these genes affect lifespan in people.

Oxidative stress seems to reduce lifespan. The free radical theory of aging was proposed by Denham Harman in the early 1950s. We now know that free radicals, produced in the cell mitochondria or introduced into the cells by physical alteration of the single oxygen molecule, the hydrogen molecule, the nitrogen molecule, and others, damage cells processes, which are conserved for life maintenance. The theory postulates that reactive oxygen species (ROS), such as superoxide and hydroxyl radicals, which are mainly generated as a result of normal cellular metabolism, give rise to damage to a wide variety of macromolecules, including DNA. Animals possess enzymes that scavenge ROS. Among the most important of such antioxidant defenses are the superoxide dismutases (SOD), which facilitate the dismutation of superoxide free radical (O_2^-.)

p66Shc regulates both lifespan (in mice) and sensitivity of cells (human or mouse cells in culture) to oxidant stress. Mice that lack p66Shc live almost one-third longer than do control animals. Certain mutations of the protein p53 lead to accelerated aging, whereas deletion of the gene for the protein p66Shc results in increased longevity. A possible function of p66Shc is to transduce signals from p53 that accelerate the rate of aging by inhibiting the expression of genes for antioxidant proteins. Removal of the p66Shc gene, which encodes an adaptor protein for cell signaling, extends lifespan by 30% in mice and confers resistance to oxidative stress. The absence of p66Shc correlates with reduced levels of apoptosis.

In *Caenorhabditis elegans,* the downregulation of insulin-like signaling induces lifespan extension (Age) and the constitutive formation of dauer larvae (Daf-c). This also causes resistance to oxidative stress (Oxr) and other stress stimuli and enhances the expression of many stress-defense-related enzymes such as Mn-superoxide dismutase (Mn-SOD) that functions to remove ROS in mitochondria. The *daf-2* gene mutation in *C. elegans*, a gene that is comparable with the human insulin-like growth factor-1 (IGF1) receptor gene, and which is involved in antioxidative action, shows a 30% increased lifespan in that species.

Sequence analysis of the IGF1 and IGF1 receptor (IGF1R) genes of female centenarians showed overrepresentation of heterozygous mutations in the IGF1R that are associated with high serum IGF1 levels and reduced activity of the IGFIR as measured in transformed lymphocytes. Thus, genetic alterations in the human IGF1R gene that result in an altered IGF signalling pathway confer an increase in susceptibility to human longevity, suggesting a role of this pathway in modulation of human lifespan. The *daf−2* receptor of *C. elegans* corresponds to the mammalian insulin/IGF1 receptor.

SOD1/SOD2 Polymorphisms – Increased Risk for Premature Aging and Cancer

The free radical theory of aging is currently the leading hypothesis for a fundamental mechanism of aging. The theory potentially unifies aging mechanisms across an array of species The SOD2 gene encodes an antioxidant enzyme, mitochondrial SOD. SOD2 polymorphisms are of interest because of their potential roles in the modulation of free radical-mediated macromolecular damage during aging. There are three types of SODs in higher eukaryotes, a copper/zinc containing cytoplasmic enzyme, SOD1; a manganese containing mitochondrial enzyme, SOD2; and a copper/zinc containing enzyme, SOD3, which is prevalent in extracellular spaces. SOD2 is constitutively expressed in most cells. *Sod2* gene dosage correlates with longevity in fruit flies and in mice. Mice that are heterozygous for a *Sod2* knockout accumulate excessive damage to mitochondrial DNA as they age. There is little understanding of the role of SODs in the modulation of longevity or health status in aging humans. Human disorders due to the SOD2 mutations have yet to be identified. However, a number of studies describe associations of SOD2 polymorphisms (particularly Ala16Val) with age-related disorders. One such study of elderly people with an Ashkenazi ethnic background suggested a possible association between Val at codon 16 of SOD2 and longevity.

Aging is controlled by different mechanisms, which influence the speed of the aging process and which are determined by inter-individual genetic variants. When we age, we register an average increase of low-density lipoprotein (LDL) cholesterol (LDL-C) and enhanced oxidation of LDL-C and atherosclerosis. Therefore, subjects over 80 years without cardiovascular disease provide a model to investigate the protective factors against atherosclerosis.

The antioxidant enzyme paraoxonase-1 (PON 1) is a component of the high-density lipoprotein (HDL) particle and mediates its anti-oxidation activity in many parts of the body. It prevents, among other things, the peroxidation of LDL complexes. Meta-analyses showed that a polymorphism (Gln>Arg Codon 192) in the PON1 gene is associated with coronary heart disease (CHD). In people with type 2 diabetes, decreased PON1 activity has been shown to be present before the manifestation of CHD. Likewise, the incidence of coronary artery spasms is increased with carriers of the Arg allele (OR = 2,52). Results of a study of Sicilians suggests that health ageing may be characterized by a low frequency of PON1 (-107)T 'risk' allele and by an high frequency of favourable genotypes such as (107)CC, influencing PON1 activity and HDL-C levels.

Mitochondrial DNA, reactive oxygen species, and aging

Mitochondria, the intracellular organelles responsible for oxidative metabolism, probably originated as separate organisms that were incorporated into eukaryotes early in evolution. The mitochondrial theory of aging states that the onset of age-related senescent changes in tissues is related to the balance between inherited healthy mitochondrial DNA and the load of age-related mutations in mitochondrial DNA. Damage or loss of mitochondrial DNA prevents post-mitotic cells from regenerating new mitochondria, thereby reducing the production of ATP and leading to cell death and aging. The degree of age-induced mutation in mitochondrial DNA varies among individuals and may be under genetic control.

The most effective environmental method of increasing lifespan is caloric restriction, which increases longevity in mice, rats, fruit flies, worms, and yeast. Caloric restriction appears to operate by slowing the aging process and the onset of diseases and disorders that are associated with advancing age, perhaps by reducing the lifelong production of harmful reactive oxygen metabolites. Another important relation between energy status of the cell and longevity is due to the genetic expression of the sirtuins, proteins that are involved in the silencing of the cell. The relationship between the NAD/NADH ratio and sirtuins gives us a new approach to the concept of caloric restriction.

Inflammation

Chronic inflammation, as manifested by high circulating levels of cytokines such as C-reactive protein (CRP), tumor necrosis factor (TNF), and interleukin (IL)-6, has been associated with several age-related diseases, including atherosclerosis, cancer, and type 2 diabetes. The inflammatory response may be an example of antagonistic pleiotropy in which genes that increase the inflammatory response to infectious organisms are also associated with harmful effects, such as atherosclerosis. Inflammation has its phylogenetic origin in the innate immune system. There is evidence that genetic cytokine variations influence the aging process, either inducing accelerated aging or increasing longevity. Aging is associated with chronic, low grade inflammatory activity leading to long-term tissue damage. Systemic chronic inflammation has been found to be related to mortality risk from all causes in older persons. Also, the genetic constitution of the organism may interact with systemic inflammation, causing defined organ-specific illnesses. Indeed, age-related diseases such as Alzheimer's disease (AD), Parkinson's disease, atherosclerosis, type 2 diabetes, sarcopenia, and osteoporosis, are initiated or worsened by systemic inflammation, thus suggesting the critical importance of unregulated systemic inflammation in the shortening of survival in humans. Accordingly, proinflammatory cytokines are believed to play a pathogenetic role in age-related diseases, and genetic variations located within their promoter regions have been shown to influence susceptibility to age-related diseases by increasing gene transcription and therefore cytokine production.

Conversely, genetic variations determining increased production of anti-inflammatory cytokines or decreased production of proinflammatory cytokines have been shown to be associated with successful aging, suggesting a role for the control of the inflammatory state in the attainment of longevity. The distribution of +874T→A interferon (IFN)-γ, -174C→G IL-6, and -1082G→A IL-10[7] SNPs has been shown to be different in centenarians than in younger people. The +874T allele, which is involved in the high production of the proinflammatory cytokine IFN-γ, was found less frequently in centenarian women than in control women. Also, the proportion of subjects homozygous for the G allele at the -174 IL-6 locus, characterized by high serum levels of the proinflammatory cytokine IL-6, was significantly decreased in centenarian men. Conversely, the presence of the -1082 GG genotype, which is thought to be associated with the high production of the anti-inflammatory cytokine IL-10, was found to be significantly increased in centenarian men in comparison with younger male subjects. These gender-related effects are difficult to explain. However, it is well known that men and women may follow different strategies to reach longevity and that the number of centenarian women is always greater than that of centenarian men, with the exception of Sardinia.

Interleukin-6 Polymorphisms (-174C→G)

The G genotype is present in approximately 38% of the population and is associated with higher IL-6 levels, which is thought to be a major predictor of disability and mortality in the elderly. The IL-6 G/G genotype has been found to be underrepresented in centenarians and, therefore, appears to be disadvantageous for longevity. This phenomenon has been observed only among males. IL-6 is a multifunctional cytokine and is involved in both the amplification of, and protection against, inflammation in response to infection and tissue injury. A polymorphism within the promoter region (G>C Pos. –174) has been suggested to modulate IL6-plama levels.

IL-6 gene expression is regulated by other cytokines, transcription factors, and several hormones, e.g. estradiol. Just like the G>A Pos. –1082 polymorphism in the IL-10 gene described below, for this IL-6 polymorphism there is also scientific evidence, that certain genotypes can be associated with an increased life expectancy.

Interleukin-10 Polymorphisms

The cytokine IL-10 physiologically limits and downregulates inflammation. Age-related diseases are initiated or worsened by systemic inflammation; conversely, genetic variations determining increased production of anti-inflammatory cytokines have been shown to be associated with successful aging. A polymorphism within the promoter region has been shown to regulate IL-10 levels. An adenine (A) at the site –1082 in the promoter region of the IL-10 gene is associated with low production of IL-10, whereas a guanine (G) as the same site is associated with high production of IL-10.

There is strong evidence to suggest that the increased expression of IL-6 combined with a decreased expression of IL-10 shorten the lifespan and accelerate the time to reach the threshold for frailty.

Methylation, Demethylation, Deacteylation, and Acetylation

The methylated CpG dinucelotides of DNA, coupled with deacetylation or acetylation of the chromatin, regulate genetic activity. Thus suggesting that the switch on and off of a particular gene is determined by this methylated or demethylated dinucleotides. Methylation is involved in cancer formation and neurotransmitter and steroid hormone elimination, as well as homocysteine formation, suggesting that methylating and de-methylating enzymes in the aging process. Genetic variants of the methylating enzymes lead to an individual expression pattern of these enzymes. The involvement of histone modification in the regulation of gene transcription has been widely demonstrated. Histone modification, specifically histone acetylation, is important in the regulation of the mammalian circadian clock. Genetics has revealed that aging may be controlled by changes in intracellular NAD/NADH ratio regulating sirtuin activity. Genetic studies using a range of organisms have indicated that enzymes called sirtuins are linked to the control of aging and lifespan. Sirtuins catalyse NAD-dependent deacetylation of histones (and other proteins) with the concomitant release of nicotimanide and O-acetyl-ADP-ribose. Other studies have suggested that metabolism of the redox couple NAD/NADH provides a link between sirtuin activity and the control of cell senescence and organism lifespan.

Aging can be delayed in various organisms by caloric restriction (CR) with adequate nutrition. CR appears to operate by slowing the aging process and the onset of diseases and disorders that are associated with advancing age, perhaps by reducing the lifelong production of harmful reactive oxygen metabolites. The effects of CR in humans remain to be determined. The pattern of gene expression among older animals that have been calorically restricted is similar in some respects to that seen among younger animals that had been fed *ad libitum* diets. Recent observations have shown that an intermittent feeding protocol, which need not involve any overall reduction in calorie intake, can also delay aging. A very interesting aspect, leading directly to the so-called skipping of dinner, has been shown to improve cardiovascular risk markers and to reduce insulin levels.

Drugs to Delay Aging

The Food and Drug Administration does not approve drugs to delay aging, because, in its opinion, aging is not a disease. Even so a number of potential anti-aging drugs are currently being studied. Sirtuin activators, which may well mimic caloric restriction, are probably the leading candidates for anti-aging drugs. The chief such drug is resveratrol, a minor ingredient of grapes and red wine. A resveratrol formulation has passed safety tests and is now being tested against diabetes and other diseases. It is possible that the life-prolonging effects of CR are due to decreasing IGF1 levels. A search of pharmacological modulators of the insulin/IGF1 signaling pathway (which resemble effects of lifespan-extending mutations or calorie restriction) could be a perspective direction in regulation of longevity. Antidiabetic biguanides are probably the most promising modulator of this pathway. Chronic treatment of female outbred SHR mice with metformin (100 mg/kg in drinking water) slowed down the age-related switch-off of estrous function, and increased mean lifespan by 37.8%, and maximum lifespan by 2.8 months (+10.3%) in comparison with control mice. However, treatment failed to influence blood estradiol concentration and spontaneous tumor incidence. Thus, antidiabetic biguanide metformin dramatically extends lifespan, even without cancer prevention in this model.

Another interesting drug is rapamycin, which inhibits the mTor signaling pathway. One study found that rapamycin significantly extended the lifespan of mice, even though the mice were already the equivalent of 60-years-old when the experiment started. Studies in mammals have led to the suggestion that hyperglycemia and hyperinsulinemia are important factors both in aging and in the development of cancer.

FURTHER READING

Ahmed N, Thornalley PJ. Advanced glycation endproducts: what is their relevance to diabetic complications? *Diabetes Obes Metab.* 2007; 9:233-245.

Ahmed N, Battah S, Karachalias N, Babeai-Jadidi R, Horanyi M, Baroti K, Hollan S, Thornalley PJ. Increased formation of methylglyoxal and protein glycation, oxidation and nitration in triosephosphate isomerase deficiency. *Biochim Biochim Acta.* 2003;1639:121-132.

Ambrosone CB, Freudenheim JL, Thompson PA, Bowman E, Vena JE, Marshall JR, Graham S, Laughlin R, Nemoto T, Shields PG. Manganese superoxide dismutase (MnSOD) genetic polymorphisms, dietary antioxidants, and risk of breast cancer. *Cancer Res.* 1999;59:602-606.

Belenky P, Racette FG, Bogan KL, McClure JL, Smith JS, Brenner C. Nicotinamide riboside promotes Sir2 silencing and extends lifespan via Nrk and Urh1/Pnp1/Meu1 pathways to NAD+. *Cell* 2007;129:473-484.

Bonawitz ND, Chatenay-Lapointe M, Pan Y, Shadel G.S. Reduced TOR signalling extends chronological life span via increased respiration and upregulated mitochondrial gene expression. *Cell Metab.* 2007;5:265-277.

Bordone L, Guarente L. Calorie restriction, sirt1 and metabolism: understanding longevity. *Nature Revs Mol Cell Biol.* 2005;6:298–305.

Cantero AV, Portero-Otin M, Ayala V, Auge N, Sanson M, Elbaz M, Thiers JC, Pamplona R, Salvayre R, Negre-Salvayre A. Methylglyoxal induces advanced glycation end products (AGEs) formation and dysfunction of PDGF receptor-(beta): implications for diabetic atherosclerosis. *FASEB J.* 2007;21:3096-3106.

Castro E, Edland SD, Lee L, Ogburn CE, Deeb SS, Brown G, *et al.* Polymorphisms at the Werner locus: II. 1074Leu/Phe, 1367Cys/Arg, longevity, and atherosclerosis. *Am J Med Genet.* 2000;95:374-380.

Castro E, Ogburn CE, Hunt KE, Tilvis R, Louhija J, Penttinen R, *et al.* Polymorphisms at the Werner locus: I. Newly identified polymorphisms, ethnic variability of 1367Cys/Arg, and its stability in a population of Finnish centenarians. *Am J Med Genet.* 1999;82:399-403.

Denu JM. Linking chromatin function with metabolic networks: sir 2 family of NAD+-dependent deacetylases. *Trends Biochem Sci.* 2003;28:41-48.

Du J, Cai S, Suzuki H, Akhand AA, Ma X, Takagi Y, Miyata T, Nakashima I, Nagase F. Involvement of MERKK1/ERK/P21Waf12/Cip1 signal transduction pathway in inhibition of IGF-1-mediated cell growth response by methylglyoxal. *J Cell Biol.* 2003;88:1235-1246.

Finkel T, Holbrook NJ. Oxidants, oxidative stress and the biology of ageing. *Nature.* 2000;408:239-247.

Fridovich I. Superoxide radical and superoxide dismutases. *Annu Rev Biochem.* 1995;64:97-112.

Gracy KN, Tang CY, Yuksel KU, Gracy RW. The accumulation of oxidized isoforms of chicken triosephosphate isomerase during aging and development. *Mech Ageing Dev.*1990;56:179-186.

Harman D. Aging: A theory based on free radical and radiation chemistry. *J Gerontol.* 1956;11:298-300.

Harman D. Free radical theory of aging. *Mutat Res.* 1992;275:257-266.

Henderson ST, Bonafe M, Johnson TE. Daf-16 protects the nematode *Caenorhabditis elegans* during food deprivation. *J Gerontol. Biol Ser A.* 2006;61:444-460.

Hipkiss AR. Caloric restriction and ageing – is glycolysis the problem? *Mech Ageing Dev.* 2006;127:8-15.

Howitz K, Bitterman KJ, Cohen HY, Lamming DW, Lavu S, Wood JG, *et al.* Small molecule activators of sirtuins extend *Saccharomyces cerevisiae* lifespan. *Nature* 2006;425:191-196.

Hekimi S, Guarente L. Genetics and the specificity of the aging process. *Science.* 2003;299:1351-1354.

Landis GN, Tower J. Superoxide dismutase evolution and life span regulation. *Mech Ageing Dev.* 2005;126:365-379.

Lin S-J, Guarente L. Nicotinamide adenine dinucleotide, a metabolic regulator of transcription, longevity and disease. *Curr Opin Cell Biol.* 2003;15:1-6.

Lin S-J, Ford E, Haigis M, Liszt G, Guarente L. Calorie restriction extends yeast life span by lowering the level of NADH. *Genes Dev.* 2004;18:12-16.

Manton KG, Corder L, Stallard E. Chronic disability trends in elderly United States populations: 1982-1994. *Proc Natl Acad Sci U S A.* 1997;94:2593-2598.

Martin B, Mattson MP, Maudsley S. Caloric restriction and intermittent feeding: two potential diets for successful brain aging. *Ageing Res Rev.* 2006;5:332-353.

Pagani F, Baralle FE. Genomic variants in exons and introns: identifying the splicing spoilers. *Nat Rev Genet.* 2004;5:389-396.

Passos JF, Saretzki G, Ahmed S, Nelson G, Richter T, Peters H, Wappler I, Birket MJ, Harold G, Schaeuble K, Birch-Machin MA, Kirkwood TBL, von Zglinicki T. Mitochondrial dysfunction accounts for the stochastic heterogeneity in telomere-dependent senescence. *PLoS Biology.* 2007;5:e110.

Schriner SE, Linford NJ, Martin GM, Treuting P, Ogburn CE, Emond M, *et al.* Extension of murine life span by overexpression of catalase targeted to mitochondria. *Science.* 2005;308:1909-1911.

Sinclair D. Toward a unified theory of caloric restriction and longevity regulation. *Mech Ageing Dev.* 2005;126:987-100.

Smith DL Jr, McClure JM, Matecic M, Smith JS. Calorie restriction extends the chronological lifespan of *Saccharomyces cerevisiae* independently of the sirtuins. *Aging Cell.* 2007;6:649-662.

Stessman J, Maaravi Y, Hammerman-Rozenberg R, Cohen A, Nemanov L, Gritsenko I, Gruberman N, Ebstein RP. Candidate genes associated with ageing and life expectancy in the Jerusalem longitudinal study. *Mech Ageing Dev.* 2005;126:333-339.

Tower J. Transgenic methods for increasing Drosophila life span. *Mech Ageing Dev.* 2000;118:1-14.

Williams MD, Van Remmen H, Conrad CC, Huang TT, Epstein CJ, Richardson A. Increased oxidative damage is correlated to altered mitochondrial function in heterozygous manganese superoxide dismutase knockout mice. *J Biol Chem.* 1998;273:28510-28515.

ABOUT THE AUTHOR

Prof. Dr. Michael Klentze is affiliated with Udayana University in Denpasar, Bali, Indonesia, and Mae Fa Luang University in Bangkok, Thailand. He serves as International Medical Director for Vitallife Corporation Ltd., in Bangkok, Thailand.

Chapter 17
Fibromyalgia: Evidence-Based Review and Emerging Pharmacological and Non-Pharmacological Therapies

Gordon D. Ko, M.D., CCFP, FRCPC, FABPMR, FABPM[1,2];
Leigh Arseneau, BSc (Hons), ND[2,3];
Mark Tsai, BSc (PT), FCAMT, CAFCI[2,4];
Bob Gottfried, PhD[2,5]

1 Sunnybrook Health Sciences Centre, University of Toronto, Ontario Canada;
2 Canadian Centre for Integrative Medicine, Markham, Ontario, Canada;
3 Naturopathic Institute of Advanced Medicine, Oshawa, Ontario, Canada;
4 Woodbine Physiotherapy, Markham, Ontario, Canada;
5 Advanced Wellness Programs, North York, Ontario, Canada.

ABSTRACT

The aim of this paper is to provide the reader with a thorough, evidence-based review of fibromyalgia, a syndrome characterized by chronic widespread muscle pain. An 8-step approach for managing fibromyalgia will be considered, and emerging pharmacological and non-pharmacological therapies will be discussed.

INTRODUCTION

The American College of Rheumatology (ACR) defines fibromyalgia (FMS) as a syndrome involving widespread muscle pain (over 3-months) and stiffness with 11 or more characteristic tender points on palpation.[1] In European literature, the term used is chronic widespread pain (CWP). The criteria for FMS diagnosis will change with the recent acceptance of the Symptom Intensity Scale (SIS) at the 73rd Annual Meeting of the American College of Rheumatology (October 2009).[2] Initial work looked at the survey criteria in which 12,799 rheumatologic patients received questionnaires. This resulted in the development of the regional pain scale (RPS) looking at 19 body sites (excluding hands and feet) and the 10 cm fatigue visual analogue scale (VAS). A score of 8 or more body sites had a sensitivity of 83.2% and specificity of 87.6% in diagnosing FMS.[3] A score of 6 cm or more on the fatigue scale also correlated with this. The new criteria were then studied on 25,417 patients with various rheumatic diseases. A score of 5.75 or higher on the SIS score (which is equal to the [VAS score + RPS score sum total divided by 2) differentiated FMS patients from those with other rheumatic conditions, identifying 95% of patients who would satisfy the survey criteria.

Using the older ACR criteria, studies show that FMS affects at least 2% of the population, predominantly females, with the most common age at presentation being 40 to 50 years.[4] Symptoms include musculoskeletal complaints ("hurt all over", stiffness, swollen feeling in tissues) and non-musculoskeletal complaints (fatigue, poor sleep, paresthesia). A number of conditions are associated with FMS, these include: irritable bowel syndrome,[5] dysmenorrhea,[6] female urethral syndrome/interstitial cystitis,[7] endometriosis,[8] non-cardiac chest pain,[9] plantar heel pain,[10] migraine headache,[11] temporomandibular joint pain,[12] sinusitis,[13] and Sjogren's syndrome.[14] A higher incidence of carpal tunnel syndrome (14.1%)[15] and Raynaud's syndrome (38%)[16] may explain some of the paresthesia complaints. Higher anxiety and depression have also been reported.[17,18]

Postulated risk factors for the development of FMS include: a family history of FMS[19]; a family history of depression and/or alcoholism in first degree relatives[20]; childhood physical and sexual abuse, eating disorders, and drug abuse[21,22]; and hypermobile joint syndrome.[23] FMS has also been documented after physical trauma[24,25] and whiplash[26] but the causal relationship has not been established in a consensus report on FMS and disability.[27] Use of dynamic MRI however may be useful in demonstrating cervical spinal cord compression[28] and ligament abnormality.[29] Physical trauma perception is associated with greater disability compensation and emotional trauma related to greater functional disability ratings and higher number of physician visits.[30] A review of psychosocial aspects concluded that the view that FMS is caused by stress or abuse is unproven and that there is no evidence that communicating such a diagnosis causes iatrogenic consequences.[31]

It has been postulated that viral infections may play an etiologic role in FMS.[32] As many as 70% of FMS patients meet the Centers for Disease Control and Prevention criteria for chronic fatigue syndrome (CFS),[33] and 70% of CFS patients meet the ACR criteria for FMS.[34] The usual routine laboratory tests such as basic hematology, ESR, muscle enzymes, rheumatoid factor, and antinuclear antibody (ANA) are all normal.[35] CFS researchers suggest that deregulation of the 2.5A synthetase Rnase L antiviral pathway may be the pathophysiological reason.[36] Recently the Canadian Blood Services banned blood donations from patients with CFS due to concerns about the latent XMRV virus.[37]

Muscle biopsy[38] and MRI spectroscopy39 studies which are controlled have proven to be non-diagnostic. Ultrastructural changes include increased DNA fragmentation (possibly due to persistent focal muscle contractions) on electron microscopy[40] and abnormal metabolism on MRI spectroscopy of paravertebral muscles.[41] Sleep study findings are abnormal[42] but also are not necessarily specific or unique to FMS.[43-45] Reduced growth hormone (GH) secretion,[46] and elevated CSF substance P,[47] homocysteine,[48] nerve growth factor levels,[49] and glutamate,[50] implicate central pain mechanisms. Unfortunately, the absence of an objective physical or readily available diagnostic test in patients with FMS has resulted in debate regarding the true existence of this condition.

Validation of the pain in FMS has emerged with definitive abnormalities on functional MRI imaging (fMRI) studies.[51-54] Neurophysiologic studies have documented the loss of descending noxious inhibitory control (DNIC)[55-58] and this has also been correlated with fMRI.[59] Further research also points to interactions between peripheral, central bulbo-spinal, and central cortical mechanisms[60] and to abnormalities in the hypothalamic-pituitary-adrenal (HPA) axis stress-response system.[61-64]

Genetic factors may predispose some individuals to a dysfunctional stress response via the HPA axis. People with a first degree relative with FMS have an 8.5-times higher risk of developing the condition themselves.[65] In addition, there is increasing evidence that early life adversity such as the death of a mother, being in institutional care or family financial hardships are linked to CWP in adult life.[66] These numerous interacting factors may be the setting in which a stressful event (which could be physical such as a viral illness, as reported by up to 30% of patients) or trauma can lead to a vulnerable health status and be a trigger for FMS in some patients.

The economic impact of FMS is significant. Chronic musculoskeletal pain is the #1 cause of disability in North America, the #2 cause of visits to the primary care physician, and the #3 cause of hospitalization (with over 250,000 spinal fusions carried out in the USA). It is estimated that the direct medical cost of FMS to the US economy is in excess of $16 billion annually.[67,68] The net cost in Canada in 1993 was estimated to exceed $700 million.[69] While a positive diagnosis of FMS may alleviate patient concerns and is associated with reduced healthcare utilization and decreased investigations,[70] many continue to question the validity of reported functional disability. A positive diagnosis also has medico-legal and work ability implications.

Randomized controlled trials (RCT) of pharmacological and non-pharmacological treatments are outlined in the tables below. Only the most recent or most comprehensive RCTs are referenced.

Table 1. Pharmacological treatments found to be effective for the treatment of FMS pain. (Bold-faced medications are discussed in more detail in this article).

Amitriptyline (10-50 mg effective for first 2-months, but not significant compared to placebo at 6-months).[71] Effects may be augmented with the addition of Fluoxetine.[72]
Botulinum toxin type-A (using a biomechanical approach)[73]
Cortef (low dose hydrocortisone)[74]
Cyclobenzaprine (10 mg qhs as effective as 10 mg tid but with less side-effects)[75] Is also helpful for morning stiffness when combined with ibuprofen[76]
Dextromethorphan (in subtype of ketamine responders)[77ab]
Dothiepin (tricyclic similar to amitriptyline)[78]
Duloxetine (FDA and Health Canada approved for FMS)[79,80,81]
Gabapentin[82]
Human growth hormone (9 and 12-month studies of FMS females with low IGF-1 levels)[83,84]
Ketamine 0.3mg/kg intravenous (IV) drip in prescreened responders)[85]
Lidocaine or xylocaine trigger point injections[86] or IV drip[87]
Milnacipran (FDA approved for FMS)[88-90]
Nabilone (oral cannabinoid)[92-94]
Paroxetine[95]
Pindolol (open trial)[96]
Pramipexole[97]
Pregabalin (FDA and Health Canada approved for FMS)[98-100]
SER282 (antidiencephalon immune serum)[101]
Sodium oxybate (commercial form of gammahydroxybutyrate)[102,103]
Somadril (carisoprodol, acetaminophen (paracetamol), caffeine)[104]
Sublingual THC (Sativex)[105,106]
Thyroid (T3) supplementation[107]
Tizanidine[108,109]
Tramadol (oral tramadol-acetaminophen)[110, 111] (IV treatment)[112]
Tropisetron (5-HT3 receptor antagonist)[113]
Tryptophan (5 hydroxytryptophan 100 mg tid)[114,115]

Review papers on pharmacological therapies concluded that the benefits of low-dose tricyclic antidepressants are short-term and have not been shown to be superior to placebo beyond 2-months of study.[116,117]

Table 2. Pharmacological treatments found to be <u>not effective for FMS pain.</u>

Acetaminophen (paracetamol)[74]
Botulinum toxin type-A injections (into the upper trapezius only)[118]
Calcitonin[119]
Chlormezanone, chlorpromazine[120]
DHEA[121]
Imipramine[122]
Lidocaine (4% injected as sphenopalatine nerve block)[123]
Lidocaine (IV 5 mg/kg), morphine (IV 0.3mg/kg)[124]
Moclobemide[125]
Non-steroidal anti-inflammatory drugs: <ul><li>ibuprofen[126] (ibuprofen + alprazolam did reduce tender point index (TPI) but not dolorimetry)[126b]</li><li>naproxen 500 mg bid[126c]</li><li>tenoxicam + bromazepam[127]</li></ul>
Prednisone 15 mg/day (most variables deteriorated)[128]
Pyridostigmine (helped with anxiety and sleep, not pain)[129]
Quetiapine (helped with other symptoms but not pain; augmented with pregabalin)[130]
Ritanserin (a 5-HT2 receptor blocker)[131]
Selective serotonin reuptake inhibitor (SSRI) drugs: <ul><li>citalopram[132]</li><li>fluoxetine (was helpful for sleep and depression but not pain at 6-weeks)[133]</li></ul>
Venlaflaxine (75 mg/day – likely sub-therapeutic)[134]
Valacyclovir[135]
Zolpidem, zopiclone (was helpful with sleep but not pain)[136]

FMS patients are high consumers of non-physician and alternative medical interventions. One study comparing those using such services found no differences in level of pain and functional impairment.[137] Another study of 111 FMS subjects found that 98% had used at least one complementary medical strategy in the preceding 6-months and that such use was correlated with lower age, higher pain, and higher disability.[138] Use of complementary therapies was seen in patients of a higher socioeconomic status and a longer duration of FMS. The most popular therapy was oral supplementation and the most popular source of advice was from magazines (40%).[139]

In September 2003, a survey of complementary and alternative medicine (CAM) use in a community education session attended by 72 FMS participants[140] found the following:

- Most common products tried:
  1. Topical rubs 66.7%
  2. Sleeping pills 66.7%
  3. TENS unit 66.7%
  4. Braces, orthotics 58.3%
  5. Diets 54.2%
  6. Over-the-counter oral medications 54.2%
  7. Glucosamine, herbals, megavitamins 50%
  8. Magnets 37.5%
  9.

- Most common CAM therapist/practitioner seen:
  1. Massage 75%
  2. Meditation/relaxation 70.8%
  3. Acupuncture 70.8%
  4. Chiropractic 58.3%
  5. Homeopathy/naturopathy 41.7%
  6. Spiritual healing/prayer 37.5%
     (The next most used therapies were craniosacral therapy, osteopathy, reflexology, and hypnosis.)

These findings were similar to the general population survey by Eisenberg[141] that rated the 5 most common CAM treatments as: relaxation, herbals, massage, chiropractic, and spiritual healing. Further clinical trials reported the following:

Table 3a. Non-physician physical therapies helpful for treating pain in FMS.

Aerobic exercise[142-144] when combined with flexibility and strength training, is superior to relaxation[145,146]
Group exercise with education and self-management[147]
Pool exercise[148-151]
Hydrotherapy, balneotherapy[152-154]
Low power laser therapy[155,156]
Strengthening exercise[157-159]
TENS (uncontrolled study)[160]
(Physical therapies found not to be helpful: Laser,[161] shape-of-sleep pillow,[162] pulsed and visible electromagnetic fields[163])

Cold exposure tends to aggravate pain in FMS.[164,165] One published RCT study found clinical effectiveness of ceramic-impregnated garments[166] for Raynaud's (many with FMS). A similar positive study was conducted for FMS.

Table 3b. Psychological therapies helpful for treating pain in FMS.

Cognitive Behavioral therapy[167,168,169]
Group therapy170 including relaxation and cognitive behavioral training[171]
Hypnotherapy[172,173]
Meditation-based stress reduction program[174]

Table 3c. Alternative medicine treatments with positive clinical trials for treating pain in FMS

Biochemical	Dietary indole supplementation (ascorbigen and broccoli powder)[175]
	Dietary supplementation of coenzyme Q10 combined with Ginkgo biloba extract[176]
	Homeopathy[177-179]
	Multimodality approach including nutrition and hormone replacement[180]
	Myers' cocktail (intravenous micronutrient therapy)[181]
	Omega 3 fatty acids[182,183]
	SAMe IV[184] PO (improved VAS pain, not TPI during last week of 6-week study[185]
	Topical agents: <ul><li>camphor, methyl salicylate, menthol lotion (uncontrolled study for a duration 20-minutes)[187]</li><li>capsaicin (35% of neck pain group with FMS)[188]</li><li>O24[189]</li></ul>
	Vegan diet[190]
Electromagnetic (autonomic nervous system)	Acupuncture[191-193]
	Copper wire bedsheet[194]
	Cranial electrotherapy and magnetic stimulation[195]
	Electromagnetic shielding fabric[196]
	Static electromagnetic fields[197]
Psychoemotional	Biofeedback-relaxation (combined with exercise best across 2 years)[198]
	Biofeedback-EMG[199-201]
	Biofeedback-EEG[202]
	Electroconvulsive therapy[203]
Structural	Chiropractic therapy (4-weeks of spinal manipulation, soft tissue therapy, passive stretching)[204ab]
	Osteopathy[205]
	Manipulation combined with ultrasound, galvanic electrical stimulation[206]
	Massage therapy[207]
	Prolotherapy (75% pain improvement; unblinded study)[208]
	Qigong[209]

In a survey of 116 physiatrists (rehabilitation medicine specialists) in Ontario, Canada, only 55% of respondents agreed that FMS is a "real disabling condition". When asked what type of alternative therapy works, 14 different types were mentioned with the top three being acupuncture, biofeedback, and chiropractic.[210]

In the earlier study[140] on FMS, patients reported different levels of effectiveness. They rated CAM therapy effectiveness on a 5-point Likert scale (-2 markedly worse, -1 mildly worse, 0 no change, +1 mildly better, +2 markedly better):

- Most effective CAM treatment used by at least 20% of surveyees (average score from Likert scale ratings):
    1. Botulinum toxin A (Botox) injections (1.6)
    2. Osteopathy/craniosacral therapy (1.4)
    3. Massage (1.3)
    4. Spiritual healing/intercessory prayer (1.3)
    5. Meditation/relaxation (1.2)
    6. Reflexology, herbals (1.1)

In contrast, medications were rated lower: over-the-counter drugs (0.5), topical rubs (0.7), sleeping pills (0.9), opioids (0.9). Common CAM therapies rated lower included acupuncture (0.5), chiropractic (0.3), glucosamine (0.25), and magnets (0.1).

RECOMMENDED 8-STEP APPROACH FOR MANAGING FIBROMYALGIA AND CHRONIC WIDESPREAD PAIN

1. Validation

Take time to listen to the patient's complaints. Incorporate a pain diagram and other useful tools[211] to capture the subjective concerns. A key question to ask is: "what worries you the most about your symptoms?" This helps to draw out the underlying fears and concerns. It also gives clues as to any secondary gain agendas (narcotic drug requests, medicolegal disability claims) that will also need to be addressed.

2. Thorough Internal Medicine/Neurological Work-Up

A thorough internal medicine/neurological work-up in order to rule out other similar and/or concomitant disorders (hypothyroidism, polymyalgia rheumatica,[212] lupus,[213] multiple sclerosis, cancer etc.) is first necessary. Prolonged morning stiffness and limited lumbar spine motion in more than one plane is more indicative of other rheumatologic diagnoses such as seronegative disease.[214] A detailed neurological exam should rule out signs of upper motor neuron dysfunction (hyperreflexia, Babinski sign, clonus, abnormal coordination and gait).[215,216]

3. Medication

For patients with severe pain, first-line medications recommended by the European League Against Rheumatism (EULAR)[217] include pregabalin (start with 75 mg qhs for 3 nights and then increase gradually to 300-450 mg/day bid or tid dosing; sensitive patients to start with 25 mg/day; warn about drowsiness, dizziness, edema, and weight gain), duloxetine (start with 30mg/day with food and titrate up to a maximum of 120 mg/day; warn about nausea, drowsiness, headache, hyperhidrosis, drug interaction risk), milnacipran (100-200 mg/day; similar warnings to duloxetine), tramadol (average dose of 150 mg/day = 4-5 Tramacet® tablets or 100-200 mg of the longer acting forms – the Contramid® delivery system is superior). Tramadol is molecularly very similar to venlafaxine acting as a serotonin-norepinephrine reuptake inhibitor (SNRI) as well as having mild mu opioid action.[218] Its use with tricyclic antidepressants, SSRIs, and SNRIs needs to be monitored carefully to avoid serotonin syndrome.[219] Strong opioids, anti-inflammatories, and corticosteroids should be avoided (unless there are co-morbid conditions such as inflammatory or malignant disease).[124,220] Cannabinoids are an emerging pharmacotherapy with RCTs supportive in FMS. Synergisms with other medications and mode of action have been reviewed in detail.[221]

4. Non-Drug Necessary Therapies

Non-drug necessary therapies (also recommended by EULAR) include active physiotherapy (aerobic and strengthening exercises, pool therapy) and psychotherapy (cognitive behavioral therapy). These should focus on the goal of exercising the body (muscles) and the brain (memory-mood). A multi-disciplinary approach (physician working together with physiotherapist/chiropractor/occupational therapist/exercise kinesiologist and with psychiatry/psychology/social worker) has been documented to be effective.[217]

5. Hope

Patients should be followed, given realistic hope and support if they elect to try non-conventional therapies. One key question to explore is: "What was happening at the onset of your symptoms?" This provides information as to a possible root cause for the constellation of FMS symptoms. For example, if the onset is after a car accident, one should look for structural problems such as spinal ligament-joint instability and neurological problems such as traumatic brain injury complicated by anterior pituitary hormonal deficiency.

One approach identifies four root sources that need healing:

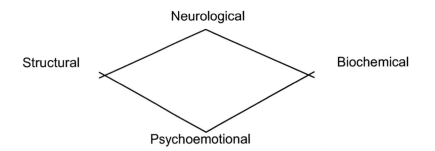

Effective emerging therapies in each area will be reviewed and presented below.

Structural Healing

Sacroiliac ligament laxity (from post-partum trauma, car accident, falls on the buttock, repetitive strains from lifting, running) can affect alignment, leading to upper body pain and FMS.[222] The sacroiliac (SI) joint plays an important role in load transfer between spine and the lower extremities. Patients usually experience significant symptoms when the SI joint is no longer able to sustain and transfer the load.[223] Pelvic stability is best described through the integrated model of function based on various anatomic and biomechanical studies. The integrated model includes four components[224]:

- Form closure (structure)
- Force closure (forces produced by myofascial action)
- Motor control (specific timing of muscle action/inaction during loading) and one that is psychological
- Emotions

Form closure contributes to SI stability through the joint surfaces and various regional ligaments such as the iliolumbar, interosseous, long dorsal, sacrotuberous, ventral sacroiliac, and sacrospinous ligaments. The sacrotuberous ligament contributes to longitudinal stability; while horizontal stability is associated with predominantly the long dorsal and interosseous ligaments.

Force closure provides stability through activation of local core muscles and global muscles in the trunk. The local system consists of muscles of the pelvic floor, transverse abdominis, diaphragm, and deep fibres of multifidus. The global muscles provide stability through three sling systems:

- Posterior oblique sling (latissimus dorsi, gluteus maximus, and thoracodorsal fascia)
- Anterior oblique sling (external oblique, contralateral internal oblique, and hip adductors)
- Longitudinal sling (biceps femoris, sacrotuberous ligament, and the erector spinae)

Furthermore motor control (the timing of specific muscle action and inaction) ensures proper coordination of the local and global system to generate stability without rigidity of posture and without episode of collapse. Emotional states of an individual can affect the neuromusculoskeletal system through consequence of psychological stress and subsequent hormonal release. For example, a negative emotion associate with past experience can lead to increased muscle hypertonicity and detrimental motor patterning thus causing excessive compression of the SI joint. Instability of the pelvis occurs when there is insufficient articular compression due to either one or a combination of:

- Stretched out ligaments as a result of general hypermobility or trauma.
- Weakness and poor coordination of local and global muscles.

Patients usually have complaints with daily activities that involve unilateral loading on one side of the pelvis. This can include high impact movement such as jumping or running. Typically, patients will have trouble with activities such as stair-climbing, turning in bed, and transferring in/out of a car. Frequently, the unstable SI joint will become subluxed, consequentially altering the biomechanical chain above and below the pelvis. This can result in widespread pain in various parts of the body due to mechanical misalignment and compensatory muscle hypertonicity (piriformis, iliopsoas, quadratus lumborum, gluteus medius/minimus). A detailed articular and myofascial manual therapy assessment can identify such problems.

Mild SI dysfunction in the form closure system can be compensated by a strong force closure system. However when the force closure system is inadequate in stabilizing an unstable SI joint (due to stretched out ligaments), prolotherapy is indicated and has been documented to be helpful.[225] This procedure involves injection of various proliferants into tendon and ligament to stimulate fibroblast proliferation. Such process will increase the strength of connective tissues in addition to decrease pain.

In vitro studies have shown that injection of chemical irritants encourages collagen proliferation.[226] In 1937, Dr. Earl Gedney achieved successful results of sclerosis in hypermobile SI joints with injection of sclerosing agent. However, it was Dr. George Hackett who perfected this technique by injecting various SI joints with saline and glucose solution.[227] Significant improvement was found post-prolotherapy in 543 patients (82% long-term success rate) who suffered from chronic low back pain. Various proliferants have been utilized over the years. These proliferants promote healing by one of three ways:

- By osmotic rupture of local cells, e.g. dextrose (12.5-25%).
- By local cellular irritation e.g. a mixture of phenol, glycerine and glucose (P2G).
- By chemotactic attraction of inflammatory mediators, e.g. sodium morrhuate (cod liver oil extract).

This involves injections into the bone-ligament interface which stimulate further fibroblast activity, collagen deposition, and ligament healing. A long-term RCT demonstrated significant improvement in both the saline and the dextrose injection groups.[228] This has led to the recommendation by Dr. Nikolai Bogduk that such injections be considered in the first-line management of chronic low back pain.[229] More recent approaches involve using platelet-rich plasma (PRP) injections. Growth factors (TGF-B, bFGF, PDGFa-b, EGF, VEGF, CTGF, cytokines) are released when injected platelets are activated. This also results in fibroblast activity and also local stem cell activation and angiogenesis. There is considerable emerging evidence reviewed for this[230,231] as well as long-term RCTs negative for Achilles tendinosis[232] and positive for tennis elbow.[233] The healing benefit of PRP is based on its effect on multiple tissues: muscles, tendon, ligament, cartilage, and skin. Results for bone have been equivocal. PRP injections have also been reported for SI joint instability with excellent results.[234,235]

Clinically, it takes 4-6 sessions of monthly injection with sodium morrhuate to achieve a satisfactory stability of the SI joint. However, much faster healing time was observed with PRP with most patients achieving the equivalent recovery time with 1-2 injections on a monthly to bimonthly basis. Prolotherapy provides strength back to the ligaments to restore form closure of the SI joint. Following PRP-prolotherapy, specific core stabilization exercises are carried out by patients to restore and maximize the force closure system. This will allow patients to achieve full recovery permanently instead of just masking the symptoms.

Psychological Healing
Neurotherapy utilizes an EEG recording system along with training software to enhance brain wave activity that is instrumental for improving concentration. Much of the research has been focused on children with attention deficit disorders.[236] Some patients also exhibit autonomic dysfunction[237] and may respond to biofeedback retraining. One of our patients resolved her "brain fog" symptoms completely after 20 sessions of neurotherapy.[238]

Biofeedback
Biofeedback is a unique, scientifically based treatment that has been used for many years to treat patients suffering from FMS and chronic pain. This therapy works by testing changes of different aspects of the autonomic nervous system (ANS) of a person including body temperature, muscle tension, blood pressure, breathing, and heart rate. By showing the person what the ANS is doing, and by training through this process of feedback to make changes, the person can gain control over different non-voluntary functions such as pain and stress response. This is accomplished by using mental technology such as deep breathing, progressive relaxation, mindfulness training, visualization, meditation, and so on. Studies have shown that individuals can benefit from this treatment modality by enhancing self-regulation, which results in less pain, reduced stress, and improved sleep.[239,240]

In addition, FMS patients can experience improvement in their cardiovascular, digestive, and respiratory systems through the use of biofeedback. Individuals suffering from anxiety and depression, secondary to FMS may also require cognitive-behavioral therapy to augment the biofeedback treatment.

Traditional biofeedback measures changes in different aspects of the ANS and feeds them back through a computer to the user, who trains to gradually make changes and enhance mind-body control. In the past few years, a new modality called Heart Rate Variability (HRV) has been successfully introduced and used in improving the function of the ANS.[241]

One of the greatest benefits of biofeedback is that it produces relatively quick results without any side effects associated with the treatment. Most patients report noticeable improvement between 6 and 12 sessions. More sessions may be required to deepen the effect and also to make sure that the changes become permanent. It is recommended, however, in between biofeedback sessions and once the biofeedback program is completed, to continue with deep breathing and visualization practices to further reinforce the positive changes.

Neurofeedback

Neurofeedback, also called EEG biofeedback, is a more advanced aspect of biofeedback. This technology measures the different types of brain waves and their ratio in the brain. The brain produces a variety of waves that control the persons different states of arousal:

- Delta – sleep state
- Theta – between sleep and awake, also a meditative state
- Alpha – relaxed state
- Beta1 – focused concentration
- Beta2 – alert state
- Beta3 – very alert, vigilant
- Beta4 – hyper vigilant

The ability to produce the right state, whenever it is necessary, is paramount to our health and well being, and neurofeedback can train the brain to improve those waves that are either deficient or in excess. For instance, FMS patients' brains produce an excessive amount of slow brain activity, which makes them feel even more tired. Low levels of Beta1 waves reduce their ability to focus clearly. Neurofeedback has been successfully used to improve physical functions, emotional control, muscle tension, and sensitivity in tender points, but it is especially useful in improving cognitive functions.[242,243]

Fibrofog also referred to as brain fog, is a mental condition related to FMS patients describing a mental state of fogginess. As a result, such individuals experience difficulties with focus, concentration, and memory (especially short-term memory). These cognitive impairments can be very debilitating and discouraging for those who are already experiencing many other symptoms on a physical and emotional level.[244] Most patients describe fibrofog as a state of fogginess or haze that prevents them from being able to think clearly and focus attentively. They forget not only where they placed things but even worse, they forget names, and important numbers that they have regularly used for most of their lives. Other problems include mental confusion, not being able to express their thoughts clearly, and language-related difficulties, as well as problems with executive functions such as prioritizing, decision making, and organizing.

Fibrofog can be associated with depression related to the pain, as well as with sleep deprivation common to FMS patients. Individuals with FMS experience excessive amount of slow brain activity. As a result, their frontal lobes, which are responsible for many of the cognitive processes including executive functions, are not fully activated, which results in cognitive impairment. This can be tested by measuring blood flow levels to the frontal lobes. Individuals with FMS have been shown to exhibit decreased blood flow in the frontal region of the brain. Working memory has also shown to be impaired in individuals with FMS. In addition, reduced levels of neurotransmitters, such as serotonin, can also contribute to a compromised   memory   capacity.

Neuro-cognitive training has shown good results in improving brain wave activity and frontal lobe activation,   which   usually   results   in   improved   cognitive   function. There are now new software-based programs that offer neuro-cognitive treatments both in the clinic and at home, and these have proven to be effective in reducing fibrofog and thus improving focus, concentration, and memory. Programs such as SharperBrain and SharperMemory have shown good results in treating the above-mentioned cognitive-related symptoms. This is an affordable home-based program that anyone can install and use on any Windows-based computer. Studies have shown that with regular practice of 3 to 5 times a week for 20 to 30-minutes, noticeable changes in cognitive capacity can occur within a few weeks of practice. More information about this program can be obtained at www.SharperPrograms.com

Biochemical Healing

We have also seen improvement in some patients with naturopathic "functional medicine" interventions. Recent reports also suggest a link between FMS and type 2 diabetes[245,246] thus supporting the recommendation of a low glycemic diet (i.e. avoiding processed refined carbohydrates and sugar). Deficiencies have been shown in omega 3 fatty acids[247] and in vitamin D.[248,249] Some (a minority) of patients have done well with the Dr. St. Amand's protocol.[250] This requires oral guaifenesin titrated to promote renal excretion of inorganic phosphate. Strict dietary changes including avoidance of salicylates (including most brands of toothpaste) is required for this to work. However, a good RCT needs to be done.[251]

The functional medical approach incorporates knowledge and understanding of the systems that are implicated in the biochemical pathogenesis of FMS. Each patient's dysfunctions are unique and therefore management of the disease requires a comprehensive and personalized approach. The initial focus is on identification of the unique underlying causes. There are five main areas: gastrointestinal abnormalities ("leaky gut" syndrome); HPA neuroendocrine dysregulation; chemical toxicity; mitochondrial dysfunction; oxidative stress. Each implicated dysfunctional system is seen as influencing the others, as part of an intricate network of biological factors contributing to the final pathology. Restoration of health will require a multifaceted approach.

Each dysfunction may be positively influenced by a variety of integrative medical options including specific nutrients, amino acids, botanicals, medical foods, and phytochemicals, but must include patient participation through modification of the primary dietary signals, adjustment of harmful lifestyle habits and exposure to environmental triggers.

Gastrointestinal Dysfunction

A well-established link is that between intestinal dysfunction and FMS. Research suggests that up to 70% of patients with FMS complain of symptoms associated with irritable bowel syndrome (IBS). Patients with IBS also tend to experience extraintestinal symptoms that overlap with FMS complaints, including increased nerve sensitivity, morning stiffness, headaches, sleep disturbances, and fatigue. Research suggests an autonomic imbalance, and the enteric nervous system may be the pathway by which both intestinal and extra-intestinal symptoms are seen. Indeed, greater intestinal membrane permeability has been observed in IBS.[252] A possible cause of this is small bowel bacterial overgrowth (SIBO). SIBO may be an underlying factor in malabsorption due to the requirement of symbiotic bacteria for healthy enterocyte activity.[253] A comprehensive, tailored gastrointestinal restoration program such as the 4R program, should be of benefit.

This strategy incorporates four steps: remove, replace, reinoculate, and repair. The removal stage eliminates food allergies and food sensitivities by using the oligoantigenic diet, which kills pathogenic microbes using various products such as berberine and carnosine. One of our younger FMS patients was 90% improved by eliminating tartrazine (in red dyes to color meats) from her diet.[238] Chinese herbals may also be helpful.[254] The replace step ensures adequate pancreatic enzymes, bile acids, and gastric hydrochloric acid. The reinoculate stage incorporates prebiotics such as arabinogalactans and soluble rice fibre with strain specific probiotics, such as *bifidobacterium lactus* Bi-07 and *lactobacillus acidophilus* NCFM for healthy, intestinal biota. Probiotics may also exert an effect on (cannabinoid) CB2 receptors in the gut wall.[255] Finally, the repair stage consists of nutrients required for a healthy epithelial mucosa including vitamin D, vitamin A, glutamine, zinc, lactoferrin and phosphatidylcholine.[256]

HPA Neuroendocrine Dysfunction

Most FMS patients (41.9%) have had significant life stress and/or have inordinate responses to daily life stressors.[257] Altered reactivity of the HPA axis, resulting in hyposecretion of adrenal androgens (e.g., cortisol) has been observed in such patients. Hyposecretion of DHEA, testosterone, and insulin-like growth factor (IGF)-1 has also been observed. This suggests that assessment of FMS should include a comprehensive lab work up of hormones and review of symptoms related to such imbalances. Treatment should be aimed at replacement of hormone deficiencies (aiming for optimal lab values and correlated with clinical symptoms and signs). Bioidentical hormone replacement preference and nutrient-hormone interactions must be considered. Derangement of ANS dysfunction may also play a role.[258] Assessment of neurotransmitter imbalance and treatment designed to support inhibitory pathways, and rebalance and retune the nervous system may be helpful. Thus, treatment aimed at re-establishing balance and supporting neuroendocrine function is paramount. Options for nervous system support include: taurine and essential fatty acids for neuronal membrane stabilization; methylcobolamine, trimethylglycine, and folate for healthy methylation; niacinamide, vitamin E, N-acetyl-cysteine, and mixed carotenoids for antioxidant support, glycine, GABA, and 5HTP for inhibitory neurotransmitter support; and L-carnitine for metabolic support.[258] Adaptogens are substances that increase the body's ability to maintain homeostasis during stressful events. Adaptogens mobilize our internal reserves to prevent our bodies from overreacting to the stressor, thus avoiding, reducing, or delaying the exhaustion phase or a hypo HPA response. *Rhodiola rosea, eleuthrococcus sensticosus, glycerrhiza glabra*, resveratrol, and turmeric (curcumin) may help balance altered HPA in FMS patients.[259]

Chemical Toxicity

Excessive xenobiotic or toxic exposure can result in prolonged firing of peripheral pain receptors, resulting in central nervous system sensitization and exaggerated stimuli response (as referenced earlier). In fact, toxin exposure has been suggested to play a significant role in the development and progression of FMS. Approximately 47% to 67% of patients have reported at least one episode of symptom exacerbation after specific chemical exposure.[260] Hence a personalized metabolic detoxification program may be beneficial. Areas to consider include: enhancing the activities of several hepatic detoxification enzymes[261]; limiting chemical exposure; maintaining a healthy pH balance; protecting from reactive oxygen species; maintaining a positive nitrogen balance; and ensuring healthy excretion through the gastrointestinal system, kidneys, lungs, and skin. Nutrients shown to enhance detoxification include: phosphatidyl choline and sulphates; amino acids such as glycine, cysteine, and glutamine; minerals such as potassium, magnesium, and selenium; antioxidants such as grape seed extract and glutathione; botanicals such as *Cynara scolymus, Curcuma longa* and *Silybum marianum*. Finally, biphasic compounds which can be included in the diet to enhance the program include epigallocatechin gallate from green tea, glucosinolates from cruciferous vegetables (broccoli, cauliflower, brussel sprouts, and cabbage), resveratrol from grapes and peanut skins, and polyphenols and anthocyanidins from berries. Sulphorafanes are the most potent inducers of phase II detoxification in the liver.[262] Exposure of toxic metals such as mercury from dental amalgams must be assessed before beginning a metabolic detoxification program.[263] Techniques to lower heavy metal load include: identification of sources and avoidance; improved excretion of heavy metals through intravenous chelation therapy; finally, zinc, *Andrographis paniculata,* and *Hummulus lupulus* may positively influence gene expression leading to increased metallothionein and improved transport and elimination of mercury.[264]

Mitochondrial Dysfunction

In the last 50 years our understanding of the importance of mitochondria function in health and its relation to an increasing number of diseases has grown. It has been theorized that underneath the elusive syndrome of FMS lies damage to the mitochondria in the muscles and nerve cells, thus leading to an energy deficient state. It is relatively unclear as to the source of the mitochondropathy, but some evidence implicates viral induced damage, reactive oxygen and nitrogen species, xenobiotics, nutrient insufficiencies, and fungal metabolites. Each of these substances alone or in combination with others may contribute to membrane leakage, DNA damage, altered electropotential, disruption of the organic acid production in the citric acid cycle, and ultimately low yield of ATP. There is also evidence that the accumulation of toxic metals such as mercury, lead, or cadmium can also produce reduced mitochondrial function and lowered bioenergetics. Irrespective of the disturbance a combination of nutrients known to maintain integrity and improve proper functioning of mitochondrial and energy production may support a higher rate of ATP synthesis. Nutrients such as lipoic acid and B vitamins serve as cofactors for cellular energy production and metabolism; amino acids like creatine allow muscle to regenerate ATP, and N-acetyl-L-carnitine helps transport nutrients (i.e., fatty acids) into the mitochondria for energy production. High dose D-ribose has been shown to be helpful.[265]

Oxidative Stress

Antioxidants such as coenzyme Q10, L-glutathione, N-acetylcysteine, and vitamins C and E help prevent oxidative damage. Substrates and nutrients that act as co-factors and influence enzyme kinetics may be of benefit, these include: malic acid,[186] pantothenic acid, niacinamide, and magnesium. A properly balanced metabolic detoxification program can have a favorable effect on the body's acid-alkaline balance, which in turn helps to regulate cellular mitochondrial function.

It is further postulated that chronic overstimulation of the ANS while the patient is at rest contributes to a weakened autonomic response to physical challenge, contributing to the increased fatigue, decreased tissue oxygenation, and reduced threshold for pain seen in FMS patients; suggesting overlap and the importance of considering the neuroendocrine system when treating the gastrointestinal system, i.e. the network approach. Furthermore, lack of amino acid absorption and transport in the gastrointestinal system may lead to deficiencies in neurotransmitter precursors and neuropeptides. Several studies suggest that patients with FMS have a defect in amino acid homeostasis, in particular, deficiencies in L-tryptophan, L-leucine, L-isoleucine, and L-valine. Researchers hypothesize that the amino acid deficiencies seen in patients with FMS may be the result of defective intestinal amino acid transport mechanisms. L-tryptophan deficiency is a good example of how reduced amino acid transport may be related to FMS symptoms. L-tryptophan is a precursor to 5-hydroxytryptamine, or serotonin. Serotonin is highly concentrated in the brainstem and is active throughout the central nervous system. The largest concentration of serotonin outside the brain is in the digestive system. Known as a "neuromodulator," serotonin is involved in the configuration of emotional, cognitive, and motor functions, as well as circadian and neuroendocrine rhythms. Research suggests that decreased L-tryptophan and the resulting low serotonin levels play a pathophysiologic role in FMS. Replacing suboptimal amino acids, such as neurotransmitter precursors and branched chain amino acids intravenously, utilizing techniques to increase the absorptive capabilities and restoring the integrity of mucosa may be of benefit.

Dietary modification has also shown to improve quality of life in a subset of patients. In one study, 30 patients participating in a dietary intervention were told to consume a diet consisting of 24% fat, 65% carbohydrate, and 11% protein from fresh fruit, green salad, carrot juice, dehydrated barley grass juice, omega-3 fatty acid dietary supplements, and minimal amounts of animal products. After 7-months, 19 of the 30 patients responded favourably with significant improvements in quality of life, including pain, range of motion, and flexibility. The researchers concluded that this form of dietary intervention may play a significant role in helping patients with FMS. Another beneficial modification of the diet showed that certain food additives such as monosodium glutamate and/or aspartame when removed from the diet caused complete or nearly complete resolution of symptoms in a subset of FMS patients. Other implicated nutrients that may be suboptimal in these patients include specific trace minerals such as magnesium and zinc. Addition of specific B vitamins in high doses intravenously showed significant reduction in symptoms. Other nutrients have been found to be low including alpha lipoic acid and co-enzyme Q10, but not in all patients, thus suggesting different underlying mechanisms for each FMS patient. A widely used intravenous antioxidant therapy is the Myers' cocktail. A randomized, double-blind, placebo controlled pilot study of 8-weeks, revealed significant improvement in tender points, pain, depression, and quality of life measures with the administration of the intravenous Myers' cocktail.[181]

The use of CAM must be monitored for adverse effects and potential interactions with medications. As a general rule of thumb, all herbal products should be stopped (blood thinning effect) prior to any surgery or extensive and/or deep soft tissue injections.

Neurological Healing

Traumatic brain injury (TBI) can result in hypopituitarism and hormonal deficiencies. This is summarized extensively in chapter 5 of Dr. Mark Gordon's textbook *The Clinical Application of Interventional eEndocrinology*.[266] In particular, adult GH deficiency following TBI is a condition recognized by the American Association of Clinical Endocrinologists.[267] The incidence of TBI in the USA is 1.5-2 million people per year. Of that, some 80,000 people will sustain a chronic disabling condition. It is believed that 2.5-6.5 million persons are living with TBI sequelae. The male-to-female ratio is greater than 2:1. It is estimated that 30-50% of patients who survive TBI will have endocrine complications. Prior TBI is also very common (lifetime prevalence of 53%) among homeless people and is associated with poorer health.[268] It is likely that there is overlap in symptomatology between TBI and FMS but this has yet to be studied.

Autopsy studies in TBI demonstrate a high prevalence of hypothalamic and pituitary abnormalities including anterior lobe infarct and necrosis (9-38% of cases), posterior lobe hemorrhage (12-45%), and traumatic lesions of the hypothalamic-pituitary stalk (5-30%). The latter may lead to disruption of the portal blood supply from the hypothalamus via the hypophyseal portal veins. Edema of the pituitary within the bony sella turcica compromises blood supply, thus leading to anterior lobe ischemia and necrosis. Anterior pituitary hormones (GH, thyrotropin, corticotrophin, and gonadotropins) are released by the neuropeptide-releasing hormones from the hypothalamus. Posterior pituitary hormones (vasopressin, oxytocin) are produced by the hypothalamus and are carried by long axons into the posterior pituitary where they are then released. The posterior lobe supply is not affected by pituitary stalk trauma because it is supplied by the inferior hypophyseal arteries (arising from the internal carotid artery below the diaphragma sella). The most common acute endocrine complication following TBI (33% of cases) is syndrome of inappropriate antidiuretic hormone (SIADH), which can lead to life-threatening seizures and coma from dilutional hyponatremia. Criteria for this diagnosis includes low serum osmolality, hyponatremia, and inappropriately concentrated urine (urine sodium > 25 mEq/L).

The most common chronic endocrine complication involves the anterior pituitary hormones particularly GH.[269] Endocrine work up should include hormonal assays – a.m. cortisol, free and total testosterone, TSH, T3, T4, FSH, LH, estrogen (females) – and IGF-1, which is a screening assay for GH deficiency. Primary adrenal insufficiency presenting with psychiatric symptoms (depression, confusion, apathy, and even psychosis) can also be a rare complication.[270] Treatment involves bioidentical hormone replacement therapy which may be required long-term (at 12-month follow-up, the only anterior pituitary hormone that continued to decrease was GH).[271] Randomized trials have been published on effective treatment of FMS with GH (earlier table). Progesterone has also been found to be neuroprotective.[272] In menopausal patients, bioidentical hormone replacement therapy may resolve symptoms all together.[273]

6. Risk Factors for Poor Treatment Outcomes

High scores (> 21/63 on the Beck depression inventory) indicate a major depression which should first be treated.[274] Studies suggest that patients with FMS or CFS differ from those with depression.[275] Pain and depression have different pathways on fMRI.[276] High catastrophizers (Pain Catastrophizing Scale) also should be screened out (focus more on psychological interventions first).[277] Axis one psychiatric disorders including "hysteria-conversion disorders" should also be excluded.[278] Patients involved in stressful disability claim appeals and litigation, ideally should have such issues resolved prior to initiating treatment. More detailed evaluation should first be completed.

7. Pre-Screening for Injection Treatments (PRP and/or Botox in Structural Therapy)

Relative contraindications to injection and acupuncture treatments include: needle phobia, lack of motivation, unwilling to comply, coagulopathy or on blood thinners, pregnancy, unstable medical or psychiatric condition. Marked skin allodynia (pre-treatment with a neuropathic pain drug and/or topical local anesthetic is advised prior to any injections)

Contraindications to Botulinum toxins include patients with flu symptoms, who are on aminoglycosides or have neuromuscular junction disorders (myasthenia gravis, eaton-lambert syndrome, myopathies). It is also recommended not to inject into atrophic, flaccid muscles. The same applies also to Botulinum-toxin B (Myobloc®) and the new equivalent German Botulinum-toxin A (Xeomin®).

Contraindications to PRP injections include: low platelet count (<105/uL); low hemoglobin (<10 g/dL); low blood pressure – hemodynamic instability; dysfunctional platelets and clotting (hemophiliac); consistent use of NSAIDs within 48-hours of PRP procedure[279]; corticosteroid injection at treatment site within 2-weeks of PRP procedure; corticosteroid by mouth or IV within 2-weeks of PRP; concurrent or recent fever or illness; septicemia; active history of *Pseudomonas*, *Enterococcus*, or *Klebsiella* infections (PRP in one study was shown to potentially stimulate these pathogens); cancer – especially hematopoetic or of bone; and rash at injection site.

If all of the above are satisfied, then a further optional screening step is a test TrP injection(s) with preservative-free hydroxide-buffered 1% procaine or lidocaine. This has the advantage (over regular anesthetics) of a much lower likelihood of post-injection soreness/allergic reaction. Patients return after 1-week with a completed pain diary. If there is increased pain or no pain reduction, then Botox injection should not be done in the same sites. If there is a significant reduction in pain (VAS decreases over 2 points or by 30%),[280] Botox would be indicated. Informed consent and follow-up with validated outcome measures are necessary.[281]

8. Long-Term Management of Fibromyalgia

There is no universal "magic bullet" for the treatment of FMS. It is a syndrome characterized by central sensitization, loss of DNIC, and neuroendocrine dysfunction. Hallmark symptoms are widespread pain, loss of restorative sleep, fatigue, and comorbid syndromes. Studies suggest that 67% of patients had preceding migraine prior to onset of their FMS[282] and that 25% of chronic low back pain patients will evolve into FMS.[283,284] If poorly managed, the persistence of widespread pain may be associated with higher mortality rates.[285-287] Co-existent major depression may also be associated with accelerated brain grey matter atrophy.[288]

Symptoms may last on average 15 years.[289] Review papers suggest that positive outcomes occur not only with age[290] but also with an adequate physical activity level[291] and coping skills.[292] Excess major negative life events and permanent disability pensions are associated with a negative outcome.[293] Younger age of onset and less sleep disturbance are associated with a more favorable outcome.[294] Effective management is best with an interdisciplinary approach[295-297] emphasizing lifestyle improvement, for example FMS smokers have been found to have more pain, numbness, global severity, and functional difficulties than non-smokers.[298] Weight loss also helps symptoms.[299] A self-help approach known as TENSQ (Toxin elimination; Exercise-stamina, strength, skills; Nutrition; Sleep hygiene; Quiet time) is available for patients and physicians on the website resource www.DrKoPRP.com.

CONCLUDING REMARKS

This review has summarized not only published peer-review literature on pain management in the area of FMS, but also presented 22-years of clinical experience in managing such patients. Evidence-based guidelines support the first-line use of pregabalin, duloxetine, milnacipran, and tramadol for severe pain. There is emerging evidence for pharmaceutical cannabinoids and gamma-hydroxy-butyrate. Cognitive-behavioral therapy and meditation stress-reduction approaches are helpful for coping with (not reducing) pain. The key functional goal is exercise (aerobic and strengthening) for the body and the mind. Aquatic exercise in particular, has advantages over land-based and home exercises for FMS.[300,301] Though, most non-drug studies are of poorer quality, it must be realized that CAM clinical trials are often difficult to implement in a true blinded fashion[302] and with the needed multidisciplinary-multimodal approach.[303] Research is all the more needed, noting that CAM use is amongst the highest in this difficult-to-treat group of patients.

Validation and hope for such patients is predicated on careful, comprehensive history and physical examination (looking for signs of structural, biochemical, psychoemotional, and neurological dysfunction), and correlative investigations. Emerging hopeful therapies include platelet-rich plasma prolotherapy for ligamentous deficiency, functional medicine with diet, nutrition, and detoxification changes, neurotherapy (EEG biofeedback) for brain function and bioidentical hormone replacement (particularly human GH in the post-TBI subgroup). From an evidence-based perspective, there is obviously a need to conduct further randomized controlled double-blinded studies for the various subgroups in FMS. It is hoped that this review paper will stimulate such research for the long-term pain relief and healthy aging of all our patients.

REFERENCES

1. Wolfe F, Smythe HA, Yunus MB, et al. The American College of Rheumatology 1990 criteria for classification of fibromyalgia: report of the multicenter criteria committee. Arthritis Rheum. 1990;33:160-172.
2. Wolfe R, Rasker JJ. The symptom intensity scale, fibromyalgia and the meaning of fibromyalgia-like symptoms. J Rheumatol. 2006;33:2291-2299.
3. Katz RS, Wolfe F, Michaud K. Fibromyalgia diagnosis, a comparison of clinical, survey and American College of Rheumatology criteria. Arthritis Rheum. 2006;54:169-176.
4. Wolfe F, Ross K, Anderson J, et al. The prevalence and characteristics of fibromyalgia in the general population. Arthritis Rheum. 1995;38:19-28.
5. Sivri A, Cindas A, Dincer F, Sivri B. Bowel dysfunction and irritable bowel syndrome in fibromyalgia patients. Clinical Rheumatol. 1996;15:283-286.

6. Yunus MB, Masi AT, Aldag JC. A controlled study of primary fibromyalgia syndrome: clinical features and association with other functional syndromes. *J Rheumatol* 1989; 16 suppl 19:62-71.

7. Paira SO. Fibromyalgia associated with female urethral syndrome. *Clinical Rheumatol.* 1994;13:88-89.

8. Sinaii N, Cleary SD, Ballweg ML, *et al.* High rates of autoimmune disorders, fibromyalgia, chronic fatigue syndrome and atopic diseases among women with endometriosis: a survey analysis. *Hum Reprod.* 2002;17:2715-2724.

9. Mukerji B, Mukerji V, Alpert MA, Selukar R. The prevalence of rheumatologic disorders in patients with chest pain and angiographically normal coronary arteries. *Angiology* 1995;46:425-430.

10. Harvey CK. Fibromyalgia. Part II. Prevalence in the podiatric patient population. *J Amer Podiatric Med Assoc.* 1993;83:416-417.

11. Nicolodi M, Sicuteri F. Fibromyalgia and migraine, two faces of the same mechanism. *Advances in Experimental Medicine & Biology.* 1996;398:373-379.

12. Plesh O, Wolfe F, Lane N. The relationship between fibromyalgia and temporomandibular disorders: prevalence and symptom severity. *J Rheumatol.* 1996;23:1948-1952.

13. Cleveland CH. *Jr Allergy Proc.* 1992;13:263-267.

14. Bonafede RP, Downey DC, Bennett RM. An association of fibromyalgia with primary Sjogren's syndrome: a prospective study of 72 patients. *J Rheumatol.* 1995;22:133-136.

15. Perez-Ruiz F, Calabozo M, Alonso-Ruiz A *et al.* High prevalence of undetected carpal tunnel syndrome in patients with fibromyalgia syndrome. *J Rheumatol.* 1995;22:501-504.

16. Lapossy E, Gasser P, Hrycaj P, *et al.* Cold-induced vasospasm in patients with fibromyalgia and chronic low back pain in comparison to healthy subjects. *Clinical Rheumatol.* 1994;13:442-445.

17. Martinez JE, Ferraz MB, Fontana AM, Atra E. Psychological aspects of Brazilian women with fibromyalgia. *J Psychosomatic Res.* 1995;39:167-174.

18. Kraj NJ, Norregaard J, Larsen JK, Danneskiold-Samsoe B. A blinded controlled evaluation of anxiety and depressive symptoms in patients with fibromyalgia, as measured by standardized psychometric interview scales. *Acta Psychiatrica Scandinavica.* 1994;89:370-375.

19. Buskila D, Neumann L, Hazanov I, Carmi R. Familial aggregation in the fibromyalgia syndrome. *Seminars Arthritis Rheum.* 1996;26:605-611.

20. Katz RS, Kravitz HM. Fibromyalgia, depression, and alcoholism: a family history study. *J Rheumatol.* 1996; 23:149-154.

21. Boisset-Pioro MH, Esdaile JM, Fitzcharles MA. Sexual and physical abuse in women with fibromyalgia syndrome. *Arthritis Rheum.* 1995;38:235-241.

22. Taylor ML, Trotter DR, Csuka ME. The prevalence of sexual abuse in women with fibromyalgia. *Arthritis Rheum.* 1995;38:229-234.

23. Gedalia A, Press J, Klein M, Buskila D. Joint hypermobility and fibromyalgia in schoolchildren. *Ann Rheum Dis.* 1993;52:494-496.

24. Wolfe F. Post-traumatic fibromyalgia: a case report narrated by the patient. *Arthritis Care Res.* 1994;7:161-165.

25. Waylonis GW, Perkins RH. Post-traumatic fibromyalgia. A long-term follow-up. *Amer J Phys Med Rehabil.* 1994;73:403-412.

26. Buskila D, Neumann L, Vaisberg G, Alkalay D, Wolfe F. Increased rates of fibromyalgia after cervical spine injury: a controlled study of 161 cases of traumatic injury. *Arthritis Rheum.* 1997;40:446-452.

27. Wolfe F and the Vancouver Fibromyalgia Consensus group: Special report: the fibromyalgia syndrome: a consensus report on fibromyalgia and disability. *J Rheumatol.* 1996;23:534-539.

28. Holman AJ. Positional cervical spinal cord compression and fibromyalgia: a novel comorbidity with important diagnostic and treatment implications. *J Pain.* 2008;9:613-622.

29. Lindgren KA, Kettunen JA, Paatelma M, Mikkonen RHM. Dynamic kine magnetic resonance imaging in whiplash patients and in age-and sex-matched controls. *Pain Res Manage.* 2009;14:427-432.

30. Aaron LA, Bradley LA, Alarcon GS *et al.* Perceived physical and emotional trauma as precipitating events in fibromyalgia. *Arthritis Rheum.* 1997;40:453-460.

31. Nielson WR, Merskey H. Psychosocial aspects of fibromyalgia. *Curr Pain Headache Rep.* 2001;5:330-337.

32. Tyler AN. Influenza A virus: a possible precipitating factor in fibromyalgia? *Alternative Med Review.* 1997;2:82-86.

33. Buchwald D, Garrity D. Comparison of patients with chronic fatigue syndrome, fibromyalgia and multiple chemical sensitivities. *Arch Intern Med.* 1994;154:2049-2053.
34. Goldenberg DL, Simms RW, Geiger A, Komaroff AK. High frequency of fibromyalgia in patients with chronic fatigue seen in a primary care practice. *Arthritis Rheum.* 1990; 33:381-387.
35. Yunus MB, Hussey FX, Aldag JC. Antinuclear antibodies and connective tissue disease features in fibromyalgia syndrome:a controlled study. *J Rheumatol.* 1993;20:1557-1560.
36. Nijs J, De Meirleir K, Coomans D, *et al.* Deregulation of the 2.5A synthetase Rnase L antiviral pathway by Mycoplasma spp. In subsets of Chronic Fatigue Syndrome. *J Chronic Fatigue Syndrome.* 2003;11:37-50.
37. Neilson L. Highlights of Quest Newsletter No. 83, Spring 2010. (April 11, 2010) www.mefmaction.net.
38. Drewes AM, Andreasen A, Schroder HD, *et al.* Pathology of skeletal muscle in fibromyalgia: a histo-immuno-chemical and ultrastructural study. *Br J Rheumatol.* 1993;32:479-483.
39. Simms RW,Roy SH, Hrovat M, *et al.* Lack of association between fibromyalgia syndrome and abnormalities in muscle energy metabolism. *Arthritis Rheum.* 1994;37:794-800.
40. Sprott H, Salemi S, Gay RE *et al.* Increased DNA fragmentation and ultrastructural changes in fibromyalgia muscle fibres. *Ann Rheum Dis.* 2004;63:245-251.
41. Sprott H, Rzanny R, Reichenbach JR, *et al.* 31P magnetic resonance spectroscopy in fibromyalgic muscle. *Rheumatology (Oxford).* 2000;39:1121-1125.
42. Moldofsky H, Scarisbrick P, England R, Smythe H. Musculoskeletal symptoms and non-REM sleep disturbance in patients with "fibrositis syndrome" and healthy subjects. *Psychosom Med.* 1975;37:341-351.
43. Chervin RD, Teodorescu M Kushwaha R, *et al.* Objective measures of disordered sleep in fibromyalgia. *J Rheumatol.* 2009;36:2009-2016.
44. Hyyppa MT, Kronholm E. Nocturnal motor activity in fibromyalgia patients with poor sleep quality. *J Psychosomat Res.* 1995;39:85-91.
45. Rains JC, Penzien DB. Sleep and chronic pain. Challenges to the alpha-EEG sleep pattern as a pain specific sleep anomaly. *J Psychosom Res.* 2003;54:77-83.
46. Paiva ES, Deodhar A, Jones KD, Bennett R. Impaired growth hormone secretion in fibromyalgia patients: evidence for augmented hypothalamic somatostatin tone. *Arthritis Rheum.* 2002;46:1344-1350.
47. Russell IJ, Orr MD, Littman B, *et al.* Elevated cerebrospinal fluid levels of substance P in patients with the fibromyalgia syndrome. *Arthritis Rheum.* 1994;37:1593-1601.
48. Regland B, Andersson M, Abrahamsson L, *et al.* Increased concentrations of homocysteine in the cerebrospinal fluid in patients with fibromyalgia and chronic fatigue syndrome. *Scand J Rheumatol.* 1997;26:301-307.
49. Giovengo SL, Russel IJ, Larson AA. Increased concentration of nerve growth factor in cerebrospinal fluid of patients with fibromyalgia. *J Rheumatol.* 1999;26:1564-1569.
50. Harris RE, Sundren PC, Craig AD, *et al.* Elevated insular glutamate in fibromyalgia is associated with experimental pain. *Arthritis Rheum.* 2009;60:3146-3142.
51. Gracely RH, Petzke F, Wolf JM, Clauw DJ. Functional magnetic resonance imaging evidence of augmented pain processing in fibromyalgia. *Arthritis Rheum.* 2002; 46: 1333-1343.
52. Mailis-Gagnon A, Giannoylis I, Downar J, *et al.* Altered central somatosensory processing in chronic pain patients with "hysterical" anesthesia. *Neurology* 2003; 60:1501-1507.
53. Glesecke T, Gracely RH, Grant MA, *et al.* Evidence of augmented central pain processing in idiopathic chronic low back pain. *Arthritis Rheum.* 2004;50:613-623.
54. Cook DB, Lange G, Ciccone DS *et al.* Functional imaging of pain in patients with primary fibromyalgia. *J Rheumatol.* 2004;31:364-378.
55. Kosek E, Hansson P. Modulatory influence on somatosensory perception from vibration and heteroropic noxious conditioning stimulation (HNCS) in fibromyalgia patients and healthy subjects. *Pain* 1997;70:41-51.
56. Julien N, Goffaux P, Arsenault P, Marchand S. Widespread pain in fibromyalgia is related to a deficit of endogenous pain inhibition. *Pain* 2005;114:295-302.
57. Abeles AM, Pillinger MH, Solitar BM, Abeles M. Narrative review: the pathophysiology of FM. *Ann Intern Med.* 2007;146:726-734.

58.   Zautra AJ, Fasman R, Davis MC, Craig AD. The effects of slow breathing on affective responses to pain stimuli: an experimental study. *Pain* 2010;149:12-18.

59.   Jensen KB, Kosek E, Petzke F, *et al*. Evidence of dysfunctional pain inhibition in fibromyalgia reflected in rACC during provoked pain. *Pain* 2009;144:95-100.

60.   Staud R, Nagel S, Robinson ME, Price DD. Enhance central pain processing in fibromyalgia patients is maintained by muscle afferent input: a randomized, double-blind, placebo-controlled study. *Pain* 2009;145:96-104.

61.   Adler GK, Kinsley BT, Hurwitz S, *et al*. Reduced hypothalamic-pituitary and sympathoadrenal responses to hypoglycemia in women with fibromyalgia syndrome. *Am J Med.* 1999;106:534-543.

62.   Riedel W, Schlapp U, Leck S, *et al*. Blunted ACTH and cortisol responses to systemic injection of corticotropin-releasing hormone [CRH] in fibromyalgia: role of somatostatin and CRH-binding protein. *Ann NY Acad Sci.* 2002;96:483-490.

63.   Calis M, Gokce C, Ates F *et al*. Investigation of the hypothalamo-pituitary-adrenal axis by 1 microg ACTH test and metyrapone test in patients with primary fibromyalgia syndrome. *J Endocrinol Invest.* 2004;27:42-46.

63b.   Cohen H, Neumann L, Kotler M, Buskila D. Autonomic nervous system derangement in fibromyalgia syndrome and related disorders. *Isr Med Assoc J.* 2001;3:755-760.

64.   McBeth J, Silman AJ, Gupta A, *et al*. Moderation of psychosocial risk factors through dysfunction of the hypothalamic-pituitary-adrenal stress axis in the onset of chronic widespread musculoskeletal pain: findings of a population-based prospective cohort study. *Arthritis Rheum.* 2007;56:360-371.

65.   Arnold LM, Hudson JI, Hess EV, *et al*. Family study of fibromyalgia. *Arthritis Rheum.* 2004;50:944-952.

66.   Jones GT, Power C, Macfarlane GJ. Adverse events in childhood and chronic widespread pain in adult life: Results from the 1958 British Birth Cohort Study. *Pain.* 2009;143:92-96.

67.   Russell IJ. Fibromyalgia syndrome. In: Mense S, Simons DG, eds. *Muscle Pain: Understanding its Nature, Diagnosis, and Treatment.* Baltimore, MD: Lippincott Williams & Wilkins; 2001:289-237.

68.   Berger A, Dukes E, Martin S, *et al*. Characteristics and healthcare costs of patients with fibromyalgia syndrome. *Int J Clin Pract.* 2007;61:1498-1508.

69.   White KP, Speechley M, Harth M, Ostbye T. The London fibromyalgia epidemiology study: direct health care costs of fibromyalgia syndrome in London, Canada. *J Rheumatol.* 1999;26:885-889.

70.   Hughes G, Martinez C, Myon E, Taïeb C, Wessely S. The impact of a diagnosis of fibromyalgia on health care resource use by primary care patients in the UK: an observational study based on clinical practice. *Arthritis Rheum.* 2006;54:177-183.

71.   Carette S, Bell MJ, Reynolds WJ, *et al*. Comparison of amiptriptyline, cyclobenzaprine and placebo in the treatment of fibromyalgia: a randomized, double-blind clinical trial. *Arthritis Rheum.* 1994;37:32-40.

72.   Goldenberg D, Mayskliy M, Mossey C, *et al*. A randomized double-blind crossover trial of fluoxetine and amitriptyline in the treatment of fibromyalgia. *Arthritis Rheum.* 1996;39:1852-1859.

73.   Ko GD, Whitmore S, Huang D, McDonald R. Effective pain palliation in fibromyalgia patients with Botulinum Toxin type-A: case series of 25. *J Musculoskel Pain.* 2007;15:55-66.

74.   McKenzie R, O'Fallon A, Dale J, *et al*. Low-dose hydrocortisone for treatment of chronic fatigue syndrome: a randomized clinical trial. *J Amer Med Assoc.* 1998; 280:1061-1066.

75.   Santandrea S, Montrone F, Sarzi-Puttini P, *et al*. A double-blind crossover study of two cyclobenzaprine regimens in primary fibromyalgia syndrome. *J Int Med Res.* 1993;21:74-80.

76.   Fossaluzza V, De Vita S. Combined therapy with cyclobenzaprine and ibuprofen in primary fibromyalgia syndrome. *Int J Clin Pharm Res.* 1992;12:99-102.

77.   Staud R, Vierck CJ, Robinson ME, Price DD. Effects of the N-methyl-D-aspartate receptor antagonist dextromethorphan on temporal summation of pain are similar in fibromyalgia patients and normal control subjects. *J Pain.* 2005;6:323-332.

77b.   Cohen SP, Verdolin MH, Chang AS, *et al*. The intravenous ketamine test predicts subsequent response to an oral dextromethorphan treatment regimen in fibromyalgia patients. *J Pain.* 2006;7:391-398.

78.   Caruso I, Sarzi Puttini PC, *et al*. Double-blind study of dothiepin versus placebo in the treatment of primary fibromyalgia syndrome. *J Int Med Res.* 1987;15:154-159.

79. Arnold LM, Lu Y, Crofford LJ, *et al*. A double-blind, multicenter trial comparing duloxetine to placebo in the treatment of fibromyalgia pataients with or without major depressive disorder. *Arthritis Rheum*. 2004;50:2974-84.

80. Russell IJ, Mease PJ, Smith TR, *et al*. Efficacy and safety of duloxetine for treatment of fibromyalgia in patients with or without major depressive disorder: results from a 6-month, randomized, double-blind, placebo-controlled, fixed-dose trial. *Pain* 2008;136:432-444.

81. Chappell AS, Littlejohn G, Kajdasz DK, *et al*. A 1-year safety and efficacy study of duloxetine in patients with fibromyalgia. *Clin J Pain*. 2009;25:365-375.

82. Arnold LM, Goldenberg DL, Stanford SB *et al*. Gabapentin in the treatment of fibromyalgia: a randomized, double-blind, placebo-controlled, multicenter trial. *Arthritis Rheum*. 2007;56:1336-1344.

83. Bennett RM, Clark SC, Walczyk J. A randomized double-blind placebo-controlled study of growth hormone in the treatment of fibromyalgia. *Amer J Med*. 1998;104:227-231.

84. Cuetracasas G, *et al*. Growth hormone as concomitant treatment in severe fibromyalgia associated with low IGF-1 serum levels: a pilot study. *BMC Musculoskel Disorders*. 2007:30:119.

85. Graven-Nielsen T, Kendall SA, Henriksson KG, *et al*. Ketamine reduces muscle pain, temporal summation, and referred pain in fibromyalgia patients. *Pain* 2000;85:483-491.

86. Hong CZ, Hsueh TC. Difference in pain relief after trigger point injections in myofascial pain patients with and without fibromyalgia. *Arch Phys Med Rehabil*. 1996;77:1161-1166.

87. Raphael J, Southall J, Treharne G, Kitas G. Efficacy and adverse effects of intravenous lignocaine therapy in fibromyalgia syndrome. *BMC Musculoskelet Disord*. 2002;3:21.

88. Mease PJ, Clauw DJ, Gendreau RM, *et al*. The efficacy and safety of milnacipran for treatment of fibromyalgia. A randomized, double-blind, placebo-controlled trial. *J Rheumatol*. 2009;36:398-409.

89. Clauw DJ, Mease P, Palmer RH, *et al*. Milnacipran for the treatment of fibromyalgia in adults: a 15-week, multicener, randomized, double-blind, placebo-controlled, multiple-dose clinical trial. *Clin Ther*. 2008; 30:1988-2004.

90. Goldenberg D, Clauw DJ, Palmer RH, Mease P. One-year durability of response to milnacipran treatment for fibromyalgia. *Arthritis Rheum*. 2007;56(9 Suppl):S603.

91. Samborski W, LezaÅ„ska-Szpera M, Rybakowski JK. Effects of antidepressant mirtazapine on fibromyalgia symptoms. *Rocz Akad Med Bialymst*. 2004;49:265-269.

91b. Hrycaj P, Stratz T, Mennet P, Muller W. Pathogenetic aspects of responsiveness to ondansetron in patients with primary fibromyalgia syndrome: a preliminary study. *J Rheumatol*. 1996;23:1418-1423.

92. Skrabek RQ, Galimova L, Ethans K, Perry D. Nabilone for the treatment of pain in fibromyalgia. *J Pain*. 2008;9:164-173.

93. Ko G, Hum A, Eitel M, Tumarken E. A retrospective chart review of add-on nabilone in the clinical management of fibromyalgia. *Pain Res Manage*. 2009;14:152.

94. Ware MA, Fitzcharles MA, Joseph L, Shir Y. The effects of nabilone on sleep in fibromyalgia : results of a randomized controlled trial. *Anesth Analg*. 2009

95. Ataoglu S, Ataoglu-A, Erdogan-F, *et al*. Comparison of paroxetine, amitriptyline in the treatment of fibromyalgia. *Turk J Med Sci*. 1997;27:535-539.

96. Wood PB, Kablinger AS, Caldito GS. Open trial of pindolol in the treatment of fibromyalgia. *Ann Pharmacother*. 2005;39:1812-1816.

97. Holman AJ, Myers RR. A randomized, double-blind, placebo-controlled trial of pramipexole, a dopamine agonist, in patients with fibromyalgia receiving concomitant medications. *Arthritis Rheum*. 2005;52:2495-2505.

98. Crofford LJ, Rowbotham MC, Mease PJ, *et al*. Pregabalin for the treatment of fibromyalgia syndrome: results of a randomized, double-blind, placebo-controlled trial. *Arthritis Rheum*. 2005;52:1264-1273.

99. Mease PJ, Russell IJ, Arnold LM, *et al*. A randomized, double-blind, placebo-controlled, phase III trial of pregabalin in the treatment of patients with fibromyalgia. *J Rheumatol*. 2008;35:502-514.

99b. Arnold LM, Russell IJ, Diri EW, *et al*. A 14-week, randomized, double-blinded, placebo-controlled monotherapy trial of pregabalin in patients with fibromyalgia. *J Pain*. 2008;9:792-805.

100. Crofford LJ, Mease PJ, Simpson SL, *et al*. Fibromyalgia relapse evaluation and efficacy for durability of meaningful relief (FREEDOM): a 6-month, double-blind, placebo-controlled trial with pregabalin. *Pain* 2008;136:419-431.

101. Kempenaers C, Simenon G, Vander Elst M, *et al*. Effect of an antidiencephalon immune serum on pain and sleep in primary fibromyalgia. *Neuropsychobiology* 1994;30:66-72.

102. Scharf MB, Baumann M, Berkowitz DV. The effects of sodium oxybate on clinical symptoms and sleep patterns in patients with fibromyalgia. *J Rheum.* 2003;30:1070-1074.

103. Russell IJ, Perkins AT, Michalek JE. Oxybate SXB-26 FM Syndrome Study Group. Sodium oxybate relieves pain and improves function in FM syndrome: a randomized, double-blind, placebo-controlled, multicenter clinical trial. *Arthritis Rheum.* 2009;60:299-309.

104. Vaeroy H, Abrahamsen A, Forre O, Kass E. Treatment of fibromyalgia: a parallel double blind trial with carisoprodol, paracetamol and caffeine (Somadril comp) versus placebo. *Clin Rheumatol.* 1989;8:245-350.

105. Ko G, Wine W, Tumarkin E. Case series of fibromyalgia patients with neuropathic pain improved with the sublingual cannabinoid Sativex. *European J Pain.* 2007;11:145-146.

106. Nurmikko TJ, Serpell MG, Hoggart B, *et al.* Sativex successfully treats neuropathic pain characterized by allodynia: a randomized, double-blind, placebo-controlled clinical trial. *Pain* 2007;133:210-220.

107. Lowe JC, Garrison RL, Reichman AJ, *et al.* Effectiveness and safety of T3 therapy for euthyroid fibromyalgia: a double-blind, placebo-controlled, response driven crossover study. *Clin Bulletin Myofasc Therapy.* 1997;2:31-58.

108. McLain D. An open label dose finding trial of Tizanidine for treatment of fibromyalgia. *J Musculoskel Pain.* 2002;10:7-18.

109. Russell IJ, Michalek JE, Xiao Y, *et al.* Therapy with a central alpha 2-adrenergic agonist (tizanidine) decreases cerebrospinal fluid substance P and may reduce serum hyaluronic acid as it improves the clinical symptoms of the fibromyalgia syndrome. *Arthritis Rheum.* 2002;46:S614.

110. Bennett RM, Kamin M, Karim R, Rosenthal N. Tramadol and acetaminophen combination tablets in the treatment of fibromyalgia pain: a double-blind, randomized, placebo-controlled study. *Am J Med.* 2003;114:537-545.

111. Bennett RM, Schein J, Kosinski MR, *et al.* Impact of fibromyalgia pain on health-related quality of life before and after treatment with tramadol/acetaminophen. *Arthritis Rheum.* 2005;53:519-527.

112. Biasi G, Manca S, Manganelli S, Marcolongo R. Tramadol in the fibromyalgia syndrome: a controlled clinical trial versus placebo. *Int J Clin Pharm Res.* 1998;18:13-19.

113. Muller W, Stratz T. Results of the intravenous administration of tropisetron in fibromyalgia patients. *Scand J Rheumatol.* 2000;29 (Suppl 113):59-62.

114. Puttini PS, Caruso J. Primary fibromyalgia syndrome and 5-hydrdoxy-L-tryptophan: a 90 day open study. *J Int Med Res.* 1992;20:182-189.

115. Caruso I, Puttini S, Cazzola M, Azzolini V. Double-blind study of 5-hydroxytryptophan versus placebo in the treatment of primary fibromyalgia syndrome. *J Int Med Res.* 1990;18:201-209.

116. Nishishinya B, Urrutia G, Walitt B, *et al.* Amitriptyline in the treatment of fibromyalgia: a systematic review of its efficacy. *Rheumatol* 2008;47:1741-1746.

117. Tofferi JK, Jackson JL, O'Malley PG. Treatment of fibromyalgia with cyclobenzaprine: a meta-analysis. *Arthritis Rheum.* 2004;51:9-13.

118. Paulson GW, Gill W. Botulinum toxin is unsatisfactory therapy for fibromyalgia. *Movement Disorders.* 1996;11:459.

119. Bessette L, Carette S, Fossel AH, Lew RA. A placebo controlled crossover trial of subcutaneous salmon calcitonin in the treatment of patients with fibromyalgia. *Scand J Rheum.* 1998;27:112-116.

120. Patrick M, Swannell A, Doherty M. Chlormezanone in primary fibromyalgia syndrome: a double blind placebo controlled study. *Brit J Rheumatol.* 1993;32:55-58.

120b. Moldofsky H, Lue FA. The relationship of alpha and delta EEG frequencies to pain and mood in "fibrositis" patients treated with chlorpromazine and L-tryptophan. *Electroencephalgr Clin Neurophysiol.* 1980;50:71-80.

121. Kuratsune H, Yamaguti K, Sawada M, *et al.* DHEA-S deficiency in chronic fatigue syndrome. *Int J Mol Med.* 1998;1:143-146.

121b. Scott LV, Svec F, Dinan. A preliminary study of dehydroepiandrosterone response to low-dose ACTH in chronic fatigue syndrome and in healthy subjects. *Psychiatry Res.* 2000;97:21028.

121c. Finckh A, Berner IC, Aubry-Rozier B, So AK. A randomized controlled trial of dehydroepiandrosterone in postmenopausal women with fibromyalgia. *J Rheumatol.* 2005;32:1336-1340.

122. Wysenbeck AJ, Nor F, Lurie Y, *et al.* Impramine for the treatment of fibrositis: a therapeutic trial. *Ann Rheum Dis.* 1985;44:752-753.

123. Janzen VD, Scudds R. Sphenopalatine blocks in the treatment of pain in fibromyalgia and myofascial pain. *Laryngoscope* 1997;107:1420-1422.

124. Sorensen J, Bengtsson A, Ahlner J, *et al*. Fibromyalgia: are there different mechanisms in the processing of pain: A double blind crossover comparison of analgesic drugs. *J Rheumatol.* 1997;24:1615-1621.

125. Hannonen P, Malminiemi K, Yli-Kerttula U, *et al*. A randomized double-blind placebo-controlled study of moclobemide and amitriptyline in the treatment of fibromyalgia in females without psychiatric disorder. *Brit J Rheumatol.* 1998;37:1279-1286.

126. Yunus MB, Masi AT, Aldag JC. Short term effects of ibuprofen in primary fibromyalgia syndrome: a double blind, placebo controlled trial. *J Rheumatol.* 1989;16:527-532.

126b Russell IJ, Fletcher EM, Michalek JE, *et al*. Treatment of primary fibrositis/ fibromyalgia syndrome with ibuprofen and alprazolam: a double-blind, placebo-controlled study. *Arthritis Rheum.* 1991;34:552-560.

126c. Goldenberg DL, Felson DT, Dinerman H. A randomized controlled trial of amitriptyline and naproxen in the treatment of patients with fibromyalgia. *Arthritis Rheum.* 1986;29:1371-1377.

127. Quijada-Carrera J, Valenzuela-Castano A, Povedano-Gomez J, *et al*. Comparison of tenoxicam and bromazepan in the treatment of fibromyalgia: a randomized, double-blind, placebo-controlled trial. *Pain* 1996;65:221-225.

128. Clark S, Tindall E, Bennett RM. A double-blind crossover trial of prednisone versus placebo in the treatment of fibrositis. *J Rheumatol.* 1985;12:980-983.

129. Jones KD, Burckhardt CS, Deodhar AA, *et al*. A six-month randomized controlled trial of exercise and pyridostigmine in the treatment of fibromyalgia. *Arthritis Rheum.* 2008;58:612-622.

130. Hidalgo J, Rico-Villademoros F, Calandre EP. An open-label study of quetiapine in the treatment of fibromyalgia. *Prog Neuropsychopharmacol Biol Psychiatry.* 2007;31:71-77.

130b. Calandre EP, Morillas-Arques P, Rodriguez-Lopez CM *et al*. Pregabalin augmentation of quetiapine therapy in the treatment of fibromyalgia:an open-label, prospective trial. *Pharmacopsychiatry* 2007;40:68-71.

131. Olin R, Klein R, Berg PA. A randomized double-blind 16 week study of ritanserin in fibromyalgia syndrome: clinical outcome and analysis of autoantibodies to serotonin, gangliosides and phospholipids. *Clin Rheum.* 1998;17:89-94.

132. Norregaard J *et al*. A randomized controlled trial of citalopram in the treatment of fibromyalgia. *Pain* 1995;61:445-449.

133. Wolfe F, Cathey MA, Hawley DJ. A double-blind placebo controlled trial of fluoxetine in fibromyalgia. *Scand J Rheumatol.* 1994;23:255-259.

134. Zijsltra TR *et al*. *Arthritis Rheum.* 2002;46:S105.

135. Kendall SA, Schaadt ML, Graff LB, *et al*. No effect of antiviral (valacyclovir) treatment in fibromyalgia: a double blind, randomized study. *J Rheumatol.* 2004;31:783-784.

136. Fitzcharles MA, Esdaile JM. Nonphysician practitioner treatments and fibromyalgia Moldofsky H, Lue FA, Mously C, Roth-Schechter B, Reynolds WJ. The effect of Zolpidem in patients with fibromyalgia: a dose ranging, double blind, placebo controlled, modified crossover study. *J Rheumatol.* 1996;23:529-533.

136b Gronblad M, Nykanen J, Donttinen J, *et al*. Effect of zopiclone on sleep quality,   morning stiffness, widespread tenderness and pain and general discomfort in primary   fibromyalgia patients. A double-blind randomized trial. *Clin Rheumatol.* 1993;12:186-   191.

137. syndrome. *J Rheumatol.* 1997;24:937-940.

138. Nicassio PM, Schuman C, Kim J, *et al*. Psychosocial factors associated with complementary treatment use in fibromyalgia. *J Rheumatol.* 1997;24:2008-2013.

139. Dimmock S, Troughton PR, Bird HA. Factors predisposing to the resort of complementary therapies in patients with fibromyalgia. *Clin Rheumatol.* 1996;15:478-482.

140. Jokic M. University of Toronto, 4th year Human Biology HMB499 Research Project report. 2004;23-26.

141. Eisenberg DM, Davis RB, Ettner SL, *et al*. Trends in alternative medicine use in the United States, 1990-1997. *JAMA* 1998;280:1569-1575.

142. Busch AJ, Barber KA, Overend TJ, Peloso PM, Schachter CL. Exercise for treating fibromyalgia syndrome. *Cochrane Database Syst Rev.* 2007;4:CD003786.

143. Burckhardt CS, Mannerkorpi K, Hedenberg L, Bjelle A. A randomized controlled trial of education and physical training for women with fibromyalgia. *J Rheumatol.* 1994;21:714-720.

144. Richards SC, Scott DL. Prescribed exercise in people with fibromyalgia: parallel group randomized controlled trial. *BMJ* 2002;325:185.

145. Martin L, Nutting A, MacIntosh BR, *et al.* An exercise program in the treatment of fibromyalgia. *J Rheumatol.* 1996;23:1050-1053.

146. Wigers SH, Stiles TC, Vogel PA. Effects of aerobic exercise versus stress management in fibromyalgia. A 4.5 year prospective study. *Scand J Rheumatol.* 1996;25:77-86.

147. Rooks DS, Gautam S, Romeling M, *et al.* Group exercise, education and combination self-management in women with fibromyalgia: a randomized trial. *Arch Intern Med.* 2007;167:2192-2200.

148. Mannerkorpi K, Nyberg B, Ahlmen M, Ekdahl C. Pool exercise combined with an exercise program for patients with fibromyalgia syndrome. A prospective randomized study. *J Rheumatol.* 2000;27:2473-2481.

149. Cedraschi C, Desmeules J, Rapiti E, *et al.* Fibromyalgia: a randomized, controlled trial of a treatment programme based on self management. *Ann Rheum Dis.* 2004;63:290-296.

150. Munguia-Izauierdo D, Legaz-Arrese A. Assessment of the effects of aquatic therapy on global symptomatology in patients with fibromyalgia syndrome: a randomized controlled trial. *Arch Phys Med Rehabil.* 2008;89:2250-2257.

151. Mannerkorpi K, Nordeman L, Ericsson A, Arndorw M; GAU Study Group. Pool exercise for patients with fibromyalgia or chronic widespread pain: a randomized controlled trial and subgroup analyses. *J Rehabil Med.* 2009;41:751-760.

152. Ammer K, Melnizky P. Medicinal baths for treatment of generalized fibromyalgia. *Forschende Komplementarmedizin.* 1999;6:80-85.

152b Karagulle MZ, Karagulle M. Balneotherapy and spa therapy of rheumatic diseases in Turkey: a systematic review. *Forsch Komplementarmed Klass Naturheilkd.* 2004;11: 33-41. [German].

153. Gunther V, Mur E, Kinigadner U, Miller C. Fibromyalgia: the effect of relaxation and hydrogalvanic bath therapy on the subjective pain experience. *Clinical Rheumatol.* 1994;13:573-578.

154. Ardia F, Ozgen M, Aybek H, *et al.* Effects of balneotherapy on serum IL-1, PGE2 and LTB4 levels in fibromyalgia patients. *Rheumatol Int.* 2007;27:441-446.

155. Gur A, Karakoc M, Nas K, *et al.* Efficacy of low power laser therapy in fibromyalgia: a single-blind, placebo-controlled trial. *Lasers Med Sci.* 2002;17:57-61.

156. Gur A, Karakoc M, Nas K, *et al.* Effects of low power laser and low dose amitriptyline therapy on clinical symptoms and quality of life in fibromyalgia. *Rheumatol Int.* 2002;22:188-193.

157. Rooks DS, Silverman CB, Kantrowitz FG. The effects of progressive strength training and aerobic exercise on muscle strength and cardiovascular fitness in women with fibromyalgia: a pilot study. *Arthritis Care & Research.* 2002;47:22-28.

158. Bircan C, Karasel SA, Akgün B, El O, Alper S. Effects of muscle strengthening versus aerobic exercise program in fibromyalgia. *Rheumatol Int.* 2008;28:527-532.

159. Hakkinen A, Hakkinen K, Hannonen P, Alen M. Strength training induced adaptations in neuromuscular function of premenopausal women with fibromyalgia: comparison with healthy women. *Ann Rheum Dis.* 2001;60:21-26.

159b. Tomas-Carus P, Gusi N, Häkkinen A, Häkkinen K, Raimundo A, Ortega-Alonso A. Improvements of muscle strength predicted benefits in HRQOL and postural balance in women with fibromyalgia: an 8-month randomized controlled trial. *Rheumatology (Oxford).* 2009;48:1147-1151.

160. Kaada B. Treatment of fibromyalgia by low-frequency transcutaneous nerve stimulation stimulation. *Tidsskrift for Den Norske Laegeforening.* 1989;109:2992-2995. [Norwegian].

161. Matsutani LA, Marques AP, Ferreira EA, Assumpção A, Lage LV, Casarotto RA, Pereira CA. Effectiveness of muscle stretching exercises with and without laser therapy at tender points for patients with fibromyalgia. *Clin Exp Rheumatol.* 2007;25:410-415.

161b Thorsen H, Gam AN, Jensen H, *et al.* Low energy laser treatment effect in localized fibromyalgia in the neck and shoulder regions. *Ugeskrift for Laeger.* 1991;153:1801-1804. [Danish].

162. Ambrogio N, Cuttiford J, Lineker S, Li L. A comparison of three types of neck support in fibromyalgia patients. *Arthritis Care & Research.* 1998;11:405-410.

163. Thomas AW, Graham K, Prato FS *et al.* A randomized, double-blind, placebocontrolled clinical trial using a low-frequency magnetic field in the treatment of musculoskeletal chronic pain. *Pain Res Manag.* 2007;12:249-258.

163b Pearl SJ, Lue F, MacLean AW, *et al.* The effects of bright light treatment on the symptoms of fibromyalgia. *J Rheumatol.* 1996;23:896-902.

164. Carli G, Suman AL, Biasi G, Marcolongo R. Reactivity to superficial and deep stimuli in patients with chronic musculoskeletal pain. *Pain* 2002;100:259-269.

165. Berglund B, Harju EL, Kosek E, Lindblom U. Quantitative and qualitative perceptual analysis of cold dysesthesia and hyperalgesia in fibromyalgia. *Pain* 2002;96:177-187.

166. Ko GD, Berbrayer D. Effect of ceramic-impregnated "thermoflow" gloves on patients with Raynaud's syndrome: randomized placebo-controlled study. *Altern Med Rev.* 2002;7:327-334.

167. Hadhazy VA, Ezzo J, Creamer P, Berman BM. Mind-body therapies for the treatment of fibromyalgia. A systematic review. *J Rheumatol.* 2000;27:2911-2918.

167b. Williams DA, Cary MA, Groner KH, *et al.* Improving physical functional status in patients with fibromyalgia: a brief cognitive behavioral intervention. *J Rheumatol.* 2002;29:1280-1286.

168. Redondo JR, Justo CM, Moraleda FV, *et al.* Long-term efficacy of therapy in patients with fibromyalgia: a physical exercise-based program and a cognitive-behavioral approach. Arthritis Rheum. 2004;51:184-192.

169. Bennett R, Nelson D. Cognitive behavioral therapy for fibromyalgia. *Nat Clin Pract Rheumatol.* 2006;2:416-424.

170. Bennett RM, Burckhardt CS, Clark SR, *et al.* Group treatment of fibromyalgia: a 6 month outpatient program. *J Rheumatol.* 1996;23:521-528.

171. Keel PJ, Bodoky C, Gerhard U, Muller W. Comparison of integrated group therapy and group relaxation training for fibromyalgia. *Clin J Pain.* 1998;14:232-238.

172. Haanen HC, Hoenderdos HT, van Romunde LK *et al.* Controlled trial of hypnotherapy in the treatment of refractory fibromyalgia. *J Rheumatol.* 1991;18:72-75.

173. Grondahl JR, Rosvold EO. Hypnosis as a treatment of chronic widespread pain in general practice: a randomized controlled pilot trial. *BMC Musculoskelet Disord.* 2008;9:124.

174. Kaplan KH, Goldenberg DL, Galvin-Nadeau M. The impact of a meditation-based stress reduction program on fibromyalgia. *Gen Hosp Psychiatry.* 1993;15:284-289.

174b Grossman P, Tiefenthaler-Gilmer U, Raysz A, Kesper U. Mindfulness training as an intervention for fibromyalgia: evidence of postintervention and 3-year follow-up benefits in well-being. *Psychother Psychosom.* 2007;76:226-233.

174C Sephton SE, Salmon P, Weissbecker I, *et al.* Mindfulness meditation alleviates depressive symptoms in women with fibromyalgia: results of a randomized clinical trial. *Arthritis Rheum.* 2007;57:77-85.

175. Bramwell B, Ferguson S, Scarlett N, Macintosh A. The use of ascorbigen in the treatment of fibromyalgia patients: a preliminary trial. *Altern Med Rev.* 2000;5:455-462.

176. Lister RE. An open, pilot study to evaluate the potential benefits of coenzyme Q10 combined with Ginkgo biloba extract in fibromyalgia syndrome. *J Int Med Res.* 2002;30:195-199.

177. Fisher P, Greenwood A, Huskisson EC, *et al.* Effect of homeopathic treatment in fibrositis (primary fibromyalgia). *Br Med J.* 1989;299:365-366.

178. Gemmell HA, Jacobson BH, Banfield K. Homeopathic rhus toxicodendron in the treatment of fibromyalgia. *Chiropr J Aust.* 1991;21:2-6.

179. Bell IR, LewisII DA, Brooks AJ, *et al.* Improved clinical status in fibromyalgia patients treated with individualized homeopathic remedies versus placebo. *Rheumatology* 2004;43:577-582.

180. Teitelbaum J, Bird B, Greenfield R, *et al.* Effective treatment of chronic fatigue syndrome and fibromyalgia: a randomized, double-blind, placebo-controlled, intent to treat study. *J Chronic Fatigue Syndrome.* 2001;8.

181. Ali A, Njike VY, Northrup V *et al.* Intravenous micronutrient therapy (Myers' Cocktail) for fibromyalgia: a placebo-controlled pilot study. *J Altern Complement Med.* 2009;15:247-257.

182. Ozgocmen S, *et al.* Effect of omega-3 fatty acids in the management of fibromyalgia syndrome. *Int J Clin Pharmacol Therap.* 2000;38:362-363.

183. Ko G, Nowacki N, Arseneau L, Eitel M, Hum A. Omega 3 fatty acids for neuropathic pain: case series. *Clin J Pain.* 2010;26:168-172.

184. Volkmann H, Norregaard J, Jacobsen S, *et al*. Double-blind, placebo-controlled cross-over study of intravenous S-adenosyl-L-methionine in patients with fibromyalgia. *Scand J Rheumatol.* 1997;26:206-211.

185. Jacobsen S, Danneskiold-Samsoe B, Andersen RB. Oral S-adenosylmethionine in primary fibromyalgia. Double-blind clinical evaluation. *Scand J Rheumatol.* 1991;20:294-302.

186. Russell IJ, Michalek JE, Flechas JD, Abraham GE. Treatment of fibromyalgia syndrome with Super Malic: a randomized, double blind, placebo controlled, crossover pilot study. *J Rheumatol.* 1995;22:953-958.

187. Romano TJ, Stiller JW. Usefulness of topical methyl salicylate, camphor, and menthol lotion in relieving pain in fibromyalgia syndrome patients. *Amer J Pain Management.* 1994;4172-174.

188. Mathias BJ, Dililngham TR, Zeigler DN, *et al*. Topical capsaicin for chronic neck pain: a pilot study. *Am J Phys Rehabil.* 1995;74:39-44.

189. Ko GD, Hum A, Traitses G, Berbrayer D. Effects of topical O24 essential oils on patients with Fibromyalgia syndrome: a randomized, placebo-controlled pilot study. *J Musculoskel Pain.* 2007;15:11-20.

190. Kaartinen K, Lammi K, Hypen M, *et al*. Vegan diet alleviates fibromyalgia symptoms. *Scand J Rheumatol.* 2000;29:308-313.

191. Deluze C, Bosia L, Zirbs A, *et al*. Electroacupuncture in fibromyalgia: results of a controlled trial. *Br Med J.* 1992;305:1249-1252.

191b Berman BM, Ezzo J, Hadhazy V, Swyers JP. Is acupuncture effective in the treatment of fibromyalgia? Evidence-based clinical review. *J Fam Pract* 1999;48:213-218.

191c Sprott H, Frank S, Hein G. Pain treatment of fibromyalgia by acupuncture. *Rheumatology International.* 1998;18:35-36.

192. Singh BB, Wu WS, Hwang SH, *et al*. Effectiveness of acupuncture in the treatment of fibromyalgia. *Altern Ther Health Med.* 2006;12:34-41.

193. Martin DP, Sletten CD, Williams BA, Berger IH. Improvement in fibromyalgia symptoms with acupuncture: results of a randomized controlled trial. *Mayo Clin Proc.* 2006;81:749-757.

194. Biasi G, Badii F, Magaldi M,*et al*. A new approach to the treatment of fibromyalgia syndrome. The use of Telo Cypro. *Minerva Medica.* 1999;90:39-43.

195. Lichtbroun AS, Raicer MM, Smith RB. The treatment of fibromyalgia with cranial electrotherapy stimulation. *J Clin Rheumatol.* 2001;7:72-78.

195b Fregni F, Gimenes R, Valle AC, *et al*. A randomized, sham-controlled, proof of principle study of transcranial direct current stimulation for the treatment of pain in fibromyalgia. *Arthritis Rheum.* 2006;54:3988-3998.

195c Sampson SM, Rome JD, Rummans TA. Slow-frequency rTMS reduces fibromyalgia pain. *Pain Med.* 2006;7:115-118.

196. Bach GL, Clement DB. Efficacy of Farabloc as an analgesic in primary fibromyalgia. *Clin Rheumatol.* 2007;26:405-410.

197. Alfano AP, Taylor AG, Foresman PA, *et al*. Static magnetic fields for treatment of fibromyalgia: a randomized controlled trial. *J Altern Compl Med.* 2001;7:53-64.

198. Buckelew SP, Conway R, Parker J, *et al*. Biofeedback / relaxation training and exercise interventions for fibromyalgia: a prospective trial. *Arthritis Care & Research.* 1998;11:196-209.

199. Sarnoch H, Adler F, Scholz OB. Relevance of muscular sensitivity, muscular activity and cognitive variables for pain reduction associated with EMG biofeedback in fibromyalgia. *Perceptual & Motor Skills.* 1997;84:1043-1050.

199b Ferraccioli G, ghirelli L, Scita F, *et al*. EMG-biofeedback training in fibromyalgia syndrome. *J Rheumatol.* 1987;14:820-825.

200. van Santen M, Bolwijn P, Verstappen F, *et al*. A randomized clinical trial comparing fitness and biofeedback training versus basic treatment in patients with fibromyalgia. *J Rheumatol.* 2002;29:575-581.

201. Drexler AR, Mur EJ, Gunther VC. Efficacy of an EMG-biofeedback therapy in fibromyalgia patients. A comparative study of patients with and without abnormality in [MMPI] psychological scales. *Clin Exp Rheumatol.* 2002;20:677-682.

202. Mueller HH, Donaldson CCS, Nelson DV, Layman M. Treatment of fibromyalgia incorporating EEG-driven stimulation: a clinical outcomes study. *J Clin Psychol.* 2001;57:933-953.

203. Usui C, Doi N, Nishioka M, *et al*. Electroconvulsive therapy improves severe pain associated with fibromyalgia. *Pain* 2006;121:276-280.

204. Blunt KL, Rajwani MH, Guerriero RC. The effectiveness of chiropractic management of fibromyalgia patients: a pilot study. *J Manipulative & Physiological Therapeutics*. 1997;20:389-399.

204b Schneider M, Vernon H, Ko G, *et al*. Chiropractic management of fibromyalgia syndrome: a systematic review of the literature. *J Manipulative Physiol Ther*. 2009;32:25-40.

205. Field T, Diego M, Cullen C, *et al*. Fibromyalgia pain and substance P decrease and sleep improves after massage therapy. *J Clin Rheumatol*. 2002;8:72-76.

206. Gamber RG, Shores JH, Russo DP, Jimenez C, Rubin BR. Osteopathic manipulative treatment in conjunction with medication relieves pain associated with fibromyalgia syndrome: results of a randomized clinical pilot project. *J Am Osteopath Assoc*. 2002;102:321-325.

207. Citak-Karakaya I, Akbayrak T, Demirtark F, *et al*. Short and long-term results of connective tissue manipulation and combined ultrasound therapy in patients with fibromyalgia. *J Manipulative Physiol Ther*. 2006;29:524-528.

208. Reeves KD. Treatment of consecutive severe fibromyalgia patients with prolotherapy. *J Orthopaedic Medicine*. 1994;16:84-89.

209. Haak T, Scott B. The effect of Qigong on Fibromyalgia: A controlled randomized study. *Disabil Rehabil*. 2007;Jun 15:1-9.

210. Ko GD, Berbrayer D. Complementary and alternative medicine: Canadian physiatrists' attitudes and behavior. *Arch Phys Med Rehabil*. 2000;81:662-667.

211. Bennett RM, Friend R, Jones KD, *et al*. The revised fibromyalgia impact questionnaire [FIQR]: validation and psychometric properties. *Arthritis Res Ther*. 2009;11:R120.

212. Helfgott SM, Kieval RL. Polymyalgia rheumatica in patients with a normal erythrocyte sedimentation rate. *Arthritis Rheum*. 1996;39:304-307.

213. Middleton GD, McFarlin JE, Lipsky PE. The prevalence and clinical impact of fibromyalgia in systemic lupus erythematosus. *Arthritis Rheum*. 1994;37:1181-1188.

214. Fitzcharles MA, Boulos P. Inaccuracy in the diagnosis of fibromyalgia syndrome: analysis of referrals. *Rheumatology (Oxford)*. 2003;42:263-267.

215. Heffez DS, Ross RE, Shade-Zeldow Y, *et al*. Clinical evidence for cervical myelopathy due to Chiari malformation and spinal stenosis in a nonrandomized group of patients with fibromyalgia. *Eur Spine J*. 2004;13:516-523.

216. Chaudhuri A, Behan PO. Fatigue in neurological disorders. *Lancet* 2004;363:978-988.

217. Carville SF, Arendt-Nielsen S, Bliddal H, *et al*. EULAR, EULAR evidence-based recommendations for the management of fibromyalgia syndrome. *Ann Rheum Dis*. 2008;67:536-541.

218. Markowitz JS, Patrick KS. Venlafaxine-tramadol similarities. *Medical Hypotheses*. 1998;51:167-168.

219. Wedge MK. The truth behind tramadol and antidepressants: an interaction of concern? *Can Pharm J*. 2009;142:71-73.

220. Harris RE, Clauw DJ, Scott DJ, *et al*. Decreased central mu-opioid receptor availability in fibromyalgia. *J Neuroscience*. 2007;27:10000-10006.

221. Ko GD, Wine W. Chronic pain and cannabinoids. *Practical Pain Management*. 2005;5:28-39.

222. Badgley LE. Disordered sacroiliac joint pain. *Practical Pain Management*. 2009;9:17-19.

223. Vleeming A, Snijders CJ, Stoeckart R, *et al*. The role of the sacroiliac joints in coupling between spine, pelvis, legs and arms. In: Vleeming A, Monney V, Dorman T, Snijders C, Stoeckart R, eds. *Movement, Stability and Low Back Pain*. Edinburgh: Churchill Livingstone;1997.

224. Lee, DG. *The Pelvic Girdle – An Approach to the Examination and Treatment of the Lumbopelvic-Hip Region*. 3rd ed. Toronto; Churchill Livingstone; 2004.

225. Ko G. Prolotherapy: a shot against chronic pain. *Parkhurst Exchange*. 2008;105:67-70.

226. Dorman T. Pelvic mechanics and prolotherapy. In: Vleeming A, Monney V, Dorman T, Snijders C, Stoeckart R, eds. *Movement, Stability, and Low Back Pain: The Essential Role of the Pelvis*. New York, NY: Churchill Livingstone; 1997:501-522.

227. Hackett GS. *Ligament and Tendon Relaxation Treated by Prolotherapy*, 3rd Edition. Illinois: Hemwall G Institute; 1958.

228. Yelland M, Glasziou P, Bogduk N, *et al*. Randomised controlled trial of prolotherapy injections, saline injections and exercises in the treatment of chronic low back pain. *Spine* 2004;29:9-16.

229. Bogduk N. Management of chronic low back pain. *Med J Aust*. 2004;180:79-83.

230. Sampson S, Gerhardt M, Mandelbaum B. Platelet rich plasma injection grafts for musculoskeletal injuries: a review. *Curr Rev Musculoskelet Med.* 2008;1:165-174.
231. Mishra A, Woodall J Jr, Vieira A. Treatment of tendon and muscle using platelet-rich plasma. *Clin Sports Med.* 2009;28:113-125.
232. DeVos RJ, Weir A, VanSchie HTM, *et al.* Platelet-rich plasma injection for chronic Achilles tendinopathy: a randomized controlled trial. *JAMA* 2010;303:144-149.
233. Peerbooms JC, Sluimer J, Bruijn DJ, Gosens T. Positive effect of an autologous platelet concentrate in lateral epicondylitis in a double-blind randomized controlled trial: platelet-rich plasma versus corticosteroid injection with a 1-year follow-up. *Am J Sports Med.* 2010;38:255-262.
234. Alderman D, Sweeting RC. Prolotherapy for sacroiliac joint laxity. *Practical Pain Management* 2009(May): 44-46.
235. Ko GD, Whitmore S, Hein T, Tsai M, Lawson G, MacDonald R. Case series of low back pain patients with sacroiliac joint laxity effectively treated with platelet-rich plasma. *Clin J Pain* 2010 [In press].
236. Monastra VJ, Monastra D, George S. The effects of stimulant therapy, EEG Biofeedback, and parenting style on the primary symptoms of attention deficit hyperactivity disorder. *Applied Psychophysiology & Biofeedback.* 2002;27:231-249.
237. Martinez-Lavin, M, Hermosillo AG, Rosas M, Soto ME. Circadian studies of autnomic nervous balance in patients with fibromyalgia: a heart rate variability analysis. *Arthritis Rheum.* 1998;41P:1966-1971.
238. Ko GD, Whitmore S, Gottfried B, *et al.* Fibromyalgia/ Chronic Pain syndrome:an Alternative Medicine perspective. *Critical Reviews in Physical and Rehabilitation Medicine.* 2005;17:1-30.
239. Corrado P, Gottlieb H, Abdelhamid MH. The effect of biofeedback and relaxation training on anxiety and somatic complaints in chronic pain patients. *Amer J Pain Management.* 2003;13:133-139.
240. Ferrari R, Fipaldini E, Birbaumer N. Individual characteristics and results of biofeedback training and operant treatment in patients with chronic pain. *Psicoterapia Cognitiva e Comportamentale.* 2006;12:161-179.
241. Hassett AL, Radvanski DC, Vaschillo EG, *et al.* A pilot study of the efficacy of heart rate variability (HRV) biofeedback in patients with fibromyalgia. *Applied Psychophysiology and Biofeedback.* 2007;32:1-10.
242. Thornton K. Improvement/rehabilitation of memory functioning with neurotherapy/QEEG biofeedback. *Journal of Head Trauma Rehabilitation.* 2000;15:1285-1296.
243. Raymond J, Varney C, Parkinson LA, Gruzelier JH. The effects of alpha/theta neurofeedback on personality and mood. *Brain Res Cogn Brain Res.* 2005;23:287-292.
244. Glass JM, Review of cognitive dysfunction in fibromyalgia: A Convergence on Working Memory and Attentional Control Impairments. *Rheum Dis Clin North Am.* 2009;35:299-311.
245. Wolak T, Weitzman S, Harman-Boehm I, *et al.* Prevalence of fibromyalgia in type 2 diabetes mellitus. *Harefuah* 2001;140:1006-1009,1119-11120.
246. Ostuni P, Botsios C, Sfriso P, *et al.* Fibromyalgia in Italian patients with primary Sjogren's syndrome. *Joint Bone Spine.* 2002;69:51-57.
247. Puri BK. The use of eicosapentaenoic acid in the treatment of chronic fatigue syndrome. *Prostaglandins Leukot Essent Fatty Acids.* 2004;70:399-401.
248. Plotnikoff GA, Quigley JM. Prevalence of severe hypovitaminosis D in patients with persistent, nonspecific musculoskeletal pain. *Mayo Clin Proc.* 2003;78:1463-1470.
249. Huisman AM, White KP, Algra A, *et al.* Vitamin D levels in women with systemic lupus erythematosus and fibromyalgia. *J Rheumatol.* 2001;28:2535-2539.
250. St. Amand RP, Marek CC. *What Your Doctor May Not Tell You About Fibromyalgia.* New York, NY: Warner Books; 1999.
251. St. Amand RP, Potter C. The use of uricosuric agents in fibromyalgia: theory, practice, and a rebuttal to the Oregon study of guaifenesin treatment. *Clin Bull Myofascial Therapy.* 1997;2:5-12.
252. Zhou Q, Zhang B, Verne GN. Intestinal membrane permeability and hypersensitivity in the irritable bowel syndrome. *Pain* 2009;146:41-46.
253. Noback S, Johansson ML, Molin G, *et al.* Alteration of intestinal microflora is associated with reduction in abdominal bloating and pain in patients with irritable bowel syndrome. *Amer J Gastroenterology.* 2000;95:1231-1238.

254. Bensoussan A, Talley NJ, Hing M, *et al*. Treatment of irritable bowel syndrome with chinese herbal medicine: a randomized controlled trial. *JAMA* 1998;280:1585-1589.

255. Rousseaux C, Thuru X, Gelot Z, *et al*. Lactobacillus acidophilus modulates intestinal pain and induces opioid and cannabinoid receptors. *Nat Med*. 2007;13:35-37.

256. Rigden S, Barrager E, Bland JS. Evaluation of the effect of a modified entero-hepatic resuscitation program in chronic fatigue syndrome patients. *Functional Medicine Research Report*. 1997;103:1-11.

257. Bennett RM, Jones J, Turk DC, *et al*. An internet survey of 2596 people with fibromyalgia. *BMC Musculoskel Disorders*. 2007;8:27-38.

258. Rossini M, Di Munno O, Valentini G, *et al*. Double-blind, multicenter trial comparing acetyl l-carnitine with placebo in the treatment of fibromyalgia patients. *Clin Exp Rheumatol*. 2007;25:182-188.

259. Xu Y, *et al*. Curcumin reverses the effects of chronic stress on behavior, the HPA axis, BDNF expression and phosphorylation of CREB. *Brain Research*. 2006;1122:56-64.

260. Bell IR, Baldwin CM, Schwartz GE. Illness from low levels of environmental chemicals: relevance to chronic fatigue syndrome and fibromyalgia. *Am J Med*. 1998;105(Suppl 3A):74S-82S.

261. Lamb JJ. A case study evaluating the effects of a medical food program for liver detoxification in a patient with fibromyalgia. *Metagenics Inc*. 2007; May:119FM507.

262. Kostova-Dinkova, AT, *et al*. Extremely potent triterpenoid inducers of the phase 2 response: Correlations of protection against oxidant and inflammatory stress. *PNAS* 2005;102:4585-4589.

263. Kotter I, *et al*. Mercury exposure from dental amalgam fillings in the etiology of primary fibromyalgia: a pilot study. *J Rheumatol*. 1995;22:2194-2195.

264. Sato M, Kondoh M. Recent studies on metallothionein: protection against toxicity of heavy metals and oxygen free radicals. *Tohoku J Exp Med*. 2002;196:9-22.

265. Teitelbaum JE, St. Cyr JA, Johnson C. The use of D-ribose in chronic fatigue syndrome and fibromyalgia: a pilot study. *J Alternative Complementary Med*. 2006;12:857-862.

266. Gordon ML. *The Clinical Application of Interventional Endocrinology*. Beverly Hill, CA: Phoenix Books Inc.

267. Cook DM, Yuen KCJ, Biller BMK, *et al*. American Association of Clinical Endocrinologists medical guidelines for clinical practice for growth hormone use in growth hormone-deficient adults and transition patients—2009 update. *Endocrine Practice*. 2009;15(Suppl2):1-29.

268. Hwang SW, Colantonio A, Chiu S, *et al*. The effect of traumatic brain injury on the health of homeless people. *CMAJ* 2008;179:779-784.

269. Aimaretti G, *et al*. Hypopituitarism and growth hormone deficiency after traumatic brain injury. *Growth Horm IGF Res*. 2004;14(SupplA):S114-117.

270. Powner DJ, Boccalandro C. Adrenal insufficiency following traumatic brain injury in adults. *Curr Opin Crit Care*. 2008;14:163-166.

271. Schneider HJ, *et al*. Prevalence of anterior pituitary insufficiency 3 and 12-months after traumatic brain injury. *Eur J Endocrinol*. 2006;154:259-265.

272. Singh M. Mechanisms of progesterone-induced neuroprotection. *Ann N Y Acad Sci*. 2005;1052:145-151.

273. Teitelbaum J, Bird B, Greenfield R, *et al*. Effective treatment of chronic fatigue syndrome and fibromyalgia: a randomized, double-blind, placebo-controlled, intent to treat study. *J Chronic Fatigue Syndrome*. 2001;8:3-24.

274. Burckhardt CS, O'Reilly CA, Bennett RM, *et al*. Assessing depression in fibromyalgia patients. *Arthritis Care Res*. 1994;7:35-39.

275. Panerai AE, Vecchiet J, Panzeri P, *et al*. Peripheral blood mononuclear cell beta-endorphin concentration is decreased in chronic fatigue syndrome and fibromyalgia but not in depression. *Clin J Pain*. 2002;18:270-273.

276. Giesecke T, Gracely RH, *et al*. The relationship between depression, chronic pain and experimental pain in a chronic pain cohort. *Arthritis Rheum*. 2005;52:1577-1584.

277. Gracely RH, Geisser ME, Giesecke T, *et al*. Pain catastrophizing and neural responses to pain among persons with fibromyalgia. *Brain* 2004;127:835-843.

278. Mailis A, Papagapiou M, Umana M, Cohodarevic T, *et al*. Unexplainable non-dermatomal somatosensory deficits in patients with chronic non-malignant pain in the context of litigation/compensation: a role for involvement of central factors? *J Rheumatol*. 2001;28:1385-1393.

279. Elder CL, Dahners LE, Weinhold PS. A cyclooxygenase-2 inhibitor impairs ligament healing in the rat. *Amer J Sports Med.* 2001;29:801-805.
280. Farrar JT, Young JP, LaMoreaux L, *et al.* Clinical importance of changes in chronic pain intensity measured on an 11-point numerical pain rating scale. *Pain* 2001;94:149-158.
281. White KP, Harth M. An analytical review of 24 controlled clinical trials for fibromyalgia syndrome. *Pain* 1996;64:211-219.
282. Hudson JI, Goldenberg DL, Pope HG, *et al.* Comorbidity of fibromyalgia with medical and psychiatric disorders. *Amer J Med.* 1992;92:363-367.
283. Lapossy E, Maleitzke R. Hrycaj P, *et al.* The frequency of transition of chronic low back pain to fibromyalgia. *Scand J Rheumatol.* 1995;24:29-33.
284. Huppe A, Brockow T, Raspe H. Chronic widespread pain and tender points in low back pain: a population-based study. *Z Rheumatol.* 2004;63:76-83.
285. McBeth J, Symmons DP, Silman AJ, *et al.* Musculoskeletal pain is associated with a long-term increased risk of cancer and cardiovascular-related mortality. *Rheumatology* 2009;48:74-77.
286. Macfarlane GJ, McBeth J, Silman AJ. Widespread body pain and mortality: prospective population based study. *BMJ* 2001;323:1-5.
287. McBeth J, Silman AJ, Macfarlane GJ. Association of widespread body pain with an increased risk of cancer and reduced cancer survival. *Arthritis Rheum.* 2003;1686-1692.
288. Hsu MC, Harris RE, Sundgren PC, *et al.* No consistent difference in gray matter volume between individuals with fibromyalgia and age-matched healthy subjects when controlling for affective disorder. *PAIN* 2009;143:262-267.
289. Kennedy M, Felson DT. A prospective long-term study of fibromyalgia syndrome. *Arthritis Rheum.* 1996;39:682-685.
290. Cronan TA, Serber ER, Walen HR, Jaffe M. The influence of age on fibromyalgia symptoms. *J Aging Health.* 2002;14:370-384.
291. Busch A, Schachter CL, Peloso PM, Bombardier C. Exercise for treating fibromyalgia syndrome *Cochrane Database Syst Rev.* 2002;3:CD003786.
292. Baumgartner E, Finckh A, Cedraschi C, Vischer TL. A six year prospective study of a cohort of patients with fibromyalgia. *Ann Rheum Dis.* 2002;61:644-645.
293. Wigers SH. Fibromyalgia outcome: the predictive values of symptom duration, physical activity, disability pension, and critical life events: a 4.5 year prospective study. *J Psychosom Res.* 1996;41:235-243.
294. Fitzcharles MA, Costa DD, Poyhia R. A study of standard care in fibromyalgia syndrome: a favorable outcome. *J Rheumatol.* 2003;30:154-159.
295. Turk DC, Okifuji A, Sinclair JD, Starz TW. Interdisciplinary treatment for fibromyalgia syndrome: clinical and statistical significance. *Arthritis Care Res.* 1998;11:186-195.
296. King SJ, Wessel J, Bhambhani Y, *et al.* The effects of exercise and education, individually or combined, in women with fibromyalgia. *J Rheumatol.* 2002;29:2620-2627.
297. Gustafsson M, Ekholm J, Broman L. Effects of a multiprofessional rehabilitation programme for patients with fibromyalgia syndrome. *J Rehabil Med.* 2002;119-127.
298. Yunus MB, Arslan S, Aldag JC. Relationship between fibromyalgia features and smoking. *Scand J Rheumatol.* 2002;31:301-305.
299. Shapiro JR, Anderson DA, Danoff-Burg S. A pilot study of the effects of behavioral weight loss treatment on fibromyalgia symptoms. *J Psychosom Res.* 2005;59:275-282.
300. Assis MR, Silva LE, Alves AM, *et al.* A randomized controlled trial of deep water running: clinical effectiveness of aquatic exercise to treat fibromyalgia. *Arthritis Rheum.* 2006;55:57-65.
301. Evcik D, Yigit I, Pusak H, Kavuncu V. Effectiveness of aquatic therapy in the treatment of fibromyalgia syndrome: a randomized controlled open study. *Rheumatol Int.* 2008;28:885-890.
302. Ernst E. Obstacles in research in complementary and alternative medicine. *Med J Aust.* 2003;179:279-280.
303. van Wilgen CP, Bloten H, Oeseburg B. Results of a multidisciplinary program for patients with fibromyalgia implemented in the primary care. *Disabil Rehabil.* 2007;29:1207-1213.

ABOUT THE AUTHOR

Primary author Dr. Gordon Ko is the medical director for the Fibromyalgia Integrative management clinic at Sunnybrook Health Sciences Centre, University of Toronto and for the Canadian Centre for Integrative Medicine (Markham), where he heads up a multidisciplinary team including pain MDs, EMG (including quantitative sensory testing for neuropathic pain), physiotherapy, chiropractic, naturopathy, osteopathy, biofeedback-psychotherapy. Besides completing residencies in Family practice, Emergency medicine and Physical Medicine & Rehabilitation, he also completed American board certifications in PM&R, IME, Naturopathic Medical Association, Pain Medicine (subspecialty 2004) and Anti-Aging and Regenerative Medicine (diplomate exams 2007). He continues to teach medical students/residents, lecture and author peer-reviewed papers as Associate professor, School of Health and Human Resources, Rutherford University and Lecturer, Division of Physiatry, Department of Medicine, University of Toronto. Dr. Ko has trained over 50 physicians one-on-one in injection (ultrasound/EMG-guided Botox) and pharmacotherapeutic (pregabalin, cannabinoid, opioid) with functional medicine approaches.

Chapter 18
Alternative Therapies in the Treatment of Cardiac Injury: A Case Report with Recovery Regimens for Non-Ablatable Atrial Fibrillation and Greatly Enlarged Left Atrium

Hans J. Kugler, Ph.D.;

with Ulrich Friedrichson, M.D., Ph.D.; Fouad Ghaly, M.D.; and Paul Ward, PED

ABSTRACT

Two side-impact accidents left a 68-year-old patient with a damaged heart for which orthodox medicine had no treatment. This paper details how the multifactorial approach (MFA) –combining key essential requirements for optimum health, with an emphasis on rebuilding the muscles of the heart and the revascularization of regenerated heart muscles – enabled the patient to achieve a full recovery.

Keywords: multifactorial approach; alternative therapies; cardiac injury; left atrium; A-Fib

INTRODUCTION

Patient: 68-year-old Caucasian male, impact-induced (2 severe car accidents) atrial fibrillation (non-reversible; shock, chemical, ablation), left atrium 6.8 (<4.0 is normal), ejection fraction 28% (>50% is normal), 4/6 heart murmur. Besides "three drugs and a pacemaker/defibrillator," mainstream medicine has no treatment protocol for such a patient, and absolutely none for a full recovery. Using the multifactorial approach (MFA) – combining key essential requirements for optimum health, with an emphasis on rebuilding the muscles of the heart and the revascularization of regenerated heart muscles – , we achieved a full recovery. Heart rhythm has been 100% sinus for 3 years now, ejection fraction 80%, left atrium 3.7 (normal again), and 1/6 heart murmur. The key alternative modalities that were combined included: resistance exercise (weight-lifting), organ-specific embryonic cell extracts (heart, mesenchyme, and muscle), EECP (enhanced external counter pulsation), small amounts of human growth hormone (HGH), meditation, breathing techniques, and a number of nutrients that are heart-specific and anti-inflammatory.

Addendum: 62-year-old male patient, extremely poor state of health (bronchitis, poor skin color, congestive heart failure, coronary artery disease, heart irregularities uncontrollable with pacemaker, ejection fraction 18%, on priority list for heart transplant) followed the same recovery protocol in two 4-months segments. He is now off the heart transplant list, his ejection fraction has nearly tripled, his pacemaker now effective, and he is "in good health with lots of smiles" back working on his farm, lifting bails of hay for weight-training exercises.

ALTERNATIVE THERAPIES IN THE TREATMENT OF CARDIAC INJURY: A CASE REPORT
History

In October 2003, while not in motion, the patient's car was impacted on the left by another car. ECG at the accident site had some unusual spikes and the paramedics suggested a follow-up with regular ECG. During the follow-up visit kidney contusion (blood in urine), severe back muscle spasms, and torn tissues in the left shoulder were diagnosed. Heart murmur (4/6) manifested itself a few weeks later. Initial treatment focused on severe muscle spasms and kidney damage. Patient was not put on muscle relaxants because of previous impact-induced heart injuries and atrial fibrillation (A-Fib). Doctor prescribed EECP plus a strong supplementation program.

About 2 years prior to the 2003 accident, the patient was involved in a severe multiple car accident that resulted (besides torn muscles and connective tissues, left shoulder dislocation, and twisted back) in a heart injury resulting in A-Fib, 28% ejection fraction (>50% is normal), left atrium 6.8 (<4.0 is normal). A literature search showed several cases of accident-induced A-Fib; one case pinpointed the car accident as the cause of the A-Fib 3 years after the accident. The A-Fib, which was irreversible with shock or chemical cardioversion, was ablated and the patient stayed in sinus rhythm and was recovering well up to the point of the second car accident.

Just prior to the October 2003 accident:
- An ECG was taken on 9.03.03 which was completely normal (sinus).
- No heart murmur was present.
- No history of chronic A-Fib or any related symptoms prior to the accidents.
- Passed aviation medical 4 weeks prior to the accident.

After the second car accident, the patient's heart condition steadily declined over the next 1½ years. Starting with a "borderline" ECG (11/2003), mini ECGs (printouts while getting EECP treatments) kept deteriorating; heart murmur 4/6 (4 on a scale of 1-6) manifested itself. Various attempts to control A-Fib with single drugs (Coreg, amiodarone) failed; drug combinations were also ineffective. Cardioversion (08/2005) was unsuccessful; sinus rhythm held for only 3 days. Ablation (09.2005) was also unsuccessful; sinus rhythm held for only 5 days.

Following unsuccessful ablation, the patient was advised that nothing else could be done regarding reversing the A-Fib, 4/6 heart murmur, 28% ejection fraction, and left atrium 6.8. Examining doctors judged the second accident as far more serious than the first because of the additional heart murmur and unsuccessful ablation. Patient was advised: "3 to 4 drugs and a pacemaker/defibrillator for the rest of your life."

The patient, who had research experience in the field of aging and the biomedical field,[1-4] and having published studies based on the MFA to optimum health and longevity,[5-8] was unwilling to accept defeat and, after 3 second opinions, consulted with various experts in cardiology and related fields regarding a possible recovery protocol. The most basic advice – "think outside the box!" – required a closer look at what was inside the box, namely pharmaceutical drugs:

- US pharmaceutical drug consumption versus ranking of health world-wide:
  - 1976: Prof. E. Charskin, Alabama University School of Medicine: "U.S. outranked by some third world nations that can't afford pharmaceutical drugs, but that have a climate for agriculture and livestock."
  - 2005: John Abramson, MD, Harvard Medical School, writes that the drop in the US health system ranking (at this time 15th to 23rd worldwide) is inversely proportional to the tremendous increase in pharmaceutical drug consumption.[9]
  - 2008: Prof. Andrew Weil, MD, Arizona School of medicine: US now ranked # 37 in the world – out-done by underdeveloped countries.
- # 1 cause of death in the US is medicine itself; much of this is connected directly to pharmaceutical drug consumption.[10]
- Unnecessary prescribing of $15+ billion of antidepressant drugs annually. Research suggests that depression is caused by a lack of physical activity, and that it can be classified as an exercise deficiency because it is easily treated with an exercise regimen that follows American College of Sports Medicine (ACSM) guidelines. In 2008 the antidepressant drug industry began to admit that treatment of depression is not very effective by recommending the addition of a second drug to treatment regimens. What kind of health care program would agree to people consuming billions of dollars worth of drugs (with potentially severe side effects, including thoughts of suicide) when a simple activity program can eliminate the problem?
- The effectiveness, or lack thereof, of HAART (highly active antiretroviral therapy) drugs. A study of 20,000 European and N-American AIDS patients, showed that taking these drugs for up to 1 year had zero effects on the death rate from AIDS, and that taking these drugs longer than 1 year actually increased the death rate from AIDS.[11] In the light of these data one can only suspect that the $60 to 100 billion drug company profits are the only reasons for keeping the "HIV causes AIDS" hypothesis alive.

These drug data bring to mind an Albert Einstein quote: "The definition of insanity is doing the same thing over and over again and expecting different results."

Leaders in alternative and anti-aging medicine agree that "the regenerative power of a healthy body is immense." According to Professor E Charaskin of Alabama School of Medicine, "health" is defined as a state of homeostasis, determined by at least 60 variables that can be grouped together as essential health practices, including exercise, nutrition, environment (toxins in the body), and stress management. He believes that combining these factors will produce synergistic effects on the overall state of health and recovery

The cardiac experts consulted agreed that the MFA could be the basis for a recovery program. In its most basic form, the MFA acknowledges that combining several positive single modalities will have a bottom-line synergistic effect. All of the modalities incorporated in the heart recovery protocol had previously been tried separately, and with some positive effects. Would combining them give the, synergistically enhanced, hoped for results?

There was also unanimous agreement among the cardiac experts that, for such a recovery protocol to be successful, the heart rhythm must get converted to sinus rhythm, and be kept in sinus rhythm, before the recovery protocol that focuses on rebuilding and strengthening the heart muscles could begin.

Recovery Protocol: The Major Modalities and Reasons for Employing and Combining Them

Cardioversion to restore sinus rhythm (and keep the heart in sinus rhythm) was the critical first stage of treatment. Once this was achieved the patient began the recovery program, this included:

- Cell extracts: A refinement of Dr. Niehans Zelltherapie injectable (5 ml, i.m.), organ-specific extracts (contain low molecular weight peptides, nucleic acids, and growth factors) from embryonic sheep and porcine tissues, combined with oral cell extracts that are available in the US.[12] Injectable mesenchyme has been shown to increase healing,[13] and heart extract has been shown to strengthen the heart and heart rhythms.[14] Ulrich Friedrichson, MD, PhD reported that muscle extract has been shown effective in the recovery of muscle injuries, and in training and muscle development in athletes (personal communication, November 9, 2005).
- Super circuit weight training: Weight training has been shown to increase heart muscle in general, and build atrium walls specifically.[15-18] The weight-training exercise program used was designed by Dr. Paul Ward, PED, Olympic trainer.[15]
- EECP (enhanced external counter pulsation): Left atrium muscle needs to be revascularized if there is any hope of rebuilding it. EECP, besides greatly improving heart functions, has been shown to revascularize heart muscle.[19,20]
- Niacin-based detox: Since rebuilding heart muscle is vital for recovery, estrogen effects and immune suppression, caused by exposure to BPA (bis-phenol-A) and other organic pollutant exposure from plastics was unacceptable. A niacin-based detox program (1½ g of non-flushing niacin taken one hour before inducing sweating) was therefore practiced 2 to 3 times per week.
- Human growth hormone (HGH): 6 mg/month of HGH was used to support for the above modalities.
- Meditation and optimum breathing techniques: There are numerous references in the scientific literature that show a connection with breathing and heart functions.[18,21]
- Nutrition and nutritional supplements: A quality diet – with an emphasis on avoiding trans fats, high-fructose corn syrup, and chemical pollutants – was supported with blueberries, strawberries, and pomegranate juice/concentrate. A basic supplementation program as recommended by Dr. Melvyn Werbach, MD: consisting of B-complex, multi-minerals, antioxidants,[22-24] and extra niacin.[25-27] In addition:
  - Fish oil: Biochemistry of lipid metabolism and anti-inflammatory action show a high priority for fish oil, later supported with data that showed a reduction of arrhythmias with fish oil.[28-30]
  - Acetyl carnitine: Increases the activity of cytochrome oxidase in the heart, and is thus important for mitochondrial energy metabolism.[31-33]
  - Alpha lipoic acid: Important for mitochondrial – high energy output – cell functioning.[34,35]
  - L-Arginine: Metabolized to nitric oxide, a key factor in blood pressure regulation and exercise metabolism.[36-38]
  - Turmeric: The curcumin in turmeric has a demonstrated anti-inflammatory effect, and has been shown to benefit the heart.[39,40]

175

- Vitamin D: Vitamin D deficiency, especially in the light of new (higher) vitamin D requirements, is a risk factor for heart health.[41-43]
- Coenzyme Q10: Protection from oxidative stress, and more, makes Co-Q-10 a key factor in metabolic therapy for heart disease.[44-46]
- Trimethylglycine (TMG): Decreases plasma homocysteine concentrations, increases oxygenation of tissues, and has a corrective effect on the nicotinamide coenzyme and adenine nucleotide content of the tissues.[47-49]

There were two stages to the recovery program – an initial 3-months regimen, followed by a 5-months regimen.

3-Month Treatment Regimen

After chemical cardioversion (1.0 mg ibutilide IV) the patient adhered to the following regimen:

1. To keep the heart in the right (sinus) rhythm (at least for the first weeks of training) the patient took amiodarone and Coreg (carvedilol). Amiodarone: 600 mg/day, reduced to 400 mg/day after 2-weeks, 200 mg/day after 6-weeks, and 0mg/day after 8-weeks. Coreg: 12 mg/day – steadily decreased to 0 mg/day by 3-weeks.
2. Biochemical growth factors and nutritional support:
   a. Cell extract injections: 3 per week – alternating mesenchyme, heart, muscle.
   b. HGH: 5 mg/month, cycling – 1 unit/day for 3-days, then 3-days off.
   c. Overall quality nutrition: Including pomegranate extract, strawberries and blueberries, and a basic supplementation program (B-complex, multi-minerals, antioxidants, niacin). In addition special nutrients: fish oil (4 softgels, 1,200 mg each, BID.), acetyl carnitine (2x 1,000 mg/day), arginine (2x 2,000 mg/day), turmeric (2x 2,500 mg/day), vitamin D3 (3,000 IU/day if 30 minutes of full body sun exposure was possible, otherwise 5,000 IU/day), CoQ10 (2x 120 mg/day), alpha lipoic acid (800 mg/day), TMG (1,000 mg/day).
3. EECP treatment twice per week.
4. Super circuit weight training: At start 3 times/week. 30 minutes each time. Pulse rate in lower range of [60 - 80% of (220 minus age)] maximum. Duration of exercise sessions was increased by 15 minutes each week, to a total work-out period of 2 hours (3 times/week). Heart rate: increase 5 points/week up to a maximum of 110-115. Training supported with long walks and horseback riding.
5. Emphasis on meditation, breathing techniques.

Results

Heart rhythm was 100% sinus during the entire 3-month period. Heart murmur had decreased to 1-2 by the end of the 3-month period. Echocardiogram confirmed recovery success: ejection fraction 60% (up from 28%), left atrium 5.8 (down from 6.8, normal is <4.0), and all other variables in normal range. Patient felt extremely good; exercise capacity is back to near pre-accident level, including jogging, weight-lifting, and horseback riding.

5-Month Follow-Up Regimen

Since EECP and the cell extracts at the treatment level were quite expensive, these two treatment modalities had to be greatly reduced; the recovery regimen (as above) was continued with only one EECP session and one cell extract per week. The cell extracts were gradually reduced and replaced with two types of oral cell extracts: liquid (mesenchyme and thymus, alternating, at a frequency of three 6 ml vials per week) and tablets (15 tablets 2 times/day). These adjustments did not change cardiac performance/output.

After 3-months on this reduced treatment regimen, EECP frequency and injections of the embryonic cell extracts were further reduced to one every two weeks, and were discontinued after the 4th month. All other modalities, oral cell extracts, health practices, nutritional support, and special supplements, were continued as before, for a total of 5 months.

Results

Echocardiogram after the 5-months recovery protocol showed further improvements: ejection fraction 80%, left atrium further improved to 3.7 (now in normal range), and all other variables within normal ranges. Routine examinations, besides confirming the excellent state of health, also recorded a further decrease in the heart murmur to 1-2/6. Patient felt very good, and was maintaining a strong health and fitness approach. Patient had lost 18 lbs of lean body mass in the time following the 2003 accident. However, by following the super-circuit weight training, as developed by Dr. Paul Ward,[14] he had managed to regain 12 lbs of lean body mass by December 07. ECG, blood analysis, and regular examinations have shown him to be fully recovered and in excellent health (also passed two aviation medical examinations).

Addendum

62-year-old male patient in extremely poor state of health – bronchitis, skin color waxy, pale, blood pressure 140/110, edema of lower extremities (2+ mid calf), reduced lung capacity (rhochi and rales), greatly reduced heart capacity (ejection fraction 18%, severe heart irregularities, uncontrollable with pacemaker), on priority list for a heart transplant – followed the above recovery program in two 4-month stages.

Patient's health is greatly improved: good skin color, echocardiogram shows a near tripling of ejection fraction, heart rhythm now controllable with pacemaker, off the heart transplant list, is "in good spirits, with lots of smiles," working on his ranch again, and lifting hay bails as exercise.

DISCUSSION

In previous research projects the MFA[5] yielded excellent results in longevity studies on cancer-prone animals,[6,7] in the reversal of two prostate cancer case histories,[8] and in longevity studies on humans.[50,51] In the heart recovery described above, several of the modalities used had previously been used separately, with good indications. When, after the 2003 accident, all of these modalities were combined correctly, real success was achieved.

An explosion of data, demonstrating the importance of key nutrients in respect to heart health, was published previous to the time when our recovery protocol was designed; some data regarding the importance of these nutrients came from "the horses mouth" even before they were published, and that also included data regarding correct dosages. A good example is vitamin D. After becoming aware of ongoing research that linked vitamin D and heart health, the dose was increased to effectively 7,000 IU/day (including the sunshine-produced vitamin D). Another example is fish oil, which was originally used at a dosage of 2,000 mg/day, was increased to 10 g/day, after becoming aware of data that showed great reductions in arrhythmias and even atrial fibrillation with fish oil use. Similar reasoning led to a reduction in vitamin E (from 400 IU/day to the 100 IU contained in the basic vitamin and mineral supplement).

With high energy-output cells, like those of the heart, mitochondrial functioning is essential – that is why acetyl-carnitine and alpha lipoic acid were included in the regimen. Besides the references quoted above, a Pub Med search for "mitochondrial functioning and heart" will yield nearly 100 references.

Regarding the supplements and other modalities like EECP, cell extracts and weight-training, we stayed on the aggressive side because we were dealing with a serious condition and many experts pointed out that (in their opinion) our chance for success was minimal or non-existent, thus we felt that we had to take our chance with truly aggressive levels. It is important to note that for every modality used and increased to maximum levels, we explored the literature (and consulted experts) to evaluate if the suggested level could do any harm; only when the answer to this question was a clear "no," then the aggressive level was followed. This was one of the reasons why HGH was kept at a lower level.

Can we answer the question: What specifically made this protocol successful? The answer is clear: Synergism via the MFA. Each modality that was incorporated had good science supporting its use – when used in combination, the modalities enhanced each other. The patient's true belief also impacted the effectiveness of all the supplements and modalities – that this *would be a success*, with consistent visualizing of 1) optimum health, 2) passing aviation medicals, and 3) flying bigger and faster airplanes. In essence, he planned tomorrow as if there were no problems at all today; all of his future and specific goals that required health and delivered happiness were seen and felt as a *fait accompli*.

There was one key point of observation, a profound state of feeling well and recovered, which the patient termed "achieved homeostasis". He kept a record of how it felt immediately after applying specific modalities, and his notes showed that this feeling of "achieved homeostasis" followed the day when he took cell extracts or EECP, and the second day after weight lifting in the gym. Breathing techniques, combined with meditation, were also high on the list of modalities that contributed to the feeling of "achieved homeostasis".

The successful recovery of another heart patient gave additional credence to the overall program

Our lasting results point towards the need for research in several areas: After an ablation there is a period of "burning in the circuits", and drugs like amiodarone (even though with numerous negative side-effects) are quite effective in achieving success. Present ablation success rates are 70-80%. Future research needs to find out which of the modalities we used are helpful in burning in the circuits, and which ones are effective in giving lasting results.

Mainstream medicine also has no recovery protocol for a severely enlarged left atrium; most likely the great enlargement of the left atrium was due to an injury incurred during the accident and the delay in diagnosis/treatment. This area looks most promising for future research; since all the modalities that were used in our recovery program are non-drug, and carry no risk for subjects, even the most basic research protocol would quickly pinpoint priorities and the degree of effectiveness of the modalities used.

The need for more research is underlined again with initial findings (follow-up observations by Fouad Ghaly, MD) that suggest greater improvements in heart functions when a patient is given a choice to combine EECP with any one, or more, of the alternative modalities discussed above.

In retrospect, we wondered why, after the first accident, it took more than one year to diagnose A-fib. Examinations usually took place in the morning. The night before patient took 5-HTP and GABA (gamma amino butyric acid) for better sleep. GABA is chemically related to the cardioversion drug ibutilide. GABA can also hydrolyze in the body, via a nucleophilic substitution reaction, to GHB (gamma hydroxybutyric acid), which has a strong sedative effect. Could GABA have slowed down heart rhythm (possibly in sinus) in the morning when examinations usually took place?

REFERENCES

1. Kugler H. BS in Physiology, University of Munich Medical School under Nobel Laureate A. Butenandt (1959), and PhD (1969) under F. Ramirez, Stony Brook, New York.
2. Kugler H. Associate Professor (Chemistry, Longevity studies) at Roosevelt University, Chicago, Illinois. (1969-72).
3. Kugler H. Director of Research, International Academy of Anti-Aging Medicine (IAAM), Redondo Beach, California. (2004-present).
4. Kugler H. Director, HK Stem Cell Research, Torrance, California. (2007-present).
5. Kugler H. The Multi-Factorial Theory on Aging. *American Laboratory.*1975;17:43-45.
6. Kugler H. The Multi-Factorial Approach to optimum longevity. Presented at: International Academy of Preventive Medicine Meeting; 1976; Denver, Colorado.
7. Kugler H. The scientific basis for designing your personal anti-aging program. In: Klatz, R, Goldman R, eds. *Anti-Aging Medical Therapeutics*. Chicago. IL: A4M: 1999;9-19.
8. Kugler H. The Multi-Factorial Approach to cancer. Presented at: A4M Meeting; 2001; Las Vegas, Nevada.
9. Abramson J. *Overdosed America: The Broken Promise of American Medicine.* New York, NY: HarperCollins; 2004.
10. Null G, Dean C, Feldman M, Rasio D, Smith D. *Death by Medicine.* Life Extension Magazine. 2006; August. Available at: http://www.lef.org/magazine/mag2006 /aug2006_report_death_01.htm Accessed March 4th, 2010.
11. May MT, Sterne JA, Costagliola D, Sabin CA, Phillips AN, Justice AC, *et al*; Antiretroviral Therapy (ART) Cohort Collaboration. HIV treatment response and prognosis in Europe and North America in the first decade of highly active antiretroviral therapy: a collaborative analysis. *Lancet.* 2006;368:451-458.
12. Cell extracts: liquid EXTRA-CELL mesenchym and thymus (www.Douglaslabs.com), tablets CARDIO-PLUS (www.standardprocess.com).
13. Schmid F. *Mikrooekologische Therapie.* 4th ed. Luebeck, Germany: Verlag Schmidt-Roemhild; 1997.
14. Neumeyer, G. Therapie mit Thymus und Milzpeptiden. Presentation at: Internationaler Kongress der Internationalen Gesellschaft fuer Organfiltrate; 1993; Mannheim, Germany.
15. Ward P. *The Encyclopedia of Weight Training.* Laguna Hills, CA: QPT Publications; 1997: 158-14.

16. Dickerman RD, Schaller F, McConathy WJ. Left ventricular wall thickening does occur in elite power athletes with or without anabolic steroid use. Cardiology 1998;90:145-148.
17. Oakley D. The athlete's heart. *Heart* 2001;86:722-726.
18. Thornton J. The biology of exercise. *Men's Health*. 2007;Dec:156-194.
19. Braverman D. *Heal Your Heart with EECP: The Only Noninvasive Way To Overcome Heart Disease.* Waterville, ME: Thorndike Press; 2006.
20. Nichols WW, Estrada JC, Braith RW, Owens K, Conti RC. Enhanced External Counterpulsation Treatment Improves Arterial Wall Properties and Wave Reflection Characteristics in Patients With Refractory Angina. *J Am Coll Cardiol.* 2006;48:1208-1214.
21. Calais-Germain B. *Anatomy of Breathing.* Vista, CA: Eastland Press; 2003.
22. Werbach M. *Textbook of Nutritional Medicine.* Tarzana, CA: Third Line Press; 1999.
23. Werbach M. Nutritional influences on illness: the influence of minerals on congestive heart failure. *Townsend Letter.* 2007; July.
24. Werbach M. Nutritional influences on illness: the influence of vitamins on congestive heart failure. *Townsend Letter.* 2008.
25. Hausenloy DJ, Yellon DM. Targeting residual cardiovascular risk: raising high-density lipoprotein cholesterol levels. *Heart.* 2008;94:706-714.
26. Abdel-Maksoud M, Sazonov V, Gutkin SW, Hokanson JE. Effects of modifying triglycerides and triglyceride-rich lipoproteins on cardiovascular outcomes. *J Cardiovasc Pharmacol.* 2008;;51:331-351.
27. Schaefer EJ, Asztalos BF. Increasing high-density lipoprotein cholesterol, inhibition of cholesteryl ester transfer protein, and heart disease risk reduction. *Am J Cardiol.* 2007;100(11 A):n25-31.
28. Roos B, Geelen A, Ross K, Rucklidge G, Reid M, Duncan G, Caslake M, Horgan G, Brouwer IA Identification of potential serum biomarkers of inflammation and lipid modulation that are altered by fish oil supplementation in healthy volunteers. *Proteomics.* 2008;8:1965-1974.
29. Booker CS, Mann JI. Trans fatty acids and cardiovascular health: translation of the evidence base. *Nutr Metab Cardiovasc Dis.* 2008;18:448-456.
30. Davis W. Averting arrhythmias with omega-3 fatty acids. *Life Extension.* 2008:14:60-68.
31. Lesnefsky EJ, He D, Moghaddas S, Hoppel CL. Reversal of mitochondrial defects before ischemia protects the aged heart. *FASEB J.* 2006;20:1543-1545.
32. King KL, Okere IC, Sharma N, Dyck JR, Reszko AE, McElfresh TA, Kerner J, Chandler MP, Lopaschuk GD, Stanley WC. Regulation of cardiac malonyl-CoA content and fatty acid oxidation during increased cardiac power. *Am J Physiol Heart Circ Physiol.* 2005;289:H1033-1037.
33. Bian F, Kasumov T, Thomas KR, Jobbins KA, David F, Minkler PE, Hoppel CL, Brunengraber H. Peroxisomal and mitochondrial oxidation of fatty acids in the heart, assessed from the 13C labeling of malonyl-CoA and the acetyl moiety of citrate. *J Biol Chem.* 2005;280:9265-9271.
34. Sethumadhavan S, Chinnakannu P. L-carnitine and alpha-lipoic acid improve age-associated decline in mitochondrial respiratory chain activity of rat heart muscle. *J Gerontol A Biol Sci Med Sci.* 2006;61:650-659.
35. Wenzel P, Hink U, Oelze M, Schuppan S, Schaeuble K, Schildknecht S, Ho KK, Weiner H, Bachschmid M, Münzel T, Daiber A. Role of reduced lipoic acid in the redox regulation of mitochondrial aldehyde dehydrogenase (ALDH-2) activity. Implications for mitochondrial oxidative stress and nitrate tolerance. *J Biol Chem.* 2007;282:792-799.
36. Seddon MD, Chowienczyk PJ, Brett SE, Casadei B, Shah AM. Neuronal nitric oxide synthase regulates basal microvascular tone in humans *in vivo. Circulation.* 2008;117:1991-1996.
37. Ally A, Kabadi S, Phattanarudee S, Patel M, Maher TJ. Neuronal nitric oxide synthase (nNOS) blockade within the ventrolateral medulla differentially modulates cardiovascular responses and nNOS expression during static skeletal muscle contraction. *Brain Res.* 2007;1150:21-31.
38. Giles TD. Aspects of nitric oxide in health and disease: a focus on hypertension and cardiovascular disease. *J Clin Hypertens (Greenwich).* 2006;8 (12 Suppl 4):2-16.
39. Davis JM, Murphy EA, Carmichael MD, Zielinski MR, Groschwitz CM, Brown AS, Gangemi JD, Ghaffar A, Mayer EP. Curcumin effects on inflammation and performance recovery following eccentric exercise-induced muscle damage. *Am J Physiol Regul Integr Comp Physiol.* 2007;292:R2168-2173.
40. Jacob A, Wu R, Zhou M, Wang P. Mechanism of the anti-inflammatory effect of curcumin: PPAR-gamma activation. *PPAR Res.* 2007;2007:89369.
41. Mitka M. Vitamin D deficits may affect heart health. *JAMA.* 2008;299:753-754.

42. [No authors listed] Boosting vitamin D may reduce your heart risk. Research shows that the vitamin helps fight inflammation, lower blood pressure, and may also play a role in controlling cholesterol. *Heart Advis.* 2007;10:9.

43. Mancuso P, Rahman A, Hershey SD, Dandu L, Nibbelink KA, Simpson RU. 1,25-Dihydroxyvitamin-D3 treatment reduces cardiac hypertrophy and left ventricular diameter in spontaneously hypertensive heart failure-prone (cp/+) rats independent of changes in serum leptin. *J Cardiovasc Pharmacol.* 2008;51:559-564.

44. Ochoa JJ, Quiles JL, Huertas JR, Mataix J. Coenzyme Q10 protects from aging-related oxidative stress and improves mitochondrial function in heart of rats fed a Belardinelli R, polyunsaturated fatty acid (PUFA)-rich diet. *J Gerontol A Biol Sci Med Sci.* 2005;60:970-975.

45. Muçaj A, Lacalaprice F, Solenghi M, Seddaiu G, Principi F, Tiano L, Littarru GP. Coenzyme Q10 and exercise training in chronic heart failure. *Eur Heart J.* 2006;27:2675-2681.

46. Hadj A, Pepe S, Marasco S, Rosenfeldt F. The principles of metabolic therapy for heart disease. *Heart Lung Circ.* 2003;12 Suppl 2:S55-62.

47. Schwab U, Törrönen A, Meririnne E, Saarinen M, Alfthan G, Aro A, Uusitupa M. Orally administered betaine has an acute and dose-dependent effect on serum betaine and plasma homocysteine concentrations in healthy humans. *J Nutr.* 2006;136:34-38. Erratum in: *J Nutr.* 2007;137:1124.

48. Olthof MR, Verhoef P. Effects of betaine intake on plasma homocysteine concentrations and consequences for health. *Curr Drug Metab.* 2005;6:15-22.

49. Cureton T. TMG supplementation increases oxygen-carrying capacity of the blood. Presented at: National Meeting of Health and Tennis Corporation; October, 1995; Honolulu, HI.

50. Breslow L, Bellow N. Relationship of physical health status and health practices. *Preventive Medicine.* 1972;1:409-421.

51. Jones H. Optimal development and prevention of degenerative diseases." Presented at: Conference of the Holistic Health and Nutrition Institute; 1977; Mill Valley, CA

ABOUT THE AUTHOR

Primary author Dr. Hans J. Kugler is a well-known scientific researcher and author. He is president and founder of HK Stem Cell Research, and served as past president and board member of the National Health Federation. A victim of an extreme car accident in 2003, Dr. Kugler is in-person evidence of the importance of being your own health advocate and seeking answers "outside of the box": the accident ruptured parts in his heart, and numerous treatment attempts failed; Dr. Kugler developed his own recovery protocol with the help of cardiac experts from around the world. He is now fully recovered, back to fitness training, and is once again flying airplanes.

Chapter 19
The Viral Crisis: Natural Anti-Viral Agents
Shari Lieberman, Ph.D., CNS, FACN

ABSTRACT

The viral crisis represents a major threat to public health. Viruses develop drug resistance just like bacteria, and antibiotic resistance to viruses is a worldwide problem. The need for safe, effective antiviral drugs has become paramount. Virucidal resistance has occurred in herpes simplex I and II as a result of acyclovir resistance. There are very limited antiviral treatments in conventional medicine against the vast majority of viruses that affect humans. However, there are several antiviral plant compounds with well-documented human and animal clinical research that have been shown to be extremely effective against viruses such as: HIV, measles, herpes simplex I and II, herpes zoster, cytomegalovirus, Epstein-Barr virus, influenza and hepatitis A, B, and C, without inducing resistance. Additionally, many of these virucidal compounds also exhibit anti-fungal effects against *Candida albicans* and antibacterial effects against bacteria such as *Staphylococcus aureus* and *Streptococcus*. Plants and plant compounds that have exhibited profound virucidal activity against the aforementioned viruses, bacteria, and yeast include glycyrrhizin, monolaurin, and several *Phyllanthus* species. The aim of this paper is to discuss the clinical application and mechanism of action of these plants and plant compounds. .

INTRODUCTION

The viral crisis represents a major threat to public health. Viruses develop drug resistance just like bacteria, and antibiotic resistance to viruses is a worldwide problem. The need for safe, effective antiviral drugs has become paramount. Virucidal resistance has occurred in herpes simplex I and II as a result of acyclovir resistance. There are very limited antiviral treatments in conventional medicine against the vast majority of viruses that affect humans. However, there are several antiviral plant compounds with well-documented human and animal clinical research that have been shown to be extremely effective against viruses such as: HIV, measles, herpes simplex virus (HSV) 1 and HSV-2, herpes zoster, cytomegalovirus (CMV), Epstein-Barr virus (EBV), influenza and hepatitis A, B, and C, without inducing resistance. Additionally, many of these virucidal compounds also exhibit anti-fungal effects against *Candida albicans* and antibacterial effects against bacteria such as *Staphylococcus aureus* and *Streptococcus*. Plants and plant compounds that have exhibited profound virucidal activity against the aforementioned viruses, bacteria, and yeast include Glycyrrhizin, monolaurin, several *Phyllanthus* species. The aim of this paper is to discuss the clinical application and mechanism of action of these plants and plant compounds.

NATURAL ANTIVIRAL AGENTS
Glycyrrhizin: A Natural Antiviral for the Treatment of Hepatitis C

Hepatitis C is occurring at epidemic proportions all over the world – there are more than 3.9 million people infected in the United States (four-times those infected with HIV), and more than 170 million people worldwide. Chronic hepatitis C develops in approximately 85% of people infected, and is the most common cause of chronic liver disease, cirrhosis of the liver, and liver cancer in the Western hemisphere. Research has shown that people with chronic hepatitis C infection have a 17-fold increased risk of dying from liver disease and a 6-fold increased risk of dying from liver cancer. In the United States, chronic hepatitis C infection kills 8,000 to 10,000 people each year, and the Centers for Disease Control and Protection (CDC) expect that figure to triple by 2010.[1]

Thus, it can be seen that hepatitis C poses a major threat to society. Unfortunately, conventional medicine has not really made great progress with treating hepatitis C. The current standard method of treatment for hepatitis C infection is a combination of interferon (INF) and other antiviral drugs, such as ribavirin. INF treatment is only successful in a minority of patients. Of those patients who do exhibit viral clearance 30-70% relapse within a few months, and a sustained response of at least six months occurs in just 10-15% of patients. When INF is used in combination with ribavirin the results are better, with 28% to 66% of patients showing a sustained response for 12-months. It is important to note that this treatment only decreases the risk of progression to hepatocellular carcinoma in sustained virological responders.

INF is associated with numerous side effects, including: myalgia, fatigue, fever, headache, nausea, leukopenia, thrombocytopenia, alopecia, irritability, depression, thyroid abnormalities, pulmonary complications, and retinal damage. In fact, these side effects are so serious that many patients cannot work, or even function, during treatment. The side effects of INF combined with ribavirin are far worse – ribavirin causes hemolytic anemia and is also a teratogen.

In short, the side effects of conventional hepatitis C treatment are so bad, and potentially serious, you have to wonder if the treatment is actually worse than the disease. Indeed, after taking into account the success rate of conventional treatment and its side effects, it is difficult to see why doctors are still using this line of treatment, particularly when there is an effective alternative treatment available.

Glycyrrhizin (GL), a conjugate of glycyrrhetinic acid (GA) and glucuronic acid, is by far the most antiviral substance I have ever used in my practice. It has been used in Japan for more than 20 years under the name Stronger Neonimphagen C (SNMC). Oral GL is metabolized in the intestine to GA, whilst intravenous GL is metabolized into GA when excreted through the bile into the intestines. It has been shown to be effective in the treatment of:

- Hepatitis A, B, and C
- HIV – it is actually superior to AZT
- Herpes – I, II, zoster, and possibly 6
- Lichen planus
- Influenza
- Cytomegalovirus
- Cancer

My own personal experience with GL has shown that it is also effective in the treatment of chronic fatigue, EBV, condyloma, and many other types of viral illnesses. Moving back to hepatitis C, research by Okuno et al showed that GL also helps to boost the efficacy of conventional INF and ribavirin.[2] Thus, GL can benefit patients who opt for conventional treatment and for those who feel that conventional treatment is not for them.

How does GL work? The mechanism of action of GL is well established. Research has shown that GL has both direct and indirect antiviral properties. Directly, it inhibits some RNA transcriptases, including HIV. Indirectly, it decreases cell membrane permeability (and thus can reduce hepatocyte injury), inactivates viruses, and inhibits viral proliferation. It is a potent free radical scavenger, and increases levels of endogenous INF, T-cells, and natural killer (NK) cells – which may help to explain why it is also effective at treating cancer. It also inhibits the cytolytic reactivity of the complement system.[3] GL does not inhibit (in fact, it may actually enhance) immune adherence, which is vital for protecting the body against invading pathogens. Last, but most certainly not least, GL inhibits the arachidonic acid cascade (phospholipase A_2), and thus has anti-inflammatory properties

So, GL has numerous benefits and is proven to be effective against hepatitis C. How do you go about treating patients with GL? A 20 ml ampoule of SNMC contains 40 mg GL, 400 mg glycine, and 20 mg L-cysteine. 2 ml ampoule are also available, but the dose of GL (4 mg) is simply too low for treating hepatitis C. The typical therapeutic intravenous dose is 40-60 ml, however research suggests that 100 ml/day may be optimal. The oral dose is 200 mg/day. SNMC also contains aminoacetic acid and L-cysteine in order to prevent pseudoaldosteronism (aldosterone suppression caused by a rise in renal cortisol). Pseudoaldosteronism is rarely reported at therapeutic doses, and on the rare occasion that it is an issue, it is easily treated with the mineralocorticoid receptor antagonist spironolactone. Ensuring that patients eat a healthy, potassium-rich diet may help to reduce the risk of pseudoaldosteronism.

Medical Literature Review of SNMC in Treating Hepatitis C

Iino et al conducted a comparative study to determine the efficacy of different doses of SNMC in treating patients with chronic hepatitis B or hepatitis C.[4] Participants were randomly assigned to receive 100 ml/day SNMC for 3 weeks (group A, n=44) or 40 ml/day SNMC for 3 weeks (group B, n=46). Nearly half (49%) of participants had previously been treated with IFN therapy, with no improvement in alanine aminotransferase (ALT) levels – remember, ALT is the best prognostic predictor with respect to liver cancer risk, not viral load. Participants were rated "markedly improved" if ALT levels dropped to <1.2 times the normal upper limit, and "improved" if ALT dropped to <1.2 - 1.5 the normal upper limit. In group A, 23 of 44 (52.3%) of participants were rated "improved" or better, compared with just 12 of 46 (26.1%) participants in group B. The authors concluded: "Group A showed significant improvement compared to group B, thus documenting the greater efficacy of administering SNMC at 100 ml/day compared to only 40 ml/day."

Arase *et al* retrospectively collected data on hepatitis C patients treated with SNMC.[5] The study involved 84 patients who had received 100 ml/day SNMC for 8 weeks and then a maintenance dose of 2-7 times a week for 2-16 years, and a control group of 109 patients who were treated with herbs or nutritional supplements. Results showed that ALT fell to normal levels in 35.7% of the SNMC group compared to just 6.4% in the control group. Furthermore, the 15-year rate of cumulative cirrhosis was 21% in the SNMC group compared to 37% in the control, and the 15-year rate of liver cancer was 12% in the SNMC group compared to 25% in the control group. The authors concluded: "The long-term administration of SNMC for chronic HCV was considered to be effective in the reduction of liver carcinogenesis. The reason why SNMC administration reduces hepatocarcinogenesis is believed to be related to the suppression of the necroinflammatory reaction in the liver and the protection against histologic aggravation."

Watanabe *et al* reported on a patient with chronic active hepatitis C.[6] In 1986, the patient's aspartate aminotransferase (AST) level was elevated at 63 and ALT was significantly elevated at 94, a laparoscopy revealed pre-cirrhosis of the liver. By 2000, his AST level had risen to 323 and his ALT to 348, at this point he was given the GL-containing herbal supplement Sho-Saiko-To, which is a widely used prescription drug in Japan. Although Sho-Saiko-To contains GL it does not contain levels comparable to those in SNMC. In 1992 his AST had fallen to 57 and his ALT to 61. Laparoscopy revealed liver cirrhosis and his viral load was high (HCV RNA 100 kcopies/ml). At this point he was given INF for 24-weeks, however he did not respond to treatment. In 1997, he began treatment with SNMC (60 ml three times a day), which lasted for two years. By 1999, his AST was 30, his ALT was 39, and his viral load was low (HCV RNA 3.2 kcopies/ml). The decision was then made to retry INF therapy and he was treated for 16-weeks. A sustained response was obtained and he has been HCV RNA-negative ever since.

Patients with chronic hepatitis C who were non-responders, or who were unlikely to respond (genotype 1/cirrhosis) to INF were included in a study of SNMC by van Rossum *et al.*[7] Participants were treated with intravenous glycyrrhizin 6 x 200 mg/week, 3 x 240 mg/week, or 3 x 0 mg/week (placebo) for 4 weeks. The proportion of patients with ALT normalization at the end of treatment was higher in actively treated patients than in placebo, and was higher in those receiving SNMC six times each week (47%) than in those receiving treatment three times each week (26%). Many patients involved in this study asked to continue taking SNMC rather than INF, because they felt better whilst taking SNMC.

Kumada conducted a study to determine whether long-term treatment of hepatitis C with SNMC reduces the risk of cirrhosis and liver cancer.[8] The therapeutic schedule of SNMC was aimed at suppressing ALT levels (below 75 IU/L). Participants were given 40 ml (80 mg GL) of SNMC 5-6 times per week, and if ALT was lowered sufficiently they were given a maintenance dose 3 times per week. If this regimen failed, SNMC was increased to 100 ml (200 mg GL) 5-6 times/wk until patients responded, and the maintenance dose was tailored to keep ALT levels low. Results showed that liver cirrhosis occurred less frequently in patients receiving long-term SNMC treatment than in controls (28 vs. 40% at year 13). Liver cancer also developed less frequently in patients receiving long-term SNMC treatment than in controls (13 vs. 25% at year 15). The author of this study noted that there is a linear relationship between the cumulative ALT score and the increase in the stage of fibrosis, irrespective of the stage of fibrosis found in the first biopsy, thus meaning that the higher the stage of fibrosis in the first biopsy, the lower the cumulative ALT score is required for the progression to the next stage of fibrosis. Therefore, to prevent progression of fibrosis the cumulative ALT score needs to be kept increasingly lower as the stage of fibrosis increases. It was also noted that the incidence of liver cancer increases in parallel with the mean ALT score. So, keeping ALT as low as possible is key in the treatment of hepatitis C.

Glycyrrhizin for the Treatment of Other Viral Infections

As mentioned previously, GL is a potent antiviral agent that is effective at treating a number of viral infections – not just hepatitis C.

Hepatitis B

In Japan GL is routinely used to treat chronic hepatitis B. Su *et al* conducted a study of 80 patients with hepatitis B.[9] Participants were given oral doses of 7.5 g crude *Glycyrrhiza* root concentrated to contain 750 mg GL (30 days for those with acute hepatitis B, 90 days for those with chronic hepatitis B), two control groups (one acute and one chronic) received the immunostimulant Poly I:C. Results showed a significantly marked improvement on indices of liver function and negative conversion of hepatitis B surface antigen (HBsAg) and hepatitis B envelope antigen (HBeAg) in the GL group than the control group. Furthermore, indices of liver function tests returned to normal in 85% of subjects with acute hepatitis and 75% of those with chronic hepatitis who were treated with GL, compared to just 35% and 10% of those in the control groups. A daily intravenous dose of 100 - 140 ml for 4 weeks has been shown to be both safe and efficacious in the treatment of acute hepatitis B, and intravenous administration of GL for 1 year in patients with chronic hepatitis B has been shown to be successful in 30-40% of cases, which is comparable to the success rate achieved with INF.

HIV Infection

According to Fiore *et al*, SNMC (5 mg GL/Kg) has been successfully used to treat AIDS patients with high CD4/CD8 ratios. Study results showed that almost half of patients improved significantly during treatment.[10] Fiore also cites another study of patients with hemophilia A and HIV, (but who were asymptomatic), where it was shown that GL inhibits viral replication, has interferon-inducing and NK cell enhancing effects, and is extremely effective in preventing progression to full blown AIDS and improving the CD4/CD8 count.[10] GL has been shown to inhibit cell-to-cell infection by HIV1, HIV2, and T-cell lymphotropic virus type 1.[11] It also inhibits HIV replication in cultures of peripheral blood mononuclear cells from HIV-infected patients. In 31% of samples, GL inhibited more than 90% of HIV replication, including a non-synctium-inducing variant of HIV (NSI-HIV).[10]

SARS and Coronavirus

No treatment for SARS (severe acute respiratory syndrome) has been established. However, GL has been shown to inhibit SARS-associated coronavirus (SARS-CoV) replication by inhibiting absorption and penetration during the early steps of the replication cycle. GL was found to be most effective when administered both during and after the absorption period of the replication cycle.[11]

Herpes

In vitro studies show that GL is effective against varicella zoster, inactivating more than 99% when incubated with GL for 30 minutes. GL has also been shown to inactivate HSV-1 and HSV-2, and EBV *in vitro*. GL demonstrates additive effects when given alongside acyclovir and beta-interferon.

Cytomegalovirus

GL has been shown to be effective against CMV both *in vitro* and *in vivo*.[11] Numazaki investigated the therapeutic effect of GL for liver dysfunction associated with CMV infection. Intravenous SNMC was administered (GL 10-20 mg/kg/day intravenously for 8 weeks) to 4 infants. Liver dysfunction in all 4 cases improved and CMV disappeared from urinary samples after administration of GL intravenously by the age of 12 months. Another 6 infants were treated with Glycyron (25 mg GL supplemented with 25 mg methionine and 25 mg glycine) orally for 12 weeks. Liver dysfunction normalized and CMV disappeared by the age of 16 months after administration of GL orally. No side effects were noted during the treatment with GL. Numazaki concluded that GL therapy is a "suitable treatment for improving liver dysfunction in immunocompetent infants and children associated with CMV infection."[11]

Upper Respiratory Tract Infection

Yanagawa *et al* conducted a study to assess the tolerability, efficacy, and cost of GL in improving the severity and duration of signs and symptoms of upper respiratory tract infections (URTIs).[12] Of the 41 study participants, 15 were assigned to treatment with intravenous GL and 26 were assigned to treatment with an intravenous placebo. Results showed that GL therapy was associated with a shorter hospitalization, lower-grade fever, and lower cost of therapy compared to placebo.

Phyllanthus for the Treatment of Hepatitis B

Phyllanthus niruri, amarus, and *urinaria*, are commonly used in Ayurvedic medicine. *Phyllanthus amarus* has a history of use for the treatment of hepatitis B. Wang *et al* conducted a study of 123 patients with hepatitis B.[13] Participants were randomly assigned to receive *Phyllanthus amarus* (n=11), *Phyllanthus. niruri* (n=42), *Phyllanthus urinaria* (n=35), or placebo (n-35). Those assigned to the

Phyllanthus amarus group were treated with 500 mg t.i.d. for 3 months, while those assigned to the *Phyllanthus niruri* and *Phyllanthus urinaria* groups were treated with 300 mg t.i.d. in month 1, 600 mg t.i.d. in month 2, and 900 mg t.i.d. in month 3. Results showed that those treated with *Phyllanthus urinaria* were more likely to lose detectable HBeAg from their serum and were more likely to seroconvert their hepatitis B e-antibody status from negative to positive to those in the other groups.

Liu *et al* conducted a systematic review of 22 randomized trials of *Phyllanthus* for the treatment of chronic hepatitis B infection.[14] Combined results revealed that:

- *Phyllanthus* had a positive effect on clearance of HBsAg.
- There was no significant difference between *Phyllanthus* and INF in terms of clearing HBsAg, HBeAG, and hepatitis B virus (HBV) DNA.
- *Phyllanthus* used in combination with IFN was more effective at clearing HBeAg and HBV DNA than INF alone.
- *Phyllanthus* had a significant effect on antiviral activity
- *Phyllanthus* was more effective at normalizing ALT levels than IFN.
- *Phyllanthus amarus* and *Phyllanthus urinaria* had a positive affect on HBsAg and HBeAg, however only *Phyllanthus urinaria* had a positive effect on HBV DNA.

Huang *et al* conducted an *in vitro* study on 25 compounds isolated from Phyllanthus to determine which compounds were effective against the hepatitis B virus. Results showed that niranthin, nirtetralin, hinokinin, and geraniin were effective at suppressing the expression of both HBsAg and HBeAg. Niranthin exhibited the best anti-HBsAg activity, while the most potent anti-HBeAg activity was observed with hinokinin.

Lauric Acid and Monolaurin

Lauric acid is the most active antiviral and antibacterial substance in human breast milk. Monolaurin is the glycerol ester of lauric acid, and is more biologically active than lauric acid, it is nontoxic and is designated as GRAS by the Food and Drug Administration. *In vitro* studies have shown that monolaurin is able to inactivate or kill numerous viruses (influenzavirus, pneumovirus, paramyxovirus (Newcastle), morbillivirus (rubella) coronavirus (avian infectious), bronchitis virus, HSV-1, HSV-2, CMV, HIV…), gram-positive bacteria (anthrax, listeria, *Staphylococcus aureus*, *Streptococcus* (groups A, B, F, and G), *Clostridium perfringens*…), gram negative bacteria (*Chlamydia pneumoniae*, *Neisseria gonorrhoeae*, *Helicobacter pylori*…), yeast, fungi, and molds. A number of protozoa, including *Giardia lamblia*, are also inactivated or killed by monolaurin.[16] It is not effective against polio virus, coxsackie virus, encephalomyocarditis virus, rhinovirus and rotaviruses. Monolaurin has a number of antiviral modes of action, it:

- Binds to the lipid-protein envelope of the virus and inactivates the virus
- Inhibits the replication of viruses by interrupting the binding of virus to host cells
- Prevents the uncoating of viruses necessary for replication and infection
- Removes all measurable infectivity by directly disintegrating the viral envelope
- Binds to the viral envelope, thus making the virus more susceptible to host defenses

CONCLUDING REMARKS

GL, monolaurin, and *Phyllanthus* are natural products, which I have used extensively, and with great success, in my practice for more than 25 years. There are no known adverse effects associated with monolaurin and *Phyllanthus*. GL has been linked to pseudoaldosteronism, however this is a rare complication, even so it is important to regularly monitor blood pressure in patients undergoing treatment with oral or intravenous GL, as well as to encourage them to eat a potassium-rich diet. No viral, bacterial, or fungal resistance has ever been seen with any of these natural compounds. They may be used alone, or in combination with each other. In fact, these compounds may be synergistic, thus combining low doses of these compounds may be more effective than using higher doses of single compounds since they have different mechanisms of action.

REFERENCES

1. Wong JB, McQuillan GM, McHutchison JG, Poynard T. Estimating future hepatitis C morbidity, mortality, and costs in the United States. *Am J Public Health.* 2000;90:1562-1569.
2. Okuno T, Arai K, Shindo M. [Efficacy of interferon combined glycyrrhizin therapy in patients with chronic hepatitis C resistant to interferon therapy]. *Nippon Rinsho.* 1994;52:1823-1827. [Japanese]
3. Fujisawa Y, Sakamoto M, Matsushita M, Fujita T, Nishioka K. Glycyrrhizin inhibits the lytic pathway of complement--possible mechanism of its anti-inflammatory effect on liver cells in viral hepatitis. *Microbiol Immunol.* 2000;44:799-804.
4. Iino S, Tango T, Matsushima T, et al. Therapeutic effects of stronger neo-minophagen C at different doses on chronic hepatitis and liver cirrhosis. *Hepatol Res.* 2001;19:31-40.
5. Arase Y, Ikeda K, Murashima N, Chayama K, Tsubota A, Koida I, Suzuki Y, Saitoh S, Kobayashi M, Kumada H. The long term efficacy of glycyrrhizin in chronic hepatitis C patients. *Cancer.* 1997;79:1494-1500.
6. Watanabe M, Uchida Y, Sato S, Moritani M, Hamamoto S, Mishiro T, Akagi S, Kinoshita Y, Kohge N. Report of a case showing a recovery from liver cirrhosis to chronic hepatitis, type C, after glycyrrhizin injection for 2 years and a sustained response by the following interferon therapy. *Am J Gastroenterol.* 2001;96:1947-1949.
7. van Rossum TG, de Jong FH, Hop WC, Boomsma F, Schalm SW. 'Pseudo-aldosteronism' induced by intravenous glycyrrhizin treatment of chronic hepatitis C patients. *J Gastroenterol Hepatol.* 2001;16:789-795.
8. Kumada H. Long-term treatment of chronic hepatitis C with glycyrrhizin [stronger neo-minophagen C (SNMC)] for preventing liver cirrhosis and hepatocellular carcinoma. *Oncology.* 2002;62 Suppl 1:94-100.
9. Su XS, Chen HM, Wang LH, Jiang CF, Liu JH, Zhao MQ, Ma XH, Zhao YC, Han DW. Clinical and laboratory observation on the effect of glycyrrhizin in acute and chronic viral hepatitis. *J Tradit Chin Med.* 1984;4:127-132.
10. Fiore C, Eisenhut M, Krausse R, Ragazzi E, Pellati D, Armanini D, Bielenberg J. Antiviral effects of Glycyrrhiza species. *Phytother Res.* 2008;22:141-148.
11. Numazaki K. Glycyrrhizin therapy for viral infections. *African J Biotech.* 2003;2:392-393.
12. Yanagawa Y, Masatsune O, Fujimoto E, Shono S, Okuda E. Effects and cost of glycyrrhizin in the treatment of upper respiratory tract infections in members of the Japanese maritime self-defense force: preliminary report of a prospective, randomized, double-blind, controlled, parallel-group, alternate day treatment assignment clinical trial. *Curr Ther Res.* 2004;65:26-33.
13. Wang M, Cheng H, Li Y, Meng L, Zhao G, Mai K. Herbs of the genus *Phyllanthus* in the treatment of chronic hepatitis B: observations with three preparations from different geographic sites. *J Lab Clin Med.* 1995;126:350-352.
14. Liu J, Lin H, McIntosh H. Genus *Phyllanthus* for chronic hepatitis B virus infection: a systematic review. *J Viral Hepat.* 2001;8:358-366.
15. Huang RL, Huang YL, Ou JC, Chen CC, Hsu FL, Chang C. Screening of 25 compounds isolated from *Phyllanthus* species for anti-human hepatitis B virus in vitro. *Phytother Res.* 2003;17:449-453.
16. Lieberman S, Enig MG, Preuss HG. A review of monolaurin and lauric acid: natural virucidal and bactericidal agents. *Alternative & Complementary Therapies.* 2006;12:310-314.

ABOUT THE AUTHOR

Dr. Shari Lieberman earned her PhD in Clinical Nutrition and Exercise Physiology from The Union Institute, Cincinnati, OH and her MS degree in Nutrition, Food Science and Dietetics from New York University. As a Certified Nutrition Specialist (CNS) and a Fellow of the American College of Nutrition (FACN); she was in private practice as a clinical nutritionist for more than 20 years. Dr. Lieberman established two fully accredited Masters Programs, one at the University of Bridgeport, Connecticut and another at New York Chiropractic College, the latter for which she served as Founding Dean of the MS Degree in Clinical Nutrition. She also served as a board member and chair of the exam committee for the Certification Board for Nutrition Specialists, and immediate past President of the American Association for Health Freedom. The fields of nutrition and preventative medicine mourn the passing of Dr. Lieberman in July 2009.

Chapter 20
Adult Stem Cells: Current Clinical Applications and Future Potential Treatments

Dipnarine Maharaj, MBChB, M.D., FRCP (Glasg), FRCP (Edin), FRCPath, FACP
Medical Director, South Florida Bone Marrow Stem Cell Transplant Institute
(Boynton Beach, FL USA)

ABSTRACT

Stem cells have the potential to be one of the most effective agents against aging available to medicine. This paper will discuss some of the many medical applications of adult stem cells in medicine today. The aims of this paper are to discuss:
1. The different types of stem cells (adult and embryonic).
2. The current indications for stem cell transplantation in the treatment of hematologic malignancies.
3. The use of bone marrow adult stem cells for transplantation in a novel outpatient setting.
4. How adult stem cells can be used as an agent for regenerative medicine.

INTRODUCTION

Stem cells have the power and potential to be one of the most effective agents against aging available to medicine today. A stem cell is an unspecified cell that can both self-renew (produce an exact clone of itself) and differentiate into mature tissues, such as the heart, lung, liver, etc. Adult stem cells are collected from bone marrow (bone marrow stem cells), peripheral blood (peripheral blood stem cells), and cord blood (cord blood stem cells). Embryonic stem cells are collected from a fertilized egg or from an embryo, and can form any of the 200 different tissue types present in the body. It is important to remember that embryonic stem cells are a foreign tissue, and thus carry the risk of all the complications associated with an allogeneic or an unrelated donor transplant if these cells are transplanted into an individual. This paper is concerned with adult stem cells.

ADULT STEM CELLS

Adult stem cells are obtained from tissues after birth. They can differentiate into a range of tissues, albeit a far narrower range than embryonic stem cells. Adult stem cells exhibit plasticity and can repair tissues by replenishing specialized cells. Adult stem cells are found in the bone marrow (the stem cell niche). If we can understand what goes on within the stem cell niche and the signals that go back and forth between the stem cells and the cells of the bone marrow, we will have a much better understanding of how to be able to use stem cells to treat patients much more effectively.

There are stem cells niches in every organ, but we know the most about the stem cell niche in the bone marrow. There are two types of niches in the bone marrow: the osteoblastic niche and the vascular niche. The osteoblastic niche is formed by subendooseal cells in the bone. Other cells present in the osteoblastic niche include osteoblasts, osteoclasts, and mesenchymal cells. Interestingly, there are also neuronal cells within the osteoblastic niche. The purpose of the osteoblastic niche is to store stem cells for the purpose of self-renewal. The vascular niche contains cells that originated in the osteoblastic niche. These cells were activated while in the osteoblastic niche, and this enabled them to migrate to the vascular niche. Activation gives the cells the powers of mobilization and homing. These powers enable the cells to respond accordingly to signals. For example, if the body undergoes trauma, the body sends out signals instructing the stem cells in the vascular niche to move into the circulation and home in on the injured tissues.

Harvesting Adult Stem Cells

Adult stem cells can be harvested from the bone marrow and from peripheral blood. A bone marrow harvest is performed under general anesthetic. Approximately 600-700 ml of bone marrow is harvested from the posterior iliac crest. The aim is to obtain a minimum of at least 1-2 x 10^6 CD34 cells/kg. So, if you take a 100 kg individual, we are looking to harvest at least 100 million stem cells. Why do we need so many cells? We require such a large number of cells simply because experience has shown that that is the number of stems cells you need to be able to repopulate the bone marrow. There has been some discussion that this can be done with fewer cells, however I do not agree. From my own experience, I have found that having fewer cells can lead to bone marrow failure or delayed engraftment. Once the stems cells are actually extracted from the bone marrow, they are filtered, mixed with the cryoprotectant DMSO, and frozen at −196°C.

We now know that it is also possible to harvest adult stem cells from peripheral blood. In order to obtain stem cells in this way, patients are first treated with a growth factor drug that stimulates the release of stem cells into the bloodstream. The blood is then obtained via apheresis, a process whereby blood is removed from the patient, passed through the apparatus (which removes the stem cells), and then returned to the patient. Apheresis takes approximately 3 hours, however during that time the patient is able to read or watch television. Once the cells are collected they are mixed with a cryoprotectant, frozen, and stored. This procedure actually yields 15-20 times more stem cells than a bone marrow harvest, and is safer as no general anesthetic is required.

Current Clinical Applications – Hematological Disorders and Malignancies

Adult stem cells have been successfully used to treat blood disorders, blood cancers, and immune system disorders, for the last 50 years or so. Such treatments are routine medical procedures that provide curative protocols.

An adult stem cell transplant, or hematopoietic stem cell transplant (HSCT), is a procedure in which progenitor cells that are capable of reconstituting normal bone marrow function are administered to a patient. HSCT is usually carried out to eliminate a bone marrow infiltrative process, such as leukemia, or to correct nonmalignant disorders. In order to carry out a HSCT the patient's bone marrow is destroyed with high-dose chemotherapy and radiotherapy and the new stem cells are then transplanted into the patient.

The stem cells which are used to replace the bone marrow and restore immune function are obtained from the patient (an autologous transplant), a donor (an allogeneic transplant), or from a genetically identical individual e.g. monozygotic twins (a syngeneic transplant). In order to conduct an autologous transplant the patient has to be in complete remission and the bone marrow has to be clean of tumor cells. In the case of allogeneic transplants, the donor and the recipient are not genetically identical, but they are histocompatible. There are several different types of allogeneic transplants: HLA (human leukocyte antigen)-matched sibling, HLA-matched unrelated donor, unmatched donor, and cord blood transplant. A relatively new technique is a nonmyeloablative or "mini" allogeneic transplant. In this procedure the bone marrow is not ablated. Instead, lower doses of chemotherapy are used to create a space within the bone marrow. The donor stem cells from the normal donor are then infused into the space, thus creating a chimera – where both recipient and donor cells coexist within the bone marrow space. Ultimately, the normal cells will destroy the abnormal stem cells. Nonmyeloablative transplants are still somewhat experimental; however they are associated with a lower risk of transplant-related mortality and thus offer a potential cure to patients who are considered too high-risk for conventional allogeneic HSCT. Common indications for allogeneic HSCT include:

- Malignant disorders:
  - Acute myelogenous leukemia (AML)
  - Non-Hodgkin's lymphoma (NHL)
  - Hodgkin's disease
  - Acute lymphoblastic leukemia (ALL)
  - Chronic myeloid leukemia (CML)
  - Multiple myeloma (MM)
  - Chronic lympocytic leukemia (CLL)
- Nonmalignant disorders:
  - Aplastic anemia
  - Thalassemia major
  - Severe combined immunodeficiency
  - Myelodysplastic syndromes
  - Sickle cell anemia

What about autologous transplants? Multiple myeloma remains the most common indication, followed by lymphoma, and then leukemia. Autoimmune diseases are also considered for autologous transplant.

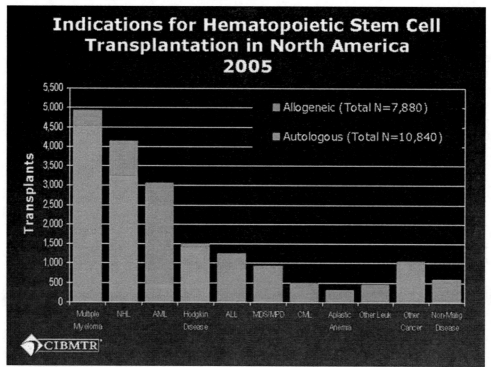

Figure 1. Indications for Hematopoietic Stem Cell Transplantation in North America (2005)

Figure 1 illustrates data taken from the Center for the International Bone Marrow Transplant Registry. The green shows the number of allogeneic transplants that were carried out for different disease types and the yellow shows the autologous transplants. From this illustration it can be seen that the most common type of HTSC for multiple myeloma is an autologous transplant, whereas for acute lymphoblastic leukemia, the most common indication is for an allogeneic transplant.

Table 1. 5-Year Disease Free Survival Rate is Dependent Upon Transplant Type

5-Year Disease Free Survival			
Disease		Autologous Transplantation	Allogeneic Transplantation
AML	1st Complete Remission	40%	55%
AML	2nd Complete Remission	30%	45%
Advanced AML		10%	20%
Multiple Myeloma		40%	35%
ALL	1st Complete Remission		40%
ALL	2nd Complete Remission		25%
HG Non-Hodgkin's Lymphoma		50%	25%
Hodgkin's Lymphoma		60%	
CML	Chronic Phase 1st Year		68%
CML	Chronic Phase >1st Year		53%

As can be seen in Table 1, different types of HTSC are better than others for specific diseases. For example, the 5-year survival rate of a patient with multiple myeloma is approximately 40% with autologous transplant. However, with allogeneic transplants it is approximately 35. So, for multiple myeloma, an autologous transplant is the treatment of choice.

Research has shown that adult stem cells decline in function as we get older, but not in number. DNA damage and epigenetic modifications present in the older individual are known to limit the regenerative potential of adult stem cells. Thus, it is important to consider the age of a patient or stem cell donor, because even though we may be collecting large number of the cells many of them may be nonfunctional, and that will obviously have an impact upon the outcome of the transplant procedure. There is an obvious way around these problems, and that is to collect and store stem cells when we are young and healthy. The storage of healthy and functional adult stem cells provides biological insurance for the treatment of blood malignancies and for future regenerative therapies.

Adult Stem Cell Transplants in the Outpatient Setting

To many people's surprise, it is entirely possible to conduct adult stem cell transplants in the outpatient setting. We conduct stem cell transplants for blood cancers on a totally outpatient basis, and we also perform evolving stem cell therapies for cardiac and neurological diseases, and immunotherapy for cancer. In addition, we offer intermediate dose (Mob/IDC) and high dose (HDC) chemotherapy in an outpatient setting – we do not offer conventional dose chemotherapy. The conventional dose of the drug Cytoxan is 750 mg. For patients receiving IDC the dose would be 9000 mg, and the dose for patients on a HDC regimen would be 12000-14000 mg.

The main benefit of offering these procedures on an outpatient basis is that it significantly lowers the likelihood that your severely immunosuppressed patient will contract a hospital-acquired infection. Figure 2 illustrates the results of a study by Williams *et al* entitled: *Hospitalized cancer patients with severe sepsis: analysis of incidence, mortality, and associated costs of care.*[1]
This study analyzed data of more than 600,000 cancer hospitalizations in the United States in 1999. The results showed that a patient's risk of developing severe sepsis was dependent upon the type of cancer they had. For example, patients with acute leukemia were 66 times more likely to develop severe sepsis than a cancer-free hospitalized patient. Basically, what this study showed is that patients with hematological malignancies are at significantly higher risk of contracting hospital acquired infections. Thus, one of the best ways of preventing hospital-acquired infections is to simply keep the patient out of the hospital by treating them as an outpatient.

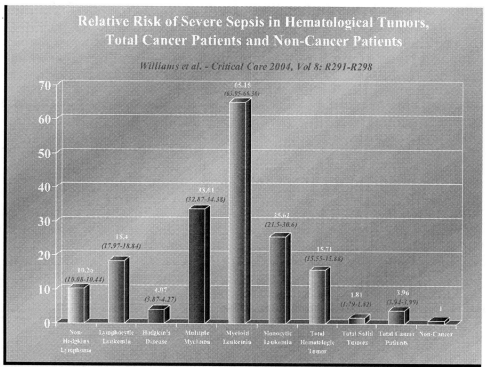

Figure 2. The Relative Risk of Severe Sepsis is Dependent upon the Type of Tumor[1]

Our own data shows that treating cancer patients as outpatients is extremely effective at reducing a patient's risk of contracting hospital-acquired infections. The incidence of severe sepsis among outpatients treated with IDC (9000 mg Cytoxan plus 1600 mg/m^2 VPB16) is 0%, and our overall incidence of infection has been very low. The incidence of mucositis, a common complication of chemotherapy, is also extremely low. In outpatients receiving HDC the incidence of sepsis is 1%, but the overall incidence of infection is extremely low.

How do we achieve this? We focus. We are proactive. We all know the complications that can occur with this type of chemotherapy, so we take steps to prevent them. Proactive intervention reduces the risk of infection and sepsis and decreases the toxicities associated with HDC. First and foremost, hand washing is very important and strictly adhered to. We use prophylactic medications to prevent the known toxicities of HDC – instead of treating nausea we simply prevent the patient from feeling nauseous in the first instance! Early intervention and treatment of complications prevents hospitalization. We also ensure that the patient is treated by the same healthcare professionals throughout their treatment. We know the patient, so we know how they have responded before and we can give them almost personalized care. Treating patients in this way benefits both the patients and the hospital. The patients benefit both physically and psychologically, as they are less likely to develop infections and they are able to go home to their families each day. The hospital benefits because reducing the risk of patient complications also reduces the number of people who are needed to care for each patient, and thus keeps costs low.

STEM CELLS AND AGING

What is aging? Aging is defined by tissue and organ function decline. This decline in function is associated with increased oxidative damage, mitochondrial dysfunction, endocrine imbalance, and genomic instability. Aging can also be defined as a decline in the responsiveness of the regenerative capacity of an organ. Every organ has stem cells; however some stem cells are more proliferative than others. For example, the stem cells of the bone marrow are highly proliferative, whereas the cells of the liver, heart and kidneys are not. So, is it possible to switch those less proliferative stem cells back on so we can get them to repair those tissues and therefore slow the process of aging? Can we rejuvenate stem cells by exposing them to a young systemic environment?

Conboy *et al* established probiotic pairings (shared circulatory system) between young and old mice, thus exposing the old mice to factors present in young serum.[2] Results showed that the stem cells from the young mice were able to migrate into the bone marrow of the old mice and aid regeneration of the bone marrow within the old mice. Further investigations revealed that the exposure of old mice to young serum restored the activation of Notch signaling, enhanced the expression of the Notch ligand (Delta), and enhanced proliferation. The findings of this study demonstrate a number of things:

1. Systemic factors in the blood moderate molecular signaling pathways that are critical to the activation of tissue-specific progenitor cells.
2. The systemic environment of a young animal promotes successful tissue regeneration.
3. The systemic environment of older animals fails to promote, or actively inhibits, tissue regeneration.
4. Aging can be reversed by the modulation of systemic factors.

CONCLUDING REMARKS

Using stem cells to treat disease is not a new concept. Adult stem cells have been successfully used to treat blood disorders, blood cancers, and immune system disorders, for nearly half a century. Today, such treatments are routine medical procedures that provide curative protocols. It is possible to conduct HSCT in an outpatient setting. This reduces the risk of the patient contracting hospital-acquired infections, increases patient satisfaction and psychological wellbeing, and reduces costs.

Stem cells are likely to prove invaluable in the field of regenerative medicine. Research has shown that it is possible to rejuvenate old stem cells by exposing them to specific factors, thus suggesting that aging is indeed reversible.

REFERENCES

1. Williams MD, Braun LA, Cooper LM, Johnston J, Weiss RV, Qualy RL, Linde-Zwirble W. Hospitalized cancer patients with severe sepsis: analysis of incidence, mortality, and associated costs of care. *Critical Care.* 2004;8:R291-R298.
2. Conboy IM, Conboy MJ, Wagers AJ, Girma ER, Weissman IL, Rando TA. Rejuvenation of aged progenitor cells by exposure to a young systemic environment. *Nature* 2005;433:760-764.

ABOUT THE AUTHOR

Dr. Dipnarine Maharaj is the Medical Director and founder of the South Florida Bone Marrow/Stem Cell Transplant Institute, one of the few completely outpatient bone marrow/stem cell transplant facilities in the country. He was also involved in the establishment of bone marrow/ stem cell transplant programs at the University of Miami and for other communities in Florida. He has been involved with clinical research studies using stem cells in the areas of cardiac regeneration, neurodegenerative diseases, and cancer treatments. Most recently, he has secured an Investigator-initiated IND from the FDA to study a novel treatment of solid tumors using only healthy white blood cells. Dr. Maharaj earned both his medical degree and research doctorate at the University of Glasgow Medical School. He is also certified in Internal Medicine by the Royal College of Physicians of the UK, and has accreditations in Hematology, specializing in oncology and bone marrow transplantation. He has been a lecturer on Internal medicine, hematology, and bone marrow transplantation at medical schools and universities in the US and Europe, and is currently Professor at the Charles E. Schmidt College of Biomedical Science, UMMSM regional campus at Florida Atlantic University. .

Chapter 21
The Effects of Whey Zoonutrient Powder and Green Phytonutrient Powder on Pre-Hypertension and Stage 1 Hypertension

John H. Maher, D.C., D.C.B.C.N., B.R.I.C.
Co-Founder and Vice-President of Education and Research,
BioPharma Scientific (San Diego, CA USA)

ABSTRACT

Cardiovascular disease is the number one cause of mortality in the US. Control of hypertension may be the cornerstone of heart disease prevention. Recently, some authorities have suggested aggressive pharmaceutical approaches even for prehypertension. Considering the side effects of pharmaceuticals and long-term compliance issues with strict diets, such as the DASH (dietary approach to stopping hypertension) diet, if nutraceuticals were proven equally efficacious in blood pressure control to either one, they might offer an attractive alternative to integrative physicians and their patients. This paper reviews two pilot studies of a multiple ingredient green phytonutrient powdered drink mix (GPP) and a whey-based phytonutrient powder drink mix (WZP) in prehypertension and stage 1 hypertension.

Results of these pilot studies demonstrate efficacy equal to or greater than the DASH diet and any one common blood pressure medication. The statistically significant results were true with GPP alone, WZP alone, and GPP plus WZP. These results add to a growing body of evidence which suggests that phytonutrient and zoonutrient nutraceuticals may have a place in the integrative management of prehypertension and hypertension.

Keywords: hypertension, prehypertension, phytonutrients, whey, zoonutrient, nutraceuticals

INTRODUCTION

Cardiovascular disease (CVD) is the number one cause of mortality in the US. Control of hypertension is considered primary in CVD Prevention. There is no clear consensus on treatment of pre-hypertension besides lifestyle modification. The question addressed in this paper is: In what instances might nutraceutical supplementation be a superior first intervention of choice as compared to pharmaceutical intervention, if lifestyle moderation is not completely successful?

If nutraceuticals can lower mild blood pressure elevations more or less as well as prescription medications there are then several reasons why they should be considered for utilization as primary interventions over pharmaceuticals as additional support to standard lifestyle modification efforts, particularly in the case of uncomplicated pre-hypertension and borderline stage I hypertension. The reasons for such a consideration for nutraceutical support over pharmaceuticals may include pharmaceuticals having more undesirable side effects and greater cost. The arguments for nutraceuticals include the potential for a wider range of other salubrious effects both in the cardiovascular system and throughout the body in general, and greater patient compliance potential among those patients who prefer "natural medicine".

Essential hypertension is high blood pressure that (as of yet) has no clear definitive cause. It describes 95% of cases of hypertension. Secondary hypertension is high blood pressure due to another condition, such as kidney disease, endocrine disorders, diabetes, prescription medications, allergic reactions, and chemical sensitivities. This paper concerns uncomplicated essential hypertension.

Hypertension Classification

The Joint National Committee on Prevention, Detection, Evaluation, and Treatment of High Blood Pressure (JNC-7)[1] has classified blood pressure as follows:
- Normal blood pressure is 120/80 mmHg
- 120-130/80-90 mmHg is pre-hypertensive (either number)
- Stage I hypertension occurs when the systolic pressure is between 140-159 mmHg and / or diastolic pressure is between 90-99 mmHg
- Stage II hypertension occurs when the systolic pressure is above 160 and / or if the diastolic pressure is above 100 mmHg

- Systolic hypertension, which shows increased pulse pressure greater than 50 while demonstrating a rising systolic as compared to a more "normal" diastolic pressure, tends to occur over age 50. It suggests loss of arteriolar flexibility and atherosclerosis and may be a most dangerous sign.

Hypertension, Pulse Pressure, and Cardiovascular Disease Risk

Individuals who are in stage I have a 31% greater risk of heart attack, almost twice the risk of stroke, and a 43% increase in death rate, compared to individuals with normal blood pressure. Starting as low as 115/75 mmHg, the risk of heart attack and stroke doubles for every 20-point jump in systolic blood pressure or every 10-point rise in diastolic blood pressure for adults age 40-70.

However, when both the blood pressure and pulse pressure scores were forced into a Cox model, only the pulse pressure score remained statistically significant (P<0.0001). This prospective data suggests that pulse pressure may improve the Framingham risk prediction among middle-aged and older individuals. [2]

Treatment Strategies

The JNC-7 guidelines are the most widely accepted treatment strategy. In pre-hypertension (120 to 139/80 to 89 mmHg) treatment starts with lifestyle modification (diet, exercise, smoking cessation, moderate alcohol, sodium restriction, and weight reduction). Employing drug therapy is recommended in prehypertension patients with diabetes mellitus or chronic kidney disease. In stage I hypertension (140 to 159/90 to 99 mmHg) thiazide-type diuretics are added to lifestyle modifications are for most patients (two medications may be considered for patients with coexisting complications). For patients with stage II hypertension, (>=160/>=100 mmHg) two-drug combinations are added to lifestyle modification for most patients. [1]

However, not all researchers agree. The startling conclusions of a meta-analysis of 147 trials on the use of blood pressure lowering drugs in the prevention of cardiovascular disease were:

- "With (few)...exceptions...all the classes of blood pressure lowering drugs have a similar effect in reducing coronary heart disease events and stroke for a given reduction in blood pressure."
- "The proportional reduction in cardiovascular disease events was the same or similar regardless of pretreatment blood pressure and the presence or absence of existing cardiovascular disease."

The authors concluded that the guidelines on the use of blood pressure lowering drugs can be simplified so that drugs are offered to people with all levels of blood pressure. They even stated that their "results indicate the importance of lowering blood pressure in everyone over a certain age, rather than measuring it in everyone and treating it in some" [3]

Other researchers state that lower blood pressure targets offer no benefits below the standard 140/90 mmHg. Their research finds that treating borderline hypertension patients to reach lower targets did drop blood pressure by a modest average of 3.9 mmHg systolic and 3.4 mmHg diastolic below the conventional goals 140/90 (P<0.001). However, this drop was not associated with significant reductions in total mortality, myocardial infarction, stroke, congestive heart failure, major cardiovascular events, and end-stage renal disease. [4]

Side Effects of Common Anti-Hypertensive Medications

Typical hypertensive drugs include diuretics, calcium channel-blockers, beta-blockers, ACE inhibitors, and specific vasodilators. All have proven efficacy. All have unwanted side effect potential.

Calcium channel blockers increase the risk of heart attack and death five-fold and may cause heartburn, swelling of the abdomen and gastrointestinal bleeding, tachycardia or bradycardia, swelling ankles or feet, fatigue, flushing, shortness of breath, difficulty swallowing, dizziness, and numbness in hands and feet.

Potential side effects of beta-blockers include: congestive heart failure, shortness of breath, heart block, fatigue, lethargy, drowsiness, depression, insomnia, headaches, dizziness, tingling in the hands and feet, wheezing, bronchial spasm, increased severity of asthma or chronic pulmonary obstructive disease, decreased sex drive, muscle fatigue, reduced HDL cholesterol, and increased LDL cholesterol and triglycerides.

Potential side effects of angiotensin-converting enzyme (ACE) inhibitors and angiotensin II receptor blockers include dry cough, upper respiratory infection, cough, sinusitis, throat inflammation, gastrointestinal disturbances, diarrhea, abdominal pain, numbness or tingling in the hands and feet, joint pain, back pain, fever, lightheadedness, headache, fatigue, and lowered resistance to viral infections.

Diuretics have several potential side effects as well, including: magnesium deficiency, potassium deficiency, electrolyte imbalance, muscle cramps, fatigue, headaches, lowered HDL cholesterol, fever, rash, irregular menstrual cycles, impotence, excessive uric acid in the blood (gout), excessive urination and thirst, and up to an 11-fold increase in the risk of developing diabetes.

The Clinical Question for the Integrative Physician

Considering both the side effects of medications and the generally more salubrious effects of minerals, vitamins, antioxidants, amino acids, herbs, and whole foods, and their concentrates and extracts, when in a clinical setting might intervention with nutraceuticals over pharmaceuticals be indicated, presuming similar efficacy?

The most effective of the highly researched non-pharmaceutical interventions are the DASH diet, exercise, weight loss, sodium restriction, and fish oil supplements. However, numerous smaller studies on nutritional supplementation have found consistent significant reduction of blood pressure in subjects with elevated blood pressure.

Dietary and Nutraceutical Treatments
Diet, Minerals, Vitamins, Antioxidant, Amino Acids, and Herbs

Dr. Mark Houston suggests for consideration the following non-pharmaceutical treatments for systolic hypertension[5]:

Diet

- DASH I and DASH II (very low sodium) diets, including 10 serving of fruits and vegetables.
- Protein: total intake (40% total calories).10-1.5 mg/kg. Non-animal sources preferred but lean or wild animal protein in moderation.
- Hydrolyzed whey protein   5 g
- Soy protein (fermented is best)   30 g
- Hydrolyzed wheat germ isolate   2-4 g
- Sardine muscle concentrate extract   3 mg
- Fats: 25% total calories
- Omega-3 fatty acids (30%) PUFA   3-4 g
  (DHA, EPA, ALA, cold water fish, flax, canola oil)

Minerals

- Sodium restriction   50-100 mmol
- Potassium   60-100 mEq
- Potassium/sodium ratio   > 5:1
- Magnesium   500-1000 mg
- Calcium   1000-1500 mg
- Zinc   25 mg

Vitamins

- Vitamin C   250-500 mg BID
- Vitamin E   400 to 800 IU QD
- Vitamin B-6   100 mg QD to BID

Antioxidants

- Co-enzyme Q-10 (QGEL®)   60 mg QD to BID
- Lipoic acid   100 to 200 mg BID

<u>Amino Acids</u>
- N-acetyl cysteine   500 mg BID
- L-arginine (Heart Bar®) (3.3 g)   3 g
- L-carnitine   1000 mg BID
- Taurine   1.0 to 1.5 g BID

<u>Herbs</u>
- Hawthorne standard extract   160-900 mg QD

Whole Foods and Concentrates

Dr. Houston also provides brief reviews of statistically significant clinical trials for phytonutrient extracts of green tea, grape seed, quercetin, resveratrol, lycopene, and chocolate, among others. He goes on to state that his meta-analysis and other nutritional/diet studies emphasize the importance of the additive or synergistic effect of multiple nutrients, whole food and whole food concentrates with their nutrient combinations in a natural complex form to reduce blood pressure and CVD.

PHYTONUTRIENTS AND ZOONUTRIENTS FOR THE TREATMENT OF HYPERTENSION: TWO CLINICAL TRIALS
Phytonutrients and the DASH Diet

The DASH diet is much like the more familiar Mediterranean diet. It features 7-10 serving of fruits and vegetables, healthy fats, and 30 grams of fiber a day. The DASH studies have established that a diet emphasizing fruits, vegetables, whole grains, poultry, fish and low-fat dairy products is the most proven efficacious non-pharmaceutical approach to hypertension. The DASH II diet is the same as its predecessor except that it restricts sodium to less than 500 mg a day as well. A study of hypertensive subjects showed that following the DASH II diet lead to an average blood pressure reduction of 11.5 mmHg systolic and 6.8 mm Hg diastolic.[6]

In an article published in the *Journal of the American Dietary Association* Dr Most states: "When compared with the control diet, the DASH diet is higher in flavonols, flavanones, flavan-3-ols, beta-carotene, beta-cryptoxanthin, lycopene, lutein, zeaxanthin, and phytosterols...It therefore is possible that the health benefits of the DASH diet are partially attributable to the phytochemicals and might extend beyond cardiovascular disease risk reduction."[7]

A peer reviewed paper I co-authored with John Zhang entitled "The effect of a fruit and vegetable mix on hypertensive subjects", presents findings of the efficacy of 24 g of a green phytonutrient powder (GPP) on pre-hypertension and borderline stage 1 hypertension.[8] The purpose of the study was to find if a product with the phytonutrition of 7-10 serving of fruits and vegetables, but without the fiber, omega-3, protein, sodium restriction, vitamins and minerals found in the DASH diet, might mimic the DASH results without any further dietary or supplemental changes. This green fruit and vegetable phytonutrient powder (GPP) consisted of micro algae (spirulina, chlorella, *Dunaliella salina*), barley grass juice powder, multiple fruit and vegetable powders of all the colors, lecithin, acerola cherry, fermented cabbage, milk thistle, plant enzymes, quinoa sprout, lemon peel, oat beta glucan, soluble rice bran, concentrated extracts of green and white tea, resveratrol, lutein, zeaxanthin, lycopene, cinnamon, raspberry, iso-quercitin-rutin 50/50 and aloe vera. GPP was formulated with liposomal nanotechnology to enhance bioavailability of lipophillic and polyphenol phytonutrients. It was naturally flavored to enhance compliance.

The daily dose of 24 g (12 g BID) comprised 100 calories, 3 g fat, 4 g protein, 4 gm fiber, and 100% daily value (DV) of vitamin A (as betacarotene) and vitamin C (from Acerola cherry) and 48 g sodium, 304 g potassium, all naturally occurring. The oxygen radical absorbance capacity (ORAC) of the daily dose was approximately 14,000 ORAC units.

After taking the supplement for 90 days, both systolic and diastolic blood pressure decreased significantly. On average, systolic blood pressure decreased 12.4 mmHg (140.4 ± 17.7 to 128 ± 14.2 mmHg). The diastolic blood pressure decreased 7.1 mmHg (90.2 ± 7.7 mmHg to 83.1 ± 7.4 mmHg). No significant blood pressure decrease was observed in the control group. It was concluded that taking the green phytonutrient-rich fruit and vegetable drink for 90 days significantly reduced blood pressure.

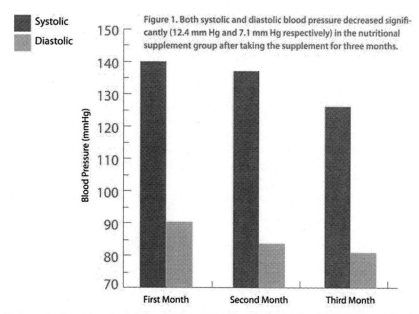

Figure 1. Both systolic and diastolic blood pressure decreased significantly (12.4 mm Hg and 7.1 mm Hg respectively) in the nutritional supplement group after taking the supplement for three months.

Figure 1. Supplementation with GPP Significantly Reduced Blood Pressure

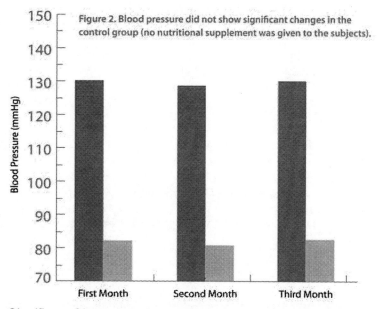

Figure 2. Blood pressure did not show significant changes in the control group (no nutritional supplement was given to the subjects).

Figure 2. No Significant Changes in Blood Pressure Were Observed in the Control Group

The results of this study supported Dr. Most's hypothesis that the efficacy of the DASH diet may largely be due to its high phytonutrient content. The most accepted current explanation is that the high antioxidant activity of phytonutrients helps to lower levels of reactive oxygen species (ROS), and thereby helps to restore endothelial function. Nonetheless, it is likely the results, if valid, come from a multitude of physiological effects of various phytonutrients, many of which are admittedly still poorly understood.

Zoonutrients for Hypertension

Phytonutrients are generally non-essential micronutrients found in plant foods that nonetheless have a salubrious effect on human health and physiology. Examples include epigallocatechin gallate (EGCG), resveratrol, lutein, and chlorophyll. Zoonutrients are similar except that they are sourced from animal foods. Examples include peptides, globulins, and enzymes.

Dairy and Whey Peptides and Cardiovascular Health

A growing body of scientific evidence reveals that whey protein contains various bioactive peptide components that may have a positive effect on cardiovascular health, protect against hypertension through angiotensin converting enzyme (ACE) inhibition and opioid-like activity. Furthermore, whey peptides may also be involved in inhibiting platelet aggregation and lowering cholesterol levels. Various studies have found that they also demonstrate antioxidant activity. Efficacy for hypertension has been well demonstrated in animal studies, but trials on human subjects are still somewhat limited.

Studies on infants have shown that di- and tri-peptides are easily absorbed in the intestine. The antihypertensive peptides from sour milk have shown to be well absorbed in the digestive system. The functional component may include various lactic acid bacteria (*Lactobacillus rhamnosus GG* and *Lactococcus lactis*) that have been shown to hydrolyze milk proteins into bioactive peptides.

Clinical Pilot Study: The Effects of Whey Zoonutrient Powder Alone and Combined with a Green Phytonutrient Powder on Subjects with Pre-Hypertension and Stage 1 Hypertension

A study was performed by John Zhang, MD, PhD of Logan College to investigate the effects, if any, of a whey-based zoonutrient powdered drink mix (WZP) both alone, and combined with phytonutrient nutritional supplementation (GPP), on the reduction of blood pressure in pre-hypertensive and hypertensive subjects.[9]

The whey-based powdered drink mix (WZP) used is made from antibiotic free, undenatured whey protein isolate (WPI) and colostrum from bovine spongiform encephalopathy (BSE) free herds not treated with growth hormone or hyper-immunization, or fed animal by-products. The whey based zoonutrient powdered drink mix (WZP) is uniquely fortified with proline rich polypeptides (PRP), which are considered to be colostrums most powerful immune-modulating peptides, along with organic selenium, reduced glutathione (protected in a liposome), soluble fiber (inulin), and lactose digesting enzymes. It is vanilla flavored and sweetened with stevia to enhance compliance. One scoop of 18 g is one serving providing 58 calories, 4 g carbohydrates (of which 3 g is soluble fiber), 12 g protein, less than 1 g fat, 73 mg sodium, 10% DV of riboflavin, 4% DV of folic acid, 3 % DV of calcium, all naturally occurring. WZP was fortified with 40 mcg organic selenium per serving (57% DV) and 50 mg of reduced glutathione.

The WZP and GPP group was consuming thereby approximately 110 calories, 14 g protein, 2 g fat, 5 g soluble fiber, and 5 g net carbohydrates twice a day.

The WZP, both alone and combined with the GPP, was tested to document their effects on prehypertension and stage 1 hypertension. The hypothesis was that WZP would be more effective in reducing blood pressure than the control (500 mg of calcium daily). Furthermore, it was hypothesized that the combined whey-based and fruit and vegetable-based supplements would be even more effective than WZP alone.

Methods
Random Selection

Subjects were assigned into one control and two experimental groups by random numbers. The first 60 numbers in the first two rows of the random table were used for the study.   Subjects   with the lowest 20 numbers were assigned in the control group, the highest 20 in the experimental group, and the middle 20 in the second experimental group. A total of three groups of subjects were recruited in the study.

Inclusion /Exclusion

Inclusion Criteria: Male or female hypertensive subjects 30-55 years old with systolic blood pressure between 130-160 mmHg, and diastolic blood pressure of 80-105 mmHg were recruited in the study.

Exclusion Criteria: Individuals with diabetes, heart, kidney, thyroid disorders, neurological diseases, and chronic disease, along with female subjects who were pregnant or breast feeding and those persons using drugs or medications were excluded.

Group Characteristics: The average age of the subjects was 24.5±4.4 years old in the three groups. All three groups had similar baseline characteristics in age, gender, blood pressure, and heart rate variability. The control group (CG) had 11 subjects (3 female), WZP group had 12 subjects (2 female) and WZP + GPP had 9 subjects (0 female).

Three Groups

The first group of subjects was the control group consuming 500 mg calcium pill per day. The second group took 2 servings (36 g) of WZP per day. The third group took 2 servings each of WZP (36 g) and GPP (24 g) products. No other changes were instituted.

Results

After taking the supplements for 90 days, both the systolic and diastolic blood pressure decreased significantly in the WZP and WZP + GPP. No significant changes were observed in the CG (Figs. 3, 4)

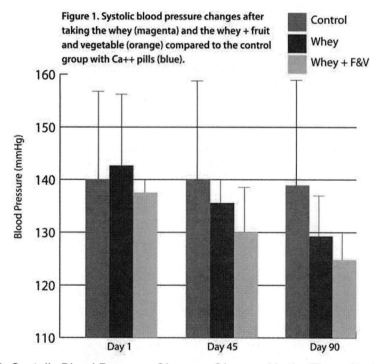

Figure 1. Systolic blood pressure changes after taking the whey (magenta) and the whey + fruit and vegetable (orange) compared to the control group with Ca++ pills (blue).

Figure 3. Systolic Blood Pressure Changes Observed in the Three Study Groups

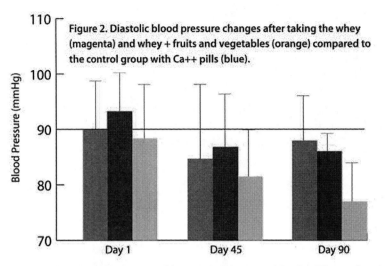

Figure 4. Diastolic Blood Pressure Changes Observed in the Three Study Groups

In the WZP group the systolic blood pressure decreased from 141.0 ±11.8 mmHg to 126.6 ±7.2 mmHg (P<0.05). The diastolic blood pressure decreased from 92.8 ±6.2 mmHg to 84.6 ±9.4 mmHg (P<0.05). This computes to an average drop of 13.4 mmHg in systolic pressure and 8.2 mmHg diastolic.

In the WZP + GPP group, the systolic blood pressure decreased from 136.3 ±3.1 mmHg to 125.4 ±5.1 mmHg (P<0.05). Diastolic blood pressure decreased from 88.5 ±7.6 mmHg to 74.6 ±7.7 (P<0.05) mmHg. This computes to an average drop of 10.9 mmHg in systolic pressure, 13.9 mmHg diastolic.

In the CG group, systolic blood pressure measured at 139.7±14.2 to 137.9±19.0 mmHg and the diastolic blood pressure from 89.8±6.9 to 87.0±7.7 mmHg, which was not significant (P>0.05).

Other Findings

After taking the supplements for 90 days, body weight increased significantly in the CG, from 190.9±20.9 pounds to 196.3±23.3 (P<0.05). The body weight in the WZP and WZP + GPP group did not show significant changes (P>0.05).

Study Conclusions

After taking the WZP and WZP+ GPP powdered drink mix supplements for 90 days, both the systolic and diastolic blood pressures decreased significantly. The body weight was increased in the control group (6 lbs) but not in the two treatment groups.

The results slightly exceed the published efficacy of the most successful dietary intervention, the DASH II diet (11.4/6.8 mmHg systolic/diastolic). The results mimic the efficacy of any one common prescription medication (12/6 mmHg systolic/diastolic). The results also mimic the efficacy of pilot studies on GPP alone (12.4 mmHg systolic and 7.1 diastolic mmHg).

The 3 study average (GPP, WZP, WZP + GPP) demonstrated a combined average drop in pressure of 12.3 mmHg systolic and 9.7 mmHg diastolic. A similar study on GPP by John Lewis, Ph.D., of the Miller School of Medicine at the University of Miami, to be published in the *Journal of the American Nutraceutical Association* in Dec 2009, demonstrated similar results.

Discussion
Considerations

It is possible that the 6 g of fiber, 80 mcg of selenium, or 100 mg of liposomal glutathione contributed largely to the results in the WZP trial, though there is little to no evidence in the literature to support this consideration. Stevia has some scientific evidence for its ability to lower blood pressure at dosages of 250 to 500 mg TID. The WZP + GPP group was consuming approximately 350 mg BID.

For control, a placebo drink would have been better than a placebo pill. The sample size was small and non heterogeneous in both studies. A longer study may well find an even greater drop in blood pressure, as can be the case with medication. Further human trials with pre-hypertensive and hypertensive subjects on larger and more diverse populations and for longer periods of time are needed.

The results for the combined group demonstrated a greater than expected drop in diastolic blood pressure, and less then expected drop in systolic blood pressure. It is thought by this author that participant numbers are too small as yet to allow for reasonable conjecture as to the potential meaning.

The serendipitous lack of weight gain/weight loss also calls for further study, as there are many similar reports with whey protein and weight loss. The relationship between lean body mass, central adiposity and blood pressure are well recognized.

Functional Food Solution?

Although various vitamins, minerals, herbs, amino acids, phytonutrients and zoonutrients used to support cardiovascular health may be taken by capsule, the question becomes which ones? How much is compliance affected as the amount of pills recommended increase?

Formulas like GPP and WZP, especially when combined, may be thought of as designed functional foods. The nutrient dense combination of GPP and WZP not only adds a very wide range of macronutrient, micronutrients, phytonutrients, and zoonutrients directly to the diet without pills, but also replaces less nutritious, pro-oxidant, pro-inflammatory, dysglycemic choices. The preparation time is minimal, as the powders are essentially instant. Additionally, the foods thus replaced may cost about the same to purchase, thereby causing minimal strain on the budget. These factors may promote greater compliance in the clinical setting.

Consider that the GPP and WZP together can form the basis of potential "heart healthy shake" meal replacement recipes. For instance, blended with 1 tsp orange flavored molecularly distilled fish oil and perhaps a ¼ tsp cinnamon in 12 ounces green tea, WZP + GPP may be also be useful for weight loss and insulin resistance (metabolic syndrome). Or WZP plus polyphenol rich baker's dark chocolate cocoa powder blended in low fat milk might be a high compliance way to lower blood pressure with a "chocolate shake".

If such "shakes" are easy to prepare and highly palatable, they might serve as nutrient dense, low calorie, convenient, high compliance meal /snack replacements. While the goal may be to see if such dietary interventions prove efficacious towards optimizing blood pressure, they may also demonstrate potential for surreptitious clinical progress in the frequently co-existent conditions of obesity or metabolic syndrome. Future studies combining WZP and GPP with a flax-based omega-3 nutraceutical drink mix powder, fortified with vegan DHA, will examine their combined effect on blood pressure, blood sugar and weight loss.

Clinical application

Clinicians need to decide if, how, and when they will consider nutraceutical supplementation or pharmaceutical intervention as needed to support lifestyle modification in cases of pre-hypertension and hypertension. Presuming similar blood pressure control, this presentation suggests that in pre-hypertension and borderline hypertension, a one to three month trial of WZP and GPP-like formulas would be the more conservative approach, or at least a "natural alternative" to offer patients who prefer such approaches. The graphic results in both studies demonstrate that at two servings a day a measurable response begins in 30 days and is clear by 60 days, with even greater benefit at 90 days. Depending on the complete clinical picture, there may be times when a trial of adding WZP and/or GPP-like formulas to the dietary lifestyle modifications is indicated.

CONCLUDING REMARKS

Cardiovascular disease is the number one cause of mortality. Optimizing blood pressure is the cornerstone of cardiovascular wellness. Any efficacious methods that demonstrate a high potential for compliance, affordability, and overall health benefits, with minimal side effects, should be worthy of investigation. The investigations herein support the hypotheses that there exist nutraceutical-rich functional food formulas and special diets that can be as efficacious as pharmaceuticals towards garnering a more optimal blood pressure. The phytonutrient and zoonutrient formulas discussed herein were not designed or intended to prevent or treat any particular disease. Indeed, they are presented as merely high compliance dietary lifestyle modifications designed for the myriads of people who wish to eat a healthier diet but for whatever reason, find it difficult to do so. This paper supports the continued investigation by integrative physicians as to the utility and suitability of phytonutrient and zoonutrient-rich drink mix powders as part of their dietary recommendations in clinical practice.

REFERENCES

1. The Seventh Report of the Joint National Committee on Prevention, Detection, Evaluation, and Treatment of High Blood Pressure. Bethesda, Md: National Institutes of Health, National Heart, Lung, and Blood Institute. 2003; NIH Publication 03-5231
2. Nawrot TS, Staessen JA, Thijs L, Fagard RH, Tikhonoff V, Wang JG, Franklin SS. Should pulse pressure become part of the Framingham risk score? *Journal of Human Hypertension.* 2004;18:279-286.
3. Law MR, Morris JK, Wald NJ. Use of blood pressure lowering drugs in the prevention of cardiovascular disease: meta-analysis of 147 randomized trials in the context of expectations from prospective epidemiological studies. *BMJ* 2009;338:b1665.
4. Arguedas JA, Perez MI, Wright JM. Treatment blood pressure targets for hypertension. *The Cochrane Database of Systematic Reviews.* 2009;3: CD004349.
5. Houston M. The Role of Vascular Biology, Nutrition, and Nutraceuticals in the Prevention and Treatment of Hypertension. *JANA* 2002;April: Supplement No. 1
6. Sacks FM, Svetkey LP, Vollmer WM, Appel LJ, Bray GA, Harsha D, *et al*. Effects on blood pressure of reduced dietary sodium and the Dietary Approaches to Stop Hypertension (DASH) diet. *N Engl J Med.* 2001;344:3-10.
7. Most MM. Estimated phytochemical content of the dietary approaches to stop hypertension (DASH) diet is higher than in the Control Study Diet. *J Am Diet Assoc.* 2004;104:1725-1727.
8. Zhang J, Maher J, Oxinos G. The effect of fruit and vegetable powder mix on hypertensive subjects: a pilot study. *Journal of Chiropractic Medicine.* 2009;8:101-106.
9. Zhang J, Maher J. The effects of whey zoonutrient powder alone and combined with a green phytonutrient powder on heart rate variability and pre-hypertension and stage 1 hypertension. *Journal of Chiropractic Education.* 2009;23:88.

ABOUT THE AUTHOR

John H. Maher, D.C., is a Diplomate of the Chiropractic Board of Clinical Nutrition, Board Certified in Integrative Medicine and past postgraduate faculty in Anti-Aging Medicine through New York Chiropractic College. Dr. Maher is co-founder of BioPharma Scientific and creator of "The SuperFood Solution™: Lifelong Wellness Made Easy".

Chapter 22
Human Longevity: A New Paradigm

Joseph C. Maroon, M.D.,
Senior Vice President A4M; Professor and Vice Chairman, Department of
Neurosurgery, Heindl Scholar in Neuroscience, University of Pittsburgh Medical Center;
Team Physician Pittsburgh Steelers
Jeff Bost PAC,
Clinical Instructor, Department of Neurosurgery, University of Pittsburgh Medical Center

ABSTRACT
This paper offers a brief introduction to the science of epigenetics, and explains how epigenetics can be used to promote health and longevity.

Keywords: Resveratrol, Genetics, Epigenetics, Red Wine, Polyphenols, Longevity, Sirtuins

INTRODUCTION
Human society has evolved at such a dramatic rate over the last 10,000 years that despite a similar facial appearance if we did somehow meet an early ancestor few would recognize any significant similarities. Early man was generally short, hungry, unkempt by today's standards, and most often did not live past the age of 30. As a society, in the last 200 years we have dramatically improved the human condition and associated human longevity through a more stable food source, immunizations, and anti-infection methods and medications. As a result, many people of the world will live well into their late 70's and early 80's in generally good health. At this point in our human timeline we are now at a cross roads of many competing influences that will either potentially continue this trend towards increased longevity or potentially reverse it.

Every moment of every day the body is rebuilding itself to survive and thereby increase our longevity. This is done daily through billions of cellular divisions. In fact, about 1% of our cells are made new each day. Entire organ systems in our bodies can be completely replaced in 6 months time. Our cells have a unique blueprint, developed through the millennium, which tells our body how to create new cells. But our decisions as to how or if we exercise, what we eat or don't eat, and to what type of environment we are exposed to has a direct influence on whether life-prolonging or life-limiting qualities are activated in each cell that is created. Our choices have the ability to either help or hurt this biological process, which, ultimately, affects our lifespan.

EPIGENETIC ACTIVATION
The actions on the body of physical activity, food quality and quantity, and environmental exposures are believed to work on either specific organ systems of our body or in the cellular protoplasm providing energy sources or toxins to be disposed of. Research now proves that the most profound effects on our bodies from these outside sources actually occur within our cellular nucleus in our genes – the blueprints of life.

What we have often been told, and many people believe, is that our fate or longevity is irrevocably linked to that of our parents. For example, a man whose father died at 60 may worry that he has reached his "genetic time limit" as he approaches his 60th year, and that he is now living on "borrowed time". This apprehension can often made worse if certain diseases, such as heart attack or stroke, were the cause of the parent's death. We are often told that we cannot escape our parent's genes for heart disease. The upshot of this is that many people in such circumstances begin to wonder why they should even bother to try and live a healthier life if their fate is already determined by their genes. However, research suggests that a person's existing genetic code only accounts for 30% of their overall longevity or lifespan, and that as much as 70% is under their control.

This fact – the 30/70 rule – requires the understanding of a whole new field of science that is just now beginning to explain how (or if) we exercise, what we eat, and to what type of environment we are exposed, to has a direct influence on whether health-producing or health-limiting genes are activated in each cell of our body. Our genetic code for either a positive effect (increased health and longevity) or for a negative effect (poor health and premature death) is linked more to factors that we can influence than those inherited from our parents.

This new discovery must be linked back to the famous discovery by Watson and Crick in 1953 – deoxyribonucleic acid, or DNA. DNA forms the basic double helix structure that can hold the complexity of all life on earth on just 23 pairs of chromosomes housed in the cell nucleus of every cell in the human body. Its most basic description can be referred to as a blueprint. When building any structure, in the case of a human cell perhaps a protein, the DNA blueprint is mostly a passive structure. It requires other cell structures and molecules called transcription factors to read the DNA blueprint and then, in turn, to construct the protein building blocks (amino acids) in their proper configuration. These other structures, that do the actual construction, can be influenced to read only certain sections of the DNA blueprint, or even to misread and place wrong sections of proteins together. The complexity of DNA blueprint reading and those things that can influence the proper reading to make those items that we need our cells for is the new science of epigenetics.

Using the science of epigenetics we now are able to explore and understand how factors such as exercise, diet, environment, and emotion can have profound effects on our health and eventual lifespan (Figure 1). What has been only recently discovered is that these listed factors can act to alter and influence many human epigenetic mechanisms that control how our genetic code is used or misused. What this means is the whilst we possess our individual DNA blueprint, as provided by our parents and all our distant ancestors from the beginnings of life on earth, the actions of epigenetic factors mean that not all aspects of the blueprint will necessarily be expressed.

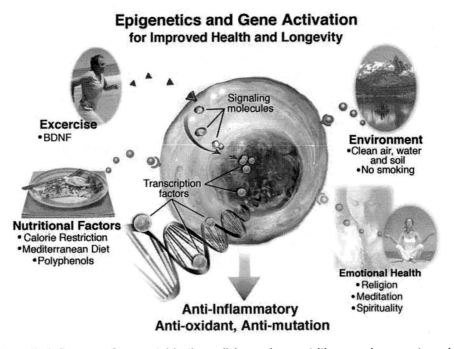

Epigenetics and Gene Activation
for Improved Health and Longevity

Signaling molecules

Excercise
•BDNF

Environment
•Clean air, water and soil
• No smoking

Transcription factors

Nutritional Factors
• Calorie Restriction
•Mediterranean Diet
• Polyphenols

Emotional Health
• Religion
• Meditation
• Spirituality

Anti-Inflammatory
Anti-oxidant, Anti-mutation

Figure 1. Epigenetic influences from outside the cell (exercise, nutrition, environment, and emotion) can activate nuclear transcription factors that can result in either very healthy (anti-inflammatory, anti-oxidant, anti-mutation) or unhealthy conditions being propagated from DNA codes.

One of the best ways to explain this concept is by an example of a discovery by scientists Lenny Guarente at MIT and David Sinclair at Harvard Medical School. In the late 1990's, the duo conducted a series of experiments on yeast cells. These experiments led them to discover that stressing the yeast cells by providing them with less sugar than they normally consumed (calorie restriction) extended the lifespan of many of the cells by as much as 60%. This discovery was not itself new, but what happened next was. Guarente and Sinclair discovered that calorie restriction activated a protein enzyme called Sir2 (silent information regulator 2), which belongs to a class of proteins known as the sirtuins. The activation of Sir2 caused the DNA structure of the yeast cells to curl up tighter, thus allowing for a more efficient cellular division. The end result of this was that the yeast cells were able to divide for a longer period and thus live longer. So, the stress of calorie restriction triggered the yeast cells to read the section of DNA blueprint code that produces additional DNA stabilizing proteins (Sir2), an action which prolonged the lifespan of the cells.

Since this discovery, all animals – including humans – have been found to possess these sirtuin activators. DNA stabilization by calorie restriction is just one pathway within animal cells that has been found to be activated by influences outside of the cell nucleus. We now know that many nutritional, activity, and environmental factors, can act on the DNA in the same epigenetic manner, to produce very healthful and life-prolonging actions.

The function of sirtuins to improve cellular division may have a profound impact on cancer and longevity itself by preserving cellular structures. Certain nutritional, activity, and environmental factors, can act on other epigenetic pathways to produce very healthy pathways that can also lead to prolonged. Similarly, there are nutritional, activity, and environmental factors that can activate pathways that can lead to disease and early death. Thus the choices are ours.

The most recent discovery related to sirtuin activation was also made by Sinclair, however this time he was working with a different researcher, Marie Lagouge, in France. In 2006, Sinclair and Lagogoue found that resveratrol, a polyphenolic phytoaxelin found in the skin of dark skinned grapes and other natural sources, activates sirtuins through the epigenetic pathway, thus replicating the epigenetic effects of calorie restriction.

Additional studies have now shown that other dietary supplements, vitamins, minerals, diet choices and exercise can epigenetically activate a protein that can influence brain cells to divide and produce new brain cells. Also environmental factors, for example some pollutants, can act epigenetically to stimulate cancer cell growth.

THE NEW HUMAN PARADIGM IN LONGEVITY

To discuss a new paradigm in human longevity we must explore how the diet choices, food quantity, and food types we now consume have been profoundly altered from the diets of our early hunter-gatherer ancestors. Their diet, which was essentially unchanged throughout millions of years of evolution, resulted to a genetic match which modern man now only remotely follows in our own diet and food choices. The foods consumed almost exclusively by early man, such as fish and seafood – rich sources of omega-3 essential fatty acids, and fruits, nuts, and berries – rich sources of health-promoting polyphenols, such as resveratrol, have all been shown to epigenetically prevent disease, and, in animals, prolong life.

Calorie restriction, practiced unintentionally by early man, has significant health benefits. Modern ethnic diets that consume high levels of omega-3's, green teas, and herb remedies such as polygonum cuspidatum (also a source of resveratrol) are also associated with improved longevity and health.

CONCLUDING REMARKS

To have a new paradigm in longevity we must both understand and practice health-enhancing measures that work on an epigenetic level to prevent illness, and not just to fight it once it occurs (sickcare). The idea of preventative medicine or "healthcare" must include choices that can lead to the best chances for a longer and healthier lifespan.

REFERENCES

Maroon, JC. *The Longevity Factor: How Resveratrol and Red Wine Activate Genes for a Longer and Healthier Life*. Simon and Schuster; 2009.

Baur JA, Sinclair DA. Therapeutic potential of resveratrol: the *in vivo* evidence. *Nat Rev Drug Discov*. 2006;5:493-506.

Baur JA, Pearson KJ, Price NL, Jamieson HA, Lerin C. Resveratrol improves health and survival of mice on a high-calorie diet. *Nature* 2006;444:337-342.

Blander G, Guarente L. The Sir2 family of protein deacetylases. *Annu Rev Biochem*. 2004;73:417-435.

ABOUT THE AUTHORS

Dr. Joseph C. Maroon is a board certified neurosurgeon at the University of Pittsburgh Medical Center, and a Professor and Heindl Scholar in Neurosurgery at the University of Pittsburgh School of Medicine. He has been the team neurosurgeon for the Pittsburgh Steelers for the last 20 years. Honored as one America's best neurosurgeons for 8 consecutive years in America's Best Doctors, he has published over 250 scientific papers, 8 books, and 40 book chapters. His two most recent books include, *Fish Oil the Natural Anti-Inflammatory* published by Basic Health Press in 2006 and *The Longevity Factor How Resveratrol and Red Wine Active Genes for a Longer and Healthier Life* published by Simon and Schuster in 2009. His research has focused on the prevention and treatment of injuries and diseases of the brain and spine. Most recently he has co-authored a paper entitled, *Evaluation of Lipid Profiles and the use of Omega-3 Essential Fatty Acids in Professional Football* – a landmark paper in this field. He currently serves as a medical advisor to Nordic Naturals and is the Head of the Medical Board at GNC. A devoted athlete he has completed over 60 triathlons – 6 of these Ironman distances (2.4 mile swim, 112 mile bike and 26.2 mile run). His last was the Hawaiian Ironman in October of 2008. Because of his athletic accomplishments and contributions to sports medicine he was inducted into the Lou Holtz Upper Ohio Valley Hall of Fame along with Joe Montana and Kareem Abdul-Jabaar.

Jeff Bost PAC has been a neurosurgical physician assistant and associate with Dr. Joseph Maroon since 1987. He and Dr. Maroon have special interest in minimally invasive spine and brain surgery and have collaborated on many scientific and medical papers and books in these areas. In 2003, both became interested in using natural products to treat pain and inflammation when it became known that certain anti-inflammatory medications, like Vioxx, could have significant and serious side effects, such as heart attacks and even death. After reviewing the available scientific literature, both became convinced that omega-3's from fish oil could offer similar anti-inflammatory relief. Following a very positive response from our neurosurgical patients we had given fish oil to use for spine pain, along with publishing several articles on the subject, Dr. Maroon and Jeff Bost co-authored a book, entitled *Fish Oil: The Natural Anti-Inflammatory*. The book is currently in its forth printing with over 75,000 copies sold. Since this time both Dr. Maroon and Jeff Bost have lectured on this subject and other natural products used to treat pain and inflammation to both national and international medical organizations and public forums. Both are considered experts in the subject and work closely with GNC as advisors on scientifically proven natural supplements.

Chapter 23
Iodine Deficiency: A Public Health Crisis
Chris D. Meletis, ND
Executive Director, The Institute for Healthy Aging (Beaverton, Oregon USA)

ABSTRACT

Health policy over the last couple of decades has recommended that we decrease salting our food due to the risk of hypertension. The consequence of not using iodized salt and the increase in bromide, fluoride, and perchlorate ingestion has set the stage for premature death, cancer, lowered IQ, hormone imbalance, and even deafness. Identifying risks for halide toxicity, testing for iodine sufficiency, and looking at other global health policies that are killing, maiming, and prematurely aging North American and Westernized societies is a health mandate that must be addressed aggressively. The aim of this paper is to discuss iodine deficiency and its impact upon public health.

IODINE DEFICIENCY – A PUBLIC HEALTH CRISIS

Iodine is a trace element required by the body for an increasing number of identified physiologic functions. This element belongs to the halogen family of elements, a group of highly reactive nonmetals that includes fluorine, chlorine, bromine, and astatine.

Most iodine intake in the United States still occurs as a result of the intake of iodized table salt. Indeed in the 1920's iodation of salt was established as a health mandate due to a growing number of iodine deficiency diseases including goiters and hormone altering thyroid disease such as hypo- and hyper-thyroidism. The genesis of this mandate arose from upper Midwest and Great Lakes region, where the incidence of goiter was as high as 30–40% in 1922, was aptly named the "goiter belt."[1]

The recommended daily allowance (RDA) of iodine for adults is 150 µg/day, for pregnant women 220 µg/day, and for lactating women 290 µg/day, and although some studies indicate that Americans' iodine intake is adequate, many other studies suggest a prevalence of sub-clinical iodine deficiency. The thinking that iodine levels are sufficient is resonant of the concept that vitamin D levels have been adequate over the years. As with the vitamin D paradigm that is now being challenged after decades of insufficiency and resultant progressive disease, iodine deficits are also contributing to further human suffering.

Blind Health Policy

The vitamin D awakening must trigger us to look at other potential nutrient deficiencies that have been created through health policy. We were told to not go in the sun, for fear of skin cancer, indeed a reasonable consideration; yet with this recommended avoidance behavior or the incorporation of using high SPF sunscreens that can block in excess over 90% of UV inducing vitamin D creation within the body, health policy set society up for increased rates of various diseases, including autoimmune disease, osteoporosis, cancer, and depression, to name a few. Likewise, blind health policy suggesting the avoidance of salt (sodium chloride) that may be protective against high blood pressure and heart disease, has led to decreased use of salt for the last couple of generations. In 1920, good health policy solved a health crisis by adding iodine to the diet; however the new health policy, without regard or warning of the public, took the iodine back out of the diet despite knowing that iodine is critical for metabolism, cognitive development, and disease prevention.

Even under the best circumstance when iodized salt is used, research suggests that only 10% of the iodide in iodized salt is bioavailable.[2] Moreover, with cautionary recommendations that Americans limit their sodium intake, an adequate intake of iodine is of concern because iodine deficiency is associated with numerous anomalies including hypothyroidism, goiter, cretinism, cognitive disorders, neurological disorders, and breast disease. Iodine deficiency is especially hazardous in pregnant women, developing fetuses, and newborn infants because of its ability to cause irreversible damage to fetuses and newborns.

The World Health Organization (WHO) has established that the mean urine iodine concentration should exceed 10 µg/dL, and should be less than 5 µg/dL in no more than 20% percent of a population. Sadly though, the United States has demonstrated clearly that we are failing to meet the minimal standards of the WHO, as discovered by The National Health and Nutrition Examination Surveys (NHANES). It was determined via the NHANES I (1971–1974) and NHANES III (1988–1994) that the median urine iodine concentration of US citizens decreased by 50%, while a low urine excretory level of iodine of less than 5 µg/dL increased by 4.5-fold in this same period. Monitoring of high-risk groups showed that 6.7% of pregnant women and 14.9% of women of childbearing age had a urine excretory level of less than 5 µg/dL of iodine.[3] Furthermore, it was demonstrated by the NHANES IV: 2001–2002 that no improvement in iodine levels has occurred since NHANES III.[4]

An Artificial Sense of Adequacy: RDA for Iodine

The minimal daily iodine recommendation (RDA) of 150 µg/day is, according to many of the leaders in the field of nutrition, overtly low, much like the RDA of 60 mg/day for vitamin C is far too inadequate for anything other than the prevention of overt scurvy. The fear of triggering autoimmune thyroid disease is scattered in the scientific literature,[5,6] however such autoimmune disease has been increasing during the same period in which iodine intake has been decreasing in the United States.[7] From a practical perspective, one must only look to the East, to be reassured on the long term safety of higher levels of iodine; in the traditional Japanese populace, the typical dietary intake of elemental iodine is said to be as high as 13.8 mg.[8]

Throughout the US and Europe physicians have prescribed iodine in a dose of 0.1–0.3 mL of Lugol's solution, a 5% solution containing 50 mg of iodine and 100 mg of potassium iodide per milliliter, thus providing 12.5-37.5 mg of the elemental iodine that is needed to treat iodine deficiency disorders and promote overall well-being.[8,9] This prescribing practice began to decrease after the use of iodized salt. Now, people have moved away from the use of iodized salt either because of health concerns, because they eat more processed food (which tends to contain excess amounts of non-iodized salt), or because of a desire to become more holistic and swap table salt for sea salt, which is not typically iodized. Thus, it makes sense that we begin to revisit the practice of prescribing iodine, while practicing cautionary medicine that includes monitoring iodine levels and thyroid function.

Metabolism of Iodine

The human body concentrates iodide in the salivary glands, breast tissue, gastric mucosa, and choroid plexus, among other sites, thus demonstrating the global importance of "sufficient" levels of iodine to more than just the thyroid gland. The body possesses a specific mechanism, the sodium/iodide transporters – protein molecules also known as "symporters" that uptake iodide from the blood into the thyroid gland and other tissues across a concentration gradient that may be as high as 50-fold, and concentrate the iodide in cells.

It has long been understood that iodide/iodine are essential for thyroxine (T4), which is converted in peripheral tissues to the hormone tri-iodothyronine (T3), which regulates growth and cellular metabolism. Additionally, vitamin A and iron deficiency, as well as the selenium deficiency noted earlier, can exacerbate iodine deficiency.[10] Intake of particular elements that compete with iodine for uptake and utilization, such as chlorine, fluorine, and bromine, may also be a factor.

Diagnosis of Iodine Deficiency

According to the WHO, median urine iodine levels should exceed 10 µg/dL in "iodine sufficient" populations. Urinary iodine excretion may also be expressed in relation to creatinine excretion, as µg of iodine per g of creatinine. There remains debate amongst researchers as to the best measure of iodine sufficiency, which should not be surprising, considering the level of entrenchment in the status quo that so many researcher adhere to as they develop and test hypotheses.12,13 The Iodine Loading test is becoming an ever growing popularity of functional testing, for this the patient is given a 50mg iodine load and their urine is collected for the next 24-hours.

The Halide Wars: Bromine, Chlorine and Fluoride

There are many competing halides that exacerbate the current inadequate dietary iodine intake. Not surprisingly, in the 1970's (when iodine levels began to drop in the US as documented by the NHANES surveys) bromine replaced iodine for use as a dough softener in bread–making. Studies of thyroid function in rats indicate that with increased intake, bromine replaces iodine in this organ.[14] Animal studies also suggest that in the presence of an iodine-deficient state, bromine may induce hypothyroid symptoms of decreased thyroxine synthesis and increased thyroid gland size, as well as decreasing iodine concentrations in the skin.[14] Studies with pregnant and lactating rats have demonstrated that increased bromine intake decreases the iodine content of mammary tissue, decreases T4 in both mothers and offspring, and decreases the body weight of offspring. Bromine also increases the renal excretion of iodine in these animals.[14] Treating rats with bromine has been shown to induce goiter and decrease the thyroid iodine concentration, while supplementation with iodine and selenium has been found to reduce the amount of bromine taken up by the thyroid by 50% compared to that in rats without such supplementation.[15]

Chlorine-Containing Anions

Perchlorate, an environmental contaminant, is a known competitive inhibitor of the iodine/sodium symporter and decreases thyroid function by inhibiting iodine uptake by the thyroid at doses of 200 mg/day or more.[16] Perchlorate is found in fireworks, explosives, solid jet and rocket fuel, and is a contaminate found in some fertilizers. Perchlorate is often consumed in plants such as lettuce and leafy greens, drinking water, and milk, as it is generally accumulated from contaminated ground water. Studies have found that the majority of dairy milk samples and all samples of breast milk tested contained perchlorate. A recent study demonstrated a mean perchlorate level in breast milk of 10.5 µg/L, suggesting that the average breast-fed infant consumes more than twice the recommended maximum daily level of perchlorate established by the National Academy of Sciences.[17]

Studies of perchlorate levels in drinking water and their relation to diseases in the United States have provided conflicting results. Several studies have measured thyroid hormone values as indicators of the health effects of perchlorate in drinking water, and have found no effect.[18] However, one study did find a statistically significant increase in newborns' TSH levels in an area where all samples of drinking water were contaminated with perchlorate, as compared to the TSH levels of newborns in an area without such contamination.[19] Some researchers suggest that the combination of perchlorate with other competitors of the iodine/sodium symporter, such as nitrates and thiocyanate, as well as the combination of perchlorate with iodine itself, increases the risk of thyroid-related disease.[20] A further study examining the incidence of attention-deficit/hyperactivity disorder (ADHD), autism, and the academic performance of fourth graders in areas with and without perchlorate contamination did not find a statistically significant difference in these conditions in the two groups. However, this study did not take into account the residence locations of mothers at the time of gestation, or their individual perchlorate exposure.[21] Also, one study showed that higher levels of perchlorate excretion were associated with increased levels of TSH and decreased levels of T4 in iodine-deficient women.[22]

Fluoride

Fluorine, often in the form of fluoride, a halogen like bromine and chlorine, is commonly added to drinking water and used as a component of dental products for decreasing the risk of caries. However, some animal studies have shown that increased intake of fluoride can decrease serum T3 and T4 levels in iodine-deficient mice.[23]

Iodine Deficiency and Thyroid Disease

There is abundant scientific and medical literature demonstrating that hypothyroidism during pregnancy can result in miscarriage, abnormal fetal growth, perinatal morbidity, and neonatal death. Of particular note, it is essential to recognize that early brain development begins around the 15th week of gestation relies on thyroxine, hence iodine status of the mother. Indeed maternal hypothyroidism and iodine insufficiency can produce fetal brain damage, cretinism, and a decreased intelligence quotient. Cretinism, a severe neuropathology caused by iodine deficiency, is marked by gross mental retardation along with varying degrees of shortness of stature, deaf-mutism, and spasticity. Because of decreased iodine retention, preterm infants, in whom renal function is not fully developed, require twice the daily intake of iodine for normal infants. To decrease these risks, the WHO in 2001 suggested an increased iodine intake for infants and an increased iodine content in infant formula.[24] However, with such a huge drop in iodine status in the US since the 1970's, would it not be prudent that not just the overtly at risk, but all children and mothers be encouraged to increase iodine levels prenatally and post-gestation?

Beyond Thyroid Disease –The Breast Health Link

Beyond thyroid function, iodine is required for the normal growth and development of breast tissue. The high level of iodine intake by Japanese women, noted earlier, has been associated with a low incidence of both benign and cancerous breast disease in this population. Evidence links iodine deficiency with an elevated risk of breast, endometrial, and ovarian cancer.[25] Antiproliferative iodolactones in the thyroid may be responsible for this effect.[26] Although autoimmune antibodies directed against thyroid peroxidase have been associated with a better prognosis in breast cancer,[27] thyroid supplementation may increase the risk of breast cancer, especially if an underlying iodine insufficiency is not addressed, though this is still a point of great debate.[28] *In vitro* studies have found that molecular iodine inhibits induction and proliferation and induces apoptosis in some human breast cancer cell lines, as well as exhibiting antioxidant activity.[29] Benign, fibrocystic breast disease is also associated with iodine deficiency. Blocking of iodine with perchlorate in the mammary tissue of rats has been found to cause histologic changes indicative of fibrocystic breast disease, as well as precancerous lesions.[30] Of clinical note, iodine supplementation has been shown to ease mastalgia. Supplementation with 3 or 6 mg/day of molecular iodine significantly decreased pain reported by patients, as well as physicians' assessments of pain, tenderness, and nodularity in benign breast disease, with a dose of 6 mg/day providing significant reduction of pain in more than 50% of patients.[31]

Brain Development and IQ – The Iodine Factor

T3 and T4 are particularly important for myelination of the developing brain, and in turn iodine is critical for thyroid hormone production, with 3 iodine molecules incorporated in T3 and 4 iodine molecules on T4. Hypothyroidism during pregnancy and lactation causes numerous neurologic and cognitive deficits. A study of schoolchildren with mild iodine deficiency found that urine iodine levels above 100 µg/L were associated with significantly higher IQ scores, while levels below 100 µg/L increased the risk of an IQ below 70.[32] The same study also found that consuming non-iodized salt and drinking milk less than once daily increased the risk of an IQ below the 25th percentile.[33] Another study found that children from severely iodine-deficient areas had IQ scores that were 12.45 points below average.[33] A small study comparing the prevalence of ADHD in children from a mildly iodine-deficient area and a moderately iodine-deficient area found that 68.7% of those from the latter area had a diagnosis of ADHD, as compared with an absence of this diagnosis in the children from the mildly iodine deficient area, and that IQ scores were lower in the moderately deficient area. Of the children with ADHD, 63.6% were born to mothers who had become hypothyroxinemic in early gestation.[34] Studies have also suggested that iodine deficiency affects hearing. Children in a mildly iodine-deficient area who had elevated serum thyroglobulin levels had higher auditory thresholds for sound of higher frequencies than did children with lower thyroglobulin levels.[35] Another comparative study examining children from a severely iodine-deficient and a mildly iodine-deficient region found that the former group had lower thyroxine levels, higher TSH levels, and lower scores on achievement motivation tests, and were slower learners than the latter group.[36] Research on endemic cretinism from congenital iodine deficiency has shown specific severe neurologic deficits including deaf-mutism and a varying degree of bilateral hearing loss, as well as dysarthria, mental deficiency, spasticity of the proximal lower extremities, rigidity, and bradykinesia. In some cases strabismus and kyphoscoliosis were also present.[37] Thus, it can be seen that subclinical cases of iodine insufficiency may also contribute to the wide myriad of the above mentioned common complaints seen in daily clinical practice.

Gastric Disease on the Rise – Iodine Correlation

There is no question that clinicians are barraged by a sheer volume of patients with gastric ailments. There is also no question that since the 1970's, when a drop in iodine sufficiency occurred in the US, stomach disease, and in particular dyspepsia, has continued to rise. Certainly there are many co-morbid factors, yet we also know that iodine deficiency has been linked to an increased risk of gastric carcinoma. One study demonstrated an increased prevalence of gastric cancer and an increased risk of atrophic gastritis in areas with a greater-than-average prevalence of iodine deficiency-related goiter. The researchers also reported that competitive inhibitors of intracellular iodine transport, such as nitrates, thiocyanate, and salt increased the risk of gastric cancer.[38] Another study found a significant correlation between decreased mean urinary iodine levels and prevalence of stomach cancer, as well as a greater frequency of severe iodine deficiency in stomach cancer than in controls.[39] There is also evidence for lower levels of iodine in cancerous gastric tissue than in surrounding normal tissue.[40]

Treatment of Iodine Deficiency

The American Thyroid Association (ATA) recommends that iodine supplementation of 150 µg/day be given to all pregnant and lactating women, and suggests that all prenatal vitamin supplements contain 150 µg of iodine.[41] Based on this recommendation; it may be possible to extrapolate this increased need to the general population. It is time to start thinking beyond the 1940's RDA approach of dosing so marginally that survival is the threshold opposed to true human thriving.

CONCLUDING REMARKS

Iodine deficiency is a worldwide concern with serious consequences to health. With the increased presence of other halogens in food and water supplies, relative iodine deficiency is a growing concern. As with vitamin D, folic acid, the omega-3 fatty acids, and other nutrients recognized as deficient in the Western diet, sub-clinical iodine deficiency may then become a thing of the past. Incorporating iodine into clinical practice makes good sense and with testing and monitoring it can be done safely and most importantly can serve as a proactive intervention to help prevent undue human suffering.

REFERENCES

1. Markel H. "When it rains it pours": Endemic goiter, iodized salt, and David Murray Cowie, M.D. *Am J Public Health.* 1987;77:219-229.
2. Abraham GE. The concept of orthoiodosupplementation and its clinical implications. *Original Internist.* 2004;11:29-38.
3. Hollowell JG, Staehling NW, Hannon WH, *et al.* Iodine nutrition in the United States: Trends and public health implications. Iodine excretion data from National Health and Nutrition Examination Surveys I and III (1971–1974 and 1988–1994) *J Clin Endocrinol Metab.* 1998;83:3401-3408.
4. Blackburn GL. National Health and Nutrition Examination Survey: Where nutrition meets medicine for the benefit of health. *Am J Clin Nutr.* 2003;78:197-198.
5. Prummel MF, Strieder T, Wiersinga WM. The environment and autoimmune thyroid diseases. *Eur J Endocrinol.* 2004;150:605-618.
6. Zois C, Stavrou I, Svarna E, *et al.* Natural course of autoimmune thyroiditis after elimination of iodine deficiency in northwestern Greece. *Thyroid* 2006;16:289-293.
7. Abraham GE, Flechas JD, Hakala JC. Orthoiodosupplementation: Iodine sufficiency of the whole human body. *Original Internist.* 2002;9:30-41.
8. Abraham GE, Brownstein D. A rebuttal of Dr. Gaby's editorial on iodine. *Townsend Letter for Doctors & Patients.* October 2005. Available at http://www.townsendletter.com/Oct2005/gabyrebuttal1005.htm Accessed on 1st April, 2007.
9. Jamieson A, Semple CG. Successful treatment of Graves' disease in pregnancy with Lugol's iodine. *Scott Med J.* 2000;45:20-21.
10. National Academies Press. Dietary Reference Intakes for Vitamin A, Vitamin K, Arsenic, Boron, Chromium, Copper, Iodine, Iron, Manganese, Molybdenum, Nickel, Silicon, Vanadium, and Zinc. 2000. Available at http://www.nap.edu/openbook.php?record_id=10026&page=268 Accessed on 1st April, 2007.
11. Gaitan E, Cooksey RC, Legan J. Antithyroid effects in vivo and in vitro of vitexin: A C-glucosylflavone in millet. *J Clin Endocrinol Metab.* 1995;80:1144-1147.
12. Simsek E, Safak A, Yavuz O, *et al.* Sensitivity of iodine deficiency indicators and iodine status in Turkey. *J Pediatr Endocrinol Metab.* 2003;16:197-202.
13. Soldin OP, Tractenberg RE, Pezzullo JC. Do thyroxine and thyroidstimulating hormone levels reflect urinary iodine concentrations? *Ther Drug Monit.* 2005;27:178-185.
14. Pavelka S. Metabolism of bromide and its interference with the metabolism of iodine. *Physiol Res.* 2004;53(suppl1):S81-S90.
15. Kotyzova D, Eybl V, Mihaljevic M, Glattre E. Effect of long-term administration of arsenic (III) and bromine with and without selenium and iodine supplementation on the element level in the thyroid of rat. *Biomed Pap Med Fac Univ Palacky Olomouc Czech Repub.* 2005;149:329-333.
16. Crump C, Michaud P, Tellez R. Does perchlorate in drinking water affect thyroid function in newborns or school-age children? *J Occup Environ Med.* 2000;42:603-612.
17. Kirk AB, Martinelango PK, Tian K, *et al.* Perchlorate and iodide in dairy and breast milk. *Environ Sci Technol.* 2005;39:2011-2017.
18. Li Z, Li FX, Byrd D, *et al.* Neonatal thyroxine level and perchlorate in drinking water. *J Occup Environ Med.* 2000;42:200-205.
19. Brechner RJ, Parkhurst GD, Humble WO, *et al.* Ammonium perchlorate contamination of Colorado River drinking water is associated with abnormal thyroid function in newborns in Arizona. *J Occup Environ Med.* 2000;42:777-782.
20. De Groef B, Decallonne BR, Van der Geyten S, *et al.* Perchlorate versus other environmental

sodium/iodide symporter inhibitors: Potential thyroid-related health effects. *Eur J Endocrinol.* 2006;155:17-25.

21. Chang S, Crothers C, Lai S, Lamm S. Pediatric neurobehavioral diseases in Nevada counties with respect to perchlorate in drinking water: An ecological inquiry. *Birth Defects Res [A] Clin Mol Teratol.* 2003;67:886-892.

22. Blount BC, Pirkle JL, Osterloh JD, Valentin-Blasini L, Caldwell KL. Urinary perchlorate and thyroid hormone levels in adolescent and adult men and women living in the United States. *Environ Health Perspect.* 2006;114:1865-1871.

23. Zhao W, Zhu H, Yu Z, *et al.* Long-term effects of various iodine and fluorine doses on the thyroid and fluorosis in mice. *Endocr Regul.* 1998;32:63-70.

24. Joint FAO/WHO Expert Consultation on Human Vitamin and Mineral Requirements, (1998: Bangkok, Thailand). *Vitamin and Mineral Requirements in Human Nutrition.* 2nd ed. Geneva: World Health Organization; 2004. Available at http://whqlibdoc.who.int/publications/2004/9241546123_chap16.pdf Accessed 1st April, 2007.

25. Stadel BV. Dietary iodine and risk of breast, endometrial, and ovarian cancer. *Lancet* 1976;1:890-891.

26. Aceves C, Anguiano B, Delgado G. Is iodine a gatekeeper of the integrity of the mammary gland? *J Mammary Gland Biol Neoplasia.* 2005;10:189-196.

27. Smyth PP. The thyroid, iodine and breast cancer. *Breast Cancer Res.* 2003;5:235-238.

28. Kapdi CC, Wolfe JN. Breast cancer: Relationship to thyroid supplements for hypothyroidism. *JAMA* 1976;236:1124-1127.

29. Shrivastava A, Tiwari M, Sinha RA. Molecular iodine induces caspase-independent apoptosis in human breast carcinoma cells involving the mitochondria-mediated pathway. *J Biol Chem.* 2006;281:19762-19771.

30. Eskin BA, Shuman R, Krouse T, Merion JA. Rat mammary gland atypia produced by iodine blockade with perchlorate. *Cancer Res.* 1975;35:2332-2339.

31. Kessler JH. The effect of supraphysiologic levels of iodine on patients with cyclic mastalgia. *Breast J.* 2004;10:328-336.

32. Santiago-Fernandez P, Torres-Barahona R, Muela-Martinez JA, *et al.* Intelligence quotient and iodine intake: A cross-sectional study in children. *J Clin Endocrinol Metab.* 2004;89:3851-3857.

33. Qian M, Wang D, Watkins WE, et al. The effects of iodine on intelligence in children: A meta-analysis of studies conducted in China. *Asia Pac J Clin Nutr.* 2005;14:32-42.

34. Vermiglio F, Lo Presti VP, Moleti M, *et al.* Attention deficit and hyperactivity disorders in the offspring of mothers exposed to mild–moderate iodine deficiency: A possible novel iodine deficiency disorder in developed countries. *J Clin Endocrinol Metab.* 2004;89:6054-6060.

35. van den Briel T, West CE, Hautvast JG, Ategbo EA. Mild iodine deficiency is associated with elevated hearing thresholds in children in Benin. *Eur J Clin Nutr.* 2001;55:763-768.

36. Tiwari BD, Godbole MM, Chattopadhyay N, *et al.* Learning disabilities and poor motivation to achieve due to prolonged iodine deficiency. *Am J Clin Nutr.* 1996;63:782-786.

37. DeLong GR, Stanbury JB, Fierro-Benitez R. Neurological signs in congenital iodine-deficiency disorder (endemic cretinism). *Dev Med Child Neurol.* 1985;27:317-324.

38. Venturi S, Venturi A, Cimini D, *et al.* A new hypothesis: Iodine and gastric cancer. *Eur J Cancer Prev.* 1993;2:17-23.

39. Behrouzian R, Aghdami N. Urinary iodine/creatinine ratio in patients with stomach cancer in Urmia, Islamic Republic of Iran. *East Mediterr Health J.* 2004;10:921-924.

40. Gulaboglu M, Yildiz L, Celebi F, *et al.* Comparison of iodine contents in gastric cancer and surrounding normal tissues. *Clin Chem Lab Med.* 2005;43:581–584.

41. Becker DV, Braverman LE, Delange F, *et al.* Iodine supplementation for pregnancy and lactation—United States and Canada: Recommendations of the American Thyroid Association. *Thyroid* 2006;16:949-951.

ABOUT THE AUTHOR

Dr. Chris D. Meletis is the executive director for The Institute for Healthy Aging, a non-profit organization dedicated to advancing and disseminating natural; medicine therapeutics that facilitate optimal wellness. He is an international author and lectures nationally on topics of family practice, nutrition, botanical medicine, and healthy aging and wellness. Many of his articles and books can be found at www.DrChrisMeletis.com.

Chapter 24
How Sunshine May Reduce Cancer By 50%
Joseph Mercola, D.O.
Founder, www.mercola.com

ABSTRACT

Vitamin D is one of the most cost effective and important health interventions at our disposal. Yet, vitamin D deficiency is pervasive in North America. This is concerning, as research continues to accumulate documenting the many benefits of vitamin D, such as reducing the risk of obesity, heart disease, osteoporosis, autoimmune disease (multiple sclerosis, rheumatoid arthritis, and type I diabetes), and lowering blood pressure. However, the most significant influence of vitamin D is likely related to its influence on cancer, with recent studies suggesting that one million people throughout the world die each year because of inadequate sun exposure, resulting in suboptimal vitamin D levels.

Since cancer incidence has increased to the point where cancer is now the number one cause of death in the US for those under 70, this demands our attention, and is moving the standard of care towards criminal and negligent malpractice if vitamin D levels are not aggressively monitored as part of most cancer treatment programs.

Although oral vitamin D therapy can be used to treat and prevent vitamin D deficiency, it is not the best approach, and is also associated with risk of potential overdose if not carefully monitored. Ideally, optimal vitamin D levels should be achieved by wise application of appropriate sun exposure.

The aim of this paper is to discuss the functions and benefits of vitamin D, and to determine the best way of preventing and treating vitamin D deficiency.

INTRODUCTION

Vitamin D is one of the most cost effective and important health interventions at our disposal. Yet, vitamin D deficiency is pervasive in North America. This is concerning, as research continues to accumulate documenting the many benefits of vitamin D, such as reducing the risk of obesity, heart disease, osteoporosis, autoimmune disease (multiple sclerosis, rheumatoid arthritis, and type I diabetes), and lowering blood pressure. However, the most significant influence of vitamin D is likely related to its influence on cancer, with recent studies suggesting that one million people throughout the world die each year because of inadequate sun exposure, resulting in suboptimal vitamin D levels.

Since cancer incidence has increased to the point where cancer is now the number one cause of death in the US for those under 70, this demands our attention, and is moving the standard of care towards criminal and negligent malpractice if vitamin D levels are not aggressively monitored as part of most cancer treatment programs.

Although oral vitamin D therapy can be used to treat and prevent vitamin D deficiency, it is not the best approach, and is also associated with risk of potential overdose if not carefully monitored. Ideally, optimal vitamin D levels should be achieved by wise application of appropriate sun exposure.

The aim of this paper is to discuss the functions and benefits of vitamin D, and to determine the best way of preventing and treating vitamin D deficiency.

VITAMIN D

Until recently it was thought that vitamin D's sole contribution to health was the prevention of rickets, osteomalacia, and osteoporosis, however we now know that this is not the case. There is now a large amount of research in the medical literature documenting the many anti-aging benefits of vitamin D. We also now know that vitamin D is not really a vitamin, it is actually a prosteroid hormone that has a powerful epigenetic influence on your body, in fact research has shown that vitamin D regulates as many as two to three thousand genes.

Vitamin D has been shown to lower inflammation – a key component of aging, prevent hypertension, and aid in the control of body weight. It plays a key role in the prevention of autoimmune diseases, including rheumatoid arthritis, multiple sclerosis, and type I and type II diabetes. Both multiple sclerosis and type I diabetes are virtually unheard of in equatorial countries, where year-round sunshine means that vitamin D deficiency is extremely rare. Vitamin D has also been linked to autism. Dr. John Cannell, a leading authority on vitamin D, believes that vitamin D deficiency has played a key role in the autism epidemic. His theory is that gestational vitamin D deficiency, caused by vitamin D deficiency in the mother, renders the unborn child highly susceptible to toxic influences that precipitate the autistic condition when they are born.[1] Vitamin D has also been shown to reduce the risk of preeclampsia. Thus, it is imperative that pregnant women and women planning to become pregnant have their vitamin D levels checked regularly, for the health of both mother and child.

Vitamin D is also a very potent antibiotic. It increases levels of several hundred antimicrobial peptides, one of the most important being cathelicidin LL-37, a key component of the innate immunity system, which plays an essential role in protecting humans against infectious diseases. It has been proposed that vitamin D may help to prevent against influenza.[2] This theory is supported by the fact the influenza epidemics are seasonal, occurring in the winter when vitamin D levels are low due to lack of sunlight. In fact, vitamin D is useful for the treatment of many infections of the upper respiratory tract. The standard dose for this is 50,000 IU for three consecutive days; however Dr Carnell has proposed that a dose of approximately 2000 IU per kilogram (up to 150,000 IU) per day may be more relevant.

The concept of using sunlight to treat disease is not new. Many people are not aware that prior to the introduction of drug therapy for tuberculosis, sunlight therapy, also known as helio or solar therapy, was the primary method of treating tuberculosis. Sunlight therapy is also useful in the treatment of lupus and psoriasis.

In short, vitamin D has been found to be of great importance in the prevention of a whole host of diseases, many of which have not been mentioned above. However, the focus of this paper is cancer, and how sunshine may reduce the risk of cancer by 50%.

CANCER AND VITAMIN D

In 1936, it was shown that when the incidence of skin cancer increases, the incidence of other cancers is decreased. Every year 7 million people die throughout the world from cancer. Dr. William Grant, a leading epidemiologist on vitamin D, believes that 2 million of these deaths – as many as 200,000 in the US – are directly caused by vitamin D deficiency. It is likely that vitamin D plays a role in the prevention of many cancers; however it has been shown to play a significant role in the prevention of breast cancer, colon cancer, lung cancer (early stage), prostate cancer, melanoma, and non-Hodgkin's lymphoma.

So, how does vitamin D reduce the risk of cancer? It appears that vitamin D helps to protect against cancer via a number of different mechanisms. A discussion of these mechanisms is beyond the scope of this paper, however to summarize: Vitamin D is believed to promote apoptosis of cancer cells, reduce the proliferation and metastatic potential of cancer cells, reduce angiogenesis, and lower inflammation.

The Importance of Sun Exposure

Interestingly, 100 years ago sun exposure was much higher than it is today, yet the incidence of skin cancer has actually increased. Why is this? One of the major reasons behind the increase in skin cancer is the increase in omega 6 fatty acids (fried food and trans fats) and the decrease of omega 3 fatty acids in the standard American diet. Another reason is that we are eating far less vegetables and fruits than our predecessors did. The recommendation is five servings a day; however the average American eats just three servings a day. Ideally, we should be eating at least ten servings each and every day. Vegetables and fruits are loaded with powerful antioxidants that help to fight against the free radicals generated by our love for eating unhealthy food that contains high levels of omega-6. So, it can be seen that a number of different factors are contributing to the rise in skin cancers that we are seeing today.

We all know that irresponsible sun exposure can increase the risk of non-melanoma skin cancer (NMSC), the most common and least dangerous type of skin cancer. Approximately 1500 people in the US die from NMSC each year. However, for every person that dies because of exposure to excess ultraviolet (UV) radiation more than 200 people die from cancers caused by insufficient UV exposure. Sunburn is dangerous. It is vital not to get a sunburn as it will increase your risk of NMSC and melanoma. However, responsible sun exposure can reduce your risk of melanoma by 15% and cancer in general by as much as 50%.

Sunscreen

There is a lot of confusion about sunscreen. It is important to realize that sunscreen filters out ultraviolet-B (UVB) radiation. As the action of UVB on your skin is vital for the photochemical production of vitamin D, this means that sunscreens will prevent, or at least drastically reduce, your skin's ability to produce vitamin. For example, using a sunscreen with a sun protection factor (SPF) of 15 or above will screen out 99.99% of UVB, thus meaning that your skin will not be able to produce any vitamin D. It is interesting to note that until very recently sunscreens did not contain filters that blocked ultraviolet-A (UVA) radiation, the type of radiation that actually causes skin damage and photoaging, and increases the risk of skin cancer. Even today, many sunscreens do not contain UVA filters. So, people have been happily slathering their skin with sunscreen that blocks out the UVB which helps your body to produce cancer-preventing vitamin D, whilst at the same time not protecting against cancer-promoting UVA. Furthermore, most sunscreens are loaded with toxic ingredients. With this in mind, it is probably not too surprising to learn that use of sunscreens has increased 18-fold since 1972 and in that same time period the incidence of melanoma has tripled.

Responsible Sunlight Exposure

The best way to ensure a plentiful supply of vitamin D is responsible sun exposure. If you have 10% of your body exposed to the sun your skin can manufacture 1000 IU per day. If half your body is exposed, your skin can make in the region of 5000 IU per day. Anything that reduces the amount of UVB radiation that penetrates into your skin (for example sunscreen, clothing, time of day, latitude, season, skin pigmentation) will have a dramatic influence on your skin's production of vitamin D. Other factors also affect how well your body can manufacture vitamin D from sunlight. Being overweight or obese and eating a poor diet, e.g. a diet high in omega 6, both impair your body's ability to manufacture the active form of vitamin D. It is important to note that older people require more exposure to sunlight in order to produce adequate amounts of vitamin D, as the older you get, the more difficult it is for your skin to synthesize active vitamin D.

UVB intensity varies with the time of day. The best time of day for sunlight exposure in terms of UVB radiation is solar noon. However, a simple test to determine whether it is possible for your skin to manufacture vitamin D is to simply stand in the sun and observe your shadow. If you are shorter than your shadow, your skin can produce vitamin D. If you are longer than your shadow it cannot.

For those people living in countries above 35° latitude in the northern hemisphere and below 35° latitude in the southern hemisphere the solar winter has a significant impact upon their skin's ability to produce vitamin D. During solar winter – from November to February in the northern hemisphere, and from May to July in the southern hemisphere – the ozone layer blocks UVB radiation from reaching the ground. So, you could stand outside stark naked all day long in solar winter and not produce any vitamin D, simply because there is not enough UVB radiation.

As most of us live in countries where there is a solar winter, this presents a major problem. Indeed, studies have shown that many people become vitamin D deficient over the winter months. So, what should you do to ensure you don't become deficient in the solar winter? Some people snowbird, however that option is obviously not available to everyone. Another option is to use a safe tanning bed, which means a tanning bed that uses electronic belts instead of magnetic belts.

How much exposure is needed? This is key. If you have light colored skin, you should expose your skin to the sun (or safe tanning bed) for as long as it takes to turn your skin the lightest shade of pink. Any additional exposure above that is unnecessary and will only serve to increase your risk of skin cancer, and cause photoaging.

It is very important to note that vitamin D is a fat-soluble vitamin. It can take as long as 48 hours after exposure to UVB for vitamin D to be fully absorbed by your body. Thus it would be ideal to avoid showering with soap after sunlight exposure in order to allow vitamin D to be absorbed into the major areas of skin covering your body.

The Hybrid Approach to Vitamin D

Many of us work 40 hours a week, and most of us work during the day, and for the vast majority of that time, we are indoors. What this means is that many of us struggle to find the time to get adequate sunlight exposure, even during the summer when UVB radiation is plentiful. Please note: being in a sunny room is no good as UVB is filtered by the glass. For those of us who simply don't have the time for adequate sunlight exposure it is vital to ensure that the body obtains a sufficient supply of vitamin D by other means.

The best way of doing this is to adopt a "hybrid" approach – a combination of sunlight exposure and oral supplementation. If, during the summer, you have the time to get two to three hours of sunlight exposure, that is great. However, if you don't manage to squeeze in the time for sunlight exposure the next week, take oral vitamin D that week instead.

The dose for oral vitamin D is 3000 IU for every 100 lbs if you are healthy. If you are treating cancer, autoimmune disease, or another serious condition, the dose is 5000 IU for every 100 lbs. If you are treating an acute infection, such as influenza and other viral upper respiratory tract infections, the dose is 2000 IU per kg (roughly 1000 IU per lb) per day for three days.

It is important to be aware that there are two types of vitamin D, vitamin D2 and vitamin D3. Vitamin D2 and foods that contain vitamin D2 (most rice milks/yogurts, almond milks/yogurts and some soy milks/yogurts) should be avoided as it prevents the conversion of vitamin D to critical hormones and inactivates the vitamin D receptor. Vitamin D3, the naturally occurring form of vitamin D in humans, should always be used for supplementation.

Should doctors be checking their patients' vitamin D levels? Yes. The assay for measuring vitamin D status is for $25(OH)D_3$. Not $1,25(OH)_2D_3$. A level of <40-50 ng/ml is deficient, whilst a level of 50-65 ng/ml is optimal in a healthy person. If you are treating a patient with cancer or autoimmune disease you should aim to get their vitamin D level to within 65-90 ng/ml. A level in excess of 100 ng/ml is too high.

CONCLUDING REMARKS

It can be seen that vitamin D is extremely important for health. Vitamin D levels should be optimized with sunlight exposure, however if that is not possible, supplementation with oral vitamin D3 or use of a safe tanning bed is recommended. However, it is important to remember the other things that are vital for good health: clean air and water, good quality sleep, stress reduction, optimizing insulin levels by cutting down on sugar, and – of course – a good diet and plenty of exercise.

REFERENCES

1. Cannell JJ. Autism and vitamin D. *Med Hypotheses.* 2008;70:750-759.
2. Cannell JJ, Vieth R, Umhau JC, Holick MF, Grant WB, Madronich S, Garland CF, Giovannucci E. Epidemic influenza and vitamin D. *Epidemiol Infect.* 2006;134:1129-1140.

ABOUT THE AUTHOR

Dr. Joseph Mercola is a pioneer in communicating natural health principles on the internet and has the most visited natural health website in the world, Mercola.com. A NY Times bestselling author, Dr. Mercola has been interviewed on national media including CNN, the Today Show, ABC Evening News, and more.

Chapter 25
Nutrigenomics: Nutrition and Genetics

Kousalya V. Nathan, Ph.D.
Visiting faculty [Hon], Department of Medicine, Chettinad University, India

ABSTRACT

Nutritional science has found its place in the 'omic' sciences with the recent unraveling of extensive human genome studies. In the past few years technological advances leading to genotyping, transcriptomics, proteomics, and metabolomics have become available to nutritional research. It is known that genetic variation and its expressions have enormous impact on degenerative and acquired diseases. Prevention is the ultimate aim of the clinical application of nutrigenomic advancements. Evolving biomedical research is increasing our understanding of disease processes that are related to nutrition and molecular genetics. The study of macromolecules important in biological inheritance and functional genomics has explored the mechanisms for inherited specific traits, expression, and variations in expression with regard to nutrition. Genome health depends on genome integrity. Macronutrients and micronutrients influence genome health. In view of recent advancements in nutrigenomics and nutrigenetics, development of gene-based designer diets for lifestyle disorders needs to be considered. This will help physicians promote lifestyle patterns along with nutrigenomics and pharmacogenomics (drug interaction) that would be compatible with the phenotypic expressions. The frontier field of nutrigenomics will lead to evidence-based dietary intervention applied towards disease prevention, health restoration, and management of chronic lifestyle diseases.

Keywords: nutrigenomics, genomics, genome health, molecular nutrition, personalized nutrition

INTRODUCTION
Nutrigenomics and Nutrigenetics

Genes define susceptibility to a disease. However lifestyle, diet, exercise, and environmental factors, determines who among the susceptible will develop the disease or condition. The term "nutrigenomics" was first used by Dr. R.O. Brennan in 1975 in his book '*Nutrigenetics – New Concepts for Relieving Hypoglycemia*". The term nutrigenetics refers to an individual's specific response to diet due to genetic variants or polymorphisms. Nutrigenomics has been defined in many ways, but it generally refers to the use of various molecular tools to explore how dietary substances interact with the genome. The ultimate goal is to determine the dietary components that are most compatible with health for a specific individual, with the ultimate aim of prevention.

The Genomic Revolution

There has been a tremendous growth in studying and understanding genetic variants (polymorphisms) and their association with chronic diseases such as cardiovascular disease, diabetes mellitus, hypertension, and cancer. These association studies have brought out the variability both in the type and frequency of the alleles, and the response to nutrients as influenced by other environmental factors e.g., smoking, dietary habits, and excess consumption of alcohol.

Genomics, genotyping, transcriptomics, proteomics, and metabolomics, along with bioinformatics, constitute the discipline of functional genomics, which is also referred to as "systems biology". The integration of systems biology into nutritional research has already begun.[1] In the last two decades, extensive nutritional research has been undertaken in a number of disciplines, including biochemistry, genetics, molecular biology, physiology, epidemiology ,and other genomic studies. Our knowledge of the mechanisms of disease processes that are related to nutrition has increased greatly since the genomic revolution. The field of biochemistry has greatly increased our understanding of the molecular processes related to metabolism and functional biochemical cycles, while molecular nutrition and molecular biology has explained many bio-regulatory processes. With the in-depth details of regulatory processes in place, nutrition science was integrated to extensive studies at the molecular level. This unraveled the use of biomarkers to draw conclusions in the nutrition and health area.[2]

Nutrigenomics in Health Promotion and Disease Prevention

The Nutrition and health relationship primarily needs to focus in maintaining and optimizing a healthy status, thereby preventing the onset of disease and disorders related to nutrition, in terms of malnutrition, imbalance of nutritional factors (more straightforwardly expressed) and chronic surplus of macronutrients. Obesity-related disorders, such as type 2 diabetes mellitus and cardiovascular diseases are clearly linked to excess calories. However one of the aims of current nutritional studies is not primarily about curing these diseases, but much more about prevention.

The complexity of the nutrition and health relationship was thus approached both from mechanistic (biochemical and biomedical research, genomic studies) research – extrapolating a disease model to a healthy situation and from functional (physiological interventions and cohort studies) research – extrapolating healthy volunteer data obtained with biomarkers to mechanisms involved in nutrition.[3]

Inter-individual differences were recognized early in nutritional research, and phenotypes were described.[4] Biochemical disorders with high nutritional relevance were linked to a genetic origin after elaborate work that took several decades to complete. Genetic disorders with pathological effects have also been described e.g. genes associated with pathological obesity,[5] as have other gene polymorphisms with consequences of human nutrition.[6]

Functional Genomics

Nutritional sciences are discovering the application of the so-called "omics" sciences. Over the past few decades, epidemiological, clinical, and mechanistic studies have indicated many relations between nutrition and health. Functional genomics technologies are not yet developed to their full potential, and while being implemented in nutritional and biomedical studies, they still need to undergo technological improvement. Studies have established associations between dietary habits and degenerative diseases, including cardiovascular diseases, diabetes mellitus, and cancer. Indeed recent research suggests that prevention or intervention of a disease may be fundamentally different from maintaining or improving good health. Bioinformatics is needed to analyze functional genomics derived data, although it is itself a scientific discipline in its infancy.[7]

What, how, when, and with whom we eat, determines a large parts of our lives. One of the ongoing trends in nutritional science is personalization of nutrition. In this chapter we will discuss the possibility of personalized preventive nutrition, which would enable us to target an individual's health at the molecular level.

NUTRIGENOMICS: MOLECULAR NUTRITION

Molecular nutrition has moved a step closer to following the prescient advice of Hippocrates, who said "Positive health requires knowledge of man's primary constitution and the powers of various foods, both those natural to them and those resulting from human skill".

This complex science can bring about organ-specific dietary responses combined with genomic technologies. From a molecular standpoint, nutrients are considered to be "signaling molecules". The signaling molecules are picked up by dietary signals from cellular sensing mechanisms and translated into gene, protein, and metabolic expressions.[8] The genomic approach has brought insight into the mechanisms of nutrition at the molecular level (i.e., what happens in our cells and organs when we eat, when we do not eat, or when we eat too much). Hence these molecular changes serve as dietary "signatures" or fingerprints giving us the clarity of the phenotype, particularly under conditions of metabolic stress, biochemical variations, cellular processes like inflammation, oxidation, methylation, and early phase of organ specific insulin resistance. Ultimately, the aim is to have a deeper knowledge of impact of the genotype in estimating the disease risk related to dietary stress, diabetes mellitus, overweight, and obesity.[9]

It is now known that most chronic diseases, such as cardiovascular disease, diabetes mellitus, metabolic syndrome, and cancer are multifactorial disorders caused by multiple genetic and environmental factors. Genetic variations in more than one susceptible gene cause multigenic or polygenic diseases. The genomic studies are more complex and complicated due to genetic variants in disease phenotype. Most genetic variations, such as single-nucleotide polymorphisms (SNP), insertions, or repeats have been found by sequencing genes coding for enzymes or transporters that are related to the disease of interest.[10]

Currently, professional nutritionists have changed their outlook towards clinical nutrition to understanding the molecular impact of macronutrients and micronutrients in promoting the long-term health of populations. This change has been driven by molecular research linking the status of particular micronutrients with altered risk of certain disease conditions. The elucidation of whole genome sequences in the Human Genome Project has under pinned the emergence of the new discipline of nutrigenomics, which explains complex relationships and interactions between genes and nutrients.[11]

Genetics deals with variation. A fundamental aspect of the genetic approach to disease is an appreciation of human variation: its nature and extent; its origin and maintenance; its distribution in families and populations; its interaction with nutrition, chemicals, the environment, and lifestyle choices, such as smoking; and its consequences for normal development, function, and homeostasis.

The study of genetic variation is largely determined by the means adopted to study the variations. SNPs refer to alterations of single bases – adenine, guanine, cystosine, thymine – in the 6-foot long string of bases that make up human DNA. In human beings, about 30% of loci have polymorphic variants, which are defined as two or more alleles with frequencies of at least 1% or more in the population. Variation in nutritional requirements and the interaction of certain nutrients with genetically determined biochemical and metabolic factors suggest different requirements for individuals. This variation (like sex differences or ethnicity) is inborn and needs to be differentiated from variations caused by the life cycle (growth, pregnancy, and old age). The mechanisms by which genes influence nutrient absorption, metabolism and excretion, taste perception, and degree of satisfaction, and the mechanisms by which nutrients influence gene expression are being mapped. Furthermore, advances in molecular and recombinant DNA technology through DNA sequencing have uncovered how uniquely we are constructed, and the extent to which genetic variations occur in human beings. The importance of the effects of genetic variation has been extensively studied and applied by pharmacologists in drug development (pharmacogenomics) and evaluation of drug metabolism and adverse reactions to drugs.[12-16]

As the science of molecular nutrition develops, one can foresee an evolution of new trends and technologies. The powerful tools of molecular biology and computational power of informatics are dramatically accelerating the progress towards the promotion of health and prevention of disease.

Personalizing Foods and Lifestyles: Is Genotype Necessary?

Genomic studies have shown how humans genetically differ in their responses to diet and how many of these differences are attributed to genetic polymorphisms. Apart from the genetic differences in humans that are attributed to varying responses to diet, there are other factors like lifestyle, environmental factors, and ethnicity that attribute to genetic variations. Life stage, lifestyle, prior nutritional and physiological variables, and even a mother's micro flora, all influence the differences in humans.

It is important to understand the measurable factors of health as a part of nutritional phenotype assessment so that personalization of nutritional requirements and guidelines at the molecular level is attainable. More accurate assessment of the inputs to human health and the consequences of those inputs measured as accurate proteomic and metabolomic analyses would bring personalized health to practice far faster than waiting for a predictive knowledge of genetic variation.

The extensive works and contribution in nutrition and genetics of the 20th century saw the identification of all the essential nutrients and the understanding of their functional importance in controlling imbalances and maintaining health. Clinical application of nutrigenomic and nutrigenetics means that diseases caused by nutrient deficiencies and malnutrition could mostly be prevented. With the growing public demand, industrialization of food processing for improved nutrient retention, nutrient enrichment, and fortification is occupying the food market, and together with optimized dietary guidelines, has ensured high-quality nutrition. Over the past 100 years, public health goals have thus been population-based agricultural production chains embedded into corresponding policies and food consumption guidelines to ensure that all individuals within a population obtain all of the essential nutrients.

As we are discovering and understanding genome health in the 21st century, the reality of diet and health is that all individuals within a population are not optimally healthy when consuming the same diets. Imbalances of dietary intakes of calories and the various macronutrients and micronutrients relative to different lifestyles are leading to metabolic imbalances and even diseases. Atherosclerosis, obesity, diabetes mellitus, hypertension, osteoporosis, allergy, metabolic syndromes, and neurodegenerative diseases are either increasing outright in subsets of the population or at least failing to decline in spite of massive improvements in medical care. The advancements leading to awareness in variations in dietary intakes of essential nutrients and its individual responses are not applied clinically to bring down the rate of birth defects, early onset of degeneration of various tissues, and diet-induced metabolic diseases during pregnancy. Humans need to understand the importance of personalized lifestyle changes to improve quality of life, reverse premature aging, and the need to adopt specific diets. Thus, a new era of health must include a personalization of diet, however it is not yet clear what scientific research is needed and what industrial processes are required, nor what economic models are capable of guiding, applying, and financing the personalization of the world's largest human enterprise – food.[17]

Diversity: Phenotypes

The physical characteristic of an organism, or the presence of a disease that may or may not be genetic, is the phenotype. Although man has evolved being able to feed on a variety of foods and to adapt to them, certain genetic adaptations and limitations have occurred in relation to diet. Because there are genetic variations among individuals, changes in the dietary patterns impact on a genetically heterogeneous population, although populations with similar evolutionary background have more similar genotypes. Therefore, to be successful, dietary inventions must be based on knowledge of the frequency of genes whose effects we are attempting to control or modify.

Data from around the world indicate that the incidence and prevalence of chronic diseases vary among individuals, families, and nations. Genetic predispositions, environmental factors, and quality of care, all contribute to these variations.[18-22]

Healthy human adults vary in height, weight, activity, cognition, strength, endurance, flexibility, body composition, eye color, hair texture, and also in their preference of foods. We are most alike at birth, but as we progress through various life stages, we diversify into individuals with strong likes and dislikes. Unfortunately, while the 20th century saw a massive scientific investment in researching the basic biological processes of the human body, detailing biochemistry from genetics to physiology, the majority of that research catalogued the commonalities of these processes across all humans. The human variables may differ genetically based on chromosomal differences, for example, male, female, or allelic polymorphisms in structural or regulatory regions of specific genes.

Environment and Epigenomics

The environment in which an individual lives includes all aspects of exogenous inputs to their phenotypes, including acute and chronic, random and volitional, and chemical and behavioral. The nature of these inputs can be described/measured by their source (e.g., geographical distribution and solar UV irradiation, population status, environmental pollution) or their effects (e.g., vitamin D formation).[23] These inputs can be either random or unavoidable (urban population) or volitional (smoking). These inputs may also be generalized to a larger population (exposure to fluoridated drinking water) or may be unique to specific individuals (chronic consumption of sweetened beverages, excess calorie intake, and consumption of fewer vegetables).[24] Environment at one stage of an individual's life can exert persistent effects on the nutritional phenotype later in life (imprinting, programming, memorization, or colonization).The explicit covalent modifications of DNA that persists through cell divisions are now recognized and are increasingly well described in the field of epigenetics.[25] The development of preferences for sensory attributes of foods – principally olfactory preferences – is persistent through much of an individuals life, guiding their lifelong food choices.

Personalized Nutrition in Action

Food personalization has been practiced for centuries with little or minimum knowledge on molecular impact. In the last decade, the scientific basis for optimizing food guidance followed by public demand and industrialization of personalized food choices has evolved to benefit people. Human beings have always used organoleptic food preferences as a key driver of their overall food choices. Food choices based on personal preferences are generally rooted to individual experience, including sensory acuity, cultural habits, religious practices, and income. Moreover, the nutrition professionals recognized long ago that different physiological events require significant adaptations to diet.

Taste

The most immediate and easily accessed basis for personalization of foods is simple taste and flavor preferences. Even though personal taste preferences have been the basis for food choices for literally thousands of years, the genetic diversity of taste and olfactory sensation in humans is now recognized to be part of the diversity of food preferences.[26]

Cultural Traditions

There is considerable diversity of foods based on core beliefs of their suitability to a particular religious or philosophy value system. Although the origins and the perpetuation of these choices (halal or kosher foods, vegetarian diets, Jain foods, and religious fasting) are not necessarily based on personal nutritional criteria they do produce nutritional consequences, whether desirable or not.[27]

Life Stage

Considerable experience by humans over the centuries has led to personalization of foods according to the different physiological needs associated with the stages of human life, for example infancy, weaning, pregnancy, lactation, aging, acute and chronic illnesses.

Life Stage Events

Many more immediate aspects of personalization of diets are associated with lifestyle choices and the events in such self-selected lifestyles. Although scientific evidence is rapidly building around these distinctive lifestyle choices and the physiological stresses that they produce, historical observational and anecdote are still the basis to a wide variety of assumptions for the value of specific foods. Foods within this category are as disparate as beverages and products for athletes before, during, and after sports events, to products associated with increased risk of deep vein thrombosis.[28]

Lifestyle Diseases

Growing lifestyle diseases such as obesity, diabetes mellitus, metabolic syndrome, and coronary artery diseases, provide another opportunity for the specific consumers who are at risk of actually experiencing gradual failure of their health to explore disease specific nutrition that revive health and quality of life. Although modern diagnostic sciences are developing sensitive methods to distinguish those who are at greater risk, a wide variety of therapeutically oriented products which are targeted either to the symptoms of the problem or to the lifestyle choice (e.g. smoking, sedentary lifestyle or high-fat diets, bingeing, junk food, excess consumption of sweetened beverages, excess calories) are of potential value.

Inherited Health Issues and Diseases

Humans have recognized the familial basis to much of health throughout recorded history, and foods have been an integral part of their solutions. Apart from familial food patterns and habits, traditional food choices are added in disease remedies as a part of personalization. From predispositions to allergies (nuts, fish, citrus foods) and intolerances (milk-lactose) to inherited errors of inborn metabolism, diet is well known to contribute to these processes and to their prevention. It is now routine in many countries for children to be tested for up to 10 metabolic diseases, not by genotyping them, but by accurate measurements of normal metabolites whose inordinate abundance in blood are a diagnostic signature of the condition.[29]

Signature Diets

As the field of nutrigenomics evolves, personalized food plans, made after understanding the genotyping and holistic investigation of the metabolism using proteomics and metabolomics to prevent diseases and to restore health at the molecular level, are anticipated.

Nutrigenomics and Genome Health

The response to specific dietary regimen and functional foods on inherited traits has an impact on genome health. This emerging area of nutrigenomics and nutrigenetics towards prevention of diseases at the DNA level has drawn the interest of scientists and nutritionists in the field of nutrigenomics. The research area of genome health is advancing due to increasing evidence of:

- DNA damage, degenerative disease, and the role of nutrition in its repair.
- The role of anti-oxidants and genome integrity.
- The metabolism of micronutrients for DNA repair and DNA replication.
- Personalized nutrition for genome stability

The genetic material and genetic code determines the occurrence of developmental defects and degenerative diseases such as cancer. DNA is under stress due to the fact that it is continuously going through major mutations (DNA expression, telomerase shortening, point mutations, chromosome breakage, and chromosome loss). Therefore, working on genome integrity would is one of the biggest challenges that the medical fraternity faces. Nutrigenomic research, although in its infancy, has already dramatically improved our understanding of the links between functional foods and genome health.[30]

Genome damage has an impact on various stages of life, from conception to old age. Human genome projects involving genome research and technology aiming at mapping and sequencing the genome of human models is providing us with the knowledge needed to understand the connection between the expression of our genes and characteristics of health or the onset of disease. Apart from genetic inheritance, gene expressions are also influenced by lifestyle practices, such as smoking, unmanaged stress, excess free radicals, chronic diseases, and malnutrition. It is known that genes control the cellular processes that regulate aging. These processes are methylation, inflammation, glycation, oxidation, and DNA repair.[31]

Genetic studies deal with variations in human polymorphisms, thus revealing the differences in DNA sequencing among individuals that may specify differences in health. Knowledge of genetic variations in individuals will form the basis for the personalized nutrition and lifestyle programs that will result in effective DNA repair and disease prevention. The control of gene expression involves various complex factors like hormonal, neuronal, lifestyle practices, nutritional factors, and nutrients. Nutrients regulate gene expression by both direct and indirect ways. Control of specific gene expressions through cis-regulatory elements is directly influenced by macronutrients such as fatty acids and their metabolites,[32] monosaccarides,[33] amino acids,[34] nucleotides,[35] and micronutrients such as vitamins and minerals.[36] The indirect influence of nutrients on gene expression is by regulating the secretion of hormones such as insulin,[37] glucagons and thyroid hormones, which, in turn, can also alter the expression of specific genes.[38] With all this detailed understanding of nutrition and nutrients, and their influence in genome health, the Center of Excellence for Nutritional Genomics at the University of California, Davis has formulated the following five tenets of nutritional genomics:

- Under certain circumstances, and in some individuals, diet can be a serious risk factor for a number of diseases.
- Common dietary chemicals can act on the human genome, either directly or indirectly, to alter gene expression or structure.
- The degree to which diet influences the balance between health and disease states may depend on a person's genetic make up.
- Some diet-regulated genes (and their normal, common variants) are likely to play a role in the onset, incidence, progression, and /or severity of chronic diseases.
- Dietary intervention based on knowledge of nutritional requirement, nutritional status, and genotype (i.e. personalized nutrition), can be used to prevent, mitigate, or cure chronic diseases.[39]

These advancements in nutrigenomics have evolved a new and futuristic concept in novel preventive medicine known as "Genome Health Clinic". These clinics are integrated centers use genome testing and nutritional intervention to prevent and treat disease, and also sustain health. These clinics work on improving the quality of life of an individual by working on gene integrity with the following goals:

- Personalization of nutritional intervention for definite results.
- Prevention of genome damage caused by micronutrient deficiency.
- Accurate diagnosis of genome instability.
- Diagnose and prevent developmental and degenerative diseases.
- Understanding of genotypes and genotoxic dietary factors (deep fried foods, excess alcohol consumption, excess sweets or white sugar, and preserved foods).[30]

Genome Health Clinics can help us face the global pandemic of diet-related chronic diseases and preventable disorders, such as type 2 diabetes mellitus, cancer, obesity, and osteoporosis. Genome analysis and research projects will create a genetic predisposition model of health and disease. The concept of genetic predisposition has arisen from the discovery that genes are not necessarily destiny. One's genes do not always predetermine health and disease, in some cases genetic outcomes are modifiable – this is particularly true in the case of diet-related diseases. By focusing on lifestyle management at the molecular level, nutrigenomics will make it possible to personalize prevention and improve quality of life.

Nutrigenomics is the corner stone of the molecular approach to health and wellness, and thereby is of great significance for food and nutrition professionals, physicians, clinical nutritionists, anti-aging physicians, and nutritional genomic practitioners. Diet-related diseases place an enormous burden upon societies, as we are now seeing rapid progress in this field, now is the time to be bold in our vision and integrate genomics into our practice.[40] This can be done by translating the research findings to practical applications in order to help subjects with chromosomal disorders or monogenic disorders that lead to developmental disorders.

Legal and Ethical Issues

Nutrigenomics has drawn the interest of nutritional researchers, genomic projects, biomedical researchers, private sectors, anti-aging physicians, and commercial investors, who are keen to develop and market personalized food products and dietary supplements.[41] This raises legal and social issues with respect to how ethical it would be to assess and understand genetic testing and associated nutritional and other personalized lifestyle programs.[42] Although the market for such products is growing rapidly, the regulatory environment has not been able to keep pace with the developments.[43] This makes it difficult to protect consumer from direct-to-consumers (DTC) marketing of nutrigenomic tests, false claims, internet nutritionists, and unproven dietary supplements.

The nutrigenomic regulatory board is slowly evolving, and it is time to strengthen the professional support capacity, as primary care physicians have minimal training in nutrigenomics and medical geneticists are in short supply to ensure the regulations are met.[44]

CONCLUD(NG REMARKS

The current developments in food science, biotechnology, genetics, and research advancements, has paved the way for the evolution of personalized "signature diets". Genomics has clearly established the proof-of-principle that humans are different with respect to optimal diets. Now, genetic variations that cause developmental or degenerative diseases can be successfully altered for optimum health. Consumers will gain value with personalization and clinicians will bridge the existing gap of disease care and health care. The extensive 'omic" studies will create a niche in taking clinical practice to its highest level of medicine – "proactive medicine".

RESOURCES OF STUDY IN NUTRIGENOMICS
Books
- DeBusk RM. Genetics: *The Nutrition Connection.* Chicago, IL: American Dietetic Association; 2003.
- Moustaid N, Berdanier CD. *Nutrient-Gene Interactions in Health and Disease.* Boca Raton, FL: CRC Press; 2001.
- Zempleni J, Hannelore D, eds. *Molecular Nutrition.* Wallingford, England: CABI Publishing; 2003.

Reviews of Nutritional Genomics
- Elliott R, Ong TJ. Nutritional genomics. *BMJ.* 2002;321:1438-1442.
- Fairweather-Tait SJ. Human nutrition and food research in the post-genomics era. *Philos Trans R Soc London B Biol Sci.* 2003;358.
- Guengerich FP. Functional genomics and proteomics applied to the study of nutritional metabolism. *Nutr Rev.* 2001;59:259-263.

Websites

- National Human Genome Research Institute. Available at: http://www.genome.gov
- US Department of Energy Genome Programs. Available at: http://www.doegenomes.org
- Center of Excellence for Nutritional Genomics at the University of California, Davis. Available at: http://nutrigenomics.ucdavis.edu
- Center for Human Nutrigenomics at Wageningen University, The Netherlands. Available at: http://www.nutrigenomics.nl

REFERENCES

1. Simopoulos AP, Ordovas JM, eds. *World Review of Nutrition and Dietetics*. Basel, Karger: 2004;93:134-152.
2. Griffith HR, Moller L, Bartosz G, Bast A, Bertoni-Freddari C, Collins A, *et al.* Biomarkers. *Mol Aspects Med.* 2002;23:101-208.
3. Simopoulos AP, Ordovas JM, eds. *World Review of Nutrition and Dietetics*. Basel, Karger: 2004;93:134-152.
4. Simopoulos AP, Childs B, eds. *World Review of Nutrition and Dietetics.* Basel, Karger: 2004;93:1-300.
5. Warden CH, Nengjin Y, Fisler J. Epistasis among genes is a universal phenomenon in obesity: Evidence from rodent models. *Nutrition.* 2004;20:74-77.
6. Simopoulos AP, Nestel PJ, eds. *World Review of Nutrition Dietetics.* Basel, Karger; 1997;80:1-171.
7. Omen BV, Stierum R. Nutrigenomics: exploiting symptoms biology in Nutrition and health arena. *Curr opin Biotechnol.* 2002;13:517-521.
8. Muller M, Kersten S. Nutrigenomics: Goals and strategies; *Nat Rev Genet.* 2003;4:315-322.
9. Afman L, Muller M. Nutrigenomics: From Molecular Nutrition to Prevention of Disease. *J Am Diet Assoc.* 2006;106:569-576.
10. Ordovas JM, Corella D. Nutritional Genomics. *Anu Rev Genomic Hum Genet.* 2004;5:71-118.
11. Simopoulos AP, Ordovas JM, eds. *World Review of Nutrition and Dietetics*. Basel, Karger; 2004;93:153-163.
12. Gonzalez FJ, Skoda RC, Kimura S, Umenom, Zanger UM, Nebert DW, *et al.* Characterization of the common genetic defect in humans deficient in debrisoquine metabolism. *Nature.*1988;331-442.
13. Evans DA. In: Kalow W, Goedde HW, Agarwal DP, eds. *Ethnic Differences in Reactions to Drugs and Xenobiotics.* New York, NY: Liss; 1986:491.
14. Evans DA, Harmer D, Downham DY, Whibley EJ, Idle JR, Ritchie J, *et al.* The genetic control of sparteine and debrisoquine in metabolism in man with new methods of analyzing Biomodal Distributions. *J Med Genet.* 1983;20:321-329.
15. Idle JR. Poor metabolizers of debrisoquine reveal their true colours. *Lancet* 1989;2:1097.
16. Wolf CR, Moss JE, Miles JS, Gough AC, Spurr NK. Detection of debrisoquine hydroxylation phenotypes. *Lancet.* 1990;336:1452.
17. Fay LB, German JB. Personalizing foods: is genotype necessary? *Curr Opin Biotechnol.* 2008;19:121-128.
18. Sing CF, Stengard JH, Kardia SLR. Genes, environment and cardiovascular disease; Anteriosclerosis. *Thromb Vasc Biol.* 2003; 23:1190-1196.
19. Simopoulus AP, Herbert V, Jacobson B. *The healing Diet; How to reduce your risks and live a longer and healthier life if you have a family history of Cancer, Heart Disease, Hypertension, Diabetes, Alcoholism, Obesity, Food Allergies.* New York, NY: Macmillan; 1995.
20. Scott J. Molecular Genetics of common diseases. *Br Med J.* 1987;295:769-771.
21. Bonne-Tamir B, Adam A. *Genetic diversity among Jews. Diseases and Markers at the DNA level.* New York, NY: Oxford University Press; 1992.
22. World Health Organization MONICA project; Registration procedures, event rates and case fatality in 38 populations from 21 countries in four continents. *Circulation* 1994;90:583-612.
23. Holick MF. Resurrection of Vitamin D deficiency and rickets. *J Clin Invest.* 2006;116:2062-2072.
24. Montonen J, Jarvinen R, Knekt P, Heliovaara M, Reunanen A. Consumption of sweetened beverages and intake of fructose and glucose predict type 2 diabetes occurrence. *J Nutr.* 2007;137:1447-1454.

25. Gluckman PD, Liilycrop KA, Vickers MH, Vickers MH, Pleasants AB, Phillips ES, et al. Metabolic plasticity during Mammalian development is directionally dependent on early nutritional status. *Proc Natl Acad Sci.* 2007;104:12796-12800.
26. Keller A, Zhuang H, Chi Q, Vashall LB, Matsunami H. Genetic variations in a human odorant Receptor alters odour perception. *Nature.* 2007;449:468-472.
27. Zirkovic AM, German JB, Sanyal AJ .Comparative review of diets for the metabolic syndrome; implications for nonalcoholic fatty liver disease. *Am J Clin Nutr.* 2007;86:285-300.
28. Murray B. The role of salt and glucose replacement drinks in the marathon. *Sports Medicine.* 2007;37:358-360.
29. Wicken B, Wiley V, Hammond J, Carpenter K. Screening newborns of inborn errors of metabolism by tandem Mass Spectrometry. *N Eng J Med.* 2003;348:2304-2312.
30. Fenech M. Genome Health Nutrigenomics and nutrigenetics diagnosis and nutritional treatment of genome damage on individual basis. *Food Chem Toxicol.* 2008;46:1365-1370.
31. Giampappa VC, Buechel FF, Karatoprak O. *The Gene Makeover – the 21st century antiaging text book.* Basic Health Publication Inc; 2007.
32. Moustaid N, Sakamoto K, Clarke SD, Beyer RS, Sul HS. Regulation of fatty acid synthase gene transcription. *Biochem J.* 1993;292:767-772.
33. Rutter GA,Tavore JM, Palmer DG. Regulation on mammalian gene expression by glucose. *News Physiology Sci.* 2000;15:149-157.
34. Jefferson LS, Kimball SR. Amino acid regulation of gene expression. *J Nutr.* 2001;131;suppl 9:2460S-2466S.
35. Sanchez-Pozo A, Gil A. Nucleotides as semi essential nutritional components *Br J Nutr.* 2002;87 (suppl):S135-S137.
36. Azzi A, Aratri E, Boscoboinik D. Vitamins and Regulation of gene expression. *Bibl Nutr Dieta.* 2001;55:177-188.
37. Patti ME. Nutrient modulation of cellular insulin action. *Ann NY Acad Sci.* 1999;892:187-203.
38. Dauncey MJ, White P, Burton KA, Katsumata M. Nutrition-hormone receptor gene interactions. Implications for developmental and disease. *Proc Nutr Soc.* 2001;60:63-72.
39. Center of Excellence of Nutritional Genomics at the University of California at Davis. Nutrigenomics. Available at: http//nutrigenomics.ucdavis.edu Accessed June 29, 2004.
40. DeBusk RM. Diet related disease, nutritional genomics and food and nutritional professionals. *J Am Diet Assoc.* 2009;109:410-413.
41. Burton H, Stewart A. Nutrigenomics: Report of the workshop hosted by the Nuffield trust and organized by the Public Health Genetics Unit, Nuffield Trust, London 2005.
42. Fogg JN, Kaput F. Nutrigenomics: an emerging scientific discipline. *Food Technol.* 2003;57:60-67.
43. Castle D. Clinical Challenges posed by new biotechnology: the case of nutrigenomics. *Post Grad Med J.* 2003;79:65-66.
44. Castle D, Ries NM. Ethical, legal and social issues in nutrigenomics: The challenges of regulating service delivery and building health professional capacity. *Mutat Res.* 2007;622:138-143.

ACKNOWLEDGEMENTS

The author gracefully acknowledges Naveen K. Visweshwariah, Ph.D. for the tremendous support and assistance in manuscript preparation.

ABOUT THE AUTHOR

Dr Kousalya V. Nathan attained her medical degree in "Natural Medicine & Yoga" from Asia's first college in India. A Ph.D. scholar at Chettinad Health City, India, she is visiting faculty [hon.] at the department of Medicine, Chettinad University, India. She is a regular feature in media for over 10 years.

Chapter 26
A Medical Model That Restores Optimal Function

Sangeeta Pati, M.D., FACOG
Medical Director, SaJune Medical Center (Orlando, FL USA)

ABSTRACT

The aim of this paper is to present a medical model which utilizes hormones, nutrients, and detoxification to restore optimal function, eliminate inflammation, prevent disease, and stay young.

INTRODUCTION

The aim of this paper is to present a medical model which utilizes hormones, nutrition, detoxification, and mind and body balancing, to restore optimal function, eliminate inflammation, prevent disease, and stay young. This model has been used to treat insomnia, panic attacks, fibromyalgia, rheumatoid arthritis, and a variety of other diseases.

My background as a gynecologist meant that I was used to treating patients with hormones, and my interest in anti-aging medicine led me to bioidentical hormones. At first I began treating my patients with bioidentical estrogens, progesterone, and testosterone; although I soon realized that it was vitally important to also consider thyroid hormone, insulin, melatonin, and pregnenolone. I then discovered that the bioidentical hormones I was prescribing would sometimes fail; investigations would usually reveal that this was due to something simple like an iodine deficiency or a vitamin D deficiency. Thus, I realized that it was vital that I also paid close attention to my patients' nutrition. Then I began to think about how we are bombarded with toxins on a daily basis, and how certain toxins can block the production and function of hormones and nutrients, and thus I realized the importance of detoxification. These thoughts led to the development of a solid restorative model for optimal health.

HORMONES

Production of progesterone drops significantly when women reach their mid-30s, this decline can cause sleep problems, anxiety, mood swings, irritability, heavy bleeding, breast cysts, ovarian cysts, fibroids, worse PMS, mid-abdominal weight gain, low sex drive, hot flashes. In fact, this drop in progesterone is the number one reason why so many women in their mid-30's are (wrongly) given a Prozac prescription, and is probably the major underlying reason why so many women in their early-40's are given a hysterectomy. Progesterone is important for osteoblast activity, thus progesterone deficiency is a major cause of bone loss. This explains why women start to lose bone mineral density in their mid-30's to early-40's, however conventional medicine still does not consider bone loss until a woman reaches her 50's.

People do not develop Xanax, Prozac, and Lipitor deficiencies as they get older. They are simply acquiring deficiencies that are related to normal glandular processes. Receptors for estrogen, progesterone, and testosterone have been found in almost every tissue and organ in the body – brain, nerve, bone, muscle, kidney, skin, and hair follicles. Therefore it is no wonder that hormone deficiencies cause symptoms in all of these organs. Declining hormone levels are also linked to a myriad of degenerative diseases, including: osteoporosis, colon cancer, heart disease, cognitive decline, Alzheimer's disease, stroke, and macular degeneration.

In most areas of medicine the answer to a deficiency is to replace the deficient substance. Cortisol deficiency is treated with bio-identical cortisol, thyroid deficiency is treated with thyroid hormone, and insulin deficiency is treated with insulin. So, why do people always think differently when it comes to sex hormone replacement? If we are looking to restore optimal function, we also need to restore sex hormones to their optimal levels.

It is important to consider the Women's Health Initiative (WHI) Study when thinking about sex hormone replacement. Dozens, maybe even hundreds, of papers trying to analyze the results of the Women's Health Initiative (WHI) study have been published. Approximately 16,000 women with an average age of 63 took part in the WHI study. The study was designed to examine the effectiveness of hormone replacement therapy (HRT). The HRT used in the study was orally administered conjugated equine estrogens (CEE) and medroxyprogesterone acetate (MPA).

Results of the study revealed an attributable risk and benefit ratio per 10,000 women of 7 more heart attacks, 18 more blood clots, 8 more strokes, 8 more breast cancers – one less case of breast cancer would have returned a non-significant risk result – six less colon cancers, and six less hip fractures.

Why did the results of the WHI Study suggest that HRT increased the risk of heart attack, blood clot, stroke, and breast cancer? From a clinical standpoint, the authors of the study made four major mistakes: they used women who were too old and who had a high rate of pre-existing disease, they used the wrong route of administration, they used the wrong ratio of hormones, and they used synthetic hormones.

HRT should be started around the time of menopause. The average age of women in the WHI Study was 63. In July 2008, the North American Menopausal Society revised their position statement on HRT in postmenopausal women. Their review of the literature, led the Advisory Panel to conclude: "Recent data support the initiation of HT [hormone therapy] around the time of menopause to treat menopause-related symptoms; to treat or reduce the risk of certain disorders, such as osteoporosis or fractures in select postmenopausal women; or both. The benefit-risk ratio for menopausal HT is favorable close to menopause but decreases with aging and with time since menopause in previously untreated women."

Deciding to administer HRT orally was another reason for the negative results of the study. There are now at least three dozen papers comparing the effect of oral estrogen and transdermal estrogen that have been published in the medical literature, and every single one has come to the conclusion that the oral estrogen significantly increases triglyceride levels and increases the risk of blood clots, heart attack, and stroke. This is because oral estrogen stimulates the production of clotting factors, triglycerides, and other inflammatory factors, as it passes through the liver (first-pass metabolism). Conversely, transdermal estrogen is delivered to the body via the bloodstream before it reaches the liver, thus meaning that transdermal estrogen does not undergo first-pass metabolism. Furthermore, studies have shown that transdermal estrogen actually decreases clotting mechanisms.

The third problem with the design of the WHI Study is that the women were treated with the wrong ratio of estrogens. At present, there are 21 known different types of estrogen; however we are concerned with the three major estrogens: estrone (E1), estradiol (E2), and estriol (E3). Just 10% of the estrogens in a premenopausal woman is E1, whereas 80% of a postmenopausal woman's estrogens is E1. Older women have higher levels of E1 because it is produced by the adrenal glands and fat cells and thus its production is unaffected by the menopause. Having high levels of E1 is undesirable because it is significantly more thrombogenic and carcinogenic than the other estrogens. Despite this, E1 was the predominant form of estrogen used in the WHI Study (CEE is approximately 50% E1).

The final flaw of the study design was the decision to use non-bioidentical hormones instead of bioidentical hormones. There is plenty of evidence in the medical literature to show that synthetic progestins significantly increase the risk of breast cancer, and are associated with increased risk of clotting, stroke, and heart attack. Bioidentical hormones were once referred to as natural. The strict definition of natural is anything that has been derived from a natural source, which means that Premarin is technically natural. A soy or yam derivative is natural but it is a derivative. So, natural does not always mean what people think. Therefore, it is much better to use the terms bioequivalent, human-equivalent, or bioidentical, to describe a substance that mimics one naturally found in the human body. Nowadays, there are plenty of bioidentical hormones available and there is no excuse not to use them.

If our aim is to restore optimal function, we need to restore sex hormones to their optimal levels. As well as restoring sex hormones it is important to consider other hormones, such as thyroid hormone. Bioidentical hormones are the key to successful HRT; synthetic hormones should be avoided at all costs. The WHI study taught us that it is vital to start HRT early (50-59), and that it is important to mimic normal estrogen ratios. Do not include E1 in HRT, and do not prescribe oral estrogen. Estrogens (bioidentical of course) should be administered transdermally. Biodentical progesterone should be used for progesterone replacement – never synthetic progestins such as MPA.

NUTRITION

Nutrient deficiencies prevent hormones from carrying out their normal actions. Iodine is a component of almost every hormone receptor. Zinc is a component of the estradiol, testosterone, and growth hormone receptor. Cobalt is essential for estrogen to function correctly. Chromium is essential for ovarian progesterone production. Vitamin B6 is needed to clear estradiol from its receptor, and methyl donors (such as folic acid) are needed for estrone metabolism. Vitamins, minerals, and co-factors are vital for countless activities and reactions in the body. Thus, if a patient does not have adequate amounts of certain nutrients, their body will not be working as well as it could be.

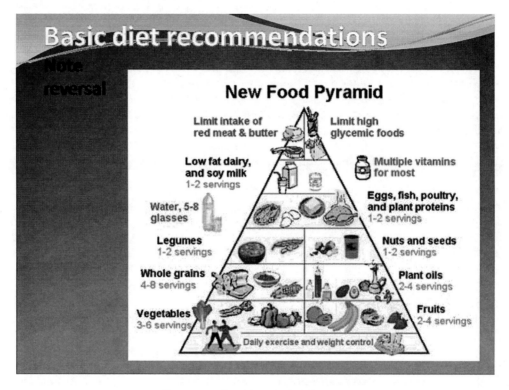

Figure 1. The New Food Pyramid

The basic dietary recommendation for patients is the reversed food pyramid. As can be seen in Fig. 1, the bottom level of the food pyramid is dedicated to fruit and vegetables. It is important to educate patients about the necessity of eating fruit and vegetables of every color as different colors contain different phytonutrients and every phytonutrient targets a different organ in the body.

Protein is an important part of the diet. Ideally, proteins should be organic, hormone-free, and antibiotic free. Why? Firstly, eggs from caged hens have a 20:1 ratio of omega-6 to omega-3, whereas organic eggs from cage-free hens have a much better omega-6 to omega-3 ratio of 2:1. Secondly, hormones present in meat and dairy products from animals treated with antibiotics and hormones have been shown to stimulate estrogen receptors in the breast tissue.

It is now possible to analyze nutrient levels simply by taking a blood sample and sending it off for functional intracellular nutritional analysis. This will give you an excellent picture of a patient's nutritional status, and will enable you to design a treatment plan if any deficiencies are detected. Patients should be retested after four months of treatment to determine whether treatment has been effective. Note: functional intracellular nutritional analysis is covered by insurance – even Medicare. Even in the absence of nutritional deficiencies it is prudent to prescribe patients a high-quality multivitamin and mineral supplement. All patients should also be prescribed 2.5 g/day omega-3 (high-quality, enteric coated), for patients with cardiovascular disease the dose should be increased to 4-5 g/day, while for patients with neurological disease the dose should be increased to 7-8 g/day.

DETOXIFICATION

American citizens are exposed to far more toxins than people living in other developed countries. Put simply, we have a lot of junk in our bodies, and this junk prevents our bodies from working properly. Most of it lies in the bowel. The bowel produces B vitamins and serotonin, and it needs to be functioning properly to do so. If you look at an infant, you will find that they often open their bowels after eating, and that is exactly what should happen. The bowel is supposed to move when you eat, so two to three bowel movements a day is healthy. The bowel is also responsible for the production of glucuronidases, which are responsible for breaking down estrogens and testosterone. A mucoid plaque can weigh up to 40 pounds. With this in mind, it is clear why we need to address the bowel.

Another site in which toxins collect is the liver. The liver activates thyroid hormone, estrogen, and testosterone, and therefore it needs to be functioning correctly if we are to stay healthy and youthful.

A major environmental toxin of the 21st century is electromagnetic radiation. Nowadays, electromagnetic radiation is everywhere, and we are bombarded by it 24 hours a day. Cell phones, computer screens, Wi-Fi zones, and cordless phone bases, are all potent emitters of electromagnetic radiation. Electromagnetic radiation has been shown to have a very significant effect on organs that are sensitive to radiation, for example, the brain, thyroid gland, and testicles. All patients should be given an organic acid and metabolic panel, so that you can determine how healthy a patient's liver and bowel are. This test will also enable you to identify exactly what is causing the dysfunction. I also carry out heavy metal testing in patients with certain conditions, such as osteoporosis, hormone resistance, neurological decline, and idiopathic hives. If you have a young patient with osteoporosis, you need to carry out heavy metal testing.

It is also a good idea to consider a patient's pH, as a tissue pH of 7.0 and above is needed for all chemical reactions to proceed. There are some very simple methods of increasing the pH, e.g. eating less meat, fish, dairy products, drinking less coffee and alcohol, deep breathing exercises, and increasing vegetable and water intake. These simple steps can have significant effects. Alkalinizing the body has proven to be particularly beneficial to patients with fibromyalgia, arthritis, intestinal disorders, and psoriasis.

IMPLEMENTING THE MEDICAL MODEL

During a patient's initial consultation we ask them to rate themselves for numerous symptoms (anxiety, PMS, heavy bleeding, insomnia, food craving, progesterone, hot flashes, vaginal dryness, urinary incontinence, bone loss, muscle loss, libido, fatigue, depression, loss of mental clarity, loss of memory, loss of concentration, depression, low mood, weight gain, constipation, coldness, etc...) on a scale of 1-10. We routinely carry out hormonal and nutritional testing, and the majority of patients are given a DEXA scan. Women are offered routine mammography. All patients are given a physical examination, and when we have the results of all the tests we write a plan of action. Patients are seen at four-week intervals until they are free of symptoms and approximately twice yearly there afterwards.

CASE STUDIES
Case Study: Typical 40-Year-Old Female Patient

A 40-year-old woman complained of insomnia and panic attacks. She rated her sleep quality at 4/10, anxiety 7/10, panic attacks, and energy at 4/10 in the morning and 2/10 in the evening. She also reported that she suffers from heavy menstrual periods, recent anemia from the bleeding, and a history of breast cysts and ovarian cysts.

She is clearly progesterone deficient. Her doctor has prescribed her Ambien, Xanax, and Provera. She had been offered an endometrial ablation for her bleeding, and was taking iron supplements. We discussed how her symptoms were caused by hormonal and nutritional imbalances. The patient was given literature and a written plan in order to ensure that she knew exactly what her program entailed.

We ordered day 21-serum testing, nutritional testing – functional intracellular analysis and serum vitamin D (25[OH]D), ferritin, and iodine. She was given a DEXA scan and a physical examination.

Laboratory testing is obviously very useful; however it is important to remember that with hormone testing, the results only tell us about hormone levels – they do not tell us whether hormone receptors are active. With this in mind, it is important to listen to the patient. Clinical symptomatology is more important than lab results. It is also important to remember that we, as anti-aging physicians, are interested in restoring levels to optimal, youthful levels. Therefore we are not interested in restoring hormone to normal lab levels. Our aim is to restore hormones to optimal levels.

The patient was started on 25 mg oral progesterone to be taken every night one hour before bedtime (with the option to increase to 75 mg if necessary). We also prescribed 3 mg of melatonin, and 10,000 mcg vitamin B12 with 400 mcg of folate to be administered intramuscularly each week. Vitamin B12 is poorly absorbed by the body due to the lack of an intrinsic factor; however it is vital for hormones and energy cycles, so it is imperative that patients have adequate levels. For these reasons we tend to give patients vitamin B12 intramuscularly.

We also prescribed the patient a daily multivitamin and mineral supplement. Not all multivitamins are equal! Multivitamin and mineral supplements should not contain preservatives, dyes, colors, or chemicals. The capsules should be vegetarian. The supplement should include active 5'phosphate forms of the B vitamins and hormone activating doses of zinc picolinate, selenium methionine, and iodine. It should contain cobalt to aid the clearance of estrone. Finally, it should contain antioxidant doses of the natural forms of vitamins A, E, and D.

Three weeks later the patient returned for her first follow-up appointment. She rated her sleeping at 8/10 – up from 4/10. She no longer suffered from anxiety and had experienced no panic attacks – a dramatic improvement on the 7/10 which she rated herself at the first appointment. She was taking 50 mg of progesterone each evening. Her energy levels had slightly improved to 6/10 in the AM (was 4/10) and 3-4/10 in the PM (was 2/10). She also reported that she had more energy in the two-three days following her intramuscular injection of vitamin B12.

By this time her laboratory results had returned. Her progesterone was just 0.5 ng/ml, however we are aiming for 5-10 ng/ml. Her estradiol (E2) was 120 pg/ml, 80-100 pg/ml is optimal for a woman of her age. Her free T3 was 230 – we are aiming for 375 to 400. All her B vitamins were low. Vitamin D was very low at 20 ng/ml, 30 mg/ml is classed as deficient, and 70 ng/ml is optimal. Her ferritin level was just 14, her zinc level was low, and her hematocrit was 34, which is also low.

On the strength of these laboratory results we prescribed 19 mcg compounded thyroid (T3 and T4), which we doubled to 38 mcg over the course of two weeks or so. We also added thyroid support (tyrosine, selenium, zinc, iodine, vitamin D3) to her program, and we increased her vitamin B12 shots from once weekly to once every three-to-four days for one month. She was also given more supplementary iron.

At her next follow-up, seven weeks on from her initial appointment, she rated her sleep at 9/10, and her energy at 6/10 in the AM and 5-6/10 in the PM. At this appointment we decided to increase her T3/T4 to 76 mcg, and we told her to add another 38 mcg two weeks later. We also reduced her vitamin B12 shots to once every four weeks.

At her next appointment at week 11, she rated her sleep at 9/10 and her energy at 8/10 in the AM and 7-8/10 in the PM. We increased her thyroid again to 152 mcg, and decreased thyroid support. By this time we had received the results of her DEXA scan, which were -1.1 for the hips and -1.5 for the spine. Her urine NTx was 54 – it should be less than 35. At this point we added bone support to her program. In our restorative model bone support includes: progesterone, because progesterone is the major bone builder and is an activator of osteoblasts; nutrients, including microcrystalline hydroxyapatite calcium (MCHC), vitamin D3 2000 IU a day for one month, vitamin K2 100 mcg, zinc, magnesium, and boron glycinate 5 mg. We also advised her to stop drinking soda and carried out heavy metal testing, which is vital when you have a young patient with bone loss. We also recommended stress management techniques and exercise – even five minutes of squat, five minutes of lunges, and five minutes of push-ups each day can make a huge difference.

At her fourth appointment at week 15, she rated her sleep at 9-10/10, and her energy at 9-10/10 in both the AM and PM. She had also lost 14 pounds in weight. Lab results showed her progesterone had increased from 0.5 ng/ml to 5.5 ng/ml, her free T3 had increased from 230 to 360, her TSH had dropped to 0.9 from 1.3, her urine NTx had dropped from 54 to 43, her hematocrit had improved from 32 to 37, and her ferritin was within normal limits. At this point we decided to discontinue the vitamin B-12 injections and move the patient to twice-yearly appointments.

Case Study: 36-Year-Old Female Patient with a Diagnosis of Fibromyalgia

A 36-year-old, previous CEO, who had been out of work for two years and had a diagnosis of fibromyalgia, complained of severe fatigue. She had a history of volatile organic acid exposure. She rated her energy level at 1-2/10 and her pain at 9/10. She was not sleeping, and complained of anxiety and panic attacks, memory loss, cognitive decline, and acid reflux. She had been prescribed prednisone, Lunesta, Xanax, and Nexium.

We presented her with a written plan and started her on 25 mg to 75 mg oral progesterone to be taken every night one hour before bedtime. We also prescribed her 10,000 mcg vitamin B12 with 400 mcg of folate to be administered intramuscularly each week and a daily multivitamin and mineral supplement. We wanted to try to take her off the Nexium as soon as possible so we began treatment with enzymes (amylase, lactase, invertase, diastase, proteases, lipases, cellulose, pectinase, and fibrinolytic enzyme – nattokinase) and probiotics (*lactobacillus – acidophilus, helveticus, platarum, casei, salvarius, rhamnosus, bacteroides – bifidum, longum, infantis,* and *streptococcus – thermophillus, boulardi*). We also prescribed far infra-red sauna sessions, breathing exercises, and yoga. Far infra-red sauna is an ideal treatment for patients who cannot exercise – it improves blood flow, enhances cellular repair, and increases the toxic content of sweat from 5 to 15%. We also conducted the usual battery of tests - day 21-serum testing, nutritional testing – functional intracellular analysis and serum vitamin D (25[OH]D), ferritin, and iodine, a DEXA scan, and a physical examination.

Three weeks later the patient returned for her first follow-up appointment. She rated her energy level at 3/10 (up from 1-2/10) and her pain at 7/10 (up from 9/10). Her sleep had improved, and she was no longer suffering from anxiety or panic attacks. Her acid reflux had slightly improved and she had managed to reduce her dose of Nexium.

Her laboratory results showed that her progesterone was 0.7ng/ml, however we are aiming for 5-10 ng/ml. Her DHEA was 10, however 40-60 is optimal for a woman of her age. Her free T3 was 178 – we are aiming for 375 to 400. Her cortisol was 5, whereas it should be 10-14. These results showed that the patient obviously needed broad support. Therefore we prescribed 50 mg progesterone, 38 mcg Thyroid (T3/T4), 10 mg DHEA, 30 mg pregnenolone twice a day, 3mg melatonin, and 5 mg hydrocortisone three times a day to replace the prednisone.

Results of the nutritional analysis revealed that she had low levels of all of the B vitamins and that her antioxidant function was extremely low – in the 23rd percentile. Therefore, we added 3-4 g of omega 3 and extra antioxidants (spirulina, chlorella, kelp, dulse, gogi, nont, mangosteen, acai) to her nutritional program.

Her urine metabolic analysis showed an ATP production defect, bowel yeast overgrowth, liver fatty acid oxidation, and DNA oxidation. Thus, we also prescribed CoQ10, ribose, L-carnitine and magnesium – all of which support ATP production, and placed her on bowel and liver detox programs.

For bowel detox we placed her on a vegan diet for four to eight weeks. Although this may sound like a very simplistic thing to do, experience has shown that it is very effective, particularly in patients that have collagen diseases or any kind of rheumatoid fibromyalgia. We also prescribed a strong probiotic in order to make the bowel move at least two to three times a day, as well as bentonite clay, psyllium husk powder, slippery elm bark, and ginger root, which all support the bowel.

After the bowel detox was completed we started the patient on the liver detox. For this we advised her not to drink alcohol. We also prescribed alpha lipoic acid, N-acetyl cysteine (NAC), methylsulfonylmethane (MSM), glycine, magnesium glycinate, malic acid, and calcium D-glucarate.

At a follow-up appointment five months later she rated her energy level at 8-9/10, her pain at 0/10, she is sleeping well, has no anxiety, her memory and cognitive function is back to normal, her acid reflux is gone, and, best of all, she has felt well enough to return to work!

In order to keep her well and prescribe a maintenance program, which includes: 75 mg progesterone, 25 mg DHEA, 76 mcg T3/T4, 3 mg melatonin, multivitamin and mineral supplement, 3-4 g omega-3, weekly IM injection of 10,000 mcg vitamin B12/ 400 mcg folate, bowel and liver detox supplements, breathing exercises, and yoga.

At this point we also decide to discontinue the hydrocortisone and move the patient to twice-yearly appointments.

CONCLUDING REMARKS

Multiple imbalances contribute to symptoms such as fatigue, weight gain, low sex drive, anxiety, and depression, which plague us as we age. Following the restorative medicine model presented in this paper will enable you to restore optimal health to your patients.

REFERENCE

Estrogen and progestogen use in postmenopausal women: July 2008 position statement of the North American Menopause Society. Menopause: *The Journal of the North American Menopause Society.* 2008;15:584-603. http://www.menopause.org/PSHT08.pdf

ABOUT THE AUTHOR

Dr. Sangeeta Pati opened holistic SaJune Medical Center in Orlando, Florida, after practicing obstetrics-gynecology in the Washington, D.C. area for 14 years. Dr. Pati helps each patient develop an aggressive preventative plan to restore optimal balance of hormones, nutrients while removing toxins. Dr. Pati graduated at the top of her medical class at the University Of Maryland School Of Medicine, Baltimore, and served a residency at Georgetown University School of Medicine, Washington, D.C. She has worked extensively in the U.S. and internationally as Medical Director for a 350-employee non-profit organization, Engenderhealth. Dr. Pati is multi-lingual and is renowned in her field, having authored numerous scientific articles and addressed audiences both domestically and internationally.

Chapter 27
Silver Sol Gel As A Broad-Spectrum Anti-Bacterial Agent
Gordon Pedersen, Ph.D.; Keith Moeller

ABSTRACT

Silver Sol Gel (Ultimate Skin and Body Care) was tested against numerous bacterial and yeast strains (*Candida albicans, Staphylococcus aureus,* methicillin-resistant *Staphylococcus aureus* (MRSA), *Pseudomonas aeruginosa, and Escherichia coli*) to determine how well it would kill a broad spectrum of disease causing pathogens. This was measured by percent reduction in pathogen, LOG reduction. Results indicate that Silver Sol Gel completely destroyed all forms of bacteria tested to a LOG 5 reduction. This is significant because an FDA category one wound care approval requires the approved product to be able to achieve a 1 log reduction (90% kill) in 7 days of contact, and a 3 log reduction (99.9% kill) within 14 days. The American Biotech Labs Ultimate Skin and Body Care product achieved a 4-5 log reduction (99.999+ kill) in the first hour of contact. The FDA further requires an approved product to be able to kill 500,000 bacteria. The Ultimate Skin and Body Care Gel was tested at 3-5 times the required amount of the pathogenic load, killing between 1,500,000 and 2, 500,000 of the deadly pathogens within the first hour.

In this study Silver Sol Gel far surpassed FDA required kill percentages by killing all yeast and bacteria tested at a significant level of 99.99900 %. This is an improvement of over 10,000-times (log 5) better kill rates than what would be required to be classified as an effective antimicrobial. It accomplished this killing in less than one hour.

Silver Sol Gel appears to be one of the best and most broad spectrum antibacterial agents and has been proven to produce no resistance. Because Silver Sol Gel kills so quickly and completely (99.99900 %) without causing bacterial resistance, it could be successfully used everyday without creating the problems of mutation and resistance created by antibiotics.

INTRODUCTION

Silver has been used as medicine and as a preservative by many cultures throughout history. Greeks used silver vessels for water purification. Pioneers trekking across the west used it to keep their water safe and prevent dysentery, colds, and flu – they actually put silver dollars in their milk containers and wooden water casks to retard the growth of bacteria. Today, silver water purification filters are used by Switzerland, international airliners, and in swimming pools, as disinfectants.[1]

Medicinal silver compounds were developed in the late 1800's and there was widespread use of silver compounds and colloids prior to 1930. By 1940 there were approximately 48 different FDA approved silver compounds marketed being used to treat virtually every infectious disease known to man. These were available in oral, injectable, and topical forms. They carried such names as: Albargin, Novargan, Proganol and Silvol.[1]

The historical facts support what we have proven in this study – that silver has germicidal properties. Since 1973, silver has been shown to have topical activity against 22 bacterial species (643 isolates) including gram positive and gram negative bacteria.[2] The gel functions as an antibiotic more or less equal to pharmaceutical drugs but is unique because bacteria do not mutate or become resistant to Silver Sol.[3] Silver Sol is approved as a homeopathic drug by the food and drug board of Ghana.

SILVER SOL GEL EFFICACY STUDY
Claims Found in United States Patent # 7135195

Silver Sol has hundreds of approved claims in the patent.[4] Some of the most significant pathogens killed include: MRSA, SARS, malaria, and anthrax. In fact, the patent covers more than 143 individual uses against bacteria, viruses (including hepatitis B, HIV, and influenza), and fungi:

- o Anti-viral patent claims – destroys reverse transcriptase and DNA polymerase types of viruses.
- o Anti-bacterial patent claims:
    - o Kills gram negative bacteria i.e. *Salmonella.*
    - o Kills gram positive bacteria i.e. *Staphylococcus aureus.*
    - o Kills nosocomial infections i.e. *Pseudomonas aeruginosa* and MRSA.

o Proven to kill a broad spectrum of both gram positive and gram negative bacteria, without destroying healthy *Lactobacillus* (flora).
o Kills *Bacillus subtilis* (99.97% in three hours).
o Kills *Yersinia pestis* (plague) (99.999999% in 6 minutes).
o Exhibits equal or broader spectrum of activity than any one antibiotic tested.[3]

It should be noted that no organism was found to be resistant to Silver Sol.[3] Furthermore, Silver Sol can be used as an internal and external disinfectant because it passes through the body unchanged, thus meaning that it produces no dangerous metabolites.

Safety
Silver Sol Gel has been rigorously tested in ingested, injected, and cytotoxic experiments. These studies have found that Silver Sol is absorbed, distributed, excreted, and passed through the body unchanged – the very definition of non-toxic).

Materials and Methods
Silver Sol Gel (24 ppm) was prepared in triplicate and placed in tubes containing 10 ml of each sample (*Candida albicans, Staphylococcus aureus, MRSA, Pseudomonas aeruginosa, Escherichia coli*). The tubes were inoculated with 0.1 ml of the test organism and mixed thoroughly. After 1-hour, 24-hours, and 7-days of exposure 1.0 ml aliquots of the test suspension were removed and added to 9 ml of neutralizer. The tubes were mixed thoroughly and serial dilutions were made in the appropriate neutralizer and assayed using a standard spread plate method. Bacterial samples were plated onto SCDA for bacteria and SDEX for yeast and incubated at 20-25 degrees Celsius for 3-5 days. Log reduction and percent neutralization were calculated using standard equations.

Results
Results showed that Silver Sol Gel completely kills *Candida albicans, Staphylococcus aureus, MRSA, Pseudomonas aeruginosa*, and Escherichia coli.

Table 1. *Results of Silver Sol Gel (Ultimate Skin and Body Care) Efficacy study*

ORGANISM	EXPOSURE TIME	PERCENT REDUCTION (%)	LOG 10 REDUCTION
Candida albicans	1-hour	>99.998544	>4.84
	24-hours	>99.998544	>4.84
	7-days	>99.998544	>4.84
Staphylococcus aureus	1-hour	>99.999133	>5.06
	24-hours	>99.999133	>5.06
	7-days	>99.999133	>5.06
MRSA	1-hour	>99.998696	>4.88
	24-hours	>99.998696	>4.88
	7-days	>99.998696	>4.88
Pseudomonas aeruginosa	1-hour	>99.999102	>5.05
	24-hours	>99.999102	>5.05
	7-days	>99.999102	>5.05
Escherichia coli	1-hour	>99.998990	>5.00
	24-hours	>99.998990	>5.00
	7-days	>99.998990	>5.00

Silver Sol Gel completely killed the bacteria and yeast at an average LOG 10 reduction of 5.0 within one hour.

CONCLUDING REMARKS

The results of this study show that Silver Sol Gel quickly and completely destroyed all the yeast (*Candida albicans*) and bacteria (*Staphylococcus aureus, MRSA, Pseudomonas aeruginosa, Escherichia coli*) tested within just one hour. It is remarkable that this substance can destroy the deadly pathogens that cause some of the most serious and life threatening diseases afflicting mankind. The results suggest that Silver Sol could be successfully used every day for prevention of disease and epidemics. Silver Sol Gel contains no alcohol so it will not dry out the skin. The topical use of this gel should safely kill all contagious pathogens tested, and especially those transferred by hand contact and poor hygiene.

REFERENCES

1. Hill JW. *Colloidal Silver Medical Uses, Toxicology & Manufacture.* 3rd ed. Clear Springs Press; 2009.
2. Carr HS, Wlodkowski TJ, Rosenkranz HS. Silver sulfadiazine: *in vitro* antibacterial activity. *Antimicrob Agents Chemother.* 1973;4:585-587.
3. de Souza A, Mehta D, Leavitt RW. Bactericidal activity of combinations of Silver–Water Dispersion™ with 19 antibiotics against seven microbial strains. *Current Science.* 2006;91:926-929.
4. Holladay RJ, Christensen H, Moeller WD, inventors. American Silver, LLC, assignee. Treatment of humans with colloidal silver composition. US patent 7 135 195. November 14, 2006.

ABOUT THE AUTHOR

Primary author Dr. Gordon Pedersen is an international best-selling author. He is the formulator of more than 150 nutritional products and is the host of the radio show "Common Sense Medicine". He now serves as the Director of the Institute of Alternative Medicine and was nominated to chair the United States Pharmacopoeia Review Board, Natural Products Committee. Dr. Pedersen received his Doctorate degree in Toxicology with emphasis in Virology from Utah State University and a Master's degree in Cardiac Rehabilitation and Wellness. Dr. Pedersen has authored a number of important protocols in virology.

Chapter 28
Swine Flu Influenza Type A/H1N1:
Protection, Vaccination, and the Cytokine Storm
Gordon Pedersen, Ph.D.

ABSTRACT

This paper will provide an overview of the current swine flu (A/H1N1) pandemic. Methods of prevention and treatment, and the problems surrounding vaccination and antiviral drugs will be considered. Cytokine storms will also be discussed.

INTRODUCTION

Influenza viruses are the respiratory viruses of greatest public health importance, particularly Influenza A.[1] The annual average U.S. winter epidemics affect 5% to 20% of the population, and every year 36,000 people die from influenza, making it the 6th leading cause of death in America.[1] The Centers for Disease Control and Prevention (CDC) estimates that it would cost America $71-166 billion if we have an influenza epidemic today. Approximately 1 out of every 1,000 swine flu patients dies from the infection. This is close to the same rate we have been seeing the past few years but antigenic drift and antigenic shift may create a new and fatal form of influenza that humans have no immunity against.[2] Antigenic drift is a variation within the HN subtype. Changes to the viral components heamagluttinin (H) and neuraminiadase (N) make large portions of the population immunologically naïve on a regular basis.[1] The problem with Type A is that it undergoes both antigenic drift and antigenic shift making it more dangerous and unpredictable.[2]

The World Health Organization declared the H1N1 Swine Flu a pandemic in June of 2009.[3] Vaccinations have not and will not provide protection because there is continuous change in the virus. In addition, many people have been injured or died from receiving vaccinations. While viruses continue to mutate, there will never be a totally effective vaccine against influenza. With these facts, the patient should always have the freedom to choose to be vaccinated or not.

Table 1. Estimated Death Toll of Historic Influenza Pandemics

Year	Flu		Deaths
1889	Russian Flu	H2H2	1,000,000
1918	Spanish Flu	H1N1	40,000,000
1957	Asian Flu	H2N2	1,500,000
1968	Hong Kong	H3N2	750,000

INFLUENZA REVIEW

The influenza virus is a member of the Orthomyxoviridae family. The genome consists of 8 segmented, negative-sense RNA strands made up of 15,000 nucleotides each. The influenza virus species is subdivided into three types; A, B and C. Types A and B have 8 RNA segments and encode 11 proteins. Subtype C has 7 RNA segments and encodes 9 proteins.

Influenza Type A is the most dangerous type. The virus can evolve quickly and produce an epidemic in weeks.[4-7] It is affected by antigenic drift and antigenic shift making it the most dangerous and likely type of influenza to mutate into a new and more fatal form.[1] Influenza Type B produces less serious disease than does Influenza Type A and is not categorized by H or N subtypes as is Influenza Type A.[1] Influenza Type C was first isolated in 1949 and is not known to be responsible for epidemics.[1]

According to the CDC, the current swine flu is characterized as Influenza type A and has 8 Single RNA strands made up of 6 human H1N1 strands with one strand of swine flu and one strand of bird flu. This genetic combination makes it very weak to pigs and birds, but it may recombine during the replication process producing a new virus that could be fatal to as much as half the world's population.

Influenza Mechanism of Action

The life cycle of the influenza viruses may be broken down into the following different stages:

- Binding to the host
- Internalization
- Fusion and un-coating
- Nuclear import of ribonucleoproteins
- Transcription
- Replication and viral protein synthesis
- Nuclear export of ribonucleoproteins
- Virus assembly and release

Neuraminidase Inhibitors

Neuraminidase inhibitors are a class of antiviral drugs that blocks the viral neuraminidase protein, thus preventing the virus from budding (reproducing). Oseltamivir (Tamiflu) a pro-drug, zanamivir (Relenza), and peramivir belong to this class.[1] These drugs work against Influenza Type A and Influenza Type B. The adamantanes amantadine and rimantidine only work on Influenza Type A. Currently, amantadine and rimantidine are not recommended, and Tamiflu has developed resistance. Relenza has some central nervous system concerns. Both Tamiflu and Relenza have been given prophylactic use directions where they can be taken for prevention in single doses (i.e. 75 mg/day) instead of the therapeutic dose (75 mg/b.i.d). This is to be continued for a period of only ten days, or a period of 7 days beyond exposure.[2]

Epidemiology

Every winter, epidemics of human influenza recur in the United States, and are associated with an annual average of 226,000 hospitalizations and 36,000 deaths, mainly caused by secondary bacterial pneumonia in the elderly and young children.[8,9] In addition, US influenza epidemics tend to originate in California, which may reflect this region's interconnectivity to Asia and Australia.[10]

February is typically the peak month of the influenza season. During the past 26 flu seasons, the peak of the influenza season has occurred in:

- November   1 season
- December   4 seasons
- January   5 seasons
- February   12 seasons
- March   4 seasons

Since the 1968 pandemic, A/H3N2 viruses have dominated most influenza seasons, including 16 of the past 20 US epidemics.[11] These viruses are associated with higher levels of morbidity and mortality,[12] higher rates of evolutionary change,[4] and greater synchrony in the timing of local epidemics across the United States than A/H1N1 viruses.[10] However, during the 2006-2007 US influenza epidemic, more viruses reported by the CDC were of the A/H1N1 (62.3%) than the A/H3N2 subtype (37.7%).[11]

People over 45 years of age seem to be less at risk from the current swine flu and suffer less severe symptoms, possibly because they have some immunity from previous H1N1 exposure. Young adults have little or no immunity according to reports from the CDC.[2]

Doctors, nurses and other healthcare providers are at the highest risk of becoming infected with influenza. Because doctors are exposed to the virus most frequently it is important to recognize the survivability of the influenza virus in open environments. Mammalian Influenza Type A can survive for up to 1 hour in mucous, while avian influenza can survive for up to 100 days in water, up to 200 days at 63°F, up to 1 day in feces, and indefinitely when frozen. Influenza is easily transmitted from human to human. The transmission rate from body fluids and hand-to-hand contact is 70%, and the airborne transmission rate is 29%. The human-to-animal transmission rate is 1%.

RECOMMENDATIONS FOR INFLUENZA PREVENTION AND TREATMENT

Doctors have the obligation to protect themselves and their patients from influenza viruses. This protection could come from many different sources including vaccination, hygiene, antiviral drugs, antibiotic drugs, nutritional supplements, air filters, water purifiers, masks, topical gels, and Silver Sol.

Table 2. Agents Capable of Destroying the Influenza Virus

• Bleach	• Quaternary ammonium compounds
• 70% ethanol	• Heat (133°F) for 60 minutes
• Aldehydes	• pH less than 2 (very acidic)
• Oxidizing agents	• Silver Sol (liquid and Gel)

Vaccination

Results indicate that U.S. children are largely serologically naïve to the novel influenza A (H1N1) virus and that vaccination with seasonal TIV (trivalent inactivated vaccine) or LAIV (live attenuated influenza vaccine) does not elicit any measurable level of cross-reactive antibody to the novel virus. This means that vaccination with recent (2005-2009) seasonal influenza vaccines is unlikely to provide protection against the novel influenza A (H1N1) virus. Results among adults suggest that some degree of preexisting immunity to the novel H1N1 strains exists, especially among adults aged 60 years and over.

It takes approximately 5 months to develop and produce a vaccine and during that time it is likely that the virus will mutate. This means that a vaccination cannot be successful and will not provide protection due to the rapid changes resulting from antigenic drift and shift.

Past epidemics provide important insights into what might happen in the potential spread of the current swine flu.[13-20] The strongest viruses survive and the most diverse seem to go extinct within a few years.[21,22] This is most likely the result of strong host-mediated selection pressure, resulting in continual evolution at key antigenic sites, a process termed 'antigenic drift'.[22,23] This antigenic evolution is observed with major changes in antigenicity occurring periodically in patterns of approximately 3 years between episodes.[24] A variety of epidemiological and evolutionary models have been developed to explain this phylogenetic pattern[25,26] and how it relates to the viral genome.[27]

Although antigenic drift is clearly a key determinant of influenza A virus evolution, this process has rarely been observed in a single locality over a single epidemic season.[28,29] Instead, multiple viral introductions appear to drive evolution at the scale of local epidemics, allowing for the co-circulation of multiple clades of the same subtype.[27,29] East and South-East Asia, appears to be important in determining large-scale epidemiological patterns.[30-32] In addition, re-assortment events between viruses of the same subtype occur frequently, and are sometimes associated with major antigenic changes in both the A/H3N2[33] and A/H1N1 subtypes.[34,35]

As mentioned earlier, during the 2006-2007 US influenza epidemic, more viruses reported by the CDC were of the A/H1N1 (62.3%) than the A/H3N2 subtype (37.7%).[11] The evolutionary dynamics of this epidemic were particularly complex, including a late-season switch in dominance from the A/H1N1 to the A/H3N2 subtype, the co-circulation of multiple antigenically distinct lineages within both A/H1N1 and A/H3N2, an A/H3N2 vaccine mismatch, and the co-circulation of amantidine-resistant and sensitive viral lineages in both subtypes.[11,36] This demonstrates how multiple risk factors combined with the fact that viruses evolve rapidly means that the viruses stay ahead of vaccines and drugs. So, vaccination and antiviral drugs are unlikely to have a great impact upon a flu pandemic, this, together with the fact that secondary bacterial infections kill nearly three-quarters of flu victims, means that we are in need of additional proven methods of prevention if we are to save more lives.

Hygiene

The CDC recommends washing the hands after any exposure, simply because most influenza is transferred by hand-to-hand contact. Patients, as well as doctors, should be encouraged to wash their hands regularly. Masks and gloves can help, but the mask must fit tightly with no leaks to be effective. A surgical mask helps protect both the persons exposed and the wearer, so if you have a fever, cough, or sneeze, a surgical mask should be worn in order to protect the patients.

People that are infected should be encouraged to stay home, stay hydrated, use hand disinfectants, and get well before exposing healthy people to the virus. Disposable tissues should be used to catch coughs and sneezes, and they should be disposed of immediately afterwards.

If there is a flu pandemic, nurse stations should be active in airports, bus terminals, and other public areas where people travel. These stations should include a rapid detection device, thermometer, hand disinfectants, preventive agents and the ability to sequester people who are ill to a safe area. Hand washing stations should also be set-up in public buildings, churches, waiting rooms, etc.

Air Filters

The CDC recommends that there should be an air filter in every room. HEPA air filters use silver to inactivate viruses and can effectively kill 99% of all bacteria and viruses in minutes.

Water Purifiers

The influenza virus can survive for up to 100 hours in water. Thus, the CDC recommends good hygiene and a water purifier. A water purifier should contain a silver filter, as they will destroy the virus. Carbon filters and reverse osmosis purifiers will not destroy or remove the virus.

Topical Disinfectants

Topical disinfectants can kill germs for 4-6 hours, and are recommended by the CDC for use between each patient. Hand disinfectants should also be used by patients as well as doctors and nurses. Patients and health care professionals should use these at least 4 times a day, or as needed. Chlorox kills viruses, but should be used sparingly because it is toxic and the gas can irritate the respiratory system. Silver Sol gel demonstrates effectiveness against some of the worst pathogens including: bird flu, methicillin-resistant *Staphylococcus aureus* (MRSA), Vancomycin-resistant *enterococcus* (VRE), *Streptococcus pneumoniae*, and other bacteria that cause pneumonia.

Silver Sol

Prescription drugs and vaccines treat and help prevent viral infection and disease but are not capable of totally controlling a dangerous new or novel virus.[37] Nutritional supplements such as vitamins, minerals, *Echinacea*, ginseng, probiotics and many others have the ability to help boost immune function and improve natural defenses, which provides some defense against disease causing viruses and the associated secondary infections. However, Silver Sol provides proven prevention and treatment against viral and bacterial infections, and there is nothing else with such broad-spectrum benefits.[38]

Silver Sol can be safely taken every day for prevention, and has been shown to provide protection against the very dangerous bird flu Influenza A virus H5N1. The combination of antibiotics with Silver Sol has been shown to enhance antibiotic function by as much as ten-fold due to the fact that Silver Sol kills the residual pathogens that the antibiotics cannot.[38] Results of the combination of 19 different prescription antibiotics and Silver Sol demonstrate safe, additive, and/or synergistic benefits across 7 different pathogenic strains (*Staphyloccocus aureus*, MRSA, *Escherichia coli*, *Pseudomonas arugenosa*, *Salmonella*, and *Streptococcus*). The results of this combination therapy result in significant pathogenic destruction while also helping to reduce bacterial resistance.[39] This can be attributed to the fact that Silver Sol does not produce resistance, nor does it destroy the beneficial intestinal probiotic bacteria.[37]

Silver Sol for Prevention, Treatment, and Combination Therapy

Different forms of silver have been used for centuries to combat viral, bacterial, and fungal infections.[12] Silver Sol has demonstrated significant antiviral benefits. These include prevention against Influenza A H5N1 (bird flu), where the animals demonstrated a 100% increase in their ability to survive a fatal H5N1 infection.[39] There are numerous forms of silver used medicinally including ionic, colloidal, and metallic forms. The colloidal silvers of the past had mediocre benefits but suffered from the problem of tissue accumulation, a condition called argyria. However, a newly patented form of silver called Silver Sol, presents a safer, and newer generation of silver. Numerous publications that demonstrate Silver Sol's unique efficacy for destroying viruses have been published. These peer-reviewed publications include in-vitro studies, animal studies, and human research publications. Silver Sol is newly patented, Environmental Protection Agency (EPA) certified, and a gel has been approved by the Food and Drug Administration (FDA).

FDA category 1 antimicrobial approval requires the approved product to be able to achieve a 1 log reduction (90% kill) in 7 days of contact, and a 3 log reduction (99.9% kill) within 14 days. Silver Sol achieved a 4-5 log reduction (99.998+ kill) in the first hour of contact. The FDA further requires an approved product to be able to kill >500,000 bacteria/ml. Silver Sol exceeded these requirements in less than 1 hour and sustained them for 28 days.

The following is a summary or studies demonstrating the benefits of Silver Sol as they apply to influenza:

- Silver Sol destroys all forms of viruses: H5N1, H1N1, H3N2, hepatitis B, Aids, SARS.
- Silver Sol prevents avian Influenza A H5N1 in mice (when taken orally twice a day).
- Silver Sol prevents H5N1 bird flu from killing mice.
- Silver Sol reduced H5N1 virus to below detectable levels in 5 hours.
- Silver Sol destroys Beijing Influenza A H1N1.
- Silver Sol destroys 98.2% of Influenza A H1N1 in 2 hours. No virus found 12 hours later.

For general prevention, two teaspoons of liquid Silver Sol should be taken orally twice a day. Silver Sol gel should be used on the hands and in the nostrils twice daily. For the treatment of flu, liquid Silver Sol should be taken in the same way as for prevention. Gel should be used on the hands and in the nostrils 4 times a day. Silver Sol liquid should also be inhaled through a nebulizer for 15 minutes twice daily. For prevention during an epidemic Silver Sol should be used as per the instructions for the treatment of flu.

Antiviral Drugs

Antiviral drugs have the ability to destroy specific viruses, but they cannot be taken for an extended period of time. They also produce side effects that mimic the flu, thus making it difficult to diagnose the severity of the disease. If taken for prevention, Tamiflu produces resistance – 18% of influenza viruses are already resistant to Tamiflu.[1] It is strongly suspected that this resistance developed as a result of healthcare professionals using Tamiflu for just 4 months as a preventive agent. This indicates that we cannot use the antiviral drugs for long periods of time. In addition, some drugs cannot be used in children. Tamiflu cannot be used in children under 13 years of age, whilst Relenza cannot be used in children under one or in adults over 65. Furthermore, antiviral drugs must be given within 48 hours of the onset of illness or the virus will run its course. Combine this with the fact that 76% of H1N1 subjects in the Spanish flu 1918, died from a bacterial infection that produced pneumonia and you have an incomplete solution to the influenza problem.

Antibiotic Drugs

Antibiotic drugs provide no solution against the virus but can be very beneficial for treating pneumonia that may develop later. It is necessary to use a broad spectrum antibiotic because there are numerous bacteria that can produce pneumonia. Silver Sol can be given with antibiotics. Using Silver Sol in combination with antibiotic drugs increases antibiotic activity against bacterial infections that can cause pneumonia by as much as ten fold.[37]

Nutritional Supplements

There are hundreds of supplements that can be of significant benefit to the immune system, and there are even some that claim to have antiviral activity. The best proven choices for nutritional supplements come in the form of immune stimulants and wellness products. The best choices include: antioxidants, vitamin C, vitamin B complex, folic acid, vitamin D (prevention), probiotics, expectorants, and Silver Sol.

THE CYTOKINE STORM

A cytokine storm (hypercytokinemia) is the systemic expression of an exaggerated immune response against pathogens. Cytokines signal immune cells such as T-cells and macrophages through intracellular communication. The activated immune cells respond by traveling to the site of infection. Normally, the immune cells maintain a healthy balance of mobilization and activation, but on occasion, activated immune cells send signals that stimulate the production of more cytokines resulting in an uncontrolled mobilization and activation of too many immune cells in one location. This can lead to a rapid accumulation of fluids in the lungs. This fluid accumulation, coupled with tissue inflammation, creates a situation where the lungs struggle to transfer needed oxygen, thus putting added pressure on the respiratory and circulatory system. Cytokine storms are not fully understood, but it appears that they may be caused by an exaggerated response that is triggered when the immune system encounters a new and highly pathogenic invader, such as the H1N1 influenza virus. The primary symptoms of a cytokine storm are high fever, swelling, redness, extreme fatigue, and nausea.

Research suggests that cytokine storms were responsible for many of the deaths during the 1918 influenza pandemic, which killed many young adults.[40-42] Research results from Hong Kong also suggest that cytokine storms were also the cause of many deaths in young people during the SARS (severe acute respiratory syndrome) epidemic in 2003.[43] Human deaths from the bird flu H5N1 virus usually involve the cytokine storm also.[44] There has also been speculation that cytokine storms could be responsible for the deaths seen in the latest flu epidemic (2009), however the CDC reports that there is insufficient information about clinical complications to determine cause.[45]

Normalizing the Cytokine Storm

There is no proven method of treating a cytokine storm; however research indicates that certain drugs may be of benefit:

- ACE inhibitors and angiotensin II receptor blockers: The rennin-angiotensin system (RAS) has been implicated in the mediation of the cytokine storm.[46] This suggests that there a potential benefit may be derived from angiotensin-converting enzyme (ACE) inhibitors and angiotensin II receptor blockers (ARB's). ACE has been implicated in inflammatory lung pathologies,[47] and has been confirmed as a useful marker for disease activity in cytokine-mediated inflammatory lung disease.[48] Marshall found that angiotensin II was associated with cytokine mediated lung injury and suggested a role for ACE inhibitors.[49] Wang published data that cytokine mediated pulmonary damage (apoptosis of the epithelial cells) in response to the pro-inflammatory cytokine TNF-alpha requires the presence of angiotensin II. This suggests that ARB's might have clinical utility against cytokine storms.[50]
- Tumor necrosis factor (TNF) inhibitors (arthritis medications) reduce inflammation by inhibiting the TNF-alpha pathway to immune cell activation. TNF-alpha blockers have been shown to reduce antibody presentation after vaccination against influenza.[51]
- Antiviral drugs, such as Tamiflu and Relenza, help to reduce the viral load that triggers the cytokine storm.
- Broad spectrum antibiotics fight secondary infection, and thus reduce inflammation and fluid retention.

CONCLUDING REMARKS

H1N1 is a serious threat to our health and way of life. The best way to fight influenza is to prevent it with good hygiene. Drugs have serious side effects, cannot be used by the entire population, and should not be used for long periods of time. Another problem is that approximately three-quarters of the people who have died from H1N1 influenza have succumbed to a secondary bacterial infection and cytokine storm in the lungs – no antiviral drug can successfully treat this situation. Vaccinations will not work long-term because the virus will continue to change due to antigenic shift and antigenic drift – this is why a new flu vaccine is developed every year.

In order to control an epidemic all types of treatment should be employed including prescription drugs, vitamins, minerals, antioxidant herbs, proper hygiene, air filtration, water filtration, and Silver Sol. Silver Sol destroys bacteria, viruses, and mold, and thus demonstrates broader spectrum of activity than any antibiotic or antiviral drug. Taken orally it can prevent viral infections, treat them and work synergistically with antibiotics to produce as much as a ten-fold increase in activity against the bacteria that cause death in influenza. Whilst Silver Sol gel can help stop the spread of virus on the body's vulnerable and contagious areas such as the hands, nose, and mouth. It is sufficiently documented and demonstrated to be a first line of defense against influenza and a significant companion to antiviral and antibacterial drug regimens topically and orally.

REFERENCES

1. Centers for Disease Control and Prevention. Update: swine-origin influenza A (H1N1) virus---United States and other countries. *MMWR* 2009;58:421.
2. Novel Swine-Origin Influenza A (H1N1) Virus Investigation Team. Emergence of a novel swine-origin influenza A (H1N1) virus in humans. *N Engl J Med.* 2009;361:2605-2615.
3. World Health Organization. Situation updates---influenza A (H1N1). Geneva, Switzerland: World Health Organization; 2009.
4. Ferguson NM, Galvani AP, Bush RM. Ecological and immunological determinants of influenza evolution. *Nature.* 2003;422:428-433.
5. Ina Y, Gojobori N. Statistical analysis of nucleotide sequences of the hemagglutinin gene of human influenza A viruses. *Proc Natl Acad Sci.* 1994;91:8388-8392.
6. Hay AJ, Gregory V, Douglas AR, Lin YP. The evolution of human influenza viruses. *Phil Trans R Soc Lond B.* 2001;356:1861-1870.
7. Jenkins GM, Rambaut A, Pybus OG, Holmes EC. Rates of molecular evolution in NA viruses: a quantitative phylogenetic analysis. *J Mol Evol.* 2002;54:156-165.
8. Leavitt, R, Pedersen G. Resistance of Silver Sol and Bacteria: A Discussion. *ABL.* 2009.
9. Viridis BioPharma. Probiotic Bacteria and Silver Sol. 2007.
10. Viboud C, Bjørnstad ON, Smith DL, Simonsen L, Miller MA, Grenfell BT. Synchrony, waves, and spatial hierarchies in the spread of influenza. *Science.* 2006;312:447-451.
11. Centers for Disease Control and Prevention. Update: influenza activity–United States and worldwide, 2006-2007 and composition of the 2007–2008 influenza vaccine. *MMWR.* 2007;56:789-794.
12. Roy R. Ultradilute material research innovations, Ag-aquasols with extraordinary bactericidal properties: role of the system. *Ag-O-H2O.* 2007;11.
13. Laver WG, Webster RG. Selection of antigenic mutants of influenza viruses. Isolation and peptide mapping of their hemagglutination proteins. *Virology.* 1968;34:193-202.
14. Sleigh MJ, Both GW, Underwood PA, Bender VJ. Antigenic drift in the hemagglutinin of the Hong Kong influenza subtype: correlation of amino acid changes with alterations in viral antigenicity. *J Virol.* 1981;37:845-853.
15. Fitch WM, Leiter JMF, Li X, Palese P. Positive Darwinian evolution in human influenza A viruses. *Proc Natl Acad Sci.* 1991;88:4270-4272.
16. Bush RM, Fitch WM, Bender CA, Cox NJ. Positive selection on the H3 hemagglutinin gene of human influenza virus A. *Mol Biol Evol.* 1999;16:1457-1465.
17. Rvachev LA. Computer modeling experiment on large-scale epidemic. *Dokl USSR Acad Sci.* 1968;2:294-296.
18. Longini IM, Fine PE, Thacker SB. Predicting the global spread of new infectious agents. *Am J Epidemiol.* 1986;123:383-391.
19. Bonabeau E, Toubiana L, Flahault A. The geographical spread of influenza. *Proc Biol Sci.* 1998;265:2421-2425.
20. Grais RF, Ellis JH, Glass GE. Assessing the impact of airline travel on the geographic spread of pandemic influenza. *Eur J Epidemiol.* 2003;19:1065-1072.
21. Buonagurio DA, Nakada S, Parvin JD, Krystal M, Palese P, Fitch WM. Evolution of human influenza A viruses over 50 years: rapid, uniform rate of change in NS gene. *Science.* 1986;232:980-982.
22. Fitch WM, Leiter JMF, Li X, Palese P. Positive Darwinian evolution in human influenza A viruses. *Proc Natl Acad Sci.* 1991;88:4270-4272.
23. Fitch WM, Bush RM, Bender CA, Cox NJ. Long term trends in the evolution of H(3) HA1 human influenza type A. *Proc Natl Acad Sci.* 1997;94:7712-7128.
24. Smith DJ, Lapedes AS, de Jong JC, Bestebroer TM, Rimmelzwaan GF, Osterhaus AD, Fouchier RA. Mapping the antigenic and genetic evolution of influenza virus. *Science.* 2004;305:371-376.
25. Ferguson NM, Galvani AP, Bush RM. Ecological and immunological determinants of influenza evolution. *Nature.* 2003;422:428-433.

26. Koelle K, Cobey S, Grenfell B, Pascual M. Epochal evolution shapes the phylodynamics of interpandemic influenza A (H3N2) in humans. *Science.* 2006;314:1898-903.
27. Rambaut A, Pybus O, Nelson MI, Viboud C, Taubenberger JK, Holmes EC. The genomic and epidemiological dynamics of human influenza A virus. *Nature.* 2008;453:615-619.
28. Lavenu A, Leruez-Ville M, Chaix ML, Boelle PY, Rogez S, Freymuth F, Hay A, Rouzioux C, Carrat F. Detailed analysis of the genetic evolution of influenza virus during the course of an epidemic. *Epidemiol Infect.* 2005:1-7.
29. Nelson MI, Simonsen L, Viboud C, Miller MA, Taylor J, George KS. Stochastic processes are key determinants of the short-term evolution of influenza A virus. *PLoS Pathog.* 2006;2:e125.
30. Viboud C, Alonso WJ, Simonsen L. Influenza in tropical regions. *PLoS Med.* 2006;3:e89.
31. Nelson MI, Simonsen L, Viboud C, Miller MA, Holmes EC. Phylogenetic analysis reveals the global migration of seasonal influenza A viruses. *PLoS Pathog.* 2007;3:e131.
32. Russell CA, Jones TC, Barr IG, Cox NJ, Garten RJ, Gregory V, et al. The global circulation of seasonal influenza A (H3N2) viruses. *Science.* 2008;320:340-346.
33. Holmes EC, Ghedin E, Miller N, Taylor J, Bao Y, St George K, et al. Whole-genome analysis of human influenza A virus reveals multiple persistent lineages and reassortment among recent H3N2 viruses. *PLoS Biol.* 2005;3:e300.
34. Nelson MI, Viboud C, Simonsen L, Bennett RT, Griesemer SB, St George K, et al. Multiple reassortment events in the evolutionary history of A/H1N1 influenza A virus since 1918. *PLoS Pathog.* 2008;4:e1000012.
35. Nelson MI, Holmes EC. The evolution of epidemic influenza. *Nat Rev Genet.* 2007;8:196-205.
36. Simonsen L, Reichert TA, Viboud C, Blackwelder WC, Taylor RJ, Miller MA. Impact of influenza vaccination on seasonal mortality in the US elderly population. *Arch Intern Med.* 2005;165:265-272.
37. Thompson WW, Shay DC, Weintraub E, Brammer L, Cox N, Anderson LJ, Fukuda K. Mortality associated with influenza and respiratory syncytial virus in the United States. *JAMA.* 2003;289:179-186.
38. De Souza A, Mehta D. Bactericidal activity of combinations of silver-water dispersion with 19 antibiotics against seven microbial strains. *Current Science.* 2006;91.
39. Pedersen G. Effect of prophylactic treatment with ASAP–AGX-32 and ASAP solutions on an avian influenza A (H5N1) virus infection in mice.
40. Osterholm MT. Preparing for the next pandemic. *N Engl J Med.* 2005;352:1839-1842.
41. [No authors listed] High stakes, high risks. *Lancet Oncol.* 2007;8:85.
42. Ferrara JL, Abhyankar S, Gilliland DG. Cytokine storm of graft-versus-host disease: a critical effector role for interleukin-1. *Transplant Proc.* 1993;25:1216-1217.
43. Huang KJ, Su IJ, Theron M, Wu YC, Lai SK, Liu CC, Lei HY. An interferon-gamma-related cytokine storm in SARS patients. *Journal of Medical Virology.* 2005;75:185-94.
44. Haque A, Hober D, Kasper LH. Confronting potential influenza A (H5N1) pandemic with better vaccines. *Emerging Infectious Diseases.* 2007;13:1512–1518.
45. Interim Guidance for Clinicians on Identifying and Caring for Patients with Swine-origin Influenza A (H1N1) Virus Infection. Centers for Disease Control and Prevention (CDC). April 29, 2009.
46. Genctoy G, Altun B, Kiykim AA, Arici M, Erdem Y, Cağlarg M, Yasavul U, Turgan C, Cağlar S. TNF alpha-308 genotype and renin-angiotensin system in hemodialysis patients: an effect on inflammatory cytokine levels? *Artif Organs.* 2005;29:174-178.
47. Moldobaeva A, Wagner EM. Angiotensin-converting enzyme activity in ovine bronchial vasculature. *J Appl Physiol.* 2003;95:2278–2284.
48. Shigehara K, Shijubo N, Ohmichi M, Kamiguchi K, Takahashi R, Morita-Ichimura S, *et al.* Increased circulating interleukin-12 (IL-12) p40 in pulmonary sarcoidosis. *Clin Exp Immunol.* 2003;132:152-157.
49. Marshall RP, Gohlke P, Chambers RC, Howell DC, Bottoms SE, Unger T, McAnulty RJ, Laurent GJ. Angiotensin II and the fibroproliferative response to acute lung injury. *Am J Physiol Lung Cell Mol Physiol.* 2004;286:L156-L164.
50. Wang R, Alam G, Zagariya A, Gidea C, Pinillos H, Lalude O, Choudhary G, Oezatalay D, Uhal BD. Apoptosis of lung epithelial cells in response to TNF-alpha requires angiotensin II generation de novo. *J Cell Physiol.* 2000;185:253-259.
51. Gelinck LB, van der Bijl AE, Beyer WE, Visser LG, Huizinga TW, van Hogezand RA, Rimmelzwaan GF, Kroon FP. The effect of anti-tumour necrosis factor alpha treatment on the antibody response to influenza vaccination. *Annals of the Rheumatic Diseases.* 2008;67:713–716.

ABOUT THE AUTHOR

Dr. Gordon Pedersen is an international best-selling author. He is the formulator of more than 150 nutritional products and is the host of the radio show "Common Sense Medicine". He now serves as the Director of the Institute of Alternative Medicine and was nominated to chair the United States Pharmacopoeia Review Board, Natural Products Committee. Dr. Pedersen received his Doctorate degree in Toxicology with emphasis in Virology from Utah State University and a Master's degree in Cardiac Rehabilitation and Wellness. Dr. Pedersen has authored a number of important protocols in virology.

Chapter 29
Parent Essential Fatty Acids, Oxygenation, and Cancer Prevention:
A New Solution

Brian Scott Peskin, BSEE
Professor, Cambridge International Institute for Medical Sciences
(www.cambridgemedscience.org)

ABSTRACT

Despite 50 years of intensive cancer research increasingly focused on genetic causes, no single unifying cause for cancer has been universally recognized; only that there is a significant correlation between the level of tumor hypoxia and prognosis. With the exception of Nobel Laureate Otto Warburg's seminal experiments and discoveries, little work has been done to investigate and advance the causal relationship between hypoxia and cancer initiation. Over 70 years ago, Warburg (with independent confirmation by American scientists) conclusively established that cells could always be made cancerous by subjecting them to intermittent hypoxic periods, and that once done it was irreversible. While modern biochemistry does not address cancer's prime cause of cellular hypoxia, physiology does. It can now be shown that Warburg's findings of a critical 35% intermittent reduction in intracellular oxygen levels initiating cancer is linked to the incorporation of adulterated, non-oxygenating, or inappropriate polyunsaturated fatty acids, specifically termed parent essential oils (PEOs), into the phospholipids of both cell and mitochondrial membranes. Such incorporation causes physiologic changes in membrane properties that impair oxygen transmission into the cell. Trans fats, partially oxidized PEO entities, and inappropriate physiologic "parent" omega-6: omega-3 ratios are all potential sources of unsaturated fatty acids that can disrupt the normal membrane structure. A solution to protect against cellular hypoxia; i.e., cancer's prime cause is given.

Keywords: essential fatty acids, parent essential oils, EFAs, PEOs, Warburg, cancer, hypoxia

INTRODUCTION

Tragically, even with enormous budgets, brilliant minds, and an earnest desire to end the cancer plague, little of significance has been accomplished in the last 35 years to reduce cancer's spread. Today, the average American will contract cancer in his or her lifetime despite the plethora of lifestyle and nutritional changes that have been advocated by cancer specialists and eagerly followed by the public. Could the cancer research community be looking in the wrong place?

New Hope – It's Not Genetic

Most physicians currently believe cancers are caused by the activation of oncogenes – genes that predispose the individual toward cancer. That is incorrect. This theory was called into question by its discoverer Dr. Robert A Weinberg of the Massachusetts Institute of Technology (MIT). He reversed himself over 10 years ago in 1998. After discovering that "[F]ewer than one DNA base in a million appears to have been miscopied," he concluded that is not enough of a defect to mutate the cell! Weinberg's exact words: "Something was very wrong. The notion that a cancer developed through the successive activation of a series of oncogenes had lost its link to reality."[1] Nearly a decade later, in 2007, Dr. Weinberg then stated, "The connection between inflammation and cancer has moved to center stage in the research arena." He even called this discovery a "rewriting of the textbook."[2] (For other references in regard to this topic, see Lewis and Pollard,[3] Balkwill *et al*,[4] and de Visser *et al*[5]).

Furthermore, over 35 years ago, Professor Henry Harris and coworkers took normal tissue cells and fused 3 types of cancer cells to them. It was thought that the cancer cells would take over the normal cells and "convert" them into cancer. Surprisingly, they grew normally, showing cancer is genetically recessive, not dominant as everyone thought.[7] Most cancer researchers are not aware of this critically important information.

Shocking, yet unknown to many cancer researchers were statements made in 2005 by the heads of the world's largest cancer research center in Houston, Texas, when they announced that cancer's prime cause is not genetic. Dr. John Mendelsohn, president of the M.D. Anderson Cancer Center, stated:

"Any claims that this [genetic research] is going to be the key to curing cancer are not appropriate."[7] As in Dr. Weinberg's 2007 revelation detailing the inflammation/cancer connection, no genetics are required to explain cancer's prime cause. In 2008, a significant article in *Scientific American* stated: "But the oncogene/tumor suppressor gene hypothesis has also failed, despite two decades of effort, to identify a particular set of gene mutations that occurs in every instance of any of the most common and deadly kinds of human cancer."[8] Note: This includes even BRCA 1 and BRCA 2, and that in 2006, researchers actually measured the number of mutations in a cancerous cell and it was a mere "65-475 mutations per 100 million nucleotides" – not nearly enough mutations in a cell to cause cancer! This new field is termed epigenetics and theorizes that the cellular environment alone – nothing to do with genetics – is the basis for cellular disorders, such as cancer. In a 2009 article, it was made clear that precancerous stem cells can remain benign or malignant depending on the environment, and that "some sort of signal or cue from their immediate environment directs them to become benign or malignant."[9] Mina Bissell, PhD, pioneered the view that a cell's environment is as important as its genes in determining the formation and progression of tumors. Bruce Lipton, PhD, has advanced this line of reasoning focusing on the cell's bi-lipid membrane. We will bring this concept to fruition, and provide a completely epigenetic basis for cancer based on a widespread cellular environmental assault few of us are aware of that gives little notice.

The great news we can take from this announcement is that even if cancer apparently "runs in your family," there is real hope because it has nothing to do with genes. But first, some popular but clinically worthless anti-cancer recommendations need to be addressed.

Popular Anticancer Recommendations Often "Called into Question"

Many people diligently follow the experts' recommendations, hoping to beat cancer. The inability of the medical and dietary professions to curb the rising level of cancer over the last 60 years bears exploring. Although many of their recommendations may sound plausible, they aren't effective in clinical practice, nor should they be; they don't have a specific metabolic pathway directly inhibiting cancer's development. Consider the following list of recommendations along with the date of their findings being questioned or even reversed as reported in the world's foremost medical journals that many cancer researchers never saw: Fruits and vegetables protect us from cancer (called into question 2001)[10]; mammography detects initial cancer growth (called into question 2000)[11]; fiber protects against colon cancer (called into question 1999 and 2001)[12,13]; fish oil alone prevents cancer (called into question 2000)[14]; omega-3 alone prevents cancer (called into question 2006)[15,16]; soy is a positive anticancer addition to our diet (called into question as early as 1946 and 1960)[17,18]; low-fat diets are the anticancer answer (called into question 2006).[19] Are there anticancer recommendations that have withstood the test of time never having to be reversed or called into question? The answer is an emphatic *yes*.

DR OTTO WARBURG'S AMAZING ANTICANCER DISCOVERY

Nobel Prize winner, Otto Warburg, MD, PhD, has often been called the greatest biochemist of the 20th century; the sheer number and magnitude of his discoveries qualify him as the most accomplished biochemist of all time. Despite this, much of his seminal work on cancer has been overlooked. No scientist or researcher has ever disproved the validity, correctness, or applicability of Warburg's important discoveries as they relate to the prevention and cure of cancer. In fact the opposite is true – none of his findings have been called into question.

The Prime Cause of Cancer

We have become so accustomed that seemingly every discovery in the battle to defeat cancer is, after a time, called into question that the following might be hard to believe. Otto Warburg discovered, then clearly and simply stated that the prime cause of cancer is oxygen deprivation at the cellular level. "We find by experiment about 35% inhibition of oxygen respiration already suffices to bring about such a transformation during cell growth," he stated at a 1966 conference of Nobel laureates in Lindau, Germany.[20] It is that simple. Just one-third less cellular oxygen than normal and you contract cancer. Based on meticulous experiments that he and many other scientists verified numerous times, Dr Warburg discovered that the prime cause of cancer is sustaining a 35% inhibition of cellular respiration.[20] In America, seminal experiments in 1953 and 1955 confirmed that decrease of sustained cellular oxygen always induces cancer, and its converse, that cancer occurs in environments of significantly decreased oxygen. You won't immediately feel the harmful effect of decreased cellular oxygenation, and you won't know it is happening. Yet if cellular oxygen levels can be kept above this deprivation threshold, cancer cells will not be able to form. It really is that simple.

Exercising supplies additional oxygen to the blood; however, this doesn't address transfer of oxygen through the cell membrane – the critical factor. This is why elite athletes still develop cancer. Warburg stated: "To be sure, cancer development takes place even in the presence of free oxygen gas in the atmosphere, but this oxygen may not penetrate in sufficient quantity into the growing body cells, or the respiratory apoenzymes of the growing body cells may not be saturated with the active groups." Warburg addressed the danger of impaired cellular oxygen transfer even in the presence of oxygen. We will soon see how the environments of each of our 100 trillion cells' membranes play in oxygen transfer, and in transferring this oxygen to the mitochondria, how one special factor significantly impairs oxygen transfer.[21]

Dr Warburg's discovery has been verified over and over again (never called into question), both as to how normal cells turn cancerous and in showing that cancer doesn't develop in sufficiently oxygenated areas. It is important to emphasize that two American physicians conclusively proved this in 1953, and two more investigators confirmed this finding in 1955. Goldblatt and Cameron published in the *Journal of Experimental Medicine* that once damage is too great to the cell, then no amount of oxygen will return the cell's respiration back to normal: it is forever doomed to a cancerous life.[22] However, they confirmed it is possible to prevent a "respiration impacted" precancerous cell from becoming permanently cancerous if oxygen deficiency is stopped early enough. This is wonderful news. In 1955, Malmgren and Flanigan confirmed the oxygen/cancer cause in an ingenious experiment with tetanus spores.[23] Consequently, prevention is the ultimate solution to conquering cancer.

Greater Oxygen Deprivation = Worse Prognosis

Numerous articles in cancer journals confirm the decreased oxygen/increased cancer prognosis: "Tumor hypoxia adversely affects the prognosis of carcinoma of the head and neck."[24] "[A]nalysis showed significantly lower survival and recurrence-free survival for patients with a median pO_2 of ≤ 10 mm Hg compared to those with better oxygenated tumors (median pO2 > 10 mm Hg). [M]edian pO_2 and the clinical stage according to the FIGO are independent, highly significant predictors of survival and recurrence-free survival."[25] "Tumor oxygenation predicts for the likelihood of distant metastases in human soft tissue sarcoma."[26] Greater cellular oxygen deprivation/hypoxia is directly correlated with a worse prognosis, shorter lifespan, and greater risk of metastases. The greater the cellular oxygen deprivation, the worse the patient's prognosis. There is no question…lower oxygen equals more virulent cancer.

How Can Tissue Become Oxygen Deficient? The Secret of PEO-Containing Oils

The body requires special fats, which, among other important functions, make it possible for sufficient oxygen to reach the cells via the cell membranes – the key to cancer prevention. These special fats are highly oxygen-absorbing entities called essential fatty acids, or EFAs, and must be eaten every day, because your body can't manufacture them on its own. There are two "parent" forms of EFAs that allow your body to make whatever it needs from them, i.e. the various types of EFA "derivatives." Supplemental EFA-derivatives, such as EPA and DHA are not required because the body makes them as needed in very small amounts. Parent omega-6 is termed linoleic acid (LA), and parent omega-3 is termed alpha-linolenic acid (ALA). I call these two parent EFAs parent essential oils (PEOs) in order to clearly differentiate these from the non-essential "derivatives" that are manufactured by the body "as needed."

Parent Omega-6 Increases Oxygen Transfer Like Little "Oxygen Magnets"

Campbell *et al* found that LA (parent omega-6), can associate with oxygen and dissociate the oxygen at relatively high oxygen pressure in cellular membranes. These researchers also found that fatty acids (in particular, LA) effect the permeability of cell membranes to molecular oxygen by increasing cellular oxygenation by up to 50%, thus helping you remain cancer-free.[27] They concluded that interference with the movement of oxygen can occur at any cell membrane in any tissue. That's why regardless of where the cancer occurs, the prime cause is the same – the cancerous tissue is the most oxygen impaired. This simple truth bears repeating. Warburg unequivocally showed all cancers occur for the same reason. American researchers confirmed the fact. Moreover, PEO deficiency can cause substitution into the cell membranes of non-oxygenating fats that impair oxygen transport, exacerbating the cancer causing state. Is there more confirmation in the medical texts of PEO's oxygenating ability? Yes. Several medical textbooks and published medical papers, to name a few, all confirm oxygenating ability (Figure 1).[28-31]

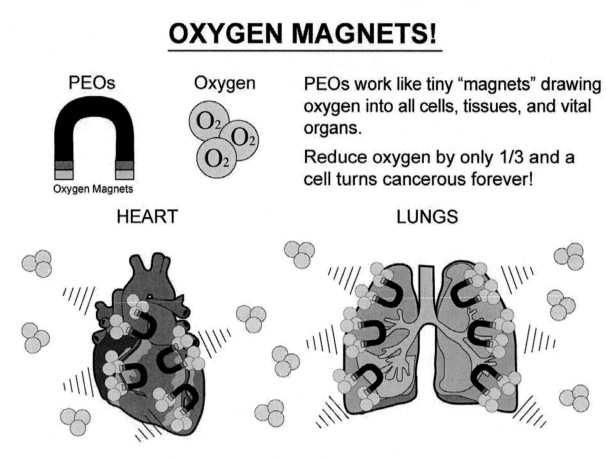

OXYGEN MAGNETS!

PEOs

Oxygen

Oxygen Magnets

PEOs work like tiny "magnets" drawing oxygen into all cells, tissues, and vital organs.

Reduce oxygen by only 1/3 and a cell turns cancerous forever!

HEART

LUNGS

Figure 1: Parent essential oils work like tiny oxygen "magnets."

What are the Tissue Parent Omega-6/3 Ratios?

It is necessary to understand the PEO composition of various tissues and organs, such as your brain, skin, heart, and muscle, to discover the overall PEO requirement of the body. A little-known but vital fact about muscle structure is that muscle contains from 5.5 to 7.5-times more parent omega-6 than parent omega-3, depending on the degree of physical condition.[32] Extremely fit individuals require less omega-6 because their oxygen-transferring efficiency, including an increased number of cell mitochondria, is greater than in non-exercising individuals. Skin contains no omega-3, only parent omega-6, while body fat contains 20-times more parent omega-6 than omega-3.[33] Figure 2 shows the parent omega-6/-3 ratios of major organs along with the respective weights. Contrary to what many researchers think, the brain is comprised of a 100:1 parent omega-6/-3 ratio; not 1:1. Most of the plasma free fatty acid and EFAs are derived from the triglycerides stored in the adipose tissue (body fat), and organs, including the brain, use these EFAs for structural incorporation.[34]

Ratio of Tissue Composition			
Tissue	Percentage of Total Body Weight	Omega-6 PEO	Omega-3 PEO
Brain/Nervous System	3	100	1
Skin	4	1000	1
Organs and Other Tissues	9	4	1
Adipose Tissue (bodyfat)	**15-35**	**22**	**1**
Muscles	**50**	**6.5**	**1**

Reference: Spector, A.A., "Plasma Free Fatty Acids and Lipoproteins as Sources of Polyunsaturated Fatty Acid for the Brain," Journal of Molecular Neuroscience, Vol. 16, 2001, pages 159-165., "Most of the plasma free fatty acid (EFA) is derived from the triglycerides stored in the adipose tissue [bodyfat]." Note: Organs, including the brain use these EFAs for structural incorporation. "Metabolism of essential fatty acids by human epidermal enzyme preparations: evidence of chain elongation, "R.S. Chapkin, et. at., Journal of Lipid Research, Volume 27, pages 954-959, 1986, Markides, M., et al., "Fatty acid composition of brain, retina, and erythrocytes in breast- and formula-fed infants," The American Journal of Clinical Nutrition, 1994;60:189-94 and Agneta Anderson, et. al., American Journal of Endocrinological Metabolism, 279: E744-E751.

Figure 2: Tissue composition and amounts of parent essential oils.

Table 1. Percentages of linoleic acid (LA) and alpha linolenic acid (ALA) in plasma and classes of lipids. Source references[30,34]

Table 1 Percentages of Linoleic Acid (LA) and Alpha Linolenic Acid (ALA) in Plasma and Classes of Lipids				
Fatty Acid	**Plasma Unesterified**	**Plasma Triglycerides**	**Plasma Phospholipids**	**Plasma Cholesterol Esters**
LA	17	19.5	23	50
ALA	2	1.1	0.2	0.5
LA:ALA ratio	8.5:1	17.5:1	115:1	100:1

References: Sinclair HM. Essential fatty acids in perspective. Hum Nutrit 1984;38C:245-260; Spector A. Plasma free fatty acid and lipoproteins as sources of polyunsaturated fatty acid for the brain. J Mol Neurosci 2001;16:159-165.

It can also be seen in Table 1 that plasma contains significantly more parent omega-6 than parent omega-3, and that plasma cholesterol esters and plasma phospholipids contain a factor of 100 times in favor of parent omega-6 to be delivered to the cells. We also see from Figure 2 the abundance of parent omega-6 throughout. If tissues and organs are not supplied through the diet with unadulterated, fully functional parent EFAs, then either damaged EFAs or even non-EFA oils, such as omega-9 (as in olive oil), will be utilized instead causing deoxygenation of the cells.[35]

Even in the brain, LA/ALA uptake is 100-times greater in favor of omega-6.[36] Surprising, both to cancer researchers and physicians, is the fact that there is not a significant bodily storage mechanism for ALA; its main metabolic route is beta-oxidation. Even significantly raising ALA intake does not cause a significant change in adipose tissue LA/ALA storage ratios.[36]

In view of emphasis solely on supra-physiologic omega-3 recommendations that ignore the critical unadulterated parent omega-6 requirements, when the supply of PEOs, in particular, unprocessed parent omega-6, is less than the body's total requirement, the body prioritizes delivery, feeding the organs it considers most important first: the brain, heart, lungs, and kidneys. This deprives "less important" organs, such as the breast and prostate glands from receiving adequate PEOs and oxygen. Breast and prostate tissues are predominately fat requiring lots of functional parent omega-6 EFAs. Is it merely a coincidence they are both the number one cancers worldwide for the respective sexes?

Are We Overdosing on Omega-3 and Omega-3 Series Derivatives? Surprise: Derivatives Made "As Needed"

In the study of Sinclair et al,[37] we discover that the major metabolic route of ALA (parent omega-3) in the body is beta-oxidation, burning for energy – not incorporation into tissue. Therefore, overdoses will be injuriously incorporated into tissue structure. In view of this, we should proceed cautiously with omega-3 supplementation, including flax oil and fish oil.

The medical journals frequently bombard us advocating supra-physiologic doses of omega-3 derivatives, such as EPA and DHA: i.e. fish oil. This recommendation is called into question because Salem et al[38] explains why only about 5% of the parent ALA (parent omega-3) is converted into derivatives. Pawlosky and others[39] calculate that less than a mere 1% goes to derivatives. In addition, recently in 2008, Barceló-Coblijn et al[40] confirmed the effectiveness of ALA conversion and accretion into erythrocytes. This means we all make derivatives from parents "as needed," and these authors made clear that we all do. The premise that diabetics all have impaired enzymatic ability to convert LA to GLA is called into question; no one converts much. This fact is not newly published; if anyone would have cared to look, the same conclusion was also published back in 2005.[41] Here, the conversion rates were shown to be even less; less than a mere 1%. Demmelmair and colleagues[42] also stated a significant reason why derivative-conversions were so overestimated: different residence times were not considered.

High omega-3 food sources – flax seed, fish oil, seafood, etc. – can be an overload in both parent and derivative omega-3 series EFAs. Fish, especially farmed fish, contains almost entirely omega-3 derivatives. Because of this, fish oil supplements originally thought to help prevent cancer have been called into question.[14] You need to know that supraphysiological doses of omega-3 series oils cause their abnormal incorporation into cell tissue.[35,43] Health practitioners should be terrified about the pharmacological overdoses fish oil gives to patients – approximately 10-times the amount the body makes on its own. Krill Oil simply contains fewer derivatives, but still contains no PEOs. The warning that omega-3 or omega-3 series EFAs will not prevent cancer was published in 2006 but too few physicians or health professionals took note.[15]

In light of this information we have a precise explanation for the rampant rise in skin cancer. As Figure 2 highlights, our skin has no omega-3 in its structure. Could a prime factor be the supra-pharmacological omega-3 overload that the body, in desperation, dumps into the epithelial tissue? Sunlight is required for vitamin D production so sunlight, in and of itself is a necessity. Because of wrong nutritional recommendations, your skin's cellular structure is the problem.

In spite of this fact, nutritional recommendations still often advocate consumption of quantities of parent omega-3 and omega-3 series derivatives that based on human physiology and biochemistry are far too large. The problem is compounded when they overlook recommending supplementation with unadulterated, fully functional parent omega-6. Not surprisingly, skin cancer contraction rates have increased along side of the increase in fish oil supplementation.

Food Processors Ruin PEO Parent Omega-6

My decade-long research confirms that cellular hypoxia occurs primarily from consumption of adulterated polyunsaturated fatty acids (PUFAs), which are incorporated into cell membranes and interfere with cellular oxygen transmission. Natural oils in prepared foods turn rancid over time. Likewise, so do oils used in both restaurant and commercial deep fryers. Food processors, for economic reasons, must stop the oxygen transfer that results in spoiled food. They use only two approaches: remove the oil or adulterate them into entities like trans fats and interesterified fats. Their thoughtless solution to longer shelf life is a prime cause of the unstoppable cancer epidemic. As long as food processors continue to find creative but dangerous ways to reduce cellular oxygen transfer by using adulterated PUFAs (parent omega-6 oils are exclusively used), unwitting consumers should be terrified. Bans on trans fats are not sufficient – any oil used must be non-oxygen-transferring. The only plausible choice for us is to incorporate unadulterated oils in our diets by way of a dietary supplement.

How Much Omega-6 Are We Consuming?

Many nutrition researchers state that the U.S. population is consuming 15, 20, or even 30-times more omega-6 than omega-3 in its diet. However, their analysis ignores the fact that meats, such as beef and chicken contain lots of parent omega-3 (although cooking denatures some of it). This unaccounted for parent omega-3 in foods decreases the overbalanced omega-6 ratio dramatically. For example, depending on the specific diet of the animal, steak and hamburger will contain a ratio typically between 2:1 to a high of 10:1 in favor of omega-6. A grain-fed chicken produces eggs that contain a ratio of from 1:1 to as much as 10:1 in favor of omega-6. But fish, shrimp, and shellfish (not their extracted oil) – a primary protein in many people's diets – contains more omega-3 series than omega-6, usually from 2:1 to a high of 20:1 in favor of omega-3 series EFAs. Therefore, the average American's omega-6 to -3 ratio in regard to consumption can't be above 12:1. Of the 12:1 at least half (conservatively) of the parent omega-6 in most processed foods has lost its oxygenating ability. For example, margarine and most supermarket cooking oils (even olive oil contains few PEOs) have no appreciable oxygenating ability and consequently will remain unspoiled even when kept outdoors for years. They are so unappealing that given a choice no animal will even attempt to eat them – nor will they oxidize and become rancid. Tragically, widespread commercial use of preservatives and other deoxygenating additives have become the norm.

Rethinking EFA Supplementation Ratios and Amounts

The current message to eat more omega-3 or more fish is overly simplistic. What dieticians should be telling us is to replace the adulterated omega-6 (e.g. trans fatty acids/hydrogenated fats, etc.) with unadulterated, organic, minimally processed sources, such as organically processed oils, nuts and seeds, while adding moderate supplementation of omega-3.

We are warned about "overdosing" on omega-6 in our diets and told that we must take lots of oils containing omega-3 to compensate. However, in 2009 this recommendation was changed by the American Heart Association because omega-6 series EFAs contain anti-inflammatory compounds, such as precursors including the powerful prostaglandin PGE_1, and the body's powerful "natural blood thinner" prostacyclin (platelet anti-aggregate and anti-adhesive).[44]

Because the body requires significantly less parent omega-3 than parent omega-6 overall (Figure 2), and because little of the parent omega-3 we eat is damaged (for example, we don't fry or cook with omega-3, nor do commercial food processors use it), a key to better health is to increase supplemental sources of undamaged parent omega-6 instead of exclusively taking excess omega-3 supplements, which the tissues don't want.

My research strongly supports the use of an unprocessed, organic supplement with a ratio of greater than 1:1 up to 2.5:1 of parent omega-6 to parent omega-3. With this ratio, a suggested use is 725 mg per 40 lb of body weight (e.g. a 160-lb person requires 3 g on a daily basis). For complete details of how this specific ratio is arrived at, please read *"The Scientific Calculation of the Optimum Omega-6/-3 Ratio"* available at www.BrianPeskin.com (click on "PEO Report").

How Well Does This Omega-6:3 Ratio Work?

In my research, I commissioned and directed an experiment with mice to study this relationship between cancer growth rates and supplementation with Peskin Protocol PEOs. Mice metabolize EFAs like humans.[33] The experiment showed that, in spite of tumor implantation with 2 million cancer cells at once, there was a statistically significant 24% reduction in tumor size (growth) in the longer 4-week pretreated mice compared to the control mice that received no PEO supplementation (Figure 3). In the last 10 days of the experiment, there was a 42.8% lower growth volume of the tumors in the 4-week pretreated mice compared to the untreated mice. These results clearly show the increasing value of a longer pretreatment period of PEOs.

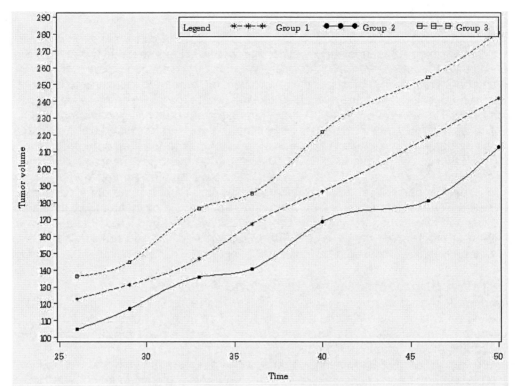

Figure 3. Tumor volumes in mice between groups from 26 to 50 days. Group 2 was pretreated with PEO formulation for 4 weeks prior to tumor implantation. Group 1 was pretreated for 2 weeks prior to tumor implantation. Group 3 was the control.

CONCLUDING REMARKS

My experiment conclusively shows that PEO-based oils are able to modify the internal structure of cells in an epigenetic fashion, thus making them more cancer resistant; the desired anti-cancer/increased cellular oxygenation solution is accomplished per Warburg's findings.

REFERENCES

1. Weinberg RA. *One Renegade Cell: How Cancer Begins*. New York, NY: Basic Books; 1998:64.
2. Stix G. A Malignant flame. *Sci Am*. July 2007:60-67.
3. Lewis CE, Pollard JW. Distinct role of macrophages in different tumor microenvironments. *Cancer Res*. 2006;66:605-612.
4. Balkwill F, Charles KA, Mantovani A. Smoldering and polarized inflammation in the initiation and promotion of malignant disease. *Cancer Cell*. 2005;7:211-217.
5. de Visser KE, Eichten A, Coussens LM. Paradoxical roles of the immune system during cancer development. *Nat Rev Cancer*. 2006;6:24-37.
6. Harris H, Miller OJ, Klein G, Worst P, Tachibana T. Suppression of malignancy by cell fusion. *Nature*. 1969;223:363-368.
7. Berger E. Cancer: Looking Beyond Mutations. *Houston Chronicle*. June 27, 2005:1.
8. Gibbs WW. Untangling the roots of cancer. *Sci Am*. 2008;289:56-65.
9. Singer E. Interpreting the genome. *Technol Rev*. January/February 2009:48-53.
10. Smith-Warner SA, Spiegelman D, Yaun SS, *et al*. Intake of fruits and vegetables and risk of breast cancer: a pooled analysis of cohort studies. *JAMA*. 2001;285:769-776.
11. Epstein S, Bertell R, Seaman B. Dangers and unreliability of mammography: Breast examination is a safe, effective, and practical alternative. *Int Journal Health Services*. 2001;31:605-615.
12. Fuchs CS, Giovannucci EL, Colditz GA, *et al*. Dietary fiber and the risk of colorectal cancer and adenoma in women. *N Engl J Med*. 1999;340:169-176.
13. Levin B. Dietary intake and occurrence of colorectal adenoma. *Lancet*. 2000;356:1286-1287.

14. Calder PC. Omega-3 polyunsaturated fatty acids, inflammation and immunity. Pare presented at: The International Society for the Study of Fatty Acids and Lipids (ISSFAL) 4th Congress; June 4-9, 2000; Tsukuba, Japan.

15. MacLean CH, Newberry SJ, Mojica WA, *et al*. Effects of omega-3 fatty acids on cancer risk. *JAMA*. 2006;295:403-415.

16. Hooper L, Thompson RL, Harrison RA, Summerbell CD, Ness AR, Moore HJ, et al. Risks and benefits of omega-3 fats for mortality, cardiovascular disease, and cancer: systematic review. *BMJ*. 2006;332:752-760.

17. Shephard TH, Pyne GE, Kirschvink JF, McLean M. Soybean goiter: Report of three cases. *New Engl J Med*. 1960;262:1099-1103.

18. Bowman DE. Differentiation of soy bean antitryptic factors. *Proceed Soc Exp Biol Med*. 1946;63:547.

19. Prentice RL, Caan B, Chlebowski RT, *et al*. Low-fat dietary pattern and risk of invasive breast cancer: the Women's Health Initiative Randomized Controlled Dietary Modification Trial. JAMA. 2006;295:629-642.

20. Warburg O. The prime cause and prevention of cancer (Lindau Lecture). Revised. Würzburg, Germany: Konrad Triltsch, 1969. Accessed August 11, 2006. (English Edition, Dean Burk, National Cancer Institute, Bethesda, Maryland, USA.) Retrieved from: http://www.hopeforcancer.com/OxyPlus.htm.

21. Peskin B. *The Hidden Story of Cancer*. Houston, TX: Pinnacle Press; 2008.

22. Goldblatt H, Cameron G. Induced malignancy in cells from rat myocardium subjected to intermittent anaerobiosis during long propagation *in vitro*. *J Exp Med*. 1953;97:525-552.

23. Malmgren, RA, Flanigan CC. Localization of the vegetative form of *Clostridium tetani* in mouse tumors following intravenous spore administration. *Cancer Res*. 1955;15:473-478.

24. Brizel DM, Sibley GS, Prosnitz LR, Scher RL, Dewhirst MW. Tumor hypoxia adversely affects the prognosis of carcinoma of the head and neck. *Int J Radiat Oncol Biol Phys*. 1997;38:285-290.

25. Hockel M, Knoop C, Schlenger K, *et al*. Intratumoral P02 predicts survival in advanced cancer of the uterine cervix. *Radiother Oncol*. 1993;26:45-50.

26. Brizel DM, Scully SP, Harrelson JM, Layfield LJ, Bean JM, Prosnitz LR, et al. Tumor oxygenation predicts for the likelihood of distant metastases in human soft tissue sarcoma. *Cancer Res*. 1996;56:941-943.

27. Campbell IM, Crozier DN, Caton RB. Abnormal fatty acid composition and impaired oxygen supply in cystic fibrosis patients. *Pediatrics*. 1976;57:480-486.

28. Murray RK, Granner DK, Mayes PA, Rodwell VW. *Harper's Illustrated Biochemistry*. 26th ed. New York, NY: McGraw Hill; 2003:93,191,418.

29. Meisenberg G, Simmons WH. *Principles of Biomedical Chemistry*. 1st edition. St. Louis, MO: Mosby; 1998:226.

30. Sinclair HM. Essential fatty acids in perspective. *Hum Nutrit*. 1984;38C:245-260.

31. Sinclair HM. Prevention of coronary heart disease: the role of essential fatty acids. *Postgrad Med J*. 1980;56:579-584.

32. Andersson A, Sjödin A, Hedman A, Olsson R, Vessby B. Fatty acid profile of skeletal muscle phospholipids in trained and untrained young men. *Am J Physiol Endocrinol Metab*. 2000;279:E744-E751.

33. Chapkin RS, Ziboh VA, Marcelo CL, Voorhees JJ. Metabolism of essential fatty acids by human epidermal enzyme preparations: evidence of chain elongation. *J Lipid Res*. 1986;27:945-954.

34. Spector AA. Plasma free fatty acid and lipoproteins as sources of polyunsaturated fatty acid for the brain. *J Mol Neurosci*. 2001;16:159-165.

35. Lands WEM, Morris A, Libelt B. Quantitative effects of dietary polyunsaturated fats on the composition of fatty acids in rat tissues. *Lipids*. 1990;25:505-551.

36. Watkins, PA, Hamilton JA, Leaf A, Spector AA, Moore SA, Anderson RE, et al. Brain uptake and utilization of fatty acids: Applications to peroxisomal biogenesis diseases. *J Mol Neurosci*. 2001;16:87-92;discussion 151-157.

37. Sinclair AJ, Attar-Bashi NM, Li D. What is the role of alpha-linolenic acid for mammals? *Lipids*. 2002;37:1113-1123.

38. Salem N, Lin Y, Brenna JT, Pawlosky RJ. Alpha-linolenic acid conversion revisited. PUFA Newsletter, December 2003. Retrieved October 12, 2007. Available at: http://www.fatsoflife.com/pufa/article.asp?edition=arch&id=162&nid=1.

39. Pawlosky RJ, Hibbeln JR, Novotny JA, Salem N Jr. Physiological compartmental analysis of alpha-linolenic acid metabolism in adult humans. *J Lipid Res.* 2001;42:1257-1265.
40. Barceló-Coblijn G, Murphy EJ, Othman R, Moghadasian MH, Kashour T, Friel JK. Flaxseed oil and fish-oil capsule consumption alters human red blood cell n-3 fatty acid composition: a multiple-dosing trial comparing 2 sources of n-3 fatty acid. *Am J Clin Nutr.* 2008;88:801-809.
41. Hussein N, Ah-Sing E, Wilkinson P, Leach C, Griffin BA, Millward DJ. Long-chain conversion of [13C]linoleic acid and alpha-linolenic acid in response to marked changes in their dietary intake in men. *J Lipid Res.* 2005;46:269-280.
42. Demmelmair H, Iser B, Rauh-Pfeiffer A, Koletzko B. Comparison of bolus versus fractionated oral applications of [^{13}C]-linoleic acid in humans. *Eur J Clin Invest.* 1999;29:603-609.
43. Burns CP, Luttenegger DG, Dudley DT, Buettner GR, Spector AA. Effect of modification of plasma membrane fatty acid composition on fluidity and methotrexate transport in L1210 murine leukemia cells. *Cancer Res.* 1979;39:1726-1732.
44. Harris WS, Mozaffarian D, Rimm E, *et al.* Omega-6 fatty acids and risk for cardiovascular disease: a science advisory from the American Heart Association Nutrition Subcommittee of the Council on Nutrition, Physical Activity, and Metabolism; Council on Cardiovascular Nursing; and Council on Epidemiology and Prevention. *Circulation.* 2009;119:902-907.

ABOUT THE AUTHOR

This article is based on the book *The Hidden Story of Cancer.* Internationally published in peer-reviewed medical journals, Professor Brian Peskin presents a uniquely penetrating and compelling approach to medicine. He earned his Bachelor of Science degree in Electrical Engineering from Massachusetts Institute of Technology (MIT) in 1979, and is chief research scientist at the Cambridge International Institute for Medical Science (www.CambridgeMedScience.org).

Chapter 30
The Failure of Statins: A New Physiologic Solution to Cardiovascular Disease

Brian Scott Peskin, BSEE
Professor, Cambridge International Institute for Medical Sciences
(www.cambridgemedscience.org)

ABSTRACT

During the last half of the 1990s, almost half of all Americans and European mortalities were from heart disease. In 2006, atherosclerotic coronary artery disease (CAD) became the number one killer of Americans, with cancer running a close second. By 2010, most American deaths will be either from heart disease or cancer. If we go back in time, heart disease did not always present such a dismal picture. In the nineteenth century, heart disease was much rarer, and during the period 1910-1920, in the wards of the Massachusetts General Hospital, coronary heart disease was considered rare. As the decades passed, a variety of factors were suggested as the culprits, including the Western diet, and by the late 1970s, LDL-cholesterol was considered to be one of the primary causes of heart disease. This belief led to the development of many pharmaceutical interventions, including the statin family of drugs. Surprisingly, statins have a number needed to treat (NNT) of 100, meaning that statins fail to prevent cardiovascular disease (CVD) in clinical practice 99% of the time – an amazing 99% failure rate. The insight to prevention of CVD lies in the pathophysiology of the cholesterol structure; in particular, the esterified adulterated parent omega-6 component. A simple, clinical solution is presented.

Keywords: cholesterol, essential fatty acids, parent essential oils (PEOs), LDL

THE FAILURE OF STATINS

A medical school student getting a grade of 90% would warrant an A; a 60% grade would likely rate a D, and a 50% grade an F – failure. Shockingly, most physicians think that statins are excellent at preventing cardiovascular disease (CVD), rating them as an "A" grade medication. On the contrary, statins are anything but effective as demonstrated by their miniscule success rate of 1% in preventing CVD.

NNT (number needed to treat): The Only Effective Measure of a Drug's Success

If you treat 100 patients with a drug and all 100 improve, the drug's number needed to treat (NNT) is 1 (100 patients/100 successes). If you treat 100 patients and only 1 patient responds positively the NNT would be 100 (100 patients treated/1 positive response). This is an awful result and equivalent to a 99% failure rate. Dr. Nortin M. Hadler, Professor of Medicine at the University of North Carolina at Chapel Hill states: "Anything over an *NNT of 50 is worse than a lottery ticket...*"[1]

Study	Design	Outcomes (NNT)	Drug Failure Rate
1997 AFCAPS/TexCAPS[a]	Compared 20-40 mg lovastatin to placebo in patients on a low saturated fat, low cholesterol diet	**NNT:** acute major coronary event: 65	**98.5%**
2008 ENHANCE[b]	Compared 80 mg simvastatin + placebo to 80 mg simivastatin + 10 mg ezetimibe	Change in intima media thickness of carotid artery: 0.0058 mm (p = 0.29; not significant)	**Dual drug not Better**
2008 JUPITER[c]	Compared 20 mg rosuvastatin to placebo in patients with elevated CRP	**NNT:** Any MI: 240; any stroke: 287; any death: 182	**99.6%**
1998 MIRACL[d]	Compared 80 mg atorvastatin to placebo in patients with unstable angina or non-Q-wave MI	**NNT: new/worsening congestive heart failure** requiring re-hospitalization: **556**	**99.8%**

Figure 1. Failure Rates of Recent Statin Trials (MI = myocardial infarction, AFCAPS/TexCAPS[2], ENHANCE[3], JUPITER[4], MIRACL[5])

Of significant importance is the fact that the 2008 JUPITER study[4] was used to try and gloss over the fact that numerous attempts to prove the "cholesterol theory" (the lower the patient's low density cholesterol [LDL-C], the greater the prevention of CVD) have failed, by attempting to make the case that the real mode of action of statin drugs was C-reactive protein (CRP) reduction. However, there is one tragic flaw: CRP is not a reliable prognostic indicator of cardiovascular events; there are better markers. An article entitled *Largest-Ever Meta-Analysis Finds CRP Is Unlikely to Be Causal for CVD*,[6] reports that scientists of the Cambridge-based Emerging Risk Factors Collaboration (ERFC)[7] found that "although CRP concentration was linearly associated with CHD (coronary heart disease), stroke, and vascular mortality, as well as nonvascular mortality, statistical adjustment for conventional cardiovascular risk factors resulted in considerable weakening of associations." Note: The JUPITER Study had an NNT of 240 (99.6% failure rate) that was not disclosed – instead, a hazard ratio (an estimate of relative risk) of 0.52 was published, thus making the trial appear much more successful than it actually was.

Statin Failures – Nothing New

Numerous medical journals have consistently published the ineffectiveness of statins to prevent or lower CVD. Here are a few examples warning of this failure. Kuhn *et al* wrote: "Blood cholesterol by itself is a poor predictor of individual risk of coronary heart disease. Few people identified purely on the basis of cholesterol levels will benefit from treatment [cholesterol lowering drugs]..."[8] Krumholz *et al* concluded: "Our findings do not support the hypothesis that hypercholesterolemia (high LDL-C levels) or low HDL-C (high-density lipoprotein cholesterol, or "good" cholesterol) are important risk factors for all-cause mortality, coronary heart disease mortality, or hospitalization for myocardial infarction or unstable angina in this cohort."[9] In 2005, on the subject of "bad" cholesterol, Colpo commented, "No tightly controlled clinical trial has ever conclusively demonstrated that LDL cholesterol reductions can prevent cardiovascular disease or increase longevity. The concept that LDL is "bad cholesterol" is a simplistic and scientifically untenable hypothesis."[10] Two years later, Mudd *et al* reiterated the pointlessness of lowering cholesterol and suggested that apolipoprotein b was a much better marker of CDV: "Despite more aggressive interventions by lowering LDL-C levels, the majority of CAD (coronary artery disease) events go undeterred [not prevented]...Measurement of apolipoprotein (apo)B has been shown in nearly all studies to outperform LDL-C and non-HDL-C as a predictor of CAD events and as an index of residual CAD risk."[11] Also in 2007 an extremely large meta-analysis of 61 prospective studies that comprised 900,000 adults found no association of cholesterol with stroke.[12] Indeed, one article wrote that the researchers seemed to be "baffled by findings indicating lower cholesterol levels were not linked to reduced stroke deaths." One of the researchers, Dr. Sarah Lewington of the University of Oxford (Britain) was quoted as saying "I think all we can say is that we don't really understand what's going on here."[13] Even in the accompanying editorial to the research study, the two authors were puzzled: "Because most of the benefit of statins in preventing cardiovascular events can be ascribed to the LDL reduction, it is puzzling that LDL cholesterol is not associated with stroke risk."[14] At the very least these studies should constitute a big red flag: all that is statin does not glitter.

Confusion at Best – Statistics are Misunderstood by Most Physicians

If there are one million patients in each of two arms of a placebo-controlled clinical trial, and in the drug arm there is one patient contracting the illness and in the placebo case two patients contracted the illness, what is the drug's effectiveness? It is zero (1/1,000,000 = 0) calculated as (2-1)/ 1,000,000. However, according to the pharmaceutical presentation, they would claim the drug's effectiveness as not zero but amazingly as fifty percent (50%), calculated as (2-1)/2. Something is unnerving here because there is no indication of sample size.

As an illustrative example, if you earn $5000 a week, a raise of $1 a week brings total salary to $5001; hardly interesting and insignificant. However, an additional $1 per week to someone earning $10 per week would make a very significant difference. You get the same relative risk with a sample size of 10 or 1,000,000 patients. This frequently used method is termed "relative risk." When testing a new pharmaceutical, when the drug does not work well the study's director always wants to use "relative risk." However, the proper statistical analysis to use is termed "absolute risk" because it always includes sample size. Because so few drugs work well and their NNTs are often above 50, making them highly ineffective, if absolute risk was used to measure their effectiveness, no one would use them because it would be so obvious that they are failures. Relative risk or a hazard ratio disguises this failure.

Direct Effect, Not Surrogate Markers

Most antibiotics have an NNT of 1.1, meaning that for every 11 patients treated, 10 patients are cured of the ailment. This is a wonderful success rate. Insulin directly decreases the blood sugar level of each patient who takes it, thus the NNT of insulin is 1. Likewise for thyroid stimulating hormone (TSH), the NNT is 1. These drugs directly control the end result; i.e. more insulin = lower blood glucose. To the contrary, for each patient prescribed statins, the LDL-C will decrease, however, that decrease is irrelevant to decreased CVD (per above chart); hence the statin NNT of 100. Note: An NNT does not include contraindications, the negative drug side effects. That is a completely separate issue. In the case of statins, there are many contraindications. For example, cerivastatin (Baychol, Lipobay) was recalled in 2001 because of rhabdomyolysis, a potentially life-threatening condition.

NNT: Absolute Risk – The Only Correct Measure of Drug Effectiveness

NNT is the reciprocal of absolute risk. Drug companies will not often disclose absolute risk and the associated NNT unless forced to. An absolute risk of 0.01 (a highly ineffective drug) translates to an NNT of 100 and vice versa.

Focus on the Physiology

Studies are always open to (mis)interpretation and mistakes in statistical analyses. Incredibly, 50% of the world's top medical journals used incorrect statistics, which wrongly favor drug effectiveness, reporting overstated conclusions concerning effectiveness.[15,16] Even today, the situation has changed little.

Studies should be used only to confirm predicted effects of known physiology/biochemistry. "Studies" on lowering cholesterol and preventing CVD fail to show a cause-effect relationship time after time. Why? The consistent failure of statin drugs is predictable based on known physiology and biochemistry – not on ignoring or denying established medical science. How many cardiologists see fewer CVD-related patients in their offices? If statins truly worked, they would be seeing many fewer patients.

A NEW PHYSIOLOGIC SOLUTION TO CARDIOVASCULAR DISEASE

Cholesterol Is Anything But "Bad"

The pharmaceutical companies have apparently brainwashed physicians into thinking that LDL-C is bad. If LDL-C was truly bad, then you should not want any of it in your or your patient's body – not just less of it. No one wants anything bad in their body. However, if you eliminated all LDL-C, your patients would all die. Something is clearly wrong with this methodology. From a physiologic perspective, LDL-C is absolutely critical for the following reasons:

- All (100 trillion) cells contain cholesterol;
- All tissues manufacture and regulate cholesterol;
- LDL-C has a significant structural role in the brain, where it is required in high concentrations;
- It is fundamental in the control and regulation of fluidity in the lipid bi-layer of cell membranes;
- It enables nerve signal transmission
- Vitamin D manufacture requires functional cholesterol. (Note: There is a significant widespread vitamin D deficiency today. Could statins be an additional cause of this deficiency?);
- Bile for digestion requires cholesterol;
- Skin requires cholesterol for protection against water-soluble toxins;
- Skin requires cholesterol to protect against dehydration;
- LDL-C is a precursor for natural anti-inflammatory steroids;
- LDL-C is a precursor for all sexual steroid-based hormones (testosterone, estrogen, etc.);
- Most importantly, the body has no blood cholesterol sensor – because none is needed. LDL-C is a dependent variable that is regulated once other tightly controlled physiologic variables are set. The body does have blood sensors for physiologic functions that are critical; for example, blood glucose is automatically controlled to 70-90 mg/dL in everyone unless they are diabetic. This is a tightly controlled tolerance of 1 part in 1,000 (0.1%)! Sodium and calcium sensors control their physiologic tolerances to 3-4% in everyone. If the body required set LDL-C tolerances, it would have them. Therefore, the converse is true; no LDL sensor is needed.

The Structure of Cholesterol Itself Never Changes (But R Does!)

It is not the cholesterol structure that is the issue causing CVD; it is the component that cholesterol is "tied to." The cholesterol molecule (better termed "cholesteryl") is tied to a structure that does change - parent essential oils (PEOs) – the variable "R" shown in Fig. 2. This is where all of the insight lies. Cholesterol itself can become oxidized, but much more significant is the oxidized esterified component.[12,13] Note that the cholesterol ester portion of apolipoprotein B (as shown in Fig. 3) is huge compared to the free cholesterol or phospholipid components.

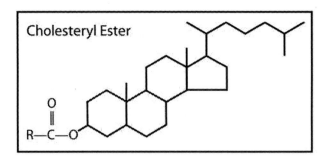

Figure 2. The Structure of a Cholesteryl Ester – An Esterol of Cholesterol

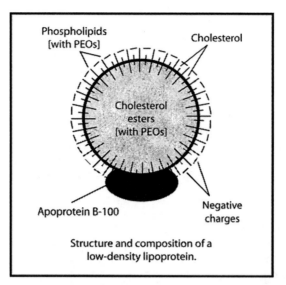

Structure and composition of a
low-density lipoprotein.

Figure 3. The Structure of Apolipoprotein B

Saturated Fat, Arterial Plaques, and Blood Lipids

There is no saturated fat in a thrombosis.[17,18] Most cardiologists are amazed when they hear this physiologic fact. Saturated fat is not causal to CVD and thrombosis, and cholesterol alone is not causal to CVD and thrombosis. Therefore, current anti-CVD recommendations of lowering LDL-C lack firm physiologic basis.

Investigators found that arterial plaques contain more than 10 different compounds, none of which are related to saturated fat. Other independent investigations confirmed this finding, but a key study in 1997 demonstrated that cholesterol esterified with nonfunctional linoleic acid (LA), a parent omega 6 fatty acid, was by far the most abundant lipid component in all types of plaque causing arterial stenosis.[19]

Percentages of Linoleic Acid (LA) & Alpha Linolenic Acid (ALA) in Plasma and Classes of Lipids				
Fatty Acid	Plasma % (Unesterified)	Plasma % Triglycerides	Plasma % Phospholipids	Plasma % Cholesterol Esters
LA (parent omega-6)	17	19.5	23	50
ALA (parent omega-3)	2	1.1	0.2	0.5
Parent omega-6: Parent omega-3 Ratio	8.5:1	17.5:1	115:1	100:1

Figure 4. Percentage of Linoleic Acid and Alpha Linoleic Acid in Plasma and Classes of Lipids[20]

Approximately 70% of the cholesterol in the lipoproteins of the plasma is in the form of cholesterol esters attached to apolipoprotein B.[21] Of dietary cholesterol absorbed, 80%-90% is esterified with long-chain fatty acids in the intestinal mucosa.[22] The majority (about 55%) of the cholesteryl ester component is linoleic acid.[23] Levels of essential fatty acid (EFA) derivatives, such as eicosapentaenoic acid (EPA) and docosahexaenoic acid (DHA), made from the only 2 parent essential oils, LA and alpha linolenic acid (ALA), are insignificant and extremely low (< 2%), so are not included in this analysis because the body makes these derivatives on an as needed basis.[24-26] The n-3 series polyunsaturated fatty acids (PUFAs) makes up only 1%-2% of fatty acids in plasma.[24-26] Even in the brain, LA/ALA uptake is 100-fold in favor of LA.[25]

Surprising to most physicians is the fact that there is no significant bodily storage mechanism for ALA (parent omega-3). In fact, most parent omega-3 is oxidized for energy. Even significantly raising ALA intake does not cause a significant change in adipose tissue LA/ALA storage ratios.[25] This means that parent omega-3 has minor physiologic use and its derivatives even less, making therapeutic use of fish oil very problematic.

The Entire Problem: Oxidized Cholesterol Carries a Poison

World leading biochemist Dr. Gerhard Spiteller concludes that it is oxidized cholesterol esters that are responsible for the initial damage to endothelial cells.[27,28] LDL-C carries these toxic compounds into the endothelial walls where they cause cell damage. Injury is not significantly caused by an increase in oxidized free cholesterol but by an increase in oxidized cholesterol esters.[27,28] This is a critical issue for cardiologists and general practitioners to understand.

Inside an Artery: The Intima

The interior of the arterial lumen consists of endothelial tissue and is termed the intima. What if the cholesterol residing in the bi-lipid membrane of the intima contained significant amounts of already oxidized or nonfunctional parent omega-6, LA, before any in vivo oxidation? This line of reasoning warrants further exploration.

We know that the intima consists of a single layer of endothelial cells containing significant LA, but no ALA.[29,30] What else could cause LA in the endothelial cells to become oxidized? Could significant amounts of *LA* already defective from routine food processing, such as trans fats, hydrogenated oils, or esterified oils, transported by LDL-C be the real culprit? Yes. Consumed, processed LA deposited in arterial intimal cell membranes leads to abnormal oxidation at the vascular injury site. Note: Even food labeled as zero trans fats can actually contain up to 0.5%, which is enough to overwhelm each cell in the body by a factor of at least 100,000.[31]

EFAs and PEOs – The Essential Difference

The term "EFA" is repeatedly used incorrectly to refer to derivatives, such as DHA and EPA, and that is incorrect because there are only 2 essential fatty acids, and they must come from the diet: parent omega-6 (LA) and parent omega-3 (ALA) – both of which are essential, thus meaning that the body cannot synthesize them. DHA from fish oil is not an EFA, as it is *not essential*: the body makes it as needed, like it does many other biological substances, such as hormones from the two PEOs. EPA from fish oil is not an EFA for the same reason.

EFA Conversion Rates are Over-Estimated: New Research

Most physicians and scientists wrongly think that most, if not all EFAs are converted to their associated derivatives. It that were true, giving patients fish oil for omega-3 derivatives would be an excellent idea. However, nothing could be further from the scientific truth because there is *no* 100% conversion of parent to derivatives. Shockingly, it is less than 5% – approximately a mere 1% of all PEOs are converted into derivatives.[32-35]

A significant new finding that few physicians are aware of was published in 2008. In this study investigators evaluated the conversion rates of [U-13 C]ALA and [U-13 C]LA to their respective long-chain n-3 fatty acids. They also compared the increase of fatty acids in the RBCs from ALA with that obtained with the use of preformed EPA and DHA from dietary fish oils. The results showed that an increase in plasma n-3 fatty acid content, especially EPA (20:5n–3) and DHA (22:6n-3) was observed after consumption of fish oil-enriched supplements. Because ALA is the direct precursor of EPA and DHA it was proposed that ALA-enriched supplements such as flax oil, might have a similar effect, and indeed consuming flax oil for 12-weeks was sufficient to elevate erythrocyte EPA and DPA content, thus demonstrating the effectiveness of ALA conversion and accretion into erythrocytes. The authors noted: "The amounts of ALA required to obtain these effects are amounts that are easily achieved in the general population by dietary modification."[36] Furthermore, Hussein *et al* observed that overall conversion rates of LA and ALA, calculated from peak [13C] LCP concentrations and adjusted for dietary influences on pool sizes of LA and ALA, were low and of similar magnitude overall for AA and EPA (just 0.18% and 0.26%). Thus, we see normal PEO conversion rates of less than a mere 1%.[35] One of the reasons that earlier work overestimated the amount of conversion to derivatives was that using the area under the curve, which is the simple, standard method of analysis, overestimates the conversion, because different residence times are not considered.[37]

Δ6-Desaturase and Δ5-Desaturase Enzymes Cannot Normally be Impaired

If Δ6-desaturase and Δ5-desaturase enzymes were impaired in the general population, as most physicians are told, we would see rampant epidemics of blindness in infants and youngsters, along with epidemics of mental and nervous system impairments due to inadequate DHA in both the retina and nervous system, including the brain. Because of epidemics of prostaglandin E1 (PGE1) deficiency, we should see rampant inflammation in these same populations. We do not. Therefore, the premise is false, and conversion rates are adequate, and PEO derivative supplements are not required. Derivatives such as DHA and EPA are made from the parent PEOs by the body as needed. Therefore, fish oil supplementation is not required for EPA and DHA manufacture and may provide harmful suprapharmacological and pathophysiologic overdoses of these substances.

Fish Oil is Not Physiologic and Cannot Work: It is Harmful

Fish oil supplementation to prevent heart disease was known to fail in 1995 and the American College of Cardiology stated that it was completely worthless in preventing or reversing heart disease. (Note: 6 g of fish oil supplement was used per day.[38,39]) It was also known that fish oil decreases the immune response; DHA and EPA, even in low doses, do this.[40] Furthermore, it was known in 2004 that fish oil is worthless in decreasing inflammation as judged by CRP levels.[41] Other detrimental physiological effects of fish oil supplements that have been reported include possible abnormalities due to overdosing issues in brain tissue,[42-44] raising blood sugar levels and causing a blunt insulin response.[45] Therefore, fish oil supplementation is awful for a diabetic.

More recently, Nair and Connolly commented that there is insufficient evidence to recommend the routine use of omega-3 (fish oil) fatty acids, and that there is weak evidence from other meta-analyses that omega-3 fatty acids prevent ventricular arrhythmia and cardiovascular mortality.[46] As Nair and Connolly's article attests, of significance importance for physicians to understand is the fact that the GISSI-Prevenzione trial[47] was not specifically designed to evaluate sudden cardiac death, which was where the observed modest reduction in mortality occurred. Nair and Connolly go on to emphasize that Health Canada currently does not approve omega-3 fatty acids [fish oil] for the prevention of cardiovascular outcomes.[46]

An additional consideration regarding fish oil supplements is that they are highly processed, requiring ultra-high heat and chemical treatment to remove impurities, making fish oil highly adulterated with impaired functionality. Therefore, the processing negatively impacts the bioavailability and functionality of the components in fish oil. Nevertheless, even if unadulterated (if obtainable), fish oil supplementation for the general population is worthless at best and physiologically harmful at worst.

Tissue Ratio of Omega-6:Omega-3

Plasma lipids have a preponderance of parent omega-6. What about tissue? The answer is that tissue has a high predominance of parent omega-6 compared to omega-3 (11:1 conservatively).

Ratio of Tissue Composition			
Tissue	Percentage of Total Body Weight	Omega-6 PEO	Omega-3 PEO
Brain/Nervous System	3	100	1
Skin	4	1000	1
Organs and Other Tissues	9	4	1
Adipose Tissue (bodyfat)	**15-35**	**22**	**1**
Muscles	**50**	**6.5**	**1**

Reference: Spector, A.A., "Plasma Free Fatty Acids and Lipoproteins as Sources of Polyunsaturated Fatty Acid for the Brain," Journal of Molecular Neuroscience, Vol. 16, 2001, pages 159-165., "Most of the plasma free fatty acid (EFA) is derived from the triglycerides stored in the adipose tissue [bodyfat]." Note: Organs, including the brain use these EFAs for structural incorporation. "Metabolism of essential fatty acids by human epidermal enzyme preparations: evidence of chain elongation, "R.S. Chapkin, et. at., Journal of Lipid Research, Volume 27, pages 954-959, 1986, Markides, M., et al., "Fatty acid composition of brain, retina, and erythrocytes in breast- and formula-fed infants," The American Journal of Clinical Nutrition, 1994;60:189-94 and Agneta Anderson, et. al., American Journal of Endocrinological Metabolism, 279: E744-E751.

Figure 5. Omega-6/Omega-3 Ratio of Different Tissues

As can be seen, physiologically, we require at least a preponderance of 11 parts of parent omega-6 for each part of parent omega-3.

A major problem is that the majority of parent omega-6 in foods is adulterated by food processors to create long shelf life. Food processors cannot have cereal or bagels smelling like spoiled fish. Without the processing to stop the oxygen transfer, they would. At least half of all ingested omega-6-containing foods are adulterated. Therefore, we require lots of fully functional, unadulterated parent omega-6 added to our diets in the form of nutritional supplements.

Statins: A Wrong Approach

Statins do reduce the amount of LDL-C. This automatically reduces the amount of nonfunctional parent omega-6 (a positive result) from processed food that reaches cell membranes. However, statins simultaneously lower the transport of vital oxygenating functional PEOs into cells (a very bad outcome). As shown in research published in 2004, over a 24-week period in which patients were given 40 mg daily of simvastatin, mean serum parent omega-3 levels dropped 34%, and parent omega-6 levels dropped 28% – both highly significant amounts.[48]

PATHWAY SUMMARY

• **PGE1** is body's most potent anti-inflammatory.

• **Prostacyclin** is body's natural "blood thinner."*

* S. Bunting, S. Moncada, and J.R. Vane, "Prostacyclin—Thromboxane A2 Balance: Pathophysiological and Therapeutic Implications," British Medical Journal, (1983), Vol. 39, No. 3, pages 271-276.

Eicosanoids: Critical prostaglandins, etc. from parent omega-6 AND omega-3: Cell-by-cell hormone analogy (PGE1 – PGE4, etc.) - very short half-life.

Very Significant in Vascular Function

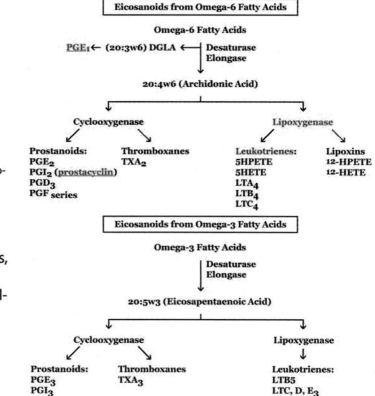

Figure 6. Eicosanoid Pathways

Note the important omega-6 pathways. PGE1 is the body's most powerful natural anti-inflammatory and prostacyclin (PGI2) is the body's natural "blood thinner," which keeps platelets separated, and stops thrombosis.

Figure 6 shows that the omega-6 series prostaglandins are more powerful than the omega-3 series prostaglandins. In the late 1980's, two significant discoveries were made. The first, was that prostaglandins are capable of limiting thrombosis.[49] The second, was that prostaglandins are capable of reversing existing thrombosis.[50] These findings are highly significant in the physiology to both reverse existing CVD and prevent patients from contracting new CVD. German physician Clause Weiss, MD, and his colleagues state: "In summary, infusion therapy with PGE1 in patients with peripheral arterial occlusive disease (PAOD) reduces thrombin formation and results in a decrease of fibrin degradation. PGE1 may thus reduce fibrin (thrombosis) deposition involved in the pathogenesis of atherosclerosis."[51] Therefore, the solution to reducing fibrin formation is adding unadulterated PEOs with a predominant LA (parent omega-6) component because they are PGE1's substrate.

It is very important to understand that PGI$_2$ production decreases significantly when blood vessels become hypoxic (decreased cellular oxygen levels).[52-55] Therefore, we need a powerful oxygenator to prevent cellular hypoxia. Fortunately, such a cellular oxygenator is available.

It is common knowledge that hypoxia is a direct cause of heart attack and stroke. By increasing consumption of fully functional parent omega-6, cellular oxygen increases. This was proven in 1976.[56] Fully functional, nonadulterated parent omega-6 in the phospholipids of the body's 100 trillion cells is the body's natural cellular oxygenator (if you have enough) – being utilized as substrates in both the cyclooxygenase and lipoxygenase pathways.

A Seminal Discovery: Oxidized Cholesterol Carries a Poison

The physiologic pathway of oxidization of LDL-C directly causing CVD cannot be stressed enough. As mentioned previously, world-leading biochemist, Dr. Gerhard Spiteller, concludes that it is oxidized cholesterol esters that are responsible for the initial damage to endothelial cells.[27,28] These harmful products are incorporated into LDL-C in the liver and this vehicle, basically a chemical transporter, deposits them on the endothelial cell walls of the vascular system (intima), where they initiate inflammation and familiar arteriosclerotic plaques develop as a result.

The LA (parent omega-6)/esterified cholesterol pathway is highly relevant for understanding why statins have an NNT of 100 – a 99% failure rate. Statins cannot fix the oxidized LA problem. The cholesterol structure in the arterial intima can contain significant amounts of oxidized or nonfunctional parent omega-6 (esterified) attributable largely to ingestion of foods containing oxidized LA or LA that is otherwise damaged in the course of routine food processing, before any in vivo oxidation! When these precious PEOs become oxidized, oxygen transfer stops, and CVD starts.

We know that the intima consists of a single layer of endothelial cells containing significant LA, but no ALA.[29,30] Consumed, processed (nonfunctional) LA deposited in arterial intimal cell membranes leads to abnormal oxidation at the vascular injury site, thus causing injurious inflammation. (Note: In this case, abnormal oxidation involves formation of a hydroperoxide from LA.) The real culprit is in our food supply, as ubiquitous "processed foods." Masquerading as harmless, they are the evil stealth villains in the CVD drama.

EFAs and Bio-Identical PEOs – the Essential Difference

The key to CVD prevention is PEOs – in particular, fully functional parent omega-6 in the esterified cholesterol. Not distinguishing between adulterated and nonadulterated PEOs, Brown and Goldstein, two 1985 Nobel Prize winners in physiology and medicine, stated in 2001: "How does elevated plasma LDL produce the complex lesions of atherosclerosis...The answer may lie in the unsaturated fatty acids [functional, unadulterated PEOs] of the cholesteryl esters and phospholipids of which LDL is composed...LDL can undergo oxidation [in the arteries]...."[57]

Although it was a major failure to distinguish between adulterated and nonadulterated essential fatty acids (PEOs), or realize that the two types would produce very different results (disease or health), Brown and Goldstein correctly showed that cholesterol itself has nothing to do with atherosclerosis; it is just a transport vehicle of tremendous amounts of the often adulterated PEOs (LA, parent omega-6 and ALA, parent omega-3).

Cause of Thrombosis (Blood Clots): The LDL Connection

Cholesterol esters are the predominant lipid fraction in all plaque types, and intimal macrophages contain substantial amounts of cholesterol esters, which are rich in PUFAs (PEOs). (Note: The intima is composed entirely of parent omega-6 – with insignificant parent omega-3.[19]) What about these oils going rancid (peroxides) in the body, such as the literature often "reiterates"? To the contrary, PEOs help protect against oxidation (Fig. 7).

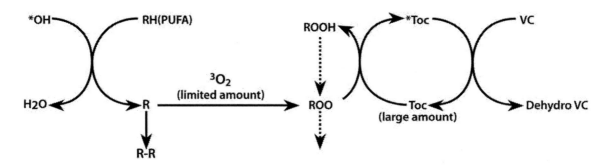

Figure 7. PEOs Act as a First Stage Scavenger of Reactive Oxygen Species In Vivo

In 2009, the American Heart Association championed a major reversal regarding omega-6 fatty acids, based on a review of the evidence.[58] "A great deal of discussion in the world of nutrition has given omega-6 fatty acids a bad reputation, which, according to the American Heart Association, is unfounded. The debate came about because one of the components of omega-6 fatty acids, called arachidonic acid, is a 'building block' for some inflammation-related molecules. This had led to concern that omega-6 consumption would lead to a greater risk of heart disease. That reflects a rather naive understanding of the biochemistry." says William S. Harris, Director of the Metabolism and Nutrition Research Center of the University of South Dakota Sanford School of Medicine and the nutritionist who led the science advisory committee that issued the report in Circulation. "Omega-6 fatty acids give rise to both pro-inflammatory compounds and anti-inflammatory compounds. To say that they are bad because they produce pro-inflammatory compounds ignores the fact that they give rise to anti-inflammatory compounds as well."[59] Years earlier, Harbige had said essentially the same thing: "Finally, the view that all n-6 PUFA are pro-inflammatory requires revision, in part, and their essential regulatory and developmental role in the immune system warrants appreciation."[60]

OXYGEN MAGNETS!

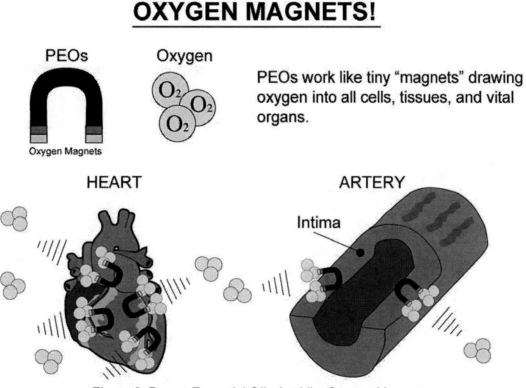

Figure 8. Parent Essential Oils Act Like Oxygen Magnets

Food processors never use omega-3 fats in frying or baking as they are far too oxygen-reactive. Most parent omega-3 in foods is, therefore, not adulterated. The problem lies exclusively in the adulterated parent omega-6 fats. This key issue needs to be properly addressed by the medical community. Because parent omega-3 oils are not processed does not mean that we don't need to understand their role in preventing CVD, as the following makes clear.

A recent cardiology journal article provides an update on the physiologic usefulness of parent omega-3. Specifically, ALA [parent omega-3] was associated with a lower risk of nonfatal acute myocardial infarction. The authors concluded: "Thus, it is possible that consumption of vegetable oils rich in α-linolenic acid could confer important cardiovascular protection in many countries where intake is low." The most significant finding was that "Fish intake was similar in cases and controls, and the variation within each group was large.... Fish or eicosapentaenoic acid [EPA] and docosahexaenoic acid [DHA] intake at the levels found in this population did not modify the observed association."[61]

It is important to note that the parent omega-3's cardio-protective result was independent of the level of fish consumption. Given all of fish oil's supposed miraculous claims, did these researchers not wonder why? However, the researchers understood that the parent omega-3 conferred benefit that the fish oil (derivatives) did not do.

There are other benefits to increased parent omega-6 (LA) consumption, such as the reduction of ventricular fibrillation (arrhythmias),[62] and for diabetic patients in terms of complications: "Erythrocyte membranes from diabetic patients show only 42% [58% *less*] of the PGE1 binding activity found in controls. These data are very important... play important roles in the long-term complications of diabetes."[63] Imagine how diabetics could be helped if more physicians, particularly endocrinologists, understood this important fact.

It is vitally important to understand that raising LA intake alone *does not* increase gamma linoleic acid (GLA), the precursor of PGE1.[64] The reason for this is likely that before widespread adulteration of cooking oils, Nature had no requirement for increasing normal physiologic rate-limited levels of PGE1. Today, that is not the case. With the widespread cooking oil adulteration, comes widespread chronic inflammation. Diabetes has become a worldwide epidemic. Unfortunately, diabetics may have impaired conversion. Therefore, any modern essential fatty acid recommendation must include gamma linoleic acid.

Don't We Get Too Much Omega-6 In Our Food?

This is true, but most, greater than 50%, is adulterated. If this were not the case, all packaged foods would quickly oxidize regardless of added antioxidants. Therefore, a substantial portion of dietary LA needs to be counted as zero because it is nonfunctional and hazardous. Some physicians wrongly think that LA promotes tumors. That conclusion is correct if the typical processed, adulterated oil is used in both human and animal studies. Furthermore, these results are often measured *in vitro* (outside the body), leading to the misunderstanding, whereas *in vivo* experiments are required.[41]

What PEO Ratio is Best?

What PEO ratio is best? A balanced physiologic blend of PEOs that allows the body to make derivatives as needed. Organic flax oil is fine for parent omega-3, but offers little parent omega-6. High linoleic (not high oleic) strains of sunflower and safflower are fine for parent omega-6, although high oleic strains cannot be used because there will not be sufficient LA.

The parent omega-6/omega-3 ratio must be 2.5:1 to 1:1 in favor of parent omega-6.[65] No omega-3-based derivative fish oil is to be used, and few derivative EFAs; only a conservative amount of GLA from evening primrose oil. Note: organic evening primrose oil produces approximately 15-times more arterial outflow of the powerful anti-inflammatory PGE1 from its GLA content than borage oil.[66] Clinicians can use this new physiologic approach to best prevent cardiovascular disease in their patients regardless of patient diet or existing complications.

REFERENCES

1. Carey J. Do cholesterol drugs do any good? *Business Week*. January 17, 2008. Available at: http://www.businessweek.com/magazine/content/08_04/b4068052092994.htm. Accessed March 16, 2010.
2. Downs JR, Clearfield M, Weis S, Whitney E, Shapiro DR, Beere PA, Langendorfer A, Stein EA, Kruyer W, Gotto AM Jr. Primary prevention of acute coronary events with lovastatin in men and women with average cholesterol levels: results of AFCAPS/TexCAPS. Air Force/Texas Coronary Atherosclerosis Prevention Study. *JAMA*. 1998;279:1615-1622.
3. Kastelein JJ, Akdim F, Stroes ES, Zwinderman AH, Bots ML, Stalenhoef AF, et al; ENHANCE Investigators. Simvastatin with or without ezetimibe in familial hypercholesterolemia. *N Engl J Med*. 2008;358:1431-1443.
4. Ridker PM, Danielson E, Fonseca FA, Genest J, Gotto AM Jr, Kastelein JJ, et al; JUPITER Study Group. Rosuvastatin to prevent vascular events in men and women with elevated C-reactive protein. *N Engl J Med*. 2008;359:2195-2207.
5. Schwartz GG, Olsson AG, Ezekowitz MD, Ganz P, Oliver MF, Waters D, et al; Myocardial Ischemia Reduction with Aggressive Cholesterol Lowering (MIRACL) Study Investigators. Effects of

atorvastatin on early recurrent ischemic events in acute coronary syndromes: the MIRACL study: a randomized controlled trial. *JAMA.* 2001;285:1711-1718.

6. Nainggolan L. Largest-ever meta-analysis finds CRP is unlikely to be causal for CVD. *Heartwire* December 21, 2009. Available at: http://www.theheart.org/article/1036519.do. Accessed March 16, 2010.

7. The Emerging Risk Factors Collaboration, Kaptoge S, Di Angelantonio E, Lowe G, Pepys MB, Thompson SG, Collins R, Danesh J. C-reactive protein concentration and risk of coronary heart disease, stroke and mortality: an individual participant meta-analysis. *Lancet.* 2010;375:132-140.

8. Kuhn H, Belkner J, Wiesner R, Schewe T, Lankin VZ, Tikhaze AK. Structure elucidation of oxygenated lipids in human atherosclerotic lesions. *Eicosanoids.* 1992;5:17-22.

9. Krumholz HM, Seeman TE, Merrill SS, Mendes de Leon CF, Vaccarino V, Silverman DI, Tsukahara R, Ostfeld AM, Berkman LF. Lack of association between cholesterol and coronary heart disease mortality and morbidity and all cause mortality in persons older than 70 years. *JAMA.* 1994;272:1335-1340.

10. Colpo A. LDL Cholesterol: 'Bad' cholesterol or bad science. *J Am Phys Surg.* 2005;10:83-89.

11. Mudd JO, Borlaug BA, Johnston PV, Kral BG, Rouf R, Blumenthal RS, Kwiterovich PO Jr. Beyond low-density lipoprotein cholesterol: defining the role of low-density lipoprotein heterogeneity in coronary artery disease. *J Am Coll Cardiol.* 2007;50:1735-1741.

12. Prospective Studies Collaboration, Lewington S, Whitlock G, Clarke R, Sherliker P, Emberson J, Halsey J, *et al.* Blood cholesterol and vascular mortality by age, sex, and blood pressure: a meta-analysis of individual data from 61 prospective studies with 55,000 vascular deaths. *Lancet.* 2007;370:1829-1839.

13. Dunham W. Cholesterol seen tied to heart disease, not stroke. *Reuters.* November 29, 2007. Available at: http://www.reuters.com/article/idUSN2922862020071129 Accessed March 16, 2010.

14. Amarenco P, Steg PG. The paradox of cholesterol and stroke. *Lancet.* 2007;370:1803-1804.

15. Glantz SA. *Primer of Biostatistics.* New York, NY: McGraw-Hill; 2002.

16. Glantz SA. How to detect, correct, and prevent errors in the medical literature. *Circulation* 1980;61:1-7.

17. Zhang WB, Addis PB, Krick TP. Quantification of 5α-cholestane-3β,5,6β-triol and other cholesterol oxidation products in fast food French fried potatoes. *J Food Sci.* 1991;56:716-718.

18. Korytowski W, Bachowski GJ, Girotti AW. Photoperoxidation of cholesterol in homogenous solution, isolated membranes, and cells: comparisons of the 5α- and 6β-hydroperoxides as indicators of singlet oxygen intermediacy. *Photochem Photobiol.* 1992;56:1-8.

19. Felton CV, Crook D, Davies MJ, Oliver MF. Dietary polyunsaturated fatty acids and composition of human aortic plaques. *Arterioscler Thromb Vasc Biol.* 1994;344:1195-1196.

20. Waddington E, Sienuarine K, Puddey I, Croft K. Identification and quantification of unique fatty acid and oxidative products in human atherosclerotic plaque using high-performance liquid chromatography. *Anal Biochem.* 2001;292:234-244.

21. Guyton A, Hall J. *Textbook of Medical Physiology.* 9th ed. Philadelphia, PA: WB Saunders; 1996:872-873.

22. Bothem KM, Mayes PA. Cholesterol synthesis, transport, and excretion. In: Murray PK, Granner DK, Mayes PA, Rodwell VW, eds. *Harper's Illustrated Biochemistry.* 27th ed. New York, NY: McGraw-Hill; 2003:235.

23. Sinclair HM. Essential fatty acids in perspective. *Hum Nutrit.*1984;38C:245-260.

24. Spector A. Plasma free fatty acid and lipoproteins as sources of polyunsaturated fatty acid for the brain. *J Mol Neurosci.* 2001;16:159-165.

25. Watkins, PA, Hamilton JA, Leaf A, Spector AA, Moore SA, Anderson RE, Moser HW, Noetzel MJ, Katz R. Brain uptake and utilization of fatty acids: Applications to peroxisomal biogenesis diseases. *J Mol Neurosci.* 2001;16:87-92.

26. Peskin BS. *The essential cardiologist: A new look at cholesterol, cancer, clogged arteries and EFAs.* Houston, TX: Pinnacle Press; 2008:26-27.

27. Spiteller G. Is atherosclerosis a multifactorial disease or is it induced by a sequence of lipid peroxidation reactions. *Ann N Y Acad Sci.* 2005;1043:355-366.

28. Spiteller G. Peroxyl radicals: Inductors of neurodegenerative and other inflammatory diseases. Their origin and how they transform cholesterol, phospholipids, plasmalogens, polyunsaturated fatty acids, sugars, and proteins into deleterious products. *Free Radical Biol Med.* 2006;41:362-87.

29. Chapkin RS, Ziboh VA, Marcelo CL, Voorhees JJ. Metabolism of essential fatty acids by human epidermal enzyme preparations: evidence of chain elongation. *J Lipid Res.* 1986;27:945-954.
30. Andersson A, Sjödin A, Hedman A, Olsson R, Vessby B. Fatty acid profile of skeletal muscle phospholipids in trained and untrained young men. *Am J Physiol Endocrinol Metab.* 2000;279:E744-E751.
31. Peskin BS. *The Hidden Story of Cancer.* Houston, TX: Pinnacle Press; 2009:255-258.
32. Salem N, Lin Y, Brenna JT, Pawlosky RJ. Alpha-linolenic acid conversion revisited. PUFA Newsletter, December 2003. Available at: http://www.fatsoflife.com/article.php?nid=1&edition =arch&id=162&issueid=31. Accessed January 12, 2010.
33. Pawlosky RJ, Hibbeln JR, Novotny JA, Salem N Jr. Physiological compartmental analysis of alpha-linolenic acid metabolism in adult humans. *J Lipid Res.* 2001;42:1257-1265.
34. Goyens PL, Spilker ME, Zock PL, Katan MB, Mensink RP. Conversion of alpha-linolenic acid in humans is influenced by the absolute amounts of alpha-linolenic acid and linoleic acid in the diet and not by their ratio. *Am J Clin Nutr.* 2006;84:44-53.
35. Hussein N, Ah-Sing E, Wilkinson P, Leach C, Griffin BA, Millward DJ. Long-chain conversion of [13C]linoleic acid and alpha-linolenic acid in response to marked changes in their dietary intake in men. *J Lipid Res.* 2005;46:269-280.
36. Barceló-Coblijn G, Murphy EJ, Othman R, Moghadasian MH, Kashour T, Friel JK. Flaxseed oil and fish-oil capsule consumption alters human red blood cell n-3 fatty acid composition: a multiple-dosing trial comparing 2 sources of n-3 fatty acid. *Am J Clin Nutr.* 2008;88:801-809.
37. Demmelmair H, Iser B, Rauh-Pfeiffer A, Koletzko B. Comparison of bolus versus fractionated oral applications of [13C]-linoleic acid in humans. *Eur J Clin Invest.* 1999;29:603-609.
38. Angerer P, Kothny W, Störk S, von Schacky C. Effect of dietary supplementation with omega-3 fatty acids on progression of atherosclerosis in carotid arteries. *Cardiovasc Res.* 2002;54:183-190.
39. Burr ML, Ashfield-Watt PA, Dunstan FD, Fehily AM, Breay P, Ashton T, Zotos PC, Haboubi NA, Elwood PC. Lack of benefit of dietary advice to men with angina: results of a controlled trial. *Eur J Clin Nutr.* 2003;57:193-200.
40. Calder P. Omega-3 polyunsaturated fatty acids, inflammation and immunity. *World Rev Nutr Diet.* 2001;88:109-116.
41. Mori T, Beilin LJ. Omega-3 fatty acids and inflammation. *Curr Atheroscler Rep.* 2004;6:461-467.
42. Bourre JM, Bonneil M, Dumont O, Piciotti M, Nalbone G, Lafont H. High dietary fish oil alters the brain polyunsaturated fatty acid composition. *Biochim Biophys Acta.* 1988;960:458-461.
43. Bourre JM, Bonneil M, Dumont O, Piciotti M, Calaf R, Portugal H, Nalbone G, Lafont H. Effect of increasing amounts of dietary fish oil on brain and liver fatty composition. *Biochim Biophys Acta.* 1990;1043:149-152.
44. Carlson SE, Salem Jr N. Essentiality of omega 3 fatty acids in growth and development of infants. In: Simopoulos AP, Kifer RR, Martin RE, Barlow S, eds. *Health effects of omega-3 polyunsaturated fatty acids in sea foods.* Basel, Switzerland: Karger; 1991:74-86.
45. Stacpoole PW, Alig J, Ammon L, Crockett SE. Dose-response effects of dietary marine oil on carbohydrate and lipid metabolism in normal subjects and patients with hypertriglyceridemia. *Metabolism.* 1989;38:946-956.
46. Nair GM, Connolly SJ. Should patients with cardiovascular disease take fish oil? CMAJ. 2008;178:181-182.
47. GISSI-Prevenzione Investigators. Dietary supplementation with n-3 polyunsaturated fatty acids and vitamin E after myocardial infarction: results of the GISSI-Prevenzione trial. *Lancet.* 1999;354:447-455.
48. Harris JI, Hibbeln JR, Mackey RH, Muldoon MF. Statin treatment alters serum n-3 and n-6 fatty acids in hypercholesterolemic patients. *Prostaglandins Leukot Essent Fatty Acids.* 2004;71:263-269.
49. Witt W, Muller B. Antithrombotic profile of iloprost in experimental models of *in vivo* platelet aggregation and thrombosis. *Adv Prostaglandin Thromboxane Leukot Res.* 1987;17A:279-284.
50. Müller B, Krais T, Stürzebecher S, Witt W, Schillinger E, Baldus B. Potential therapeutic mechanisms of stable prostacyclin (PGI2)-mimetics in severe peripheral vascular disease. *Biochim Biophys Acta.* 1988;47:S40-44.
51. Weiss C, Regele S, Velich T, Bärtsch P, Weiss T. Hemostasis and fibrinolysis in patients with intermittent claudication: effects of prostaglandin E1. *Prostaglandins Leukot Essent Fatty Acids.* 2000;63:271-277.

52. Bertele V, Cerletti C, de Gaetano G. Pathophysiology of critical leg ischaemia and mode of action of prostaglandins. *Agents Actions Suppl.* 1992;37:18-26.

53. Siegel, G., Schnalke F, Rückborn K, Müller J, Hetzer R. Role of prostacyclin in normal and arteriosclerotic human coronary arteries during hypoxia. *Agents Actions Suppl.* 1992;37:320-332.

54. Guichardant M, Michel M, Borel C, Fay L, Magnolato D, Finot PA. Effects of 9, 12, 15-octadecatrien-6-ynoic acid on the metabolism of arachidonic acid in platelets and on the platelet aggregation. *Thromb Res.* 1992;65:687-698.

55. Schrör K, Woditsch I. Endogenous prostacyclin preserves myocardial function and endothelial-derived nitric oxide formation in myocardial ischemia. *Agents Actions Suppl.* 1992;37:312-319.

56. Campbell I.M., Crozier D.N., Caton R.B. Abnormal fatty acid composition and impaired oxygen supply in cystic fibrosis patients. *Pediatrics.* 1976;57:480-486.

57. Goldstein JL, Brown MS. Molecular medicine. The cholesterol quartet. *Science.* 2001;292:1310-1312.

58. Harris WS, Mozaffarian D, Rimm E, Kris-Etherton P, Rudel LL, Appel LJ, Engler MM, Engler MB, Sacks F. Omega-6 fatty acids and risk for cardiovascular disease: a science advisory from the American Heart Association Nutrition Subcommittee of the Council on Nutrition, Physical Activity, and Metabolism; Council on Cardiovascular Nursing; and Council on Epidemiology and Prevention. *Circulation.* 2009;119:902-907.

59. WorldHealth. Concern about omega-6 fatty acids leading to greater heart disease unfounded. Available at: http://www.worldhealth.net/news/concern_about_omega-6_fatty_acids_leadin/. Accessed January 15, 2010.

60. Harbige LS. Fatty acids, the immune response, and autoimmunity: a question of n-6 essentiality and the balance between n-6 and n-3. *Lipids.* 2003;38:323-341.

61. Campos H, Baylin A, Willett WC. Alpha-linolenic acid and risk of nonfatal acute myocardial infarction, *Circulation.* 2008;118:339-345.

62. Riemersma RA, Sargent CA, Saman S, Rebergen SA, Abraham R. Dietary fatty acids and ischemic arrhythmias. *Lancet.* 1988;2:285-286.

63. Horrobin DF. *Omega-6 essential fatty acids: Pathophysiology and roles in clinical medicine.* New York, NY: Wiley-Liss;1990:510.

64. Manku MS, Morse-Fisher N, Horrobin DF. Changes in human plasma essential fatty acid levels as a result of administration of linoleic acid and gamma-linolenic acid. *Eur J Clin Nutr.* 1988;42:55-60.

65. Peskin BS. *The scientific calculation of the optimum PEO Ratio.* Houston, TX: Pinnacle Press, 2008.

66. Horrobin DF. Omega-6 essential fatty acids: Pathophysiology and roles in clinical medicine. New York: Wiley-Liss;1990:44-45.

ABOUT THE AUTHOR

Internationally published in peer-reviewed medical journals, Professor Brian Peskin presents a uniquely penetrating and compelling approach to medicine. He earned his Bachelor of Science degree in Electrical Engineering from Massachusetts Institute of Technology (MIT) in 1979, and is chief research scientist at the Cambridge International Institute for Medical Science (www.CambridgeMedScience.org).

Chapter 31
Laser Assisted Lipolysis

Agnieszka Protasewicz M.D., Ph.D.
Specialist in Orthopedics and Traumatology, Hand Surgeon,
Laser Lipolysis Physician, Poznań, Poland

ABSTRACT

Overweight and obesity are defined as abnormal or excessive fat accumulation that may impair health. Overweight and obesity lead to serious health consequences. The WHO projections indicate that at least one in three of the world's adult population is overweight and almost one in 10 is obese. Overweight is also a serious aesthetic problem. Laser-assisted lipolysis is a technique for the removal of excess fatty tissue in those areas that are usually resistant to diet and physical exercise.

268 patients with 482 areas were treated with laser lipolysis-NdYag laser. 3-4 months postoperatively 55% (n=148) patients were very satisfied with the treatment result, 36% (n=98) patients were satisfied, and 8% (n=22) were unsatisfied.

The laser beam caused lipolysis with reduced bleeding, swelling, and bruising. Furthermore, its effect on collagen tone promotes collagen retraction and skin tightening, thus avoiding the looseness that occurs with traditional liposuction.

This procedure can be used for treating areas that are typically unsuitable for traditional liposuction, or would need follow up procedures to tighten and lift the skin that was left as a result of liposuction. Laser-assisted lipolysis is the technique of choice for delicate body sculpturing not only in the submental region, but also for the treatment of gynecomastia, the abdominal region, flanks, and hips, and for smoothing asymmetry after liposuction.

Laser-assisted lipolysis is a precise method, and its advantages include: excellent patient tolerance, quick recovery time, and skin tightening. Furthermore, it is safer and less traumatic than conventional liposuction.

Keywords: laser lipolysis, laser-assisted liposuction, liposculpture, tumescent anesthesia

INTRODUCTION

Anti-aging medicine is a medical speciality founded on the application of advanced scientific and medical technologies for the early detection, prevention, treatment, and reversal of age-related dysfunction, disorders, and diseases.[1] The field of aesthetic and cosmetic dermatology, and anti aging medicine has gained remarkable interest all over the world. The main aim is to live a longer and healthier life.[1]

Overweight and obesity are defined as abnormal or excessive fat accumulation that may impair health.[2] Body mass index (BMI) is a simple index of weight-for-height that is commonly used in classifying overweight and obesity in adult populations and individuals. It is defined as the weight in kilograms divided by the square of the height in meters (kg/m^2).[2] BMI provides the most useful population-level measure of overweight and obesity as it is the same for both sexes and for all ages of adults. However, it should be considered as a rough guide because it may not correspond to the same degree of fatness in different individuals.[2]

Overweight is defined as a BMI equal to or more than 25, and obesity as a BMI equal to or more than 30 according to the and WHO.[2] There is evidence that risk of chronic disease in populations increases progressively from a BMI of 21.[2]

The WHO projections indicate that at least one in three of the world's adult population is overweight and almost one in 10 is obese. Additionally there are over 20 million children under age five who are overweight.[2] WHO's latest projections indicate that globally in 2005 approximately 1.6 billion adults (age 15+) were overweight, and at least 400 million adults were obese. WHO further projects that by 2015, approximately 2.3 billion adults will be overweight and more than 700 million will be obese.[2] Researchers at the Johns Hopkins Bloomberg School of Public Health, the Agency for Healthcare Research and Quality, and the University of Pennsylvania School of Medicine suggests that 86% of Americans could be overweight or obese by 2030, with related healthcare spending projected to be as much as $956.9 billion.[3]

Overweight and obesity lead to serious health consequences. Risk increases progressively as BMI increases. Obesity is the second leading cause of preventable deaths.[4] Annually, obesity causes at least 300,000 excess deaths in the United States. Raised body mass index is a major risk factor for chronic diseases such as: cardiovascular disease (killing 17 million people each year),[2] diabetes 2 type, gout, hypertension, musculoskeletal disorders (i.e. osteoarthritis), some cancers (endometrial, breast, and colon), hypercholesterolemia, gallbladder disease, and impaired respiratory function.[2,5] Overweight is also a serious aesthetic, social, and emotional problem.

THE IDEALS OF BEAUTY. IDEAL PROPORTIONS

In Greek mythology, Paris was called to judge who of three goddesses, Aphrodite, Hera, and Pallas Athene, was the fairest after Eris, the goddess of strife and discord, appeared at the wedding of Thetis and Peleus, and threw a golden apple inscribed 'for the prettiest one'. Each of the three goddesses attempted to bribe Paris to choose her. Hera offered him wealth and power, Athene offered honour and glory, and Aphrodite promised that Helen of Sparta (the most beautiful woman on earth) would become his wife. Paris chose Aphrodite. Paris then went on to abduct Helen from her husband Menelaus, the king of Sparta, an act that was the cause of the Trojan War.

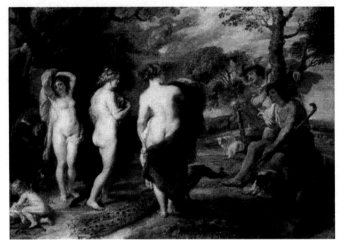

Figure 1. Judgement of Paris, Peter Paul Rubens c. 1636, National Gallery, London.

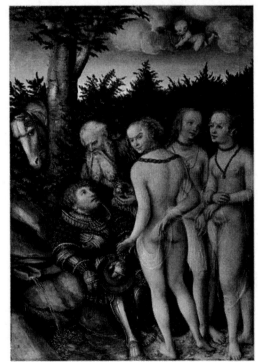

Figure 2. The Judgment of Paris Lucas Cranach the Elder(1537-40),
Royal Collection, London.

Plato the philosopher wrote: "The three wishes of every man: to be healthy, to be rich by honest means, and to be beautiful." Thus it can be seen that beauty has been an important value since ancient times. However, it is difficult to establish a universal definition of human beauty and ideal proportions as ideas of beauty have changed from era to era, and vary from culture to culture.

It is difficult to describe what is ideal beauty. Being slim has not always been synonymous with beauty. Fatness has been considered beautiful in many periods and cultures – mainly because it was a symbol of fertility or wealth (access to food). in many periods and cultures.

Leonardo da Vinci was well known for his anatomical studies and descriptions of human body proportions, however a description of ideal body proportions does not exist. Two people can be of the same weight and height, but look completely different, and one will be described as beautiful, whilst the other will not.

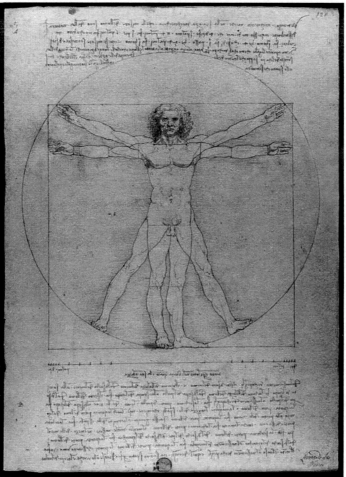

Figure 3. Leonardo da Vinci's journal, Vitruvian Man, 1492. The drawing and text are called the Canon of Proportions. Leonardo based his drawing on some hints at correlations of ideal human proportions with geometry in Book III of the Treatise De Architectura by the ancient Roman architect Vitruvius.

Today, being fat is not fashionable. Everybody wants to be slim and fit, body, and being overweight is connected with many diseases and shows our carelelessness of our health. Because today being slim is a symbol of being healthy. anti-aging therapy and cosmetic surgery became more popular for both sexes. People take care abot their health and appearance.

LIPOSUCTION

Liposuction continues to be one of the most popular procedures performed in cosmetic surgery.[6-8] According to the American Society of Aesthetic Plastic Surgeons (ASPS) the number of liposuction procedures performed in the United States was 245,000 in 2008.[9]

The purpose of liposuction (lipoplasty, fat modeling, liposculpture, or suction) is to improve the shape of the body. Some fat deposits are due to heredity, and can't be remove by exercise or dieting. It is a form of body contouring with significant attendant risks and is not a method for general weight reduction. The amount of fat removed varies by doctor, method, and patient.

History of the Traditional Techniques

Techniques for body contouring and removal of fat date back to Charles Dujarier in France, who in 1926 performed one of the first procedures (he removed subcutaneous fat using a uterine curette on a dancer's calve and knee), unfortunatelly the procedure was complicated with gangrene infection that required amputation of the operated leg.[10]

The field of modern liposuction began with the technique and instruments of Arpad and Giorgio Fischer. A technique of lipectomy for moderate degree of fatty deposition (using a blunt hollow cannula equipped with suction) was described in 1976 by Fischer. In 1978, Kesselring and Meyer published results and modifications of the technique using sharp curettage aided by suction, but this technique was not widely accepted,[11-13] and by Illouz in 1978.[14,15] Dr. Yves Gerard Illouz and Dr. Pierre-Francois Fournier started to perform liposuction using the "Illouz Method" in Paris in 1982. The "Illouz Method" featured a technique of suction-assisted lipolysis after infusing fluid (a solution of hypotonic saline and hyaluronidase) prior to aspiration into tissues using blunt cannulas and high-vacuum suction.[14,17] Illouz is considered to be the father of liposuction, and was responsible for creating worldwide publicity for the new procedure. This technique started to be used worldwide, with the first case in the United States being performed in 1982 by Martin, a Los Angeles Otolaryngologist. In 1983, Fournier described syringe liposuction.[18-20]

Liposuction was originally performed under general anasthaesia. In 1985, Klein performed liposuction in local anesthesia and then together with Lillis described the "tumescent technique" – a technique involving infiltration of a dilute solution of lidocaine with epinephrine to allow more extensive liposuction totally by local anesthesia – which significantly reduced bleeding.[21,22] The tumescent technique for local anesthesia improved the safety of large-volume liposuction (≥1500 ml of fat) by virtually eliminating surgical blood loss. It also reduced related postoperative morbidity. The common complications of hematoma and seroma formation became uncommon. Klein also described the safety of using high doses of lignocaine, he confirmed that when tumescent liposuction was performed after infiltration of 0.05% lidocaine and 1:1,000,000 epinephrine, dosages of up to 35 mg of lidocaine per kilogram of body weight were safe and effective.[21-23] In 1993 Klein started using microcannulas and multiple incisions for cannula access, he also described the way to improved postoperative care by wearing compression garments.[24-26] In 1996 Ostad *et al* published an article in which they suggest that tumescent anesthesia with a total lidocaine dose of up to 55 mg/kg is safe for use in liposuction.[27] The rate of infusion of the tumescent anesthesia was shown to be independent of plasma lidocaine levels. The tumescent technique has been the key to the safety and accuracy of modern liposuction, and has been recognized throughout the world for its importance.

In 1993, Zocchi introduced the idea of liquefying fat using ultrasonic energy to facilitate fat aspiration, this technique was also described by Lawrence and Cox as ultrasound assisted liposuction.[28]

In 1994, the use of cannulas which vibrate with great frequency, thus breaking and releasing fat cells, whilst sucking out the fat at the same time was described. The source of these vibrations are gracile pneumatic or electromotoric systems. The power assisted liposuction method and equipment was described by Flynn.[29]

LASER-ASSISTED LIPOLYSIS

To improve results, minimize risk, optimize patient comfort, and reduce the recovery period the next method for body contouring that has been developed is laser-assisted lipolysis. The use of a laser for dissolving fat was first described in 1992.[30] Technologies involving the use of laser tipped probes that induce thermal lipolysis were introduced in 1999.

The technique interstitial laser-lipolysis allows for reducing localized adipose tissue without the need to aspirate the fat, because the effect of the laser destroys the cell membrane of the fat cell. When very small areas are treated it is possible to perform the procedure without suction as the body will remove the dissolved fat by natural metabolism. At present laser assisted liposuction is used practically on all body parts with subcutaneous fat excesses.

Cellulite is another very common cosmetic complaint. During the past decades numerous treatments have been recommended for cellulite but only recently a more critical scientific approach has led to improvements in the treatment of this common and disfiguring condition. The major approaches are: skin loosening with techniques such as subcision, skin tightening with radio frequency and other approaches, and improving circulation in blood and lymphatic microvasculature using both physical treatments and pharmacotherapy. Laser-assisted lipolysis is another effective tool in body sculpturing.

Equipment and Laser Specifications

Laser-assisted lipolysis (laser lipoplasty, LipoLaser, SmartLipo) system is a FDA-approved method of removing localized areas of fat with the added benefit of skin tightening.[6-8,31-33] Photomechanical action by heating and rupturing cell membranes of adipocytes disrupts the fat which one can be easily aspired.[6,31,32] Many different varieties of laser lipolysis are available, using different wavelengths of light, and some using a continuous beam while others use a pulsed beam.[34-44]

Table 1 compares the major lipolysis laser body contouring workstations on the market today.[34-44]

Table 1. Comparison of Lipolysis Lasers.

Comparison of Lipolysis Lasers								
Wavelength	Laser type	Brand name	Manufacturer	Power Output (max)	Pulse Width (µsec)	Frequency – Maximum Rep Rate (Hz)	Delivery-fibers (µm)	Aiming Beam
924nm / 975nm	Diode Laser	Slimlipo41	Palomar	30	Continous 100	100		Diode 635nm
980 nm	Diode Laser	Lipotherme38	osyris	25	Continuous sr pulsed 0.1 at 25 seconds		600	Diode 3mW @ 635nm
980 nm	Diode Laser	Lipocontrol36	osyris	25	Continuous sr pulsed 0.1 at 25 seconds		600	Diode 3mW @ 645nm
1064 nm	Nd:Yag	Smart Lipo43	Deka	10	150	40	300	HeNe laser 1 mW @ 632.8 nm
1064 nm	Nd:Yag	Lipolite37	syneron	12	100-800	50	550	Diode 3mW @ 635nm
1064 nm	Nd:Yag	Smart Lipo42	Cynosure	6 / 12 / 18	150 / 200 / 250	40	300 SmartSense	Diode 3mW @ 635nm
1064nm / 1320nm	Nd:Yag	Smart LipoMPX44	cynosure	20 / 12	150 / 212	40 / 40	600 SmartSense	Diode 3mW @ 635nm
1064nm / 1320nm	Nd:Yag	Prolipo39	Sciton	25 (20-US)	100	50	600 1000	
1064nm / 1320nm / 980 nm	Nd:Yag / Diode Laser	Prolipoplus40	Sciton	40 / 40 / 40	150	150	600 1000	
1320nm	Nd:Yag	Coollipo35	cooltouch	15	100	50	200 320 500 CoolBlueDuet	
1444nm	Nd:Yag	Accu Sculpt34	Lutronic					

Mechanism of Action

The mechanism of action of the laser to adipose tissue may be seen on histological findings. Laser interaction with fatty tissue is achieved by the absorption of the laser energy by the receptive chromophores, which produce the heat that leads to thermal damage.[31] This damage is caused by the liberation of heat and alteration of sodium and potassium ions levels, which permits water migration into the cells until they rupture (free transport of extracellular liquid to the intracellular atmosphere).[6,7,31-33,45] Low laser energy (irradiated with 1000 J) causes reversible changes to the adipocytes known as tumefaction.[31,32] Whereas irreversible effects arise in areas receiving 3000 J, as this amount of energy causes cell membrane rupture and cytoplasmatic retraction.[6,7,31,32] The degree of tumefaction and lysis varies proportionally with the energy accumulated by the target tissue.[31] Laser energy provokes cellular death through coagulative necrosis, dependent upon time and temperature.[31] In histological findings we can also see coagulation of small vessels, microcirculation thrombosis, and reduction of bleeding.[6,7,31-33] In subdermal tissue, we notice rupture of the bands, coagulation of collagen fibers, and liberation of retracted skin and collagen tissue remodeling.[6,7,31,32] Liquefactive necrosis, or cellular lysis, is the final result of thermal damage to irradiated adipose tissue.[31] Ichikawa conducted histological evaluation in subjects treated with laser lipolysis. Scanning electron microscopy after irradiation showed greater destruction of human adipocytes than in the control, and degenerated cell membrane, vaporization, liquefaction, carbonization, and heat-coagulated collagen fibers were observed.[33]

Indications, Contraindications, and Preoperative Evaluatons

Laser-assisted lipolysis can only be performed after proper selection of the patients.[6,7,31] Selection criteria of the patients and indications for this method of treatment are similar to those for traditional liposuction: relatively healthy patient – within Class 1 or 2, and rarely 3 according to ASA classification (see Table 2),[46,47] with good physical condition (within 30% of ideal weight), localized area of lipodystrophy resistant to diet and exercise, capacity of the skin to the retraction, and patient and doctor understanding procedure limits.[6,7,21,23,24,31,48-52]

Table 2. ASA Physical Status (PS) Classification System.

The American Society of Anesthesiologists (ASA) Physical Status (PS) Classification System[46]	
ASA PS Category	Preoperative Health Status Comments, Examples
ASA PS 1	Normal healthy patient
ASA PS 2	Patients with mild systemic disease No functional limitations
ASA PS 3	Patients with severe systemic disease Some functional limitation
ASA PS 4	Patients with severe systemic disease that is a constant threat to life
ASA PS 5	Moribund patients who are not expected to survive without the operation Not expected to survive > 24 hours without surgery; imminent risk of death
ASA PS 6	A declared brain-dead patient who organs are being removed for donor purposes

Laser-assisted lypolysis is good for the treatment small areas of current moderate flaccidity[8,32] and areas with potential flaccidity, secondary treatment in areas with irregularities and/or fibrosis, "difficult" cases, so-called forbidden areas such as the upper abdomen, small areas with minimal excess of fat (e.g. peri umbilical fat),[7,8] the submental area,[8] and gynecomastia.[6,7] Almost every part of the human body can be treated using this method, however in my clinical experience, the majority of treatments are performed on the abdomen and face area.

It is important to note that laser-assisted lipolysis is not a substitute for conventional liposuction, it is a complementary method that can be used alone or in combination with conventional, ultrasound, or vibroliposuction.[8,32] It is indicated in cases when conventional liposuction is contraindicated, restricted, or will provide unwanted flaccidity,[8,31,32] and in areas in which liposuction has already been performed and which require additional sculpting.[6-8]

Like classical liposuction, laser-assisted lipolysis has also been found to be useful for non-cosmetic indications, such as hyperhidrosis of axillae[53] and lipomas.[54]

Table 3. Amount And Location of Body Areas Treated with Laser Assisted Liposuction

Author Clinical Case Study – Localisation of Treated Areas		
Location of the area treated with laser lipolysis	Number of treated areas	% treated areas
lower abdomen	93	19,6
upper abdomen	79	.16,4
chins	51	10,6
cheeks	44	9,1
outer thighs	41	8,5
love handles	39	8,1
inner thighs	34	7,1
banana fold	26	5,4
knees	22	4,6
arms	16	3,3
flanks	12	2,5
irregularities after the liposuction	7	1,5
calves	5	1
buttocks	4	0,8
ankles	4	0,8
gynecomastia	3	0,6
lipomas	2	0,4
Total	482	100
Author experience: Between 05.2007-10.2007 and 04.2008-06.2009 this technique was performed on 268 patients 221 women (82%) and 47 men (189%). 482 areas were treated. The average age was 39.6 with a range 20-68. Nd-YAG laser using wavelength of 1064nm, energy of 150 milijoules mJ, a frequency of 40Hz, and potency of 6-10W (DEKA Italy) was used. Energy was delivered via fiber optic 300 μm through a cannula. This laser also features a helium-neon (He-Ne) red aiming beam.		

Every potential patient must undergo pre-operative assessment to determine their general medical condition.[6,7] Contraindications, possible side effects, complications, and benefits must also be discussed. Preoperative evaluation involves: medical history, physical evaluation, and laboratory evaluation (liver panel, complete blood cell count with differential, INR thromboplastin and prothrombin panel, and cholesterol panel). The list of contraindications covers: systemic illness (cardiovascular, or respiratory disease, and patients with epilepsy may need to obtain a medical certificate from their general practitioner or cardiologist), tuberculosis, heart problems or failure, diabetes mellitus, uncontrolled collagen vascular disease (e.g. lupus), immunocompromised patients, pregnant or breastfeeding women, liver disease and impaired liver function (hepatitis B, hepatitis C, alcoholic liver disease – this is because fat tissue is partially eliminated via the kidney and liver, and also because patients with liver disease have a risk of developing lidocaine toxicity (lidocaine is metabolized by P450 cytochrome)), impaired kidney function, active thrombophlebitis or history of thrombophlebitis, active infection, history of pulmonary embolism or blood clots in the lungs, history of severe or multiple allergic reactions or intolerance to or problems with anesthesia, history of uncontrolled bleeding and / or poor wound healing, history of acute infections within 3 months prior to the procedure, steroids within past month, and aspirin / anticoagulant use in the past 2 weeks.

Another contraindication is unreal expectations of the patient – laser-assisted lipolysis is not a treatment for weight reduction, it is only for improvement of shape.

After consultation, every patient must sign a consent form.[6,7] Then the patient should be weighed (to determine safe maximum volume tumescent anesthesia) and a pre-operative photograph should be taken.[6,7] The area to be treated should be marked with surgical marker pen (anatomical landmarks may not be visible after administration of tumescent anesthesia and / or if the patient changes position).

Technique

Equipment, drugs, gloves, and appropriate compressive garments all need to be checked before preparing the sterile field. It is very important to remember about safety considerations during lasing. Patients and medical staff must be equipped with appropriate protective eyewear that is approved for the wavelengths in use. Reflective objects (e.g. jewelry) must be removed from the treatment room and the patient. The laser must not be operated in the presence of flammable liquids (such as alcohol) or flammable anesthetics (such as ether – anesthesia must be approved as non-flammable). A fire extinguisher should be available during each procedure.

After preparing the sterile field tumescent anesthesia is prepared (maximum lidocaine dose in the tumescent anesthesia is calculated prior to the procedure).[21-23,28] The next step is to inject the planned incision sites with lidocaine and epinephrine. I use the infiltration technique to administer the anesthetic solution – tumescent solution with lignocaine 0,15% with epinephrine at a concentration of 1:500000 – and then wait 20 minutes[7] until I make small incisions of 2-3 mm. Other authors also describe using tumescent anesthesia,[8,32] however it is also possible to use epidural or general anesthesia.[32]

The next step is to insert a 1 mm diameter cannula with fiber optic was through the incisions.[6-8,32,33] Note: The fiber must be outside the cannula. Some types of lasers use a single-use tip attached to the hand piece when the fiber optic is used. The cannula, or tip, should be inserted to the depths necessary to reach all the layers of the fatty tissue (superficial, medium, deep) and into the deep dermis.[31,32] The motion of the cannula should be kept relatively slow (as compared with conventional liposuction) as it is necessary to deliver enough accumulated energy to achieve sufficient lipolysis, and the cannula should be moved in a criss-cross pattern.[32,33] Four to ten passes (depending on the type of the laser and the treated area) are usually applied. A He-Ne aiming beam at the fiber tip provides transcutaneous illumination, and should be visible throughout the procedure, thus allowing the surgeon to identify the target.[6-8]

The total energy deposited during the procedure is dependent on the size of the treated area and tissue resistance.[7] In areas of fibrosis, or previously treated zones, the treatment time needed is usually longer.[7] It is necessary to deliver enough accumulated energy to achieve sufficient lipolysis, and in to stimulate collagen production in the subdermal area.[32] Note: The total energy deposited should be documented. In my clinical study, the average energy deposited was 7920 J per treated area – with a range of 2500-24000 J. The skin of treated areas should feel warm to the touch.[9] Palpation is used as a clinical endpoint, with successfully treated sites becoming warm, softer, and more pliable.[8,32]

After lipolysis, liquid fat may be aspirated and removed using a 2.5mm cannula using negative pressure of around 450mmHg.[6,7,32] It is possible to use syringes, pumps, or aspirators. In my clinical experience, the average amount of removed liquefied fat is 102 cc, with a range of 5-420 cc. Note: Some surgeons choose not to aspirate liquefied fat.[8]

After lipolysis has been performed, dressings should be applied to the treated areas for 2-4 days. Compression garments should be worn for 2-3 days on the face and neck, and for 7-10 days on other areas. In some case, such as treatment of areas such as the infero-lateral part of the buttocks (banana fold), additional adhesives may need to be affixed to skin. Different surgeons recommend different time periods for which compression garments and dressings should be worn. Badin and Morales recommend that dressings should be applied for one week,[32] and that compression garments should be worn on the face and neck for 3-7 days,[8] and for up to one month on other areas.[32]

There is no requirement for activity restriction, however patients should avoid sun exposure for one month following the procedure.[32]

Lymphatic drainage should begin 7-14 days after treatment, and continue twice weekly for two months.[32] If the submental area is treated it is recommended that manual lymphatic drainage and external ultrasound should be introduced on the second day.[7] However, Goldman recommended starting drainage after one week.[6] Note: It is also recommended that lymphatic drainage is carried before the procedure.

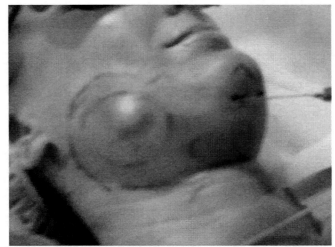

Figure. 4. Laser-assisted lipolysis of a double chin. Skin is white because it has been injected with a local anesthetic containing epinephrine to contract the blood vessels. Red light – the He-Ne beam – can be seen through the skin, thus allowing surgeon to identify the target. 1mm cannula with fiber optic is inserted underneath the skin through 2mm incision.

Results

Laser-assisted lipolysis is less traumatic than conventional liposuction.[32] It is difficult to describe the final result, however patients are usually satisfied after the procedure. Pre- and post-operative photos should be taken of the patient so that they can see the results properly. The patient should also be weighed and their BMI calculated both before and after the procedure, however improvement does not correlate with changes in body weight.[8] Kim and Geronemus tried to measure the differences in changes of fat volume using magnetic resonance imaging (MRI). Patients underwent MRI pre-procedure and at 3-month follow up, results demonstrated an average 17% reduction in fat volume, Smaller baseline volume areas had better results, for example average fat loss in the submental area was 25%.[32] The higher the total energy delivered to the tissue the higher the reduction in fat volume, thus suggesting a dose-response relationship.[32]

During my clinical study I treated 268 patients (482 areas) with laser-assisted lipolysis (NdYag laser). At follow-up 3-4 months later, 55% (n=148) patients were very satisfied with the treatment result, 36% (n=98) patient were satisfied, and 8% (n=22) were unsatisfied. Those that were unsatisfied did not have any improvement, or the result of the treatment was much smaller than they expected – 4 of them underwent additional treatment.

Apfelberg treated 51 patients, 15 were treated with laser-assisted lipolysis on one side of the treatment area and with conventional liposuction on the other side, results revealed a "slight benefit" for the laser-assisted side at both one and eight weeks for ecchymosis, pain/discomfort, and edema.[45]

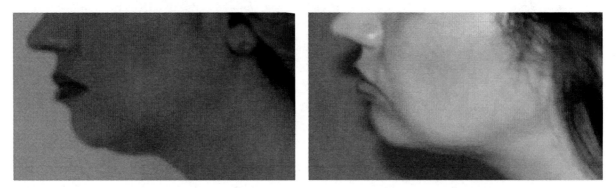

Figure 5. Preoperative submental and mandibular fat with skin flaccidity (left). Ten weeks postoperatively, good skin contour, and retraction (right). (Nd-Yag 1064nm, 6W, 40Hz, 150ms,3500J).

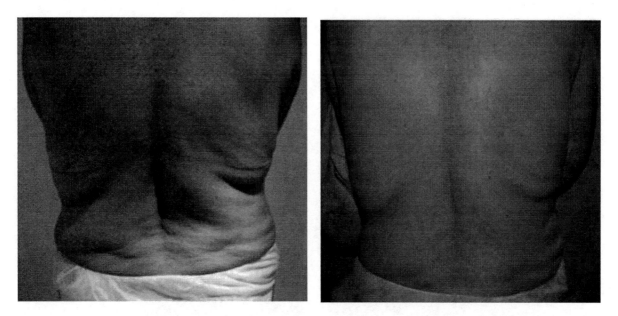

Figure 6. Patient who underwent laser-assisted liposuction of the flanks region – preoperative view (left). Postoperative view after 9 weeks (right) (Nd-Yag 1064nm, 6W, 40Hz, 150ms,2x3500J).

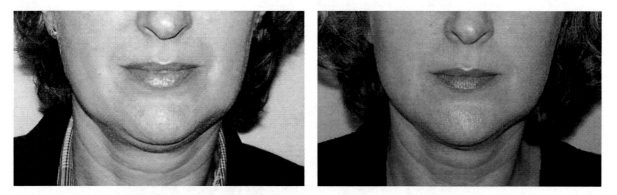

Figure 7. A Patient who underwent laser-assisted liposuction of the submental region. \
Preoperative view (left), postoperative view after 3 weeks (right). (Nd-Yag 1064nm, 6W, 40Hz, 150ms,3200J).

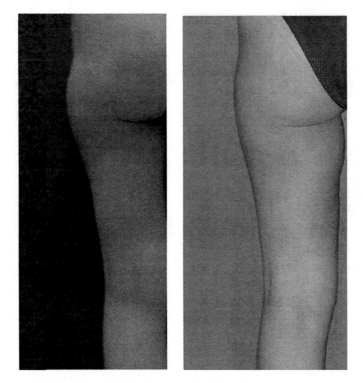

Figure 8. A Patient who underwent laser-assisted liposuction of the trochanteric and banana fold area. Preoperative view (left), postoperative view after 9 weeks (right). (Nd-Yag 1064nm, 8W, 40Hz, 150ms,6000J)

This procedure is very well tolerated by patients, and is characterized by a quick recovery time – 98% of patients return to work the day after the procedure.[6-8] According to Badin *et al*, patients are able to resume light exercise after just 7 days.[31] Other benefits include: skin tightening (skin retraction due to collagen neoformation),[7,8,33] improved local flaccidity[31] (especially at the submental area),[7] and a reduction in perioperative and postoperative bleeding.[6,7,33]

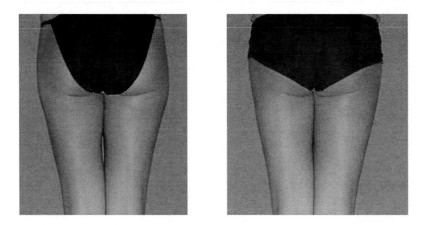

Figure 9. A Patient who underwent laser-assisted liposuction of the trochanteric and banana fold area. Preoperative view (left), postoperative view after 9 weeks (right). (Nd-Yag 1064nm, 8W, 40Hz, 150ms,5400J).

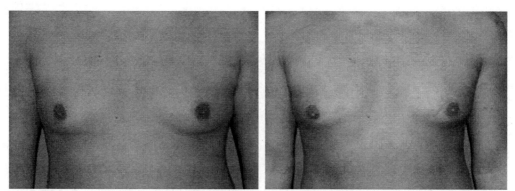

Figure 10. A Patient who underwent laser-assisted liposuction to treat gynecomastia. Preoperative view (left), postoperative view after 14 weeks (right). (Nd-Yag 1064nm, 10W, 40Hz, 150ms,2x 8200J).

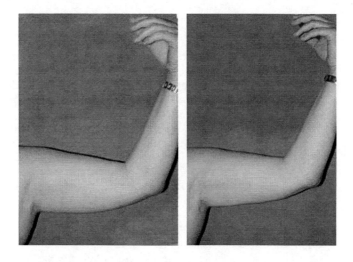

Figure 11. A Patient who underwent laser-assisted liposuction of the arms. Preoperative view (left), postoperative view after 12 weeks (right). (Nd-Yag 1064nm, 8W, 40Hz, 150ms,2x 3800J).

Complications and Side Effects

Complications and side effect are uncommon. Reported side effect and complications include: postoperative pain (minimal in the first two days, oral analgesics (e.g. acetaminophen) are required in 50% of cases), tenderness of the treated area (usually lasts 3-5 days, however tenderness persisted for as long as 4-week in 5% of cases), postoperative edema, swelling (can be minimized by using proper postoperative dressings), bleeding, bruising (postoperative ecchymosis usually disappears spontaneously within 7 days), infection (rare if proper aseptic precautions are followed), seroma, burning, scarring, pigment changes, skin contour changes, irregularities and asymmetry, pulmonary complications, allergic reaction (medication, anesthesia, or sedation), tissue hardening, numbness, asymmetry, and embolism.

Badin *et al* reported that laser-assisted lipolysis caused less swelling than conventional liposuction, and yielded good contour, even in the early postoperative period.[32] One of the problems described by Kim and Geronemus, and Badin *et al*, was under correction in early performed cases resulting from insufficient accumulated delivered energy.[8,32] Kim and Geronemus reported mild-bruising and swelling lasting 1-2 weeks, mild tingling after procedure lasting 1 month (10% of patients), hyperpigmentation (10% of cases), tenderness to palpation (20% of cases), and subcutaneous nodule which disappeared within one month (5% (n=1)).[8] Goldman described complications in less than 3% cases – 1 minor burn, 1 seroma, and 14 cases of asymmetry in total out of 1734 treated cases.[7]

Triglycerides and lipid profiles may rise postoperatively because fat is liquefied during the procedure. However, Goldman and Blugerman found no significant changes among patients treated with laser-assisted lipolysis without aspiration, 1-day, 1-week, and 1-month postprocedure.[6]

Biochemical analysis shows a higher level of triglycerides in material obtained from ultrasonically-assisted liposuction than in that obtained from the laser-assisted liposuction.[55]

During my clinical study I noticed that bruising disappeared within 5-7 days, and that swelling and edema lasted for 2-10 days postoperatively. Half of patients required painkillers after the procedure, whilst the other half did not feel any pain postoperatively. Two patients had seroma after the treatment, one of which was aspirated. Transient tissue hardening was noticed in 3 cases; however this disappeared within 6 weeks. No cases of burns were reported.

CONCLUDING REMARKS

My study showed that laser-assisted lipolysis appeared to be an effective technique for destruction of human fat tissue and improving skin tone. This procedure can be used for treating areas typically unsuitable for traditional liposuction. Laser-assisted lipolysis is the technique of choice for delicate body sculpturing not only in the submental region, but also for the treatment of gynecomastia, the abdominal region, flanks, and hips, and for smoothing asymmetry after liposuction. It is a precise method, and its advantages include: excellent patient tolerance, quick recovery time, and skin tightening. Futhermore, it is safer and less traumatic than conventional liposuction.

REFERENCES

1. Klatz R. Definition of Anti-Aging Medicine. Available at http://www.worldhealth.net/pdf/Tips_Antiaging.PDF Accessed June 28, 2009.
2. World health Organization. Available at http://www.who.int/ Accessed June 28, 2009.
3. Wang Y, Beydoun MA, Liang L, Caballero B, Kumanyika SK. Will All Americans Become Overweight or Obese? Estimating the Progression and Cost of the US Obesity Epidemic. *Obesity* 2008;16:2323-2330. doi:10.1038/oby.2008.351
4. American Obesity Association. Obesity Fact Sheets. Available at http://www.obesity.org/information/factsheets.asp Accessed June 28, 2009.
5. National Heart, Lung, and Blood Institute. Think Tank on Enhancing Obesity Research at the National Heart, Lung, and Blood Institute, Executive Summary. Available at http://www.nhlbi.nih.gov/health/prof/heart/obesity/ob_res_exsum/ob_res_exsum.pdf Accessed June 28, 2009.
6. Goldman ASD, Blugerman G. Laser lipolysis: Liposuction using Nd:YAG laser. *Rev Soc Bras Cir Plast.* 2002;17:7-27.
7. Goldman A. Submental Nd:Yag laser-assisted liposuction. *Lasers Surg Med.* 2006;38:181-184.
8. Kim KH, Geronemus RG. Laser lipolysis using a novel 1,064 nm Nd:YAG Laser. *Dermatol Surg.* 2006;32:241-248.
9. American Society of Plastic Surgeons. Top Five Surgical Cosmetic Procedures in 2008. Available at http://www.plasticsurgery.org/Media/stats/2008-top-5-cosmetic-surgery-procedures-graph.pdf Accessed June 28, 2009.
10. Glicenstein J. [Dujarier's case]. *Ann Chir Plast Esthet.* 1989;34:290-292. [French].
11. Kesselring UK. Body contouring with suction lipectomy. *Clin Plast Surg. 1984*;11:393-408.
12. Kesselring UK. Suction curette for removal of subcutaneous fat. *Plast Reconstr Surg.* 1979;63:560.
13. Kesselring UK, Meyer R. A suction curette for removal of excessive local deposits of subcutaneous fat. *Plast Reconstr Surg.* 1978;62:305-6.
14. Illouz YG. Body contouring by lipolysis: a 5-year experience with over 3000 cases. *Plast Reconstr Surg.* 1983;72:591-597.
15. Illouz YG. Illouz's technique of body contouring by lipolysis. *Clin Plast Surg.* 1984;11:409-417.
16. Illouz YG. Surgical remodeling of the silhouette by aspiration lipolysis or selective lipectomy. *Aesthetic Plast Surg.* 1985;9:7-21.
17. Illouz YG, Pfulg ME. [Selective lipectomy and lipolysis after Illouz]. *Handchir Mikrochir Plast Chir.* 1986;18:118-121. [German].
18. Fournier PF. Reduction syringe liposculpturing. *Dermatol Clin.* 1990;8:539-551.
19. Apfelberg DB. Results of multicenter study of laser-assisted liposuction. *Clin Plast Surg.* 1996;23:713-719.
20. Mandel MA. Syringe liposculpture revisited. *Aesthetic Plast Surg.* 1993;17:199-203.
21. Klein JA. The tumescent technique. Anesthesia and modified liposuction technique. Dermatol *Clin.* 1990;8:425-437.
22. Klein JA. Tumescent technique for regional anesthesia permits lidocaine doses of 35 mg/kg for liposuction. *J Dermatol Surg Oncol.* 1990;16:248-263.

23. Klein JA. Tumescent technique for local anesthesia improves safety in large-volume liposuction. *Plast Reconstr Surg.* 1993;92:1085-1098.
24. Klein JA. Tumescent liposuction and improved postoperative care using Tumescent Liposuction Garments. *Dermatol Clin.* 1995;13:329-338.
25. Klein JA. Post-tumescent liposuction care. Open drainage and bimodal compression. *Dermatol Clin.* 1999;17:881-889.
26. Klein JA. Tumescent technique for local anesthesia. *West J Med.* 1996;164:517.
27. Ostad A, Kageyama N, Moy RL. Tumescent anesthesia with a lidocaine dose of 55 mg/kg is safe for liposuction. *Dermatol Surg.* 1996;22:921-927.
28. Lawrence N, Coleman WP 3rd. Ultrasonic-assisted liposuction. Internal and external. *Dermatol Clin.* 1999;17:761-771.
29. Flynn TC. Powered liposuction: an evaluation of currently available instrumentation. *Dermatol Surg.* 2002;28:376-382.
30. Apfelberg D. Laser-assisted liposuction may benefit surgeons, patients. *Clin Laser Mon.* 1992;10:193-194.
31. Badin AZ, Gondek LB, Garcia MJ, Valle LC, Flizikowski FB, de Noronha L. Analysis of laser lipolysis effects on human tissue samples obtained from liposuction. *Aesthetic Plast Surg.* 2005;29:281-286.
32. Badin AZ, Moraes LM, Gondek L, Chiaratti MG, Canta L. Laser lipolysis: flaccidity under control. *Aesthetic Plast Surg.* 2002;26:335-339.
33. Ichikawa K, Miyasaka M, Tanaka R, Tanino R, Mizukami K, Wakaki M. Histologic evaluation of the pulsed Nd:YAG laser for laser lipolysis. *Lasers Surg Med.* 2005;36:43-46.
34. Lutronic Inc. AccuSculpt specifications. Available at http://www.lutronic.com/en/AccuSculpt-Technology/ Accessed June 28, 2009.
35. CoolTouch Inc. CoolLipo specifications. Available at http://www.cooltouch.com/CoolLipo.aspx Accessed June 28, 2009.
36. Osyris Medical USA. Lipocontrol specifications. Available at http://www.osyrismedicalusa.com/equipment/lipocontrol.php Accessed June 28, 2009.
37. Syneron Medical Ltd. Lipolite specifications. Available at http://international.syneron.com/products/specs_lipolite Accessed June 28, 2009.
38. Osyris Medical USA. Lipotherme specifications. Available at http://www.lipotherme.com/lipo_secure/physician_login.php Accessed June 28, 2009.
39. Sciton, Inc. Prolipo specifications. Available at http://www.sciton.com/public2/products/prodProlipo/prodProlipofeatures.htm Accessed June 28, 2009.
40. Sciton, Inc. Prolipoplus specifications. Available at http://www.prolipoplus.com/ Accessed June 28, 2009.
41. Palomar Medical Technologies, Inc. SlimLipo specifications. Available at http://www.palomarmedical.com/palomar.aspx?pgID=1202 Accessed June 28, 2009.
42. Cynosure, Inc. Smartlipo specifications at Cynosure page. Available at http://www.cynosure.com/products/smartlipo/specs.php Accessed June 28, 2009.
43. DEKA. Smartlipo specifications. Available at http://www.dekalaser.com/techdata.php?type=ENG_11 Accessed June 28, 2009.
44. Cynosure, Inc. Smartlipo-MPX specifications at Cynosure page. Available at http://www.cynosure.com/products/smartlipo-mpx/specs.php Accessed June 28, 2009.
45. Apfelberg DB, Rosenthal S, Hunstad JP, Achauer B, Fodor PB. Progress report on multicenter study of laser-assisted liposuction. *Aesthetic Plast Surg.* 1994;18:259-264.
46. American Society of Anesthesiologists. Physical Status (PS) Classification System. Available at http://www.asahq.org/clinical/physicalstatus.htm Accessed June 28, 2009.
47. Lawrence NL, Leonhardt J. Liposuction. In: Robinson JK, Hanke WC, Sengelmann RD, Siegel DM, eds. *Surgery of the Skin: Procedural Dermatology.* CV Mosby, St Louis, MO; CV Mosby: 2005;13,14,517.
48. Coleman WP 3rd, Glogau RG, Klein JA, Moy RL, Narins RS, Chuang TY, Farmer ER, Lewis CW, Lowery BJ; American Academy of Dermatology Guidelines/Outcomes Committee. Guidelines of care for liposuction. *J Am Acad Dermatol.* 2001;45:438-447.
49. Flynn TC, Narins RS. Preoperative evaluation of the liposuction patient. *Dermatol Clin.* 1999;17:729-734.
50. Klein J. Two standards of care for tumescent liposuction. *Dermatol Surg.* 1997;23:1194-1195.
51. Lawrence N, Coleman WP 3rd. Liposuction. *Adv Dermatol.* 1996;11:19-49.
52. Lawrence N, Coleman WP. *Liposuction* 2002;47:105-108.

53. Lillis PJ, Coleman WP. Liposuction for treatment of axillary hyperhidrosis. *Dermatol Clin.* 1990;8:479-482.
54. Pinski KS, Roenigk HH. Liposuction of lipomas. *Dermatol Clin.* 1990;8:483-492.
55. Grippaudo FR, Matarese RM, Macone A, Mazzocchi M, Scuderi N. Effects of traditional and ultrasonic liposuction on adipose tissue: a biochemical approach. *Plast Reconstr Surg.* 2000;106:197-199.

ABOUT THE AUTHOR

Dr. Agnieszka Protasewicz began her work as a hand surgeon in 2002. Dr. Protasewicz earned her medical degree *cum laude* from the University of Medical Sciences in Poznan. She presented her Ph.D thesis in 2006 (in the field of hand surgery) and obtained certification as a specialist in orthopedics and traumatology in 2009. Dr. Protasewicz is one of the most experienced clinicians in laser-assisted lipolysis in Poland, and she provides training and consultancy for other doctors who use laser-assisted lipolysis for fat reduction. Dr. Protasewicz holds the position of aesthetic medicine doctor in private practice. Areas of interest include botulinum toxin and filler injections, laser-assisted lipolysis, anti-aging, hand surgery, and microsurgery.

Chapter 32

Melatonin and Vitamin D

Ron Rothenberg, M.D.
Clinical Professor, Preventive & Family Medicine,
University of California, School of Medicine (San Diego, CA USA);
Founder, California HealthSpan Institute (Encinitas, CA USA)

ABSTRACT

This paper is concerned with melatonin and vitamin D. Melatonin is an important hormone and deficiency impacts sleep, the immune system, and cognitive function. This paper will explore the pathophysiology of melatonin, current scientific data on melatonin deficiency, and the use of melatonin from immune system to jet lag will be explored. Dosing options will be discussed. Vitamin D is also an important hormone. It serves to improve bone health and immune function. Vitamin D deficiency is associated with an increased risk of cancers, heart disease, diabetes, autoimmune disease, and multiple sclerosis. Treatment of vitamin D deficiency will reduce these risks significantly. This aims of this paper are to provide:
1. A basic understanding of the pathophysiology of vitamin D and melatonin.
2. Knowledge of the implications of vitamin D and melatonin deficiency.
3. Information on how to supplement vitamin D and melatonin.
4. Knowledge of the signs of toxicity of vitamin D.

MELATONIN

Melatonin is a hormone produced by the pineal gland, a small endocrine gland in the brain, which the French philosopher, mathematician, and physicist Rene Descartes described as the "seat of the soul". Melatonin has been evolutionarily conserved. Bacteria, fungi, plants, protozoa, invertebrates, vertebrates, and man all produce melatonin.

Melatonin helps life to connect to the cycles of the universe. It conveys information about day length, seasons, and even years. Melatonin production is inhibited by light and permitted by darkness. If light hits the retina, melatonin synthesis and secretion will come to a halt. This system helps the body to distinguish day from night and helps to regulate the sleep-wake cycle. Furthermore, the profile of melatonin synthesis and secretion is affected by the variable duration of night in summer as compared to winter. This change in duration of melatonin production each day serves as a seasonal clock.

In the past, humans were exposed to many hours of darkness during the long winter nights. However, since the dawn of artificial light, most people are only exposed to complete darkness for eight hours or less each day. There are also people, for example shift workers, who are virtually never exposed to complete darkness as they sleep while it is light outside and they work at night bathed in artificial light.

People who have little exposure to complete darkness have low melatonin levels. This does not simply mean that such people develop sleep problems, as low melatonin levels are associated with many diseases, including Alzheimer's disease, cardiovascular disease, insulin resistance, breast cancer, and other types of cancer. Many people think that melatonin only serves to regulate the sleep-wake cycle, however this is not the case, as melatonin is also a potent antioxidant and immune system enhancer.

Melatonin is a free radical scavenger. It is the most effective free radical scavenger of the hydroxyl radical that we are aware of, and is one of the few antioxidants capable of actually getting into the nucleus of the cell and protecting the DNA from injury – especially in pharmacologic concentrations. It is also know to protect against the pro-oxidation affects of iron.[1] In short, melatonin is the ultimate antioxidant in terms of protecting lipids, proteins, and DNA. It also:

- Stimulates the production of the antioxidant glutathione.
- Protects mitochondria.
- Protects against ischemia-reperfusion injury.[2]
- Protects against ionizing radiation.[2]
- Decreases levels of pro-inflammatory cytokines, such as tumor necrosis factor-alpha (TNFα), interleukin (IL)-6, and IL-1β.
- Decreases damage caused by beta amyloid (Aβ).[3]

Melatonin enhances immune function in a number of ways. It increases levels of CD4 cells and natural killer (NK) cells, counteracts stress-induced immunodepression, activates the cytokine system when needed, decreases levels of pro-inflammatory cytokines, and increases immune function in winter when there are more environmental stressors.[4] Melatonin also inhibits tumor growth.

Melatonin and Aging

Research has shown that melatonin lengthens lifespan and healthspan in rats[5] and mice.[6] It is likely that melatonin's apparent anti-aging action is due to its ability to quench free radicals and/or its ability to enhance the immune system.

Pierpaoli and Regelson found that administration of melatonin in drinking water to aging mice (15 months of age) prolonged their survival from 23.8 to 28.1 months, and preserved aspects of their youthful state.[6] More recently, Carretero et al conducted a study to determine if melatonin administration would reduce the brain mitochondrial impairment that accompanies aging. Brain mitochondria from male and female senescent prone mice aged 5 and 10 months of age were studied. Results showed that melatonin administration between 1 and 10 months of age completely prevented mitochondrial impairment.[7]

Melatonin may also protect against aging by reversing or preventing specific aging-associated metabolic changes. Research by Wolden-Hanson et al revealed that supplementation of melatonin in middle-aged male rats for 12-weeks decreased body weight (7%), intraabdominal adiposity (16%), and plasma insulin (25%), while increasing core body temperature (0.5°C), physical activity (19%), and morning plasma corticosterone levels (154%), thus restoring each of the parameters toward more youthful levels.[8]

Melatonin and Cancer

Melatonin exhibits a number of anti-cancer properties, it is anti-mitotic, it downregulates the activity of receptors (e.g. decreases estrogen binding to cells in breast cancer), it enhances the immune system, it scavenges free radicals, and is anti-angiogenic.

Melatonin is associated with an improved outcome in the treatment of glioblastoma, malignant melanoma, and breast cancer when used alongside chemotherapy and radiation. However, the doses used in these studies are very high (ranging from 20-700 mg/day). Lenoir et al found that it prevented chemically-induced breast cancer in rats.[9] While Mills et al conducted a review of randomized controlled trials of melatonin in solid tumor cancer patients and its effect on survival at 1-year. Results showed that melatonin significantly reduced the risk of death at 1-year. Furthermore, no severe adverse events were reported. The authors concluded: "The substantial reduction in risk of death, low adverse events reported, and low costs related to this intervention suggest great potential for melatonin in treating cancer."[10]

Melatonin and Inflammation

As mentioned earlier, melatonin decreases levels of pro-inflammatory cytokines. Li et al found that melatonin reduces colonic inflammatory injury by downregulating pro-inflammatory molecules. The authors of this study concluded that melatonin has significant anti-inflammatory properties and could be considered as a novel therapeutic alternative for the treatment of inflammatory bowel disease.[11] Melatonin has also been shown to reduce exercise-induced inflammation. Results of a study by Venereso et al showed that melatonin helped to protect against heart damage caused by acute exercise by impairing the production of inflammatory mediators and downregulating the NF-kappaB signal transduction pathway.[12]

Melatonin and Cardiovascular Disease

Melatonin exerts numerous benefits on the cardiovascular system. In fact, there is an inverse correlation between nocturnal melatonin levels and coronary artery disease.[13] Melatonin is known to preserve nitric oxide availability and has been suggested as a novel treatment for hypertension, especially nocturnal hypertension.[14] It has also been shown to attenuate tissue damage caused by ischemia and reperfusion, decrease ventricular tachycardia and ventricular fibrillation after reperfusion, prevent oxidation of LDL cholesterol, lower LDL cholesterol and raise HDL cholesterol levels, and protect cardiac myocyte mitochondria from free radical damage.

Melatonin and the Brain

Melatonin levels decrease with age, however patients with Alzheimer's disease have been found to have lower melatonin levels. As mentioned earlier, melatonin decreases the damage caused by the toxic protein beta amyloid, however it also prevents the formation of amyloid fibrils and has numerous other neuroprotective effects.[15]

There is also evidence to suggest that melatonin may be useful in the treatment of stroke and traumatic brain injury (TBI). Cervates *et al* reviewed the neuroprotective effects of melatonin in the treatment of ischemia/reperfusion brain injury. Numerous neuroprotective effects were documented, including: direct and indirect antioxidant activity; prevention and reversal of mitochondrial malfunction; reduction of inflammation; derangement of cytoskeleton organization, and pro-apoptotic cell signaling. Melatonin was shown to reduce infarct volume, necrotic and apoptotic neuronal death, and neurologic deficits, and increase the number of surviving neurons. The authors concluded: "The potential use of melatonin as a neuroprotective drug in clinical trials aimed to improve the outcome of patients suffering acute focal or global cerebral ischemia should be seriously considered."[16]

Melatonin Supplementation

No serious adverse effects are associated with melatonin supplementation. It commonly produces drowsiness, decreases sleep latency, and increases total sleep. Occasionally, it can cause paradoxical stimulation – some people may get wired instead of tired. This tends to occur in shift workers. It can also produce vivid dreams, which some people may like and others may not. Some patients complain that it can produce a "hangover", although this usually resolves after a couple of days. Finally, some people simply just do not like the way they feel after taking melatonin, whereas others feel well rested, bright eyed, and bushy tailed!

To help induce sleep, melatonin should be taken approximately 30 minutes before going to bed. It is best to start off on a very small dose, for example 0.5 mg. The dosage should be slowly increased until the desired effect is achieved (3-10 mg). It is important to be aware that less is more for some patients – some may sleep far better on 0.3 mg.

Melatonin can also be used to speed recovery from jet lag. The patient should set their watch to the time of their destination as soon as they get on the plane. They should then take 3-6 mg of melatonin on the airplane at the time of bedtime at their destination. It is important that they expose themselves to bright light in the AM after arrival. Finally, 3-6 mg melatonin should be taken before bedtime at their destination.

VITAMIN D

The two major forms of vitamin D are vitamin D3 (cholecalciferol) and vitamin D2 (ergocalciferol). If you wish to take vitamin D supplements, you should take vitamin D3 as it is the most bioavailable and efficacious form available. Vitamin D2 is the form of vitamin D found in food; however vitamin D2 is present in only a handful of foods (oily fish, eggs, and fortified foods) in very small amounts and it is very unlikely that adequate amounts could be obtained from the diet. Both vitamin D3 and vitamin D2 are previtamins, and are thus biologically inert. In order to convert them into calcitriol (1,25 dihydroxy vitamin D3, 1,25-dihydroxycholecalciferol, $1,25(OH)_2D$), the active form of vitamin D, they must undergo two hydroxylation reactions. Laboratory testing to determine vitamin D levels measures the serum level of calcidiol (25-hydroxy vitamin D3, $25(OH)D3$, $25(OH)D$, 25 hydroxy cholecalciferol). It is important to note that vitamin D is not technically a vitamin. Calcitriol has a similar structure to a steroid hormone; however it is actually a secosteroid hormone

You will find that vitamin D is referred to in terms of International Units (IU), micrograms (mcg), milligrams (mg), nanograms per milliliter (ng/mL), and occasionally nanomoles per liter (nmol/L). How do these measurements relate to each other?

- 1 IU = 0.025 mcg
- 1 mcg = 40 IU
- 1 mg = 40,000 IU

Nmol/L divided by 2.49 equals ng/mL, and 100 IU vitamin D3 per day will raise calcidiol levels by 1 ng/mL. Vitamin D deficiency is defined as a blood serum level of < 20 ng/mL 25(OH)D, while vitamin D insufficiency is < 32 ng/mL. The reference range for serum calcidiol used by most laboratories is 32-100 ng/mL. The optimal range is a subject of some controversy; however I would aim for 60-80 ng/mL.

As mentioned above, food is a poor source of vitamin D. The body obtains the vast majority of vitamin D from the sun. Vitamin D3 is produced photochemically when UVB radiation in sunlight reacts with the zoosterol 7-dehydrocholesterol, which is present in the skin. The previtamin vitamin D3 is then sent to the liver, where it is converted to calcidiol. The calcidiol then follows one of two pathways (Fig. 1). First and foremost, calcidiol is sent on to the kidney and converted into calcitriol, which is then used to maintain serum calcium levels. If there is any calcidiol left over, it is sent to various other tissues to bestow its beneficial effects. Indeed, we know that calcidiol is converted to calcitriol in many different cells and tissues (prostate, colon, breast, lung, monocytes, and macrophages). In these cells and tissues its function is to regulate cell growth, immune function, and gene expression.

In the past it was thought that vitamin D's only function was calcium regulation. However, we now know that that is not the case. Calcitriol targets more than 1000 genes and vitamin D receptors (VDR) are present in every single cell in the body.

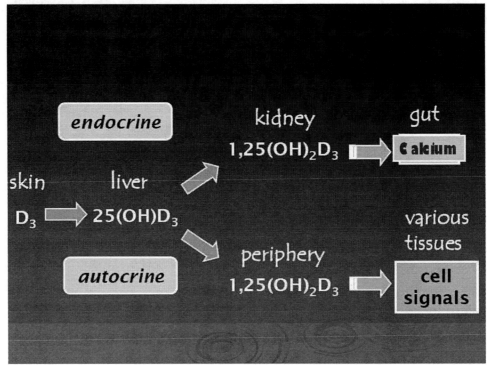

Figure 1. The Two Vitamin D Pathways

The Vitamin D Deficiency Pandemic

We are in the midst of a vitamin D deficiency pandemic. Eating a balanced diet does not provide adequate amounts of vitamin D and (for the vast majority of us) neither does spending 15 minutes in the sun each day. If you live above 35 degrees latitude, the body is unable to produce adequate amounts of vitamin D from the winter sun, and conditions in the summer are only favorable for a few hours each day. Unless you live in an equatorial country and you are able to sunbathe at noon wearing nothing but a bikini, your body will not be able to produce the vitamin D it needs from 15 minutes of exposure to the sun. Indeed, the notion that most people living in the US get adequate amounts of vitamin D is far from true.

Everyone who does not get a lot of exposure to the sun or ingests at least 2000-10,000 IU per day is at high risk for skeletal and non-skeletal consequences. Research has shown that vitamin D deficiency is present among all age groups of US citizens from children to the elderly, and especially in African-Americans.[17] Studies have shown that the prevalence of calcidiol deficiency (<20 ng/mL) is approximately 36% in young adults aged 18-29,[18] 42% of African-American women aged 15-49,[19] 41% of outpatients aged 49-83,[27] and 57% of inpatients.[20] In Europe, it is believed that between 28 and 100% of healthy adults and 70-100% of hospitalized adults have deficient calcidiol levels.[21-23]

Numerous factors have limited our ability to produce vitamin D from sunlight. Our ancestors lived naked in the sun for several million years. However, 50,000 years ago, some of us migrated north to places with far less sun. Then, we put on clothes, started working indoors, and began to live in cities where buildings block out the sun. To make matters worse, we started traveling in cars instead of walking or riding horses, and the glass windows in the cars further reduced our exposure to UVB radiation. Finally, we started to put on sunblock and actively avoid exposing our skin to sunlight in an attempt to prevent skin cancer. However, many sunblocks only screen out UVB radiation and UVB radiation does not cause melanoma – UVA radiation is the cause of melanoma. Other factors that reduce the body's ability to produce vitamin D include skin pigmentation, body fat, age (a 70-year-old can produce only a quarter of what a 20-year-old can), and drugs (anticonvulsants, corticosteroids, rifampin). All of these factors have helped to steadily reduce tissue levels of the most potent steroid hormone in our bodies, one that has powerful anti-cancer properties – vitamin D.

The really significant reductions in sunlight exposure have occurred since the Industrial Revolution. It is no coincidence that diseases like cardiovascular disease, diabetes, and cancer also became prominent at this point in history. Vitamin D deficiency is associated with heart disease, autoimmune disease, type I and II diabetes, depression, chronic pain, osteoarthritis, osteoporosis, rickets, muscle weakness, periodontal disease, infectious disease, and at least 17 types of cancer.

Benefits Associated with Vitamin D

Disease Incidence Prevention by Serum 25(OH)D Level

Serum 25(OH)D, ng/ml	6	8	10	12	14	16	18	20	22	24	26	28	30	32	34	36	38	40	42	44	46	48	50	52	54	56	58
Studies of Individuals																											
Cancers, all combined																		35%									
Breast Cancer											30%												83%				
Ovarian Cancer															12%						17%						
Colon Cancer														31%	38%				60%								
Non-Hodgkins Lymphoma														12%			18%										
Type 1 Diabetes													25%												66%		
Fractures, all combined																25%			50%								
Falls, women								72%																			
Multiple Sclerosis																			33%					46%		54%	
Heart Attack (Men)															30%												
Natural Experiments																											
Kidney Cancer															23%								49%				
Endometrial Cancer																						37%					
Rickets	50%						99%																				

**All percentages reference a common baseline of 25 ng/ml as shown on the chart.
References:
All Cancers: Lappe JM, et al. Am J Clin Nutr. 2007;85:1586-91. Breast: Garland CF, Gorham ED, Mohr SB, Grant WB, Garland FC. Breast cancer risk according to serum 25-Hydroxyvitamin D: Meta-analysis of Dose-Response (abstract).American Association for Cancer Research Annual Meeting, 2008. Reference serum 25(OH)D was 5 ng/ml. Garland, CF, et al. Amer Assoc Cancer Research Annual Mtg, April 2008,. Colon: Gorham ED, et al. Am J Prev Med. 2007;32:210-6. Diabetes: Hyppönen E, et al. Lancet 2001;358:1500-3. Endometrium: Mohr SB, et al. Prev Med. 2007;45:323-4. Falls: Broe KE, et al. J Am Geriatr Soc. 2007;55:234-9. Fractures: Bischoff-Ferrari HA, et al. JAMA. 2005;293:2257-64. Heart Attack: Giovannucci et al. Arch Intern Med/Vol 168 (No 11) June 9, 2008. Multiple Sclerosis: Munger KL, et al. JAMA. 2006;296:2832-8. Non-Hodgkin's Lymphoma: Purdue MP, et al. Cancer Causes Control. 2007;18:989-99. Ovary: Tworoger SS, et al. Cancer Epidemiol Biomarkers Prev. 2007;16:783-8. Renal: Mohr SB, et al. Int J Cancer. 2006;119:2705-9. Rickets: Arnaud SB, et al. Pediatrics. 1976 Feb;57(2):221-5.

Figure 2. Disease Incidence Prevention by Serum 25(OH)D (Calcidiol) Level

Research has shown that the incidence of many diseases could be dramatically reduced by increasing serum calcidiol levels, and by looking at Figure 2, it is easy to see why vitamin D has become of great interest in the last few years. Research shows that:

- Increasing serum calcidiol levels to 35 ng/mL could prevent 30% of myocardial infarctions in men[24] and reduce the risk of fracture in elderly people by 50%.[24]
- Increasing serum calcidiol levels to approximately 40 ng/mL could reduce the risk of cancer in postmenopausal women by 35%[26] and reduce the risk of falls in elderly people by 50%.[27]

- Increasing serum calcidiol levels to 50 ng/mL could reduce the incidence of breast cancer by as much as 80%,[28] multiple sclerosis by as much as 60%,[29] and type I diabetes by up to 50%.[30]

Why is vitamin D so beneficial? There is no clear answer at present. However, anything that has such wide-ranging benefits has to possess the ability to modulate inflammation. Indeed, studies have shown that vitamin D inhibits nuclear factor-κβ (NF-κβ)[31] – a protein that plays a key role in the inflammatory response and in the proliferation of cancer cells. It has also been shown to lower levels of the inflammatory marker CRP.[32]

Vitamin D and Cancer

Vitamin D has direct inhibitory action on the initiation and progression of various cancers. Calcitriol has been shown to have anti-proliferative, apoptotic, and anti-angiogenic properties. Cedric and Frank Garland conducted the first ecological study of cancer and solar UVB way back in 1980.[33] Their results showed that colon cancer rates were lowest in the sunniest parts of the United States, and they hypothesized that vitamin D was responsible. Figures 3 and 4 show cancer mortality rates in the United States, as can be seen the highest cancer mortality rates tend to be in the high-latitude states (with the exception of stomach cancer). Thus, suggesting that there is indeed a relationship between cancer and latitude.

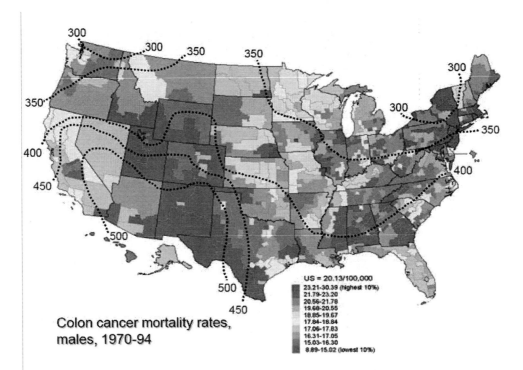

Figure 3. Relationship Between Latitude and Colon Cancer Mortality Rates in Men

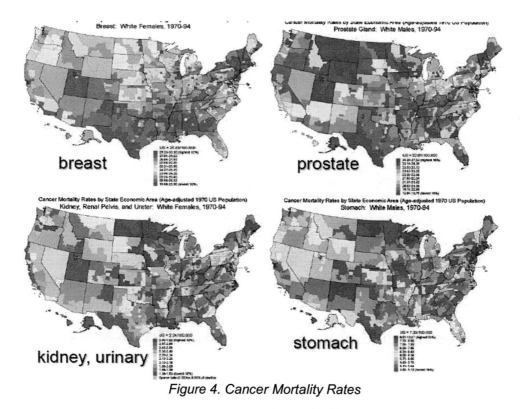

Figure 4. Cancer Mortality Rates

Giovannucci *et al* developed a vitamin D index based on vitamin D from oral intake and UVB production. They found significant inverse correlations with vitamin D and colon, esophageal, oral, pancreatic, and rectal cancer, and leukemia. Insignificant inverse correlations were found for bladder, gastric, lung, prostate, and renal cancers. Results also showed that each increment of 25 nmol/L in predicted 25(OH)D level was associated with a 17% reduction in total cancer incidence and a 29% reduction in total cancer mortality. They also estimated that male cancer deaths could be reduced by 29% with vitamin D supplementation of 1500 IU/day.[34]

Vitamin D and Cardiovascular Disease

Martin *et al* examined the association between 25(OH)D serum levels and cardiovascular disease risk factors. Results showed that hypertension, diabetes mellitus, obesity, and high serum triglyceride levels were significantly higher in those with the lowest 25(OH)D serum levels.[35] Wang *et al* studied the relationship between serum levels of 25(OH)D and cardiovascular disease. Results showed that people with a serum 25(OH)D level of <10 ng/mL were 80% more likely to develop cardiovascular disease than those with a serum 25(OH)D level of >15 ng/mL.[36] Meanwhile, Dobnig *et al* found that people with a blood serum 25(OH)D level of 17.8 ng/mL had a significantly increased risk of cardiovascular and all-cause mortality. They concluded: "Based on the findings of this study, a serum 25(OH)D level of 20 ng/mL or higher may be advised for maintaining general health."[37]

Vitamin D Supplementation and Toxicity

The idea that extreme care must be taken with vitamin D supplementation in order to avoid toxicity is totally unfounded. Maalouf *et al* conducted a study to assess the safety of vitamin D supplementation in school children aged 10-17. The children received 1400 IU/week, 14,000 IU/week, or placebo. Results showed that calcidiol levels increased from 15 to 19 ng/ml in those supplemented with 1400 IU/week and from 15 to 36 ng/mL in those supplemented with 14,000 IU/week. No toxicity was observed in either supplementation group.[38] Kimball *et al* gave 12 patients in an active phase of multiple sclerosis progressively increasing doses of vitamin D3: from 28,000 to 280,000 IU/week. The results showed that patients' serum calcidiol concentrations reached twice the top of the physiologic range without eliciting hypercalcemia or hypercalciuria, leading the authors to conclude: "The data support the feasibility of pharmacologic doses of vitamin D3 for clinical research, and they provide objective evidence that vitamin D intake beyond the current upper limit is safe by a large margin."[39] In conclusion, there have been numerous studies on vitamin D toxicity and no toxicity has been seen in doses lower than 30,000 IU/day (200 ng/mL). An excess of vitamin D causes hypercalcemia, however all known cases of vitamin D toxicity with hypercalcemia have involved intakes of 40,000 IU or more per day.

According to Bischoff-Ferrari, serum levels for 25(OH)D should be at least 75 nmol/L (30 ng/ml) for general health, while a desirable 25(OH)D level for cancer prevention is 90-120 nmol/L (36-48 ng/mL).[40]

I believe that 25(OH)D should be kept at the top of the reference range (60-80 ng/mL). No toxicity has been observed at levels of less than 150 ng/mL, even so it is a good idea to regularly check serum calcium levels to eliminate any worries concerning hypercalcemia. To achieve optimal vitamin D levels, a daily dose of 5000-15000 IU of D3 is recommended, however a weekly dose is OK. It is important to take sun exposure into consideration and to adjust the dose if necessary.

REFERENCES

1. Herrera J, Nava M, Romero F, Rodríguez-Iturbe B. Melatonin prevents oxidative stress resulting from iron and erythropoietin administration. Am J Kidney Dis. 2001;37:750-757.
2. Reiter RJ, Tan DX, Gitto E, Sainz RM, Mayo JC, Leon J, Manchester LC, Vijayalaxmi, Kilic E, Kilic U. Pharmacological utility of melatonin in reducing oxidative cellular and molecular damage. Pol J Pharmacol. 2004;56:159-170.
3. Rosales-Corral S, Tan DX, Reiter RJ, Valdivia-Velázquez M, Martínez-Barboza G, Acosta-Martínez JP, Ortiz GG. Orally administered melatonin reduces oxidative stress and proinflammatory cytokines induced by amyloid-beta peptide in rat brain: a comparative, in vivo study versus vitamin C and E. J Pineal Res. 2003;35:80-84.
4. Nelson RJ, Drazen DL. Melatonin mediates seasonal changes in immune function. Ann N Y Acad Sci. 2000;917:404-415.
5. Dilman VM, Anisimov VN, Ostroumova MN, Khavinson VK, Morozov VG. Increase in lifespan of rats following polypeptide pineal extract treatment. Exp Pathol (Jena). 1979;17:539-545.
6. Pierpaoli W, Regelson W. Pineal control of aging: effect of melatonin and pineal grafting on aging mice. Proc Natl Acad Sci U S A. 1994;91:787-791.
7. Carretero M, Escames G, López LC, Venegas C, Dayoub JC, García L, Acuña-Castroviejo D. Long-term melatonin administration protects brain mitochondria from aging. J Pineal Res. 2009;47:192-200.
8. Wolden-Hanson T, Mitton DR, McCants RL, Yellon SM, Wilkinson CW, Matsumoto AM, Rasmussen DD. Daily melatonin administration to middle-aged male rats suppresses body weight, intraabdominal adiposity, and plasma leptin and insulin independent of food intake and total body fat. Endocrinology. 2000;141:487-497.
9. Lenoir V, de Jonage-Canonico MB, Perrin MH, Martin A, Scholler R, Kerdelhué B. Preventive and curative effect of melatonin on mammary carcinogenesis induced by dimethylbenz[a]anthracene in the female Sprague-Dawley rat. Breast Cancer Res. 2005;7:R470-476.
10. Mills E, Wu P, Seely D, Guyatt G. Melatonin in the treatment of cancer: a systematic review of randomized controlled trials and meta-analysis. J Pineal Res. 2005;39:360-366.
11. Li JH, Yu JP, Yu HG, Xu XM, Yu LL, Liu J, Luo HS. Melatonin reduces inflammatory injury through inhibiting NF-kappaB activation in rats with colitis. Mediarots Inflamm. 2005;Aug:185-193.
12. Veneroso C, Tuñón MJ, González-Gallego J, Collado PS. Melatonin reduces cardiac inflammatory injury induced by acute exercise. J Pineal Res. 2009;47:184-191.
13. Dominguez-Rodriguez A, Garcia-Gonzalez M, Abreu-Gonzalez P, Ferrer J, Kaski JC. Relation of nocturnal melatonin levels to C-reactive protein concentration in patients with ST-segment elevation myocardial infarction. Am J Cardiol. 2006;97:10-12.
14. Simko F, Pechanova O. Potential roles of melatonin and chronotherapy among the new trends in hypertension treatment. J Pineal Res. 2009;47:127-133.
15. Wang JZ, Wang ZF. Role of melatonin in Alzheimer-like neurodegeneration. Acta Pharmacol Sin. 2006;27:127-133.
16. Cervantes M, Moralí G, Letechipía-Vallejo G. Melatonin and ischemia-reperfusion injury of the brain. Pineal Res. 2008;45:1-7.
17. Holick MF. High prevalence of vitamin D inadequacy and implications for health. *Mayo Clin Proc.* 2006;81:353-373.

18. Tangpricha V, Pearce EN, Chen TC, Holick MF. Vitamin D insufficiency among free-living healthy young adults. *Am J Med.* 2002;112:659-662.
19. Nesby-O'Dell S, Scanlon KS, Cogswell ME, Gillespie C, Hollis BW, Looker AC, Allen C, Doughertly C, Gunter EW, Bowman BA. Hypovitaminosis D prevalence and determinants among African American and white women of reproductive age: third National Health and Nutrition Examination Survey, 1988-1994. *Am J Clin Nutr.* 2002;76:187-192.
20. Malabanan A, Veronikis IE, Holick MF. Redefining vitamin D insufficiency [letter]. *Lancet.* 1998;351:805-806.
21. Thomas MK, Lloyd-Jones DM, Thadhani RI, Shaw AC, Deraska DJ, Kitch BT, Vamvakas EC, Dick IM, Prince RL, Finkelstein JS. Hypovitaminosis D in medical inpatients. *N Engl J Med.* 1998;338:777-783.
22. McKenna MJ. Differences in vitamin D status between countries in young adults and the elderly. *Am J Med.* 1992;93:69-77.
23. Isaia G, Giorgino R, Rini GB, Bevilacqua M, Maugeri D, Adami S. Prevalence of hypovitaminosis D in elderly women in Italy: clinical consequences and risk factors. *Osteoporos Int.* 2003;14:577-582.
24. Giovannucci E, Liu Y, Hollis BW, Rimm EB. 25-hydroxyvitamin D and risk of myocardial infarction in men: a prospective study. *Arch Intern Med.* 2008;168:1174-80.
25. Bischoff-Ferrari HA, Willett WC, Wong JB, Giovannucci E, Dietrich T, Dawson-Hughes B. Fracture prevention with vitamin D supplementation: a meta-analysis of randomized controlled trials. *JAMA.* 2005;293:2257-2264.
26. Lappe JM, Travers-Gustafson D, Davies KM, Recker RR, Heaney RP. Vitamin D and calcium supplementation reduces cancer risk: results of a randomized trial. *Am J Clin Nutr.* 2007;85:1586-1591.
27. Broe KE, Chen TC, Weinberg J, Bischoff-Ferrari HA, Holick MF, Kiel DP. A higher dose of vitamin d reduces the risk of falls in nursing home residents: a randomized, multiple-dose study. *J Am Geriatr Soc.* 2007;55:234-239.
28. Garland CF, Gorham ED, Mohr SB, Grant WB, Garland FC. Breast cancer risk according to serum s5-hydroxyvitamin D: Meta-analysis of dose-response. Presented at: American Association for Cancer Research Annual Meeting; April 12-16, 2008; San Diego, California.
29. Munger KL, Levin LI, Hollis BW, Howard NS, Ascherio A. Serum 25-hydroxyvitamin D levels and risk of multiple sclerosis. *JAMA.* 2006;296:2832-2838.
30. Hyppönen E, Läärä E, Reunanen A, Järvelin MR, Virtanen SM. Intake of vitamin D and risk of type 1 diabetes: a birth-cohort study. *Lancet.* 2001;358:1500-1503.
31. Szeto FL, Sun J, Kong J, Duan Y, Liao A, Madara JL, Li YC. Involvement of the vitamin D receptor in the regulation of NF-kappaB activity in fibroblasts. *J Steroid Biochem Mol Biol.* 2007;103:563-566.
32. Boxer RS, Dauser DA, Walsh SJ, Hager WD, Kenny AM. The association between vitamin D and inflammation with the 6-minute walk and frailty in patients with heart failure. *J Am Geriatr Soc.* 2008;56:454-461.
33. Garland CF, Garland FC. Do sunlight and vitamin D reduce the likelihood of colon cancer? *Int J Epidemiol.* 1980;9:227-231.
34. Giovannucci E, Liu Y, Rimm EB, Hollis BW, Fuchs CS, Stampfer MJ, Willett WC. Prospective study of predictors of vitamin D status and cancer incidence and mortality in men. *J Natl Cancer Inst.* 2006;98:451-459.
35. Martins D, Wolf M, Pan D, Zadshir A, Tareen N, Thadhani R, Felsenfeld A, Levine B, Mehrotra R, Norris K. Prevalence of cardiovascular risk factors and the serum levels of 25-hydroxyvitamin D in the United States: data from the Third National Health and Nutrition Examination Survey. *Arch Intern Med.* 2007;167:1159-1165.
36. Wang TJ, Pencina MJ, Booth SL, Jacques PF, Ingelsson E, Lanier K, Benjamin EJ, D'Agostino RB, Wolf M, Vasan RS. Vitamin D deficiency and risk of cardiovascular disease. *Circulation.* 2008;117:503-511.
37. Dobnig H, Pilz S, Scharnagl H, Renner W, Seelhorst U, Wellnitz B, Kinkeldei J, Boehm BO, Weihrauch G, Maerz W. Independent association of low serum 25-hydroxyvitamin d and 1,25-dihydroxyvitamin d levels with all-cause and cardiovascular mortality. *Arch Intern Med.* 2008;168:1340-1349.

38. Maalouf J, Nabulsi M, Vieth R, Kimball S, El-Rassi R, Mahfoud Z, El-Hajj Fuleihan G. Short- and long-term safety of weekly high-dose vitamin D3 supplementation in school children. *J Clin Endocrinol Metab.* 2008;93:2693-2701.
39. Kimball SM, Ursell MR, O'Connor P, Vieth R. Safety of vitamin D3 in adults with multiple sclerosis. *Am J Clin Nutr.* 2007;86:645-651.
40. Bischoff-Ferrari HA. Optimal serum 25-hydroxyvitamin D levels for multiple health outcomes. Adv Exp Med Biol. 2008;624:55-71.

ABOUT THE AUTHOR

As a pioneer in the field of Anti-Aging Medicine, Dr. Ronald Rothenberg was one of the first physicians to be recognized for his expertise to become fully board certified in the specialty. Dr. Rothenberg founded the Calfornia HealthSpan Institute in Encinitas, Califonia in 1997 with a commitment to transforming our understanding of and finding treatment for aging as a disease. Dr. Rothenberg is dedicated to the belief that the process of aging can be slowed, stopped, or even reserved through existing medical and scientific interventions. Challenging traditional medicine's approach to treating the symptoms of aging, California HealthSpan's mission is to create a paradigm shift in the way we view medicine: treat the cause. He received his MD from Columbia University, College of Physicians and Surgeons in 1970. Dr. Rothenberg performed his residency at Los Angeles County-USC Medical Center and is also board certified in Emergency Medicine. He received academic appointment to the USCD School of Medicine Clinical Faculty in 1997 and was promoted to full Clinical Professor of Preventive and Family Medicine in 1989. In addition to his work in the field of Anti-Aging Medicine, Dr. Rothenberg is an Attending Physician and Director of Medical Education at Scripps Memorial Hospital in Encinitas, California. Dr. Rothenberg travels extensively to lecture on a variety of topics, which include Anti-Aging Medicine and Emergency Medicine and is the author of Forever Ageless. He has recently been featured in the University of California MD TV series in the shows on Anti-Aging Medicine.

Chapter 33
Biochemical Foundations for Longevity
C. Norman Shealy, M.D., Ph.D.
Professor of Energy Medicine, Holos University Graduate Seminary
(www.holosuniversity.org)

ABSTRACT

Although there are hundreds of essential neurochemicals and hormones, there are three that appear to be most critical – DHEA, calcitonin, and malondialdehyde (the byproduct of free radical damage). Over the past decade, I have found four techniques for rejuvenating the body's natural production of DHEA:

- Giga frequency stimulation of 12 specific acupuncture points
- Transdermal magnesium lotion
- Natural progesterone cream
- A combination of vitamin C and MSM

Each of these raises DHEA by an average of 60% individually, and all 4 raise DHEA an average of 250% over baseline. Since exogenous DHEA administration has potential risks of flaring indolent hormonal-based cancers, the restoration of the body's ability to make DHEA is potentially much safer. Individuals with a naturally high level of DHEA are virtually immune to developing cancer.

Calcitonin is the major hormone responsible for maintenance of skeletal strength and osteoporosis is one of the leading causes of death in the elderly. Giga frequency stimulation of 13 specific acupuncture increases calcitonin levels naturally and safely.

Free radicals are the destructive contributors to aging and degeneration. Although antioxidants are tremendously useful in protecting the body, there is little evidence of total decrease in free radical production except with 10 servings of fruits or vegetables daily – the average American consumes less than 5 servings! Giga frequency stimulation of 13 specific acupuncture points reduces free radicals by an average of 85%, far greater than any other technique found in the literature.

These natural and safe approaches for rejuvenating the body's ability to make DHEA and calcitonin, and to reduce free radicals, provide a foundation for increased health and longevity.

Key Words: DHEA; calcitonin; free radicals; longevity; GigaHerz; Human DNA

INTRODUCTION

There are many thousands of chemical, neurochemical, and hormonal products produced in the human body and the balance of these is ultimately essential for life. Indeed, most illnesses are the result of imbalance of one or more of these essential indicators of a healthy metabolism. For instance, individuals who do not produce adequate cortisone will die when they have additional stress unless they have replacement cortisol. Similarly, one could argue that epinephrine, norepinephrine, sugar, insulin, ACTH, and many others are almost equally critical for optimal health. In our work over the last two decades, it appears that individuals who are able to maintain healthy levels of dehydroepiandrosterone (DHEA) and calcitonin, and keep free radical production at a minimal level, are likely to be balanced in virtually all of the other essential chemicals. In other words, stress burns out the production of DHEA long before the body decompensates by not producing adequate cortisol. Similarly, the most common cause of death in the elderly, whom may have a variety of other chemical imbalances, is a fractured hip from osteoporosis. And, of course, one of the consistent day-to-day damaging factors is excess production of free radicals.

HUMAN DNA FREQUENCY AND THE RING OF FIRE

In 1925, Georges Lakhovsky published his book, *The Secret of Life*, in France. It was not published in English until 1935 and the book is still in print. He stated that human DNA frequency is 50+ Giga Hertz (GHz). Between 1939 and 1942 he treated over 300 patients with the Lakhovsky Multiwave Oscillator at a university hospital in New York City with reports of curing many diseases. Unfortunately, he was killed in 1942 and the work was discontinued, and to my knowledge has not been repeated since then.

Meanwhile, in 1982 the Ukrainian physicists discovered that human DNA has an "eigen" (unique individual) frequency of 54 to 78 GHz. They stated that the output of the sun on the surface of the earth is 1 billionth of a watt/cm^2, and further stated that illnesses decrease the strength of DNA but not the frequency. When I visited these physicists some 15 years ago, they had applied 1 billionth of a watt/cm^2 through a 2 mm probe of random 54 to 78 GHz pulses to acupuncture points to treat many diseases. For instance, they stated that they could "cure" rheumatoid arthritis with 10 treatments. What they meant by that is that the disease would be in remission for 6 to 24 months. They reported curing peptic ulcers and indeed most diseases, including aseptic necrosis of the hip. Not having access to their equipment, I worked for several years to develop a GigaTENS unit which puts out 1 billionth of a watt/cm^2 or 75 decibels, which is the unit most often measured in the United States. This unit can be applied to specific acupuncture points, as well as used directly around areas of pain. My experiments with these frequencies began just as I was exploring methods for rejuvenation of DHEA.

RESTORING DHEA PRODUCTION
Natural Progesterone Cream
Since almost 100% of individuals have a DHEA level at age 80 of just 10% or less than what they had at age 25 or 30, it seemed important to assist individuals in rejuvenating the adrenal and/or testicular production of this critical hormone. My first research was with natural progesterone cream. I reasoned that since women almost totally lose the ability to produce progesterone when they go into menopause, it was a defect in progesterone that accelerated the loss of DHEA. In my first experiment with seven men who had low or totally deficient levels of DHEA, we asked them to use ¼ tsp. of natural progesterone cream (60 mg.) twice daily on the scrotum. Within three months, the average individual had increased DHEA production by 60%, with some individuals increasing up to 100% from their baseline. Although this is useful, it was not enough if someone started off with a DHEA of 200 ng/dl. The healthy range for DHEA at the best laboratory in the country, Nichols in Capistrano, California, is listed as 180 to 1200 ng/dl for men and 130 to 980 ng/dl for women. Incidentally, when I published my first paper on this subject, a professor of endocrinology from France wrote that there was no pathway to convert progesterone to DHEA, to which I responded, "It's a good thing my patients don't know that because they are able to do it." I was able to apply for and receive a patent on my application of progesterone to restore DHEA production.

Giga Frequency Stimulation of 12 Specific Acupuncture Points
Out of several thousand patients, I had not one patient whose DHEA level was in the upper 50% of the laboratory normal range, and half of my patients were in the totally deficient range. In searching for another method for raising DHEA, I intuitively developed a series of acupuncture points designed to activate the inherent energy of the kidneys, gonads, adrenals, thyroid, and pituitary glands, which are called the Ring of Fire. The points are:
- Kidney 3 bilaterally
- Bladder 22 bilaterally
- CV 2, 6, and 18
- Master of the Heart 6 bilaterally
- Large Intestine 18 bilaterally
- Governing Vessel 20

Just as with natural progesterone, we found that when a giga frequency stimulator was applied for 3 minutes to each of these acupuncture points, starting at Kidney 3 and working up to Governing Vessel 20, DHEA rose 30 to 100% with an average of 60% increase over baseline.

Further clinical studies with the Ring of Fire revealed that it provides excellent improvement in the following illnesses:
- Individuals suffering 1 to 4 or more migraine attacks per month had a 75% decrease in the frequency and severity of the headaches.
- 80% of individuals with diabetic neuropathy had a marked decrease in pain, 25% had some recovery of sensory loss, and 25% were able to lower their antidiabetic medication.
- 70% of individuals with rheumatoid arthritis, who had failed all conventional approaches, became essentially pain free within two weeks of stimulation of the Ring of Fire.

- 70% of individuals with depression, who had failed to respond to one or more antidepressant drugs, became free of depression.

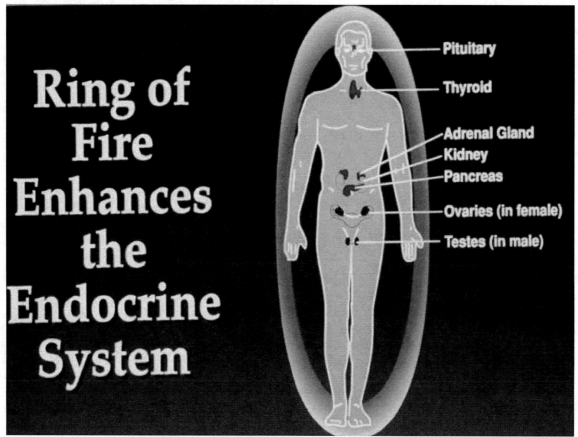

Figure 1. The Ring of Fire Acupuncture Points

A combination of vitamin C and MSM

Our next approach in attempting to restore DHEA levels was to use methylsulphonylmethane (MSM). Ten subjects were given just 1 g of MSM daily for a month, however only half of them had an increase in DHEA. When I questioned the individuals, the half who had an increase in DHEA were already taking vitamin C and the ones who did not were not taking vitamin C. So we put together a formula that I call Youth Formula, which contains 2 g of vitamin C, 1 g of MSM, 60 mcg of molybdenum, and 6 mg of beta 1,3 glucan. Each of these substances appears to enhance the body's natural ability to make DHEA, and we were able to demonstrate an average increase gain of 60% in DHEA levels with Youth Formula.

Transdermal Magnesium Lotion

Having found that 100% of my chronically depressed patients were deficient in magnesium, I had been giving them up to 10 IVs of 2 g of magnesium in a Meyer's cocktail for a number of years. Serendipitously, I found that magnesium chloride is absorbed through the skin far better than it is absorbed from the intestines. Thus, the final major DHEA rejuvenation approach has been to use transdermal magnesium chloride, although it can be used in a spray applied to the body or by soaking the feet or the body in a tub with magnesium chloride. The simplest approach is magnesium lotion, which is a 25% solution of magnesium chloride in a lotion that is easily absorbed through the skin. The use of magnesium lotion over a period of 4 to 6 weeks raises intracellular levels of magnesium back to normal and at the same time, increases DHEA significantly, an average of 60% over baseline.

Combining Techniques for a Synergistic Effect

Finally, we combined all four of these techniques and found an average increase of DHEA by 240 to 250% over baseline when all four of them are used simultaneously. Thus, these techniques work synergistically, apparently through somewhat different internal mechanisms, to restore the body's ability to make DHEA. Personally, I have been hesitant to use DHEA in most individuals because there is some evidence that taking DHEA orally can activate a dormant cancer of the prostate, uterus, ovary, or breast, probably because it does not lead to the normal "dance" between cortisol and DHEA. Ordinarily, in a stress response when cortisol is released the adrenal glands, and presumably the testicles in men, release DHEA to bring the cortisol back to normal levels. When taking DHEA orally, of course, there is no inherent balance between the two. But if the individual can produce his or her own DHEA, then this balance can be restored.

INCREASING CALCITONIN LEVELS

During the time that I was developing these other approaches, I perceived a circuit in the body that would primarily help overcome the next greatest problem, osteoporosis, and its inherent risk to the elderly. The Ring of Earth fulfills this purpose. It consists of:

- Kidney 1 bilaterally
- Bladder 54 and Bladder 60 bilaterally
- Large Intestine 16 bilaterally
- Stomach 9 bilaterally
- Small Intestine 17 bilaterally
- Governing Vessel 20

Our biochemical studies with the Ring of Earth indicated that when it was stimulated with the GigaTENS, calcitonin increased quite strikingly – an average of over 100% increase. Calcitonin, of course, is the hormone produced by the thyroid, which is responsible for maintaining adequate calcium in the skeleton itself. Calcitonin, incidentally, is also the strongest analgesic produced in the human body as it is 40 to 60 times as powerful as morphine. Individuals who have a body temperature below 98.6 during the day are relatively hypothyroid and unless their thyroid function is restored, most often by just increasing iodine intake, stimulation of the Ring of Earth will not be as effective in raising calcitonin.

REDUCING FREE RADICAL PRODUCTION

During our life from birth on, free radical production often is excessive and is one of the major underlying mechanisms for producing disease, aging, wrinkling and ultimately death. Every cell in the body is reproduced within a maximum of seven years and if each cell was reproduced into a neutral milieu relatively free of free radicals, they should be reproduced almost as in a newborn. Our next development in looking at rejuvenation and longevity was development of the Ring of Crystal. The points are:

- Spleen 4 bilaterally
- Conception Vessel 8.5
- Governing Vessel 4.5
- Conception Vessel 14.5
- Governing Vessel 7.5
- Governing Vessel 14.5
- Conception Vessel 23
- Gall Bladder 30.5 bilaterally
- Gall Bladder 11 bilaterally
- Governing Vessel 20

We found that stimulation of these thirteen points, 3 minutes per pair of points, resulted in an 85% reduction of free radicals in three days. The test we have used is measurement of malondialdehyde, which is done with the OxiData Test. It is very simple and takes only five minutes to carry out and we have repeated this in scores of individuals demonstrating the effectiveness of the Ring of Crystal.

CONCLUDING REMARKS

Looking at the American situation, the average lifespan in the US is approximately 78 years. It appears that we lose, in the country as a whole, approximately 7 years because of smoking, 7 years because of obesity, 3 or 4 years from poor nutrition, and 3 or 4 years because of lack of exercise. If individuals had avoided these unhealthy habits, the average life expectancy should increase to around 100 years of age. Purely theoretically, if we were able to restore or rejuvenate production of DHEA and calcitonin, and reduce free radical production, we might add an additional 40 years of average life. Certainly the increase in health, whether or not there is this striking increase in longevity, would be one of the most revolutionary things that could happen for the health of Americans.

In summary, we develop a peak level of DHEA at age 25. By age 80, DHEA levels are less than 10% of what they were at age 25 or 30. It appears that we can rejuvenate the body's ability to make DHEA by using GigaTENS stimulation of the Ring of Fire, natural progesterone cream, Youth Formula (a combination primarily of Vitamin C and methylsulphonylmethane), and transdermal magnesium. Stimulation of the Ring of Earth restores calcitonin production and should, over a period of decades, markedly reduce the incidence of osteoporosis and fractures. Finally, a consistent 85% reduction in free radical activity should markedly improve health and slow aging.

Considering all of these options, with good health habits, I believe that average life expectancy could be increased to 140 years, plus or minus 20 for accidents and genetics.

REFERENCES

1. Shealy CN. A review of dehydroepiandrosterone (DHEA). *Integrative Physiological and Behavioral Science.* 1995;30:308-313.
2. Shealy CN, Myss CM. The Ring of Fire and DHEA: A theory for energetic restoration of adrenal reserves. *Subtle Energies.* 1995;6:167-175.
3. Shealy CN, Borgmeyer V. Calcitonin enhancement with electrical activation of a specific acupuncture circuit. *American Journal of Pain Management.* 2003;13:29-32.
4. Shealy CN, Borgmeyer V, Thomlinson P. Reduction of free radicals by electrical stimulation of specific acupuncture points. *Subtle Energies.* 2004;13:251-259.

ABOUT THE AUTHOR

C. Norman Shealy, M.D., Ph.D. is a neurosurgeon, trained at Massachusetts General Hospital, after graduating Duke University School of Medicine. Currently he is President of Holos University Graduate Seminary (www.holosuniversity.org). In 1978, Dr. Shealy was instrumental in creating The American Holistic Medical Association, which continues to emphasize the spiritual component of healing. Dr. Shealy holds 10 patents for innovative discoveries, has published over 300 articles and 24 books.

Chapter 34
Leptin Hormone Physiology and Pathology in Obesity
Dr. Paul Ling Tai, D.P.M., FACFS, ABPS
Professor, New York College of Podiatric Medicine (New York, USA)

ABSTRACT
This paper is concerned with the obesity epidemic. The impact of obesity on health is discussed, and reasons as to why obesity is the problem it is today are considered. Particular emphasis is placed on the role of the hormone leptin in the pathology of obesity.

INTRODUCTION
The National Institutes of Health (NIH) state that as many as two-thirds of Americans are either overweight or obese. It is estimated that 77% of our children are overweight and 17% are obese – a 300% increase since 1980 – and statistics suggest that the current generation of children in America may actually have shorter life expectancies than their parents. According to an article published in *USA Today* on November 8, 2008: "The number of children who take pills for type 2 diabetes – the kind that's closely linked to obesity – more than doubled from 2002 to 2005." Facts like these, demonstrate why former US Surgeon General Dr David Satcher called obesity an "American epidemic".[1]

It is estimated that 400,000 US citizens die each year as a direct result of being overweight or obese.[2] According to Richards and Richards, people who are overweight at 40 shave 3 years off their life expectancy, while people who are obese at 40 reduce their life expectancy by 7 years, and those who are obese at 20 lose a staggering 13 years.[3]

Diseases associated with being overweight or obese include:

- Cardiovascular disease
- Hypertension
- Lung and respiratory diseases
- Renal disease
- Liver disease
- Diabetes
- Circulation failures
- Osteoarthritis
- Gastrointestinal disease
- Autoimmune disease
- Stroke
- Alzheimer's disease
- Cancer (breast, lung, pancreas, ovary, prostate, uterus)

A 30-year-long population study conducted by the National Institutes of Health investigated the short- and long-term risks of becoming overweight or obese. All participants were of normal body weight at the beginning of the study; however, by the end of the study 90% of men and 70% of women were overweight or obese.[4] The Centers for Disease Control and Prevention (CDC) estimate that at any given time 24% of men and 38% and of women are trying to lose weight.[5] As of present, effective treatment options for people who are overweight or obese are somewhat limited, expensive, and come with numerous adverse sides effects and risks.

WHY IS OBESITY THE PROBLEM IT IS TODAY?
Refined Sugars
Our modern day love of refined sugars (e.g. sucrose, fructose) may help to explain why so many people are overweight or obese. Lenoir *et al* found that when rats were allowed to choose between water sweetened with saccharin or intravenous cocaine, 94% of animals opted for the intense sweetness of saccharin. Further tests on the animals led the authors to conclude: "Our findings clearly demonstrate that intense sweetness can surpass cocaine reward, even in drug-sensitized and -addicted individuals. We

speculate that the addictive potential of intense sweetness results from an inborn hypersensitivity to sweet tastants. In most mammals, including rats and humans, sweet receptors evolved in ancestral environments poor in sugars and are thus not adapted to high concentrations of sweet tastants. The supranormal stimulation of these receptors by sugar-rich diets, such as those now widely available in modern societies, would generate a supranormal reward signal in the brain, with the potential to override self-control mechanisms and thus to lead to addiction."[6] In other words, it appears that sugar is more addictive than cocaine! This is because sugar elevates dopamine levels in the brain, which serves to intensify sugar cravings and perpetuate the addiction.

Increased Calorie Consumption

The average daily calorie intake in the US increased from 1,876 calories in 1978 to 2,043 calories by 1995.[7] Therefore; we can see that we are consuming approximately 10% more calories today than we were back in the 1970's. If we do not burn off those extra 200 calories or so a day by increasing our activity levels, the extra calories could turn into an extra 20 pounds of body fat within just 12 months. By looking at Figure 1, which compares portion sizes 20 years ago with those of today, it is not difficult to see why our average daily calorie intake has risen.

	20 Years Ago	Today
Two Slices of Pizza	500 Calories	850 Calories
Coffee w/ Milk & Sugar	45 Calories (8oz)	330 Calories (16oz)
Movie Popcorn	270 Calories(5Cups)	630 Calories (Tub)
Bagel	140 Calories(3" Dia)	350 Calories(5-6"Dia
Cheeseburgers	333 Calories	590 Calories (Burger King "Double Whopper" 1,400 Calories)
Soda	97 Calories– 8oz 145 Calories-12oz	242 Calories-20oz
Prices	$0.99/388Cal/32oz $1.09/533Cal/44oz	$1.19/776Cal/64oz

Figure 1. Portion sizes 20 years ago compared to those of today.
Adapted from the National Heart, Lung, and Blood Institute's Portion Distortion Interactive Quiz.[8]

One reason for the rise in average daily calorie seen in recent years is the trend for "supersizing". For example:

- 7-Eleven Gulp to Double Gulp Coca-Cola Classic – 37 extra cents buys 450 extra calories
- Baskin Robbins Chocolate Chip Ice Cream, Kids Scoop to Double Scoop – $1.62 extra buys 390 extra calories
- Cinnabon Minibon to Classic Cinnabon – 48 extra cents buys 370 extra calories
- McDonald's Quarter Pounder with Cheese to Medium Quarter Pounder with Cheese Extra Value Meal – $1.41 extra buys 660 extra calories
- Movie theater small to medium unbuttered popcorn – 71 extra cents buys 500 extra calories
- Subway 6-inch to 12-inch Tuna Sub – $1.53 extra buys 420 extra calories

308

Leptin

There is a type of mutant mouse called an ob/ob or obese mouse, which is always hungry and cannot stop eating. The ob/ob mouse gains weight rapidly, reaching a weight 3-times that of regular mice. Ob/ob mice also develop type II diabetes, and have great difficulty reproducing. We now know that ob/ob mice are always hungry because they possess a gene mutation that renders them unable to produce the hormone leptin,[9] which plays a key role in coordinating the metabolic, endocrine, and behavioral responses to starvation.[10] Studies have shown that when the ob/ob mouse is given leptin it stops overeating and loses weight. Leptin works exactly the same way in the human body.

LEPTIN HORMONE PHYSIOLOGY AND PATHOLOGY IN OBESITY

Leptin is secreted by white adipose tissue, the undesirable fat that accumulates on the abdomen, buttocks, and thighs. The old view of fat was that it primarily acted as a place for the body to store extra calories. However, that view has changed dramatically, and we now know that fat is a major endocrine organ.[11]

One of leptin's main roles is to communicate with the brain as to how much fat is stored in the body. When working normally, leptin levels rise when enough food has been consumed, this rise in leptin levels tells the brain to decrease appetite and increase the metabolic rate. Conversely, leptin levels drop if not enough food is consumed, thereby instructing the brain to increase appetite and decrease the metabolic rate.

There is a circadian pattern of leptin secretion, with levels being at their highest during the first few hours of sleep and at their lowest in the morning.[12] In a 24-hour period, there are as many as 32 pulses of leptin activity.[13] Research shows that these circadian changes of blood leptin levels in non-obese people are more significant than these changes in obese people.[14] Indeed, our love of refined sugars and excess consumption of food has had a serious impact on leptin's ability to communicate properly with the brain. This breakdown in communication results in leptin, insulin, epinephrine, and thyroid resistance – all of which promote weight gain.

Leptin Resistance

If a person has leptin resistance they always feel hungry, even when their leptin levels are high. This is because the hypothalamus, the part of the brain that leptin communicates with, develops resistance to leptin and does not register its signal to reduce appetite. One reason for leptin resistance is that elevated triglyceride levels in the blood (due to excess eating) decrease the transport of leptin across the blood brain barrier, effectively preventing leptin from entering the brain.[15] Other causes of leptin resistance include defects in leptin receptor signaling and blockades in downstream neuronal circuitries.[15] The upshot of leptin resistance is that the body begins to think that it is starving and so increases appetite and +decreases the metabolic rate, thus any calories consumed are sent to be stored as fat.

Insulin Resistance

Leptin resistance and insulin resistance are linked. When the brain cannot sense leptin appetite is raised, metabolic rate is lowered, and calories are sent for storage. Another function of leptin is to inhibit the biosynthesis and secretion of insulin in pancreatic beta-cells. However, research suggests that leptin resistance also renders the pancreas unable to sense leptin.[16] This causes the pancreas to keep making excess insulin, thus setting the stage for insulin resistance and, ultimately further weight gain.

Epinephrine Resistance

Repeated attempts by the brain to stimulate fat cell metabolism with epinephrine can result in chronically high epinephrine levels and can, eventually, lead to fat cells becoming resistant to epinephrine. Epinephrine resistance predisposes the individual to weight gain, especially in the abdominal area – the type of weight gain most associated with cardiovascular disease and reproductive organ cancer. It is important to note that leptin is also under short-term control of epinephrine; a quick burst of sympathetic nervous system activity depresses leptin production.[17]

Thyroid Resistance

Leptin resistance leads to, causes "false starvation" (diminished TSH secretion, suppressed T4 to T3 conversion, increase in reverse T3), which slows thyroid function even though a person is overweight.[18] Consequently, thyroid hormone will be less active everywhere in the body if there is leptin resistance. Furthermore, leptin and thyroid resistance causes the uncoupling protein UCP3 to be inactivated so there is no thermogenesis in the fat cells to burn the calories and fat away.[19]

CONCLUDING REMARKS

Our eating habits have disrupted normal leptin physiology, thus triggering leptin resistance and its associated problems of insulin resistance, epinephrine resistance, and thyroid resistance. All of these problems predispose the individual to weight gain and obesity, thus an understanding of leptin physiology and pathology is vital for any anti-aging doctor.

REFERENCES

1. Szabo L. *Number of kids on medication jumps alarmingly*. USA Today. November 2, 2008. Available at: http://www.usatoday.com/news/health/2008-11-02-kidsmedications_N.htm. Accessed September 7, 2009.
2. Mokdad AH, Bowman BA, Ford ES, Vinicor F, Marks JS, Koplan JP. The continuing epidemics of obesity and diabetes in the United States. *JAMA*. 2001;286:1195-1200.
3. Richards BJ, Richards MG. *Mastering Leptin: Your Guide to Permanent Weight Loss and Optimum Health*. 3rd ed. Wellness Resources; 2009.
4. Vasan RS, Pencina MJ, Cobain M, Freiberg MS, D'Agostino RB. Estimated risks for developing obesity in the Framingham Heart Study. *Ann Intern Med*. 2005;143:473-480.
5. Kruger J, Galuska DA, Serdula MK, Jones DA. Attempting to lose weight: specific practices among U.S. adults. *Am J Prev Med*. 2004;26:402-406.
6. Lenoir M, Serre F, Cantin L, Ahmed SH. Intense sweetness surpasses cocaine reward. *PLoS ONE*. 2007;2:e698.
7. Guthrie JF, Lin BH, Frazao E. Role of food prepared away from home in the American diet, 1977-78 versus 1994-96: changes and consequences. *J Nutr Educ Behav*. 2002;34:140-50.
8. Portion Distortion Interactive Quiz. National Heart, Lung, and Blood Institute. Available at: http://hp2010.nhlbihin.net/portion/portion.cgi?action=question&number=1. Accessed September 7, 2009.
9. Zhang Y, Proenca R, Maffei M, Barone M, Leopold L, Friedman JM. Positional cloning of the mouse obese gene and its human homologue. *Nature*. 1994;372:425-432.
10. Wilding JP. Leptin and the control of obesity. *Curr Opin Pharmacol*. 2001;1:656-661.
11. Trayhurn P, Beattie JH. Physiological role of adipose tissue: white adipose tissue as an endocrine and secretory organ. *Proc Nutr Soc*. 2001;60:329-339.
12. Sinha MK, Ohannesian JP, Heiman ML, Kriauciunas A, Stephens TW, Magosin S, Marco C, Caro JF. Nocturnal rise of leptin in lean, obese, and non-insulin-dependent diabetes mellitus subjects. *J Clin Invest*. 1996;97:1344-1347.
13. Himms-Hagen J. Physiological roles of the leptin endocrine system: differences between mice and humans. *Crit Rev Clin Lab Sci*. 1999;36:575-655.
14. Radić R, Nikolić V, Karner I, Kosović P, Kurbel S, Selthofer R, Curković M. Circadian rhythm of blood leptin level in obese and non-obese people. *Coll Antropol*. 2003;27:555-561.
15. Banks WA, Coon AB, Robinson SM, Moinuddin A, Shultz JM, Nakaoke R, Morley JE. Triglycerides induce leptin resistance at the blood-brain barrier. *Diabetes*. 2004;53:1253-1260.
16. Seufert J. Leptin effects on pancreatic beta-cell gene expression and function. *Diabetes*. 2004;53 Suppl 1:S152-158.
17. Trayhurn P, Duncan JS, Rayner DV, Hardie LJ. Rapid inhibition of ob gene expression and circulating leptin levels in lean mice by the beta 3-adrenoceptor agonists BRL 35135A and ZD2079. *Biochem Biophys Res Commun*. 1996;228:605-610.
18. Huo L, Münzberg H, Nillni EA, Bjørbaek C. Role of signal transducer and activator of transcription 3 in regulation of hypothalamic trh gene expression by leptin. *Endocrinology*. 2004;145:2516-2523.

19. Gong DW, He Y, Karas M, Reitman M. Uncoupling protein-3 is a mediator of thermogenesis regulated by thyroid hormone, beta3-adrenergic agonists, and leptin. *J Biol Chem.* 1997;272:24129-24132.

ABOUT THE AUTHOR

Dr. Paul Ling Tai is a trained Podiatric medical physician and double Board certified surgeon with expertise in natural anti-aging technologies, herbal compound engineering, research and development. Dr. Tai is Chairman and President of A4M Brasil, an AntiAging professor of Univ. Paulista, Pontifical Catholic Univ. and Univ. of UNAR; he has fourteen patents and 5 best seller books credited to his name.

Chapter 35
Beyond Weight Loss – Fat Burning Technologies

Paul Ling Tai, D.P.M., FACFS, ABPS
Chairman & President, A4M Brazil;
Professor of Anti-Aging, PUC University, Belo Horizonte, Minas Gerais, Brazil;
Professor of Anti-Aging, UNAR University, Araras, Sao Paulo, Brazil;
Co-Coordinator, Anti-Aging Department, UNIP University, Sao Paulo, Brazil

ABSTRACT
While many anti-aging enthusiasts are familiar with the hormone DHEA (dehydroepiandrosterone), far fewer are likely to be aware of its metabolite, 7-Oxo DHEA, which is responsible for many of DHEA's beneficial actions. Research shows that 7-Oxo DHEA (7-Oxo) is even more potent than its parent compound DHEA for stimulating enzymes of thermogenesis (burning calories), which increases the body's metabolic efficiency. However, 7-Oxo does not convert to androgenic hormones, such as estrogen and testosterone. Studies have also demonstrated that 7-Oxo enhances the activity of three thermogenic enzymes that stimulate fatty acid oxidation in the liver, does not accumulate in the body over time, and is free of unhealthy side effects. Results of a human, double-blind study showed that participants receiving 7-Oxo lost significantly more body weight compared than those in the placebo group (6.3 lb versus 2.1 lb). The 7-Oxo group also lost a greater percentage of body fat compared to the placebo group (1.8% versus 0.57%).

INTRODUCTION
Many published studies have documented the increasing epidemic of overweight and obesity in America. In the National Institute of Health's 30-year study of obesity, 90% of men and 70% of women who started with normal weight range ended the study as overweight or obese.[1] Americans now consume 10% (200 more calories daily) than in 1970[2] and given the lack of change in physical activity, it is equivalent to an additional 20 lbs a year.

Increasing age also plays a hand in the epidemic. Decreased activity, less muscle mass, lower hormone receptor sensitivity, leptin abnormality, lower DHEA, lower circulating thyroid hormone, and a decline in basal metabolic rate (BMR), all go hand in hand with the aging process and cause the body to burn less fat, resulting in greater incidence of obesity.

To examine this problem, we will first study the physiology of fat burning and then look at the results of a few studies which highlight the value of 7-Oxo DHEA. Finally, we will finish with a brief discussion of the natural effects of exercise in weight reduction.

FAT THERMOGENESIS
To maximize weight loss, it makes sense to first understand the physiology of fat thermogenesis and conversion to energy. Adipose tissue is divided into white and brown fat cells. The white adipose tissue (WAT) releases inflammatory compounds, called adipokines, which cause problems for the entire body. These inflammatory compounds can prevent the conversion of the reservoir thyroid hormone T4 to active thyroid hormone T3, which regulates body temperature, growth, heart rate, and many other functions of the body. These inflammatory problems are also one of the major factors in heart disease. If the body is low on these thyroid hormones (T4 and T3) then there will be three-times less uncoupling protein 3 (UCP3) activity in the fat cells and muscles, leading to an inability of the fat cells to burn.[3] The primary function of efficient leptin operation is to prevent fat from being deposited in cells that are not designed to store fat, i.e. muscle. Increased leptin and thyroid resistance will in turn cause UCP3 deactivation and a failure of thermogenesis (burning of calories and fat).

A human genomic study revealed three thermogenic pathways of fat cell metabolism. These pathways are controlled by three uncoupling proteins – UCP, UCP1, and UCP3. UCP acts upon fat cells to produce 70% heat and 30% energy, UCP1 converts brown fat into 100% heat, and UCP3 converts fat cells into 100% heat with the cooperation of leptin and thyroid hormones.

There is a domino effect in the aging process. DHEA and 7-Oxo DHEA levels in the blood drop with age. Lower DHEA results in lower enzyme activity, which results in decreased thermogenic activity. Lower thermogenic activity results in a decreased BMR, which results in weight gain.

7-Oxo DHEA

How can we prevent the dominoes from starting to fall? We suggest that the question is best approached by starting at the beginning – with DHEA. 7-Oxo DHEA stimulates three thermogenic enzymes: fatty acyl CoA oxidase, glycerol-3-phosphate dehydrogenase (GPDH), and malic enzyme. The continued activation of these enzymes at the appropriate levels is a key to maintaining BMR.

7-Oxo DHEA also lowers the efficiency of coupling phosphorylation to oxidations of Krebs cycle, which, though it is an important part of the metabolic process, also produces cell-damaging free radicals. Furthermore, 7-Oxo DHEA increases heat production by stimulating enzymes which are important for thermogenesis and promoting the utilization of fat cells for heat production. Similarly, 7-Keto DHEA lowers the efficiency of food utilization for fat synthesis by stimulating the thermogenic enzymes to make use of the supply for fat cells to raise the metabolic rate.

Scientists have been very interested in translating these new understandings of 7-Oxo DHEA and leptin into useful methods of weight loss, and have contrasted them with older, conventional methods. One common method of weight loss has been to drastically reduce calorie consumption, thus increasing the disparity between daily caloric intake and use. However, studies have shown that fasting slows thyroid function, thus preventing the production of metabolism-increasing enzymes. Another consideration is the levels of leptin in the body. Leptin is produced by fat cells, and one of its roles is to signal the brain to produce that satisfied feeling that one gets at the end of a filling meal. A recent study of obese teenagers showed that those who had the lowest leptin at the end of the weight loss period were more likely to relapse and gain their weight back.[4]

Two studies have examined the effect of 7-Oxo in weight loss. The Zenk study was conducted by Minnesota Applied Research Center and sought to determine the effect of 7-Oxo on body composition and observe its safety for weight loss.[5] This was an 8-week study in which 35 overweight, healthy volunteers ingested 100mg of 7-Oxo twice daily while on a 1,800 Kcal diet combined with a cross-training exercise program. The second study was the Kalman study.[6] This was conducted by Peak Wellness with the same objectives as the Zenk study. This was an 8-week long study in which 30 overweight, healthy volunteers ingested 100mg of 7-Oxo twice daily while also following a 1,800 Kcal diet combined with a circuit training exercise program.

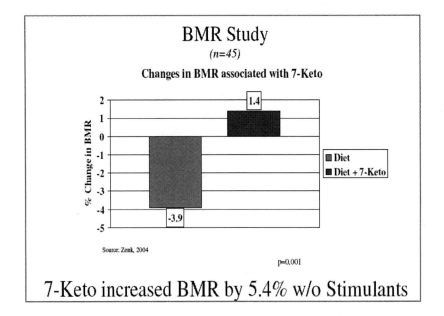

Figure 1. Results of the study by Zenk et al[5] showed that supplementation with 7-Oxo DHEA (7-keto) significantly increased BMR.

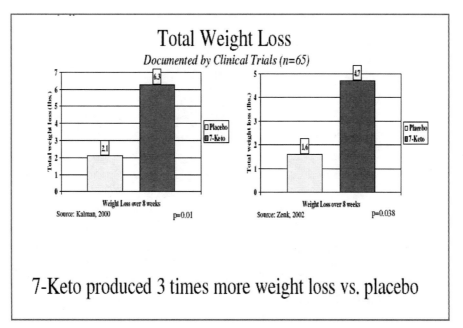

Figure 2. Results of studies by Kalman[6] and Zenk[5] showed that supplementation with 7-Oxo DHEA (7-keto) significantly increased weight loss compared to placebo.

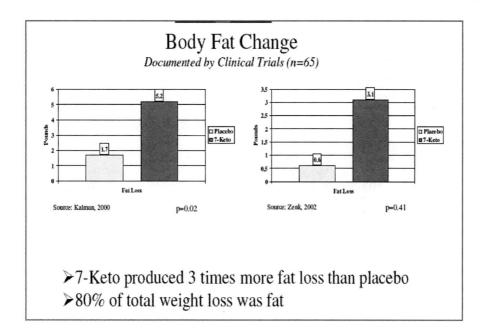

Figure 3. Results of studies by Kalman[6] and Zenk[5] showed that supplementation with 7-Oxo DHEA (7-keto) significantly increased fat loss compared to placebo.

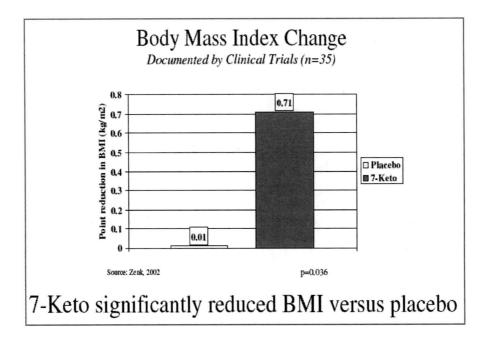

Figure 4. Results of a study by Zenk et al[5] showed that supplementation with 7-Oxo DHEA (7-keto) significantly reduced BMI.

The results in both studies speak for themselves. 7-Oxo DHEA dramatically increases weight loss, increases BMR, and promotes fat loss. Thus suggesting that 7-Oxo DHEA can confer several health benefits.

Exercise and Fat Burning
It is important to note that the subjects in the Zenk[5] and Kalman[6] studies also followed a prescribed exercise program. Thus it is important that the effects of that exercise are understood. Adhering to a few principles of exercising will greatly increase the benefits that are obtainable from exercise.

To burn the greatest amount of fat, aerobics must be performed between meals or first thing in the morning before eating. When a person has not eaten for a few hours, exercise will begin to liberate fatty acids and turn on UCP3 within 30 minutes or so. It is more important to exercise for longer time periods than to exercise harder or faster. After about 15-20 minutes, muscles will feel like they have "clicked into a gliding pace". This gliding pace is reflective of entering a fat burning mode. Exercising at too great an intensity will result in the legs feeling heavy, once this happens tiredness will begin to set in and the rate of fat burning will slow. If this happens it is vital to reduce exercise intensity. Within a few minutes of slowing down the feeling of tiredness will subside and fat burning will resume. The goal is to maintain this pace for one hour.

The fat burning enzyme UCP3 can be increased by up to seven-times the resting value by prolonged aerobic exercise.[7] A good response to exercise time will result in a ½ pound loss of body fat. Exercise frequency of at least three times a week will equate to 1-2 pounds a week of healthy fat loss. Increased UCP3 activity also improves the antioxidant status of cells.

CONCLUDING REMARKS
Results of weight loss studies suggest that DHEA and its metabolite 7-Oxo may be of great benefit to people who need to lose weight. However, further studies are needed in order to evaluate the full potential of these enzymes. Several studies show that the application of 7-Oxo DHEA is successful in affecting significantly increased weight loss. In order to reap the most benefits from 7-Oxo DHEA its use must be combined with an exercise program that maximizes fat burning.

REFERENCES

1. Vasan RS, Pencina MJ, Cobain M, Freiberg MS, D'Agostino RB. Estimated risks for developing obesity in the Framingham Heart Study. *Ann Intern Med.* 2005;143:473-480.
2. Guthrie JF, Lin BH, Frazao E. Role of food prepared away from home in the American diet, 1977-78 versus 1994-96: changes and consequences. *J Nutr Educ Behav.* 2002;34:140-50.
3. Gong DW, He Y, Karas M, Reitman M. Uncoupling protein-3 is a mediator of thermogenesis regulated by thyroid hormone, beta3-adrenergic agonists, and leptin. *J Biol Chem.* 1997;272:24129-24132.
4. Celi F, Bini V, Papi F, Contessa G, Santilli E, Falorni A. Leptin serum levels are involved in the relapse after weight excess reduction in obese children and adolescents. *Diabetes Nutr Metab.* 2003;16:306-311.
5. Zenk JL, Helmer TR, Kassen LJ, Kuskowski MA. The effect of 7-keto Naturalean on weight loss: a randomized, double-blind, placebo-controlled trial. *Current Therapeutic Research.* 2002;63:263-272.
6. Kalman DS, Colker CM, Swain MA, Torina GC, Shi Q. A randomized, double-blind, placebo controlled study of 3-acetyl-7-oxo-dehydroepiandrosterone in healthy overweight adults. *Current Therapeutic Research.* 2000;61:435-442.
7. Zhou M, Lin BZ, Coughlin S, Vallega G, Pilch PF. UCP-3 expression in skeletal muscle: effects of exercise, hypoxia, and AMP-activated protein kinase. *Am J Physiol Endocrinol Metab.* 2000;279:E622-629.

ABOUT THE AUTHOR

Dr. Paul Ling Tai is a trained Podiatric medical physician and double Board certified surgeon with expertise in natural anti-aging technologies, herbal compound engineering, research and development. Dr. Tai is Chairman and President of A4M Brasil, an AntiAging professor of Univ. Paulista, Pontifical Catholic Univ. and Univ. of UNAR; he has fourteen patents and 5 best seller books credited to his name.

Chapter 36
Detoxification and Intracellular Nutrition in Anti-Aging

Pramod Vora, BS
Holistic Educator & Health Counselor to Doctors
International Faculty Anti-Aging Medicine, SpaceAge Anti-Aging Center
(Irvine, California USA)

ABSTRACT

The subject of aesthetics and anti-aging is a very interesting and challenging one and has occupied the attention of mankind for thousands of years. We have all heard of the Egyptian Queen Cleopatra, who lived approximately 2000 years ago, and who was celebrated for her exceptional beauty, as well as her exotic beauty treatments and baths in milk, honey, saffron, and aromatic oils. Basically, she was practicing anti-aging medicine 2000 years ago!

Anti-aging medicine has, so far, centered on surgical intervention (plastic surgery) or dermatological (cosmetic) procedures to create an anti-aging effect. However, over a period of time, the body and its organs continue to age unabated with corresponding deterioration in overall appearance of the body.

The aim of this paper is to introduce a non-invasive approach of servicing and repairing various organs of the body: changing body dimension (body sculpting); creating a glowing and healthy skin; removing dark spots and irregular pigmentation; even lightening the complexion by a few noticeable shades; and creating an almost permanent effect of youth and vitality. This is unmistakably perceived by the beholder and also experienced by the subject. These are pre- and post-treatment procedures that enhance surgical and dermatological treatments which form a part of mainstream medicine today.

Use will be made of the standard reference ranges in today's pathology to derive new standards in preventive medicine called optimum values. These will form the basis of a new subject called anti-aging pathology. To illustrate the theory, clinical studies, supported by pathological evaluation of various organs of the body, will be used to prove beyond all doubt the capability of this science to anti-age the body and achieve longevity well beyond 100 years of age, coupled with aesthetic and cosmetic changes to the body. This irrefutable proof of anti-aging the body will remove the last traces of the controversy about anti-aging medicine as a valid medical science and the existence of toxins in the body. Armed with this science we are now able to prove aging as a pathologically detectable disease.

Keywords: detoxification, rejuvenation, anti-aging, nutrition, digestion, constipation, colon, detox, pathology for anti-aging

INTRODUCTION

The subject of aesthetics and anti-aging is a very interesting and challenging one and has occupied the attention of mankind for thousands of years. We have all heard of the Egyptian Queen Cleopatra, who lived approximately 2000 years ago, and who was celebrated for her exceptional beauty, as well as her exotic beauty treatments and baths in milk, honey, saffron, and aromatic oils. Basically, she was practicing anti-aging medicine 2000 years ago!

Anti-aging medicine has, so far, centered on surgical intervention (plastic surgery) or dermatological (cosmetic) procedures to create an anti-aging effect. However, over a period of time, the body and its organs continue to age unabated with corresponding deterioration in overall appearance of the body.

The aim of this paper is to introduce a non-invasive approach of servicing and repairing various organs of the body: changing body dimension (body sculpting); creating a glowing and healthy skin; removing dark spots and irregular pigmentation; even lightening the complexion by a few noticeable shades; and creating an almost permanent effect of youth and vitality. This is unmistakably perceived by the beholder and also experienced by the subject. These are pre- and post-treatment procedures that enhance surgical and dermatological treatments which form a part of mainstream medicine today.

Use will be made of the standard reference ranges in today's pathology to derive new standards in preventive medicine called optimum values. These will form the basis of a new subject called anti-aging pathology.   To illustrate the theory, clinical studies, supported by pathological evaluation of various organs of the body, will be used to prove beyond all doubt the capability of this science to anti-age the body and achieve longevity well beyond 100 years of age, coupled with aesthetic and cosmetic changes to the body. This irrefutable proof of anti-aging the body will remove the last traces of the controversy about anti-aging medicine as a valid medical science and the existence of toxins in the body. Armed with this science we are now able to prove aging as a pathologically detectable disease.

DETOXIFICATION – THE 1st STEP IN ANTI-AGING

When one looks at a machine, or for that fact, at an automobile, one knows that it must be periodically serviced to ensure trouble-free service and long life. A machine is also subject to periodic repairs where parts need to be replaced to ensure its smooth operation. The human body is also like a machine. It has various parts that need to be periodically serviced and repaired, in order to maintain it in perfect working condition for more than one hundred years.

Detoxification presupposes the presence and accumulation of large amounts of toxins in the body. This situation can be likened to an unserviced car emitting jet black smoke from the tail pipe. It then dawns on us that servicing is now due. On the other hand, or on a higher note, the concept of "nontoxification" envisages a continuous process of regular servicing, maintenance of the various organs, and periodic tune-ups of the body. Toxins are really never allowed to accumulate in the body.

The liver helps to neutralize toxic chemicals, biological poisons, and toxins produced inside the body and must be kept at peak health all the time in order to cope with this daily burden. Similarly, the main excretory organs, for example the kidneys and the colon, must be kept working at peak efficiency throughout one's life.

The foundation of anti-aging and longevity rests upon periodic cleaning out the colon, kidneys, liver, lungs, and blood of toxic waste build up and servicing and repairing these vital organs, including the heart. Keeping all the excretory organs of the body – the colon, kidneys, lungs and the skin – working at peak efficiency will ensure minimal toxic build up within the body.

To understand this concept of servicing and repairing of organs we need to understand how to properly evaluate the functioning of these organs by standard pathological tests and further continue to evolve newer pathological standards to judge if these organs are working at peak efficiency and capacity (youthful levels). This requires us to read and interpret the results of these standard pathological tests in an entirely different manner commensurate with our goal of anti-aging.

To give an example, let us take 3 commonly used parameters: creatinine, blood urea nitrogen (BUN), and serum uric acid to evaluate the functioning of the kidneys (Table 1).

Table 1. Standard Reference Ranges for Renal Function Tests

Renal Function Tests	*Standard Reference Range
Serum creatinine	0.5 to 1.5 mg/dL
Blood urea nitrogen (BUN)	4.5 to 21.0 mg/dL
Serum uric acid	3.6 to 8.2 mg/dL

* Correlate with Clinical Symptoms

In order to maintain the body in a state of perfect health and to achieve longevity, we now need to define a concept called "optimum values", which are those that are found in perfectly healthy young people (Table 2). The goal of anti-aging should be to maintain these optimum values for more than 100 years of a person's life.

Table 2. Optimum Values for Renal Function Tests

Renal Function Tests	Optimum Value	Standard Reference Range	Remarks
Serum creatinine	0.8 mg/dL	0.5 to 1.5 mg/dL	For good elimination of toxins through kidneys
Blood urea nitrogen (BUN)	12.0 mg/dL	4.5 to 21.0 mg/dL	To prevent kidney failure / disease
Serum Uric Acid	5.0 mg/dL	3.6 to 8.2 mg/dL	To help reduce aches and joint pains / arthritis

A good detoxification process of the kidneys should help a fairly healthy person to change his or her kidney profile to closely match the values given under the optimum value column. These are the values that form the standards for anti-aging pathology.

A similar analysis can be done for the liver using standard pathology tests and optimum value standards to return the liver functions back to healthy youthful levels (Table 3).

Table 3 - Optimum Values for Liver Function Tests

Liver Function Tests (LFT)	Optimum Value	Standard Reference Range	Remarks
Serum bilirubin (total)	0.8 mg/dL	up to 1.5 mg/dL	Improved liver function and toxin neutralization
SGPT (ALT) serum	20 to 24 U/L	0 to 48 U/L	
SGOT (AST) serum	15 to 20 U/L	5 to 42U/L	
GGPT (gamma GT) serum	20 to 30 U/L	12 to 64 U/L	

Table 4 illustrates optimum values that are achievable by following an elaborate detoxification process.

Table 4. Optimum Values Achievable Via Detoxification

Test Description	Optimum Value	Standard Reference Range	Remarks *
Hemoglobin Females Males	14.0 g/dL 16.0 g/dL	11.5 to 15.0 g/dL 12.5 to 17.0 g/dL	Helps to maintain good energy levels through out the day
Serum iron	125 µg/dL	60 to 180 µg/dL	For good hemoglobin values
Serum creatinine	0.8 mg/dL	0.5 to 1.5 mg/dL	For good elimination of toxins through kidneys
Blood urea nitrogen (BUN)	12.0 mg/dL	4.5 to 21.0 mg/dL	To help prevent kidney failure / disease
Serum uric acid	5.0 mg/dL	3.6 to 8.2 mg/dL	To help reduce aches, joint pains / arthritis
SGPT (ALT) serum	20 to 24 U/L	0 to 48 U/L	Improved liver function and toxin neutralization
SGOT (AST) serum	15 to 20 U/L	5 to 42U/L	Improved liver function and toxin neutralization
GGPT (gamma GT) serum	20 to 30 U/L	12 to 64 U/L	Improved liver function and toxin neutralization
Serum bilirubin (total)	0.8 mg/dL	up to 1.5 mg/dL	Improved liver function and toxin neutralization

* It is presumed that all nutritional levels of minerals and vitamins have been corrected at intracellular levels and also brought to optimum value.

Thus, we have correlated detoxification to pathology and we are now in a position to return the body back to healthy youthful levels. This is the first step to anti-aging and its periodic monitoring.

REJUVENATION – THE 2ND STEP IN ANTI-AGING

One of the most important causes of accelerated aging is poor digestion. This can be due to poor gastric acid flow, poor bile flow, poor enzyme production, or a combination of all these factors. Inefficient digestion, which is characterized by bloating, gas, burping, acid reflux, flatulence, etc. results in improper absorption of nutrition from the food we eat. We all know, that lack of proper nutrition can cause accelerated aging and even death. Hence, in rejuvenation we must look at ways and means to improve digestion, regenerate liver cells to improve liver function and bile flow, and rejuvenate the pancreas to increase the production of enzymes (e.g. protease, amylase, and lipase) to help properly digest proteins, carbohydrates, and fats.

If the digestive tract is damaged, for example by the use of antibiotics, it is important to recoat and rebuild the mucus membrane lining and also reseed the intestine and colon with healthy bacteria (probiotics) to aid digestion and naturally produce B-Complex vitamins for the body.

Luckily, all this can be done through the use of herbs and nutrition. A good detoxification and rejuvenation program will create a healthy glow on the face of the person and make them look and feel years younger than their present physical age. This is how we can create natural anti-aging. Rejuvenation can be evaluated and monitored with simple pathological tests.

Table 5. Case Study 1

Patient: Male Age: 25 years Height: 6ft Weight: 162.4 lbs (73.8 Kg.) Diet: Vegetarian			
	* 02/28/2003	** 03/24/2003	*** 05/23/2003
Total bilirubin	1.9 mg/dL	1.2 mg/dL	0.9 mg/dL
Direct bilirubin	1.2 mg/dL	0.7 mg/dL	0.6 mg/dL
Indirect bilirubin	0.7 mg/dL	0.5 mg/dL	0.3 mg/dL
SGPT (ALT)	28 IU/L	12 IU/L	13 IU/L
SGOT (AST)	20 IU/L	-	-
GGPT (gamma GT)	18 IU/L	-	-
* Prior to Herbal Liver Detoxification ** After 4 weeks of Liver Detoxification *** After 8 weeks of Liver Detoxification			

Table 6. Case Study 2

Patient: Female Age: 38 Height: 5ft 2 in Weight: 152.6 lbs (69.36 Kg) Fat = 39% (++) BP = 94 / 69 Pulse = 72 Diet: Meat Eater		
	* 04/19/2003	** 04/23/2005
Serum creatinine	0.6 mg/dL	0.7 mg/dL
Blood urea nitrogen (BUN)	18.0 mg/dL	11.0 mg/dL
Total bilirubin	0.8 mg/dL	0.3 mg/dL
Direct bilirubin	0.1 mg/dL	0.1 mg/dL
Indirect bilirubin	0.7 mg/dL	0.2 mg/dL
SGPT (ALT)	52 IU/L	20 IU/L
SGOT (AST)	24 IU/L	22 IU/L
GGTP (gamma GT)	28 IU/L	12 IU/L
Note: 8 Week detoxification was started in March 2005		
* Without prior detoxification ** After 8 weeks of whole body detoxification		

Table 7. Case Study 3

Patient: Female Age: 56 years Height: 5ft Weight: 138.4 lbs (62.9 Kg) Fat = 37% (+) Diet: Meat Eater					
	*09/13/2002	**09/16/2003	***04/11/2004	#8/06/2004	##02/23/2005
Serum creatinine	0.78 mg / dL	1.00 mg / dL	0.87 mg/dL	0.89 mg / dL	
Blood urea nitrogen (BUN)	15.02 mg /dL	18.22 mg /dL	17.34 mg /dL	12.58 mg /dL	
Total bilirubin	0.56 mg/dL	0.25 mg/dL	0.40 mg/dL	0.29 mg/dL	0.30 mg/dL
Direct bilirubin	0.23 mg/dL	0.14 mg/dL	0.14 mg/dL	0.12 mg/dL	0.17 mg/dL
Indirect bilirubin	0.33 mg/dL	0.11 mg/dL	0.26 mg/dL	0.17 mg/dL	0.13 mg/dL
SGPT (ALT)	42.37 IU/L	23.29 IU/L	21.08 IU/L	39.83 IU/L	22.0 IU/L
SGOT (AST)	29.92 IU/L	22.10 IU/L	24.30 IU/L	19.88 IU/L	21.0 IU/L
GGTP (gamma GT)	42.00 IU/L	27.30 IU/L	41.73 IU/L	52.30 IU/L	27.0 IU/L
TSH ultrasensitive	1.62 µIU/ml		2.97 µIU/ml		2.01 µIU/ml

TSH = 23.0 µIU/ml in October 2001. Eltroxin / Synthroid / thyroid hormone T4 was not administered to the patient. TSH = 2.27 µIU/ml on December 02, 2008 (Three years after discontinuing treatment with our health center and six years after TSH value was naturally brought down from a high of 23.0 µIU/ml).

*Twelve months after first detoxification
**After 8 weeks of whole body detoxification
***After 8 weeks of whole body detoxification but with substance abuse resulting in higher GGPT (gamma GT)
##After 8 weeks of whole body detoxification done annually
#Without detoxification for a whole year but with substance abuse resulting in elevated GGPT (Gamma GT)

Table 8. Case Study 4

Patient: Female Age: 37 years Height: 5ft 5 inches Weight: 155.3 lbs (70.6 Kg) Diet: Meat Eater					
	* 11/03/2000	* 12/03/2002	* 03/25/2003	* 05/08/2003	# 10/03/2003	## 12/09/2003
Hemoglobin	7.4 g/dL	8.1 g/dL	7.6 g/dL	8.9 g/dL	10.5 g/dL	11.8 g/dL
	* 09/26/2000	* 12/03/2002	* 03/19/2003	* 06/02/2003	# 10/04/2003	## 12/19/2003
Ultrasensitive TSH	3.97 µIU/ml	8.47 µIU/ml	7.53 µIU/ml	17.1 µIU/ml	7.87 µIU/ml	2.37 µIU/ml
Eltroxin / Synthroid Dose	-	50 mcg	75 mcg	75 mcg	50mcg
Detoxification					Whole Body	Whole Body
Intracellular Nutritional Therapy					Prescription Strength Iron + B - Complex (Forte)	

* The historic record shows extremely low levels of hemoglobin for a few years before detoxification. Patient confirms that low hemoglobin levels existed for over 10 years in spite of continuous iron supplementation, including ferrous sulfate, and other ferrous preparations.

*Before detoxification (detoxification was started in July 2003)
#After 12 weeks of whole body detoxification and intracellular nutrition
##After 20 weeks of whole body detoxification and intracellular nutrition

Intracellular nutrition requires the use of therapeutic doses of nutrition to be given by altering cell membrane permeability coupled with a carrier mechanism to deliver nutrition to the center of the cell where it is required.

Hemoglobin levels are measured after discontinuing nutrition for about 5 to 7 days prior to drawing blood sample. This ensures that there is proper retention of nutrition at intracellular levels and that the reading does not pertain to serum levels, which are likely to be excreted from the body a few hours after ingestion.

Table 9. Case Study 5

Patient: Female Age: 39 Height: 5ft 3 in Weight: 163.6 lbs (74.36 Kg) Fat = 42.5% (++) BP = 107 / 71 Pulse = 67 Diet: Meat Eater				
Renal Profile	* 10/12/2007	# Std. Ref. Range	** 12/03/2007	*** 04/18/2008
Blood urea nitrogen (BUN)	17.0 mg/dL	7 to 18.7 mg/dL	11.0 mg/dL	12.0 mg/dL
Serum uric acid	4.3 mg/dL	2.6 to 6.0 mg/dL	4.0 mg/dL	3.5 mg/dL
Creatinine	1.0 mg/dL	0.6 to 1.1 mg/dL	0.6 mg/dL	0.75 mg/dL
Serum total proteins	8.70 g/dL	6.4 to 8.3 g/dL	7.6 g/dL	7.75 g/dL
Serum albumin	5.4 g/dL	3.4 to 4.8 g/dL	4.9 g/dL	5.07 g/dL
Serum globulin	3.3 g/dL	1.8 to 3.6 gm%	2.7 g/dL	2.68 g/dL
A/G ratio	1.64	1.1 to 2.2	1.81	1.89
Cystatin C	1.02 mg/L	0.53 to 0.95 mg/L	0.77 mg/L	0.71 mg/L
C reactive protein	2.71 mg/L	Up to 3.0 mg/L	1.95 mg/L	0.93 mg/L
Daily protein intake RDA = 1 gm / Kg body weight	Unrestricted	Approximately 50 grams / day	10 g / day Vegetarian Source	Unrestricted protein intake
# Correlate with clinical symptoms				
Note: 8-week detoxification program was started on 15th of October 2007				
*Before starting detoxification. Note: When the program started the patient was put on a restricted protein (vegetarian) diet of 10 g/day. **After 7 weeks of whole body detoxification her protein (mixed) intake was increased to 25 g/day after noting the improvement in renal function. ***These readings were taken when there were no restrictions to protein intake.				

The above is a case study on kidney servicing, detoxification, and rejuvenation. The patient is taken from the precipice of chronic renal failure to good health, with kidney function being returned back to youthful levels in a matter of just 7 weeks.

Table 10. Case Study 6

Professional Model & Actress					
Female Age: 24 years Height: 5ft 5 in Weight: 114.4 lbs (52 Kg)					
	2/15/2007	3/20/2007	4/5/2007	5/15/2007	10/9/2007
Breast	34.0"	34.75"	34.75"	34.5"	34.5"
Waist - I	27.0"	26.0"	26.0"	27.5"	26.75"
* Waist - II	34.0"	32.0"	29.0"	29.0"	29.75"
Hips	36.5"	36.0"	35.5"	36.0"	36.0"
Full Thigh	22.0"	21.5"	21.5"	22.0"	22.0"
Mid Thigh	19.0"	19.25"	19.5"	19.25"	19.0"
Mid Arm	9.25"	9.5"	9.5"	9.5"	9.5"
Wrist	5.75"	5.75"	5.9"	5.9"	5.75"
Weight	52.818 Kg	52.00 Kg	52.00 Kg	53.454 Kg	52.272 Kg
Fat	18.8% (-)	18.0% (-)	18.0% (-)	19.4% (-)	15.3% (-)
Hydration	56.10%	56.60%	56.40%	55.70%	58.50%
Bone Mass	4.8 lbs	4.8 lbs	4.8 lbs	4.8 lbs	5.0 lbs
Avg. Daily Calories	2002	1987	1983	2010	2040
Metabolic Age	12 years	12 years	12 years	12 years	12 years
Leg Length	42.0" even				

Remarks: Happy with present weight. Would like to increase lean muscle mass, reduce water retention, and increase bone mass to 5.5 lbs. Some increase desired in mid and full thigh measurements.

Note: This patient was working out in a gym for over one year prior to detoxification.
*Waist II measurements are taken 2 inches (50 mm) below navel.
5 inches (125 mm) reduction occurred within 6 weeks of starting the detoxification program.
Maintaining the results achieved was observed over the next 6 months period with hardly any deterioration in Waist II dimensions.

Case Study 6 shows how detoxification can be used to achieve whole body sculpting. Abdominal dimension was reduced by 5 inches in a period of just 6 weeks. This was achieved by cleaning out the colon and improving digestion so that the distention in the abdominal area due to gas formation and toxic waste build up is eliminated. This is a natural method of body sculpting.

INTRACELLULAR NUTRITION – THE 3RD STEP IN ANTI-AGING

Intracellular nutrition enables us to repair and rejuvenate the various organs of the body, including the entire cardiac system.

To me, anti-aging means, the ability to live to more than 100 years, free from chronic aliments and medication of any type. To achieve this, we must look at nutrition. Not just any old nutrition, but intracellular nutrition and the ability to check and correct nutrition deficiencies in a matter of a few weeks or months. Intracellular nutrition, should allow us to repair the organs of the body, for example the heart. We should be able to correct the ECG or improve the ejection fraction of the heart, no matter what the physical age of the person. The concept of this science and the term orthomolecular medicine was coined by the Nobel Laureate Linus Pauling in 1968.

To understand why intracellular nutrition is vital it is necessary to explain a few important factors:
1. With the over cultivation of the land and the consequent falling nutritional value of the soil and hence of the food we eat, the human body has during the last 50 years progressively become malnourished. This has given rise to chronic aliments of all types. A method must be found to

correct this deficiency in a very short span of time – a few weeks or a few months. For more information on this subject read: www.space-age.com/nutri-farm-seminar.doc

2. To achieve this:
   o One must be able to administer nutrition in an organic form in therapeutic doses. Prophylactic doses presently available at the local pharmacy, chemist, or health food store are of no use.
   o The doses administered must reach intracellular levels i.e. the center of the cell where nutrition is really required and not just the serum as most prophylactic nutritional doses do. For more information on this subject read: www.space-age.com/Multivitamin-FAQs.doc

To achieve this, one must have at ones' command two technologies:
1. The capacity to alter cell membrane permeability; and
2. A carrier mechanism to carry nutrition to the center of the cell where it is required.

Imagine, a few hundred years ago, a soldier on horseback with a sword in his hand outside the thick walls of a fort. By himself, the soldier will not be able to penetrate the thick walls of the fort. Now imagine canon balls being fired at the thick walls of the fort. These canon balls will soon create an opening in the walls of the fort through which the soldier will now be able to enter the fort. The canon balls have changed the permeability of the walls of the fort, the horse is the carrier mechanism to help carry the soldier inside the fort, and the soldier is the nutrition.

Orthomolecular nutrition, when equipped with cell membrane permeability altering capabilities and further equipped with a carrier mechanism to easily carry the nutrition inside the cell to its center, is the basis of intracellular nutrition.

If we couple the principles of orthomolecular nutrition with therapeutic doses of nutrition, correctly administered in a synergetic manner at intracellular levels, we will find that it is possible to free the body of chronic aliments, such as hypertension, diabetes, hormone imbalance (and its connected diseases, e.g. hypothyroidism, prostate enlargement), and obesity, and also help to repair hardened arteries, improve the ejection fraction of the heart, and repair minor damages to various other organs of the body.

Case Study 7 (below) shows that it is possible to reduce the size of the prostate gland and prostate specific antigen (PSA) levels naturally by following a program of detoxification, rejuvenation, and intracellular nutrition.

Table 11. Case Study 7

Parameters	Std. Ref. Range	* 02/18/2005	* 05/13/2006	** 11/26/2007
Patient: Male Age: 76 Height: 5ft 4 in Weight: 123.2 lbs (56 Kg) Fat = 16.2% (0) BP = 129/ 69 Pulse = 59 Diet: Vegetarian				
PSA - prostate specific antigen	0.27 to 4.8 ng/ml (above 60 years)	1.89 ng/ml	1.28 ng/ml	0.72 ng/ml
Prostate Size	3 × 4 × 2.5 cm	4.3×4.2×3.4 cm	4.5×3.9×3.6 cm	3.3×4.0×3.5 cm
Weight	20 g (Adult)	34.4 g	34 g	24 g
Grade of Prostate enlargement		grade II	grade II	*** normal prostate
Prevoid volume		366 ml	150 ml	254 ml
Post void residue	non-significant, minimal	24 ml (7.6%) not significant	61 ml (40%) very significant	41 ml (15%) not significant.
Organic zinc (Forte) (intracellular nutrition)		none	none	60 caps of 60 mg 60 caps of 100mg
Herbal Tea				One cup of herbal tea morning and evening for 30 days

Natural treatment with herbs and intracellular nutrition began on 06/06/2006. Detoxification of various organs was done in stages.
*Readings taken prior to starting treatment with natural herbs and intracellular nutrition.
**Readings were taken after the patient underwent detoxification in June 2006 and treatment with organic zinc (Forte) and herbal tea.
***Prostate appears normal. No intravesical enlargement of prostate gland is seen.

CONCLUDING REMARKS

When we combine detoxification, rejuvenation, and intracellular nutrition we can truly achieve anti-aging in a very gentle and natural manner. The whole body will uniformly undergo anti-aging and will not only look, but will also feel, years younger, and with dedicated effort, will stay that way for many years to come.

REFERENCES

1. Grossman T. Latest advances in anti-aging medicine. *Keio J Med.* 2005;54:85-94.
2. Liska DJ. The detoxification enzyme systems. *Altern Med Rev.* 1998;3:187-198.
3. MacIntosh A, Ball K. The effects of a short program of detoxification in disease-free individuals. *Altern Ther Health Med.* 2000;6:70-76.
4. Murray M, Pizzorno J. *Encyclopedia of Natural Medicine.* Rocklin, CA: Prima Publishing; 1991:43, 50-56.
5. Rabinowitch IM. Achlorhydria and its clinical significance in diabetes mellitus. *Am J Dig Dis.* 1949;18:322-333.
6. Wintergerst ES, Maggini S, Hornig DH. Contribution of selected vitamins and trace elements to immune function. *Ann Nutr Metab.* 2007;51:301-323.
7. Lesourd B. Nutritional factors and immunological ageing. *Proc Nutr Soc.* 2006;65:319-325.
8. Resnick LM. Cellular calcium and magnesium metabolism in the pathophysiology and treatment of hypertension and related metabolic disorders. *Am J Med.* 1992;93:11S-20S.
9. Barbagallo M, Dominguez LJ, Resnick LM. Magnesium metabolism in hypertension and type 2 diabetes mellitus. *Am J Ther.* 2007;14:375-385.

ABOUT THE AUTHOR

Mr. Pramod Vora is a Holistic Educator and Health Counselor to Doctors in Preventive and Anti-Aging Medicine. His landmark research, has, for the first time, Correlated detoxification / Rejuvenation to pathologically verifiable results which prove anti-aging medicine as a valid medical science; and Used intracellular nutrition for treatment of chronic ailments like hypertension, diabetes, hormonal imbalance, etc.

Chapter 37
The Use of T3 and Herbal Medicine to Reset Body Temperature and Recalibrate Many Bodily Functions

E. Denis Wilson, M.D.
President, www.WTSmed.com

ABSTRACT

Many people in the world today suffer from intractable symptoms of chronic fatigue, including migraines, depression, easy weight gain, premenstrual syndrome, irritability, fluid retention, fibromyalgia, anxiety, panic attacks, hair loss, decreased memory and concentration, low sex drive, insomnia, constipation, and many others. Sometimes, doctors recognize the possibility that these symptoms could be due to low thyroid function. Unfortunately, many doctors have been taught that normal thyroid blood test results rule out the need for thyroid replacement therapy. This is not true! Studies suggest, and experience demonstrates, that symptomatic patients may benefit from thyroid supplementation even when their blood tests are normal.

Normal blood tests do not ensure there is adequate stimulation of the cells by the active thyroid hormone triiodothyronine (T3). Stress and chronic illness have been shown to decrease the conversion of thyroxine (T4) to T3. The effects of aging are similar to the effects of stress. The incidence of thyroid impairment increases with age. Thyroid impairment has been shown to contribute to a number of diseases, including: atherosclerosis, myocardial infarction, congestive heart failure, pulmonary failure, renal failure. The implications are staggering. Many people are living with a reversible thyroid insufficiency and impairment that might be easily corrected with simple recognition and treatment. Not only can the recognition and treatment of this problem significantly affect mortality and survival, but it can also have enormous bearing on patients' quality of life.

Low thyroid function is characterized by low body temperatures. Body temperature is a very basic physiological parameter that can have a bearing on almost every bodily function as well as the body's response to almost any form of medical treatment. When patients have low body temperatures they may not respond as expected to many conventional and alternative therapies. Wilson's Temperature Syndrome (WTS), or Wilson's Syndrome, is characterized by people with low thyroid symptoms and normal thyroid blood tests that respond well to treatment (liothyronine, herbal medicine) to normalize low body temperature. In this setting, patients often respond better to T3 alone than they do to medicines that also contain T4. When clinically hypothyroid and biochemically euthyroid patients are treated with cyclic T3 therapy their symptoms often remain improved even after the treatment has been discontinued, suggesting that their thyroid systems have been reset. The aim of this paper is to introduce WTS and to demonstrate how T3 and herbal medicine can reset body temperature and recalibrate many bodily functions.

INTRODUCTION

Many people in the world today suffer from intractable symptoms of chronic fatigue, including migraines, depression, easy weight gain, premenstrual syndrome, irritability, fluid retention, fibromyalgia, anxiety, panic attacks, hair loss, decreased memory and concentration, low sex drive, insomnia, constipation, and many others. Sometimes, doctors recognize the possibility that these symptoms could be due to low thyroid function. Unfortunately, many doctors have been taught that normal thyroid blood test results rules out the need for thyroid replacement therapy. This is not true! Studies suggest, and experience demonstrates, that symptomatic patients may benefit from thyroid supplementation even when their blood tests are normal.

Normal blood tests do not ensure there is adequate stimulation of the cells by the active thyroid hormone triiodothyronine (T3). Stress and chronic illness have been shown to decrease the conversion of thyroxine (T4) to T3. The effects of aging are similar to the effects of stress. The incidence of thyroid impairment increases with age. Thyroid impairment has been shown to contribute to a number of diseases, including: atherosclerosis, myocardial infarction, congestive heart failure, pulmonary failure, renal failure. The implications are staggering. Many people are living with a reversible thyroid insufficiency and impairment that might be easily corrected with simple recognition and treatment. Not only can the recognition and treatment of this problem significantly affect mortality and survival, but it can also have enormous bearing on patients' quality of life.

Low thyroid function is characterized by low body temperatures. Wilson's Temperature Syndrome (WTS), or Wilson's Syndrome, is characterized by people with low thyroid symptoms and normal thyroid blood tests that respond well to treatment (liothyronine, herbal medicine) to normalize low body temperature. In this setting, patients often respond better to T3 alone than they do to medicines that also contain T4. When clinically hypothyroid and biochemically euthyroid patients are treated with cyclic T3 therapy their symptoms often remain improved even after the treatment has been discontinued, suggesting that their thyroid systems have been reset. The aim of this paper is to introduce WTS and to demonstrate how T3 and herbal medicine can reset body temperature and recalibrate many bodily functions.

WILSON'S TEMPERATURE SYNDROME

Whether we are newborn, middle-aged, or elderly, male or female, tall or short, black or white, our bodies all work to maintain our body temperatures within the same very narrow range. If it is cold, we shiver to stay warm. If it is hot, we sweat to stay cool. Maintaining a normal body temperature is vital because almost all of the chemical reactions that take place in the body are catalyzed by enzymes. Enzymes depend on their shape (confirmation) for their activity, and their shape is dependent upon temperature. If the body is too hot or too cold, enzymes are unable to function optimally. Body temperature is a very basic physiological parameter that can have a bearing on almost every bodily function as well as the body's response to almost any form of medical treatment. When patients have low body temperatures they may not respond as expected to many conventional and alternative therapies.

Hypothermia and hyperthermia are rightfully treated as medical emergencies, yet if a patient presents with a body temperature a degree-and-a-half or more below normal they will, more than likely, be dismissed as being fine. Moderately-low body temperatures have been largely ignored historically. How low is low? 97.8°F (36.5°C) or lower measured orally is more than low enough to cause debilitating symptoms, however sometimes a patient will present with a body temperature of 96°F (35.5°C), 95°F (35°C), 94°F (34.4°C), or even lower. On the other hand, some people with mildly low temperatures such as 98.2°F (36.8°C) or even 98.4°F (36.9°C), can improve clinically when their body temperature is normalized to 98.6°F (37°C). People treated with T3 for low temperatures can sometimes notice a difference in a matter of hours; however symptoms usually improve within a few days, and almost certainly within a few weeks.

Probably the most exciting thing about correcting low temperature is that the temperatures and symptoms can often remain improved even after the treatment has been discontinued. Normalizing low body temperatures is one of the most dramatically effective treatment modalities there is, because the body temperature is one of the most fundamental physiologic parameters. If you address a patient's body temperature when other doctors haven't, you can often dramatically help that patient, and thus succeed where other doctors have failed. In fact, the need to correct body temperature is so great, and the results are so good, that many doctors end up treating low temperature full-time as the focus of their practices.

WTS is characterized by people with low thyroid symptoms and normal thyroid blood tests that respond well to normalization of low body temperatures; usually through the use of T3 and/or herbs. The symptoms of hypothyroidism are the symptoms of low temperature, for example:

- Fatigue
- Depression
- Weight gain
- Irritability
- Fluid retention
- Hair loss
- Dry skin, Dry hair
- Insomnia
- Irritable bowel syndrome
- Allergies
- Irregular periods
- Decreased memory
- Decreased concentration
- Muscle and joint aches
- Low sex drive
- Carpal tunnel syndrome
- Hives

People become symptomatic with hypothyroidism only when their body temperatures drop below normal and the symptoms of hypothyroidism do not improve with thyroid replacement until the body temperatures improve. This is because the thyroid system is responsible for maintaining a normal metabolic rate, or in other words, maintaining normal body temperature.

Low body temperature can also cause symptoms that are not often associated with low thyroid function, such as migraines, PMS, anxiety, panic attacks, and asthma. When low body temperatures are normalized, these symptoms often improve or resolve completely.

Hypothyroidism results in low body temperatures due to inadequate production of thyroid hormone by the thyroid gland. However, people can still suffer with debilitating low temperature symptoms even though the thyroid blood tests are normal. How can that be?

If you ask a doctor where thyroid hormone is produced he/she will likely answer, "the thyroid gland." However, it could be argued that thyroid hormone is produced in the peripheral tissues of the body. 80% of T3, the most active form of thyroid hormone, is produced outside the thyroid gland in the peripheral tissues of the body. So, although a blood test may show that normal levels of T4 have been produced by the thyroid gland, that does not mean that T4 has been adequately converted to T3, and thus made available to be utilized by the body.

It is apparent that peripheral conversion of T4 to T3 is subject to some regulatory mechanism. When people are under extreme physical or emotional stress, their conversion of T4 to T3 can drop by 50% in a matter of hours. Fasting, illness, and cortisol can also inhibit T4 to T3 conversion. Unfortunately, it appears that the system can become imbalanced because the depressed metabolic state can persist for long after the stress has passed. A typical scenario is a woman (approximately 80% of WTS patients are women) whose health was fine before experiencing a period of major stress such as childbirth, divorce, death of a loved one, or an accident. The stress results in a drop in body temperature, she develops symptoms of low body temperature, and continues feeling bad indefinitely. Childbirth is the number one cause of WTS.

What course of action should be taken if a person is suffering from persistent low body temperature and it appears that the thyroid system has become imbalanced, even though the thyroid blood tests are normal? We can do the same thing that is often done with the female hormone system when it becomes imbalanced. Just as oral contraceptives are often used temporarily to reestablish normal menstrual cycles in a woman with irregular bleeding, T3 can often be used temporarily to reestablish normal body temperature patterns with the symptoms and temperatures often remaining improved even after the T3 has been discontinued.

WTS has been presented at medical conferences for over 15 years. There is a constituency of like-minded practitioners that have been treating WTS every day for years. Despite this, WTS remains essentiality invisible to mainstream medicine. Most doctors do not recognize WTS because they are not looking for it. However, WTS is easily recognized once you are aware of it, and is easy to treat.

A legal consensus statement has established WTS as a standard of care. There are two ways that a treatment can become a standard of care: One is by randomized double-blind studies published in a peer-reviewed journal, and the other is when there is a large enough group of practitioners that agree that it is an appropriate course of treatment. WTS has reached the critical mass of signatures needed to establish a consensus statement and an uncontrolled study of WTS has been published in the *Puerto Rico Health Sciences Journal*. WTS is now taught in every naturopathic medical school, and CME certification training in WTS takes place every year.

Using T3 and Herbal Medicine to Reset Body Temperature

There are essentially three schools of thought on people that have low thyroid symptoms but normal thyroid blood tests, one is the conventional viewpoint and two are non-conventional alternatives. Conventionally, blood tests are everything – a normal blood test result means no treatment. The first alternative is centered on the belief that blood tests are not everything, and that people with normal blood test results may still benefit from empirical treatment with a T4-containing medicine, such as Synthroid, or a medicine that contains T4 and a small amount of T3, such as Armour. If this course of treatment is effective it is likely that the patient will remain on these medications for the rest of his/her life. The second alternative is also centered on the belief that blood tests are not everything, however this school of thought recommends that a patient is treated with T3 in order, to recalibrate the thyroid system, and then weaned off it after a couple of months. This second alternative is the focus of this paper.

Some doctors believe that T3 therapy is a bad idea, is not necessary, or simply does not work. However these doctors have, almost always, not read the doctor's manual for WTS, have not followed Wilson's T3 (WT3) protocol suggested by the manual, or simply haven't even tried to treat any of their patients with the WT3 protocol.

People that often respond well to treatment with T3 often noticed their symptoms developing after a major stress, such as childbirth, surgery, an accident, divorce, job change, or family stress. As mentioned previously, WTS is significantly more common in women than in men – 80% of people with WTS are women. Interestingly, people whose ancestors survived famine (Irish, Scottish, Welsh, American Indian, Russian, and Polish) are at particularly high risk of WTS, and those of mixed Irish/American Indian descent seemingly being at the greatest risk of WTS.

WTS is very common, and it can be extremely debilitating. People with low body temperatures and symptoms of low thyroid often visit numerous doctors, only to be told the same thing – that their thyroid blood tests are normal, there is nothing wrong with them, and that they do not need any treatment – if they finally find doctors who are aware of WTS and how to treat it, those doctors may just transform their lives. So, how should you go about treating a patient with WTS?

The priority of the physician treating a patient with WTS is to normalize their body temperature. There are a number of measures that can help to normalize low body temperature:

- Removing physical or emotional stress
- Removing toxins
- Correcting nutritional deficiencies
- Diet, exercise, and lifestyle changes,
- Herbs and/or treatment with T3 (WT3 protocol)

I recommend three options for treatment: herbs, the WT3 protocol, or both. Herbs carry little chance of side effects; however it can take a while to begin seeing benefits. The WT3 protocol tends to deliver a more pronounced and long-lasting effect, especially in severe cases. However, it requires discipline and can cause cardiovascular side effects – patients may also feel worse before they begin to feel better. The best option is to use both. Combining herbs with the WT3 protocol increases the benefits and decreases the side effects, while also offering the patient the best chance of success. The only downside to combination treatment is that it is more expensive (and involves more swallowing).

In some cases, thyroid herbs and cofactors are all that is need to normalize body temperature:

- Guggul, the resin of the Guggul tree (*Commiphora wightii*), increases iodine uptake and thyroid hormone production.
- The seaweeds bladder wrack and kelp provides nutrition and substrates that support thyroid function.
- Blue Flag (*Iris versicolor*) is a potent detoxifier of the thyroid gland, which is susceptible to toxins. Blue Flag used to be sold as a United States Pharmacopeia drug called Iridin in the early 1900s as a treatment for hypothyroidism.
- Zinc and selenium are important cofactors for thyroid hormone production.

If you decide to opt for the herbal approach to treat a patient they should begin to notice an improvement in their symptoms within three to four weeks. It is important to note that herbs can also be used to help patients become candidates for the WT3 protocol when otherwise they might not be. For example, Lily of the valley (*Convallaria majalis*), nightblooming cereus, Motherwort (*Leonurus cardiaca*), and Hawthorn (*Crataegus monogyna*) can help to bring down pulse rates before and during treatment, and can even normalize some abnormal EKGs. Siberian Ginseng (*Eleutherococcus senticosus*), Ashwagandha (*Withania somnifera*), Codonopsis, Astragalus, Fo-Ti (*Polygonum multiflorum*), Devil's Club (*Oplopanax horridus*), and Wild Yam (*Dioscorea villosa*) can support adrenal function and help patients to tolerate treatment with T3. Thyroid herbs can also be helpful in stopping and correcting relapses after WT3 therapy is finished.

If you choose to treat a patient with the WT3 protocol it is important that both the doctor and the patient study the *Doctor's Manual for Wilson's Temperature Syndrome*, which is available to download from http://www.wilsonsthyroidsyndrome.com/eManual/. The protocol is simple, but there is a lot to it, and it is important to study all the sections.

Patients are good candidates for treatment with the WT3 protocol if:

- They have a symptom consistent with low thyroid system function.
- They have a body temperature that averages less than 98.6°F (37°C) measured orally.
- There is no other likely explanation for their symptoms.

It is important to note that WTS cannot be diagnosed with a thyroid blood test. It is a diagnosis of exclusion. You need to take the patients history, carry out a full physical examination, and rule out other problems, such as anemia, chronic infection, liver, kidney, and blood sugar abnormalities, etc. It is also necessary to consider lifestyles factors, prescription drugs. Laboratory testing (CBC, multi-chemistry, T4, TSH, antinuclear antibody (ANA) test) and an EKG should also be conducted in order to rule out Addison disease and arrhythmias.

T3 therapy is very useful for recalibrating the thyroid system, but T3 levels must be kept steady in order to minimize side effects. Treatment begins with 7.5 mcg T3 twice a day (b.i.d.). The next step is to increase the dose by 7.5 mcg every day the average body temperature remains less than 98.6°F (37°C) – unless the patient's pulse goes over 100 or the maximum dose is reached (90 mcg b.i.d.). It is important to note that the patient's temperature may go up and then again on the way to being "captured"...this is completely normal and occurs because the body detects the exogenous T3 and thus adjusts the production of endogenous T3. We say that the temperature has been "captured" when the patient's body temperature goes up and doesn't come back down. Once the temperature has been captured, the patient should remain on that dose for a short time and then be weaned off the T3. Hopefully, the patient can be weaned off slowly enough that their temperature does not drop back down again. Body temperature and symptoms often remain improved even after the treatment has been discontinued. If the first cycle was not enough to correct the person's temperature, and usually it is not, then subsequent cycles of T3 can be repeated as needed. The aim is to bring the body temperature closer and closer to normal by using less and less medicine until the patient is able to maintain a normal temperature without the need for medicine – most patients report that they feel best when their temperature is normal and they are off T3, only a few have reported feeling better while taking T3.. The vast majority (approximately 90%) of patients who are correctly treated with the WT3 protocol are alleviated of most of their complaints, symptoms will occasionally persist however these are often easily alleviated with herbs.

The T3 used in the WT3 protocol is compounded with a sustained-release agent to be delivered over 12 hours. It is critical that the sustained-release T3 is compounded by pharmacists with the right equipment, abilities and experience, as the more homogenous the compound the steadier the release, the steadier the T3 levels, the greater the chance of benefits, and the lower the chance of side effects.

Patients need to be aware that to be treated with the WT3 protocol means that they need to commit to taking T3 every 12-hours – to the minute. They also need to take their pulse and record their heart rate daily, and pay attention to any disagreeable awareness of the heart rate. Treatment usually lasts for three to six months (approximately 70% of patients successfully finish the treatment within three months, 90% within six months, and the remainder are rarely treated for more than twelve months) during which they will need to make doctor visits at least twice a month (a course of treatment usually necessitates at least eight doctor visits). Thus it can be seen that the protocol is quite demanding, in fact as many as 20% of patients find the protocol too demanding and decide to stop treatment.

CONCLUDING REMARKS

WTS is, unfortunately, still essentiality invisible to mainstream medicine. Most doctors do not recognize WTS because they are not looking for it. However, WTS is easily recognized once you are aware of it, and is easy to treat. There is a constituency of informed practitioners that have been treating WTS every day for years, and these doctors have transformed the lives of many people simply by helping them to normalize their body temperatures.

ABOUT THE AUTHOR

Dr. E. Denis Wilson is the originator of and first to use compounded sustained-release T3. In 1988, he found that cycles of T3 (without T4) could often be used to normalize biochemically euthyroid patients' temperatures such that the temperatures and low thyroid symptoms often remain improved even after the T3 is discontinued.

Chapter 38
Vitality Weight Loss with HCG and HRT

Brian G. Wolstein, D.C.
Chief Executive Officer, Infinite Vitality (Clearwater, FL USA);
David G. Wolstein, M.D.

ABSTRACT

In America, 65% of people are overweight or obese (with obesity at over 30%), and numbers are increasing. Poor eating habits, nutritional deficiencies, lack of exercise, disease, medications, stress, depression and anxiety (causing elevated cortisol levels), blood sugar imbalance (caused by not eating breakfast and high sugar foods), and overeating caused by irregular eating habits are all contributors to weight gain and obesity.

This paper discusses the difficulties facing people who want to lose weight and explains how human chorionic gonadotrophin (HCG) can be a useful aid to weight loss.

Keywords: human chorionic gonadotrophin, HCG, obesity, weight loss, diet

INTRODUCTION

About 8000 years ago (Neolithic times), there was a time when obesity was considered a sign of health and prosperity in man and of beauty and amorousness in women. Before that, with the possible exception of some races, obesity was almost non-existent, as it still is in all wild animals and most primitive races. In America, 65% of people are overweight or obese (with obesity at over 30%), and numbers are increasing.[1] Obesity is defined by the Centers for Disease Control and Prevention (CDC) as having a Body Mass Index (BMI) of 30 or more. An adult with a BMI of 25 to 29.9 is considered overweight.[1] Obesity is increasing for several reasons. While there are some genetic factors involved, there are many environmental influences including eating patterns, inactivity, reliance on care, easy access to food, higher energy density of food, increased consumption of sugar in beverages and hidden in food products, and increased portion sizes. Poor eating habits, nutritional deficiencies, lack of exercise, disease, medications, stress, depression and anxiety (causing elevated cortisol levels), blood sugar imbalance (caused by not eating breakfast and high sugar foods), and overeating caused by irregular eating habits are all contributors to weight gain and obesity.

Many people looking for weight loss options choose to follow a diet. There are many fad diets promoted by celebrities, on TV, and in fashion magazines, which usually promote quick weight loss. These diets invariably have the opposite effect – people may experience some weight loss while following the diet, but as soon as they stop the diet, weight gain occurs. The weight lost, plus extra, is regained,[2] largely due to a slower metabolism caused by muscle loss and the rebound eating pattern after being on an extremely restrictive diet. Consider the typical over-the-counter very low-calorie diet (VLCD). Many have less than 800 calories and studies have shown that about 25% of weight lost on these diets will be from muscle tissue.[3] Low carbohydrate diets which cause ketosis result in loss of water weight and muscle, and cause emotional discomfort due to the ketosis state.[4] Once the diet is over, most people will return to their normal diet and more to make up for the restriction.

In addition to the restrictive nature of these diets, they also slow metabolism by not providing enough of the proper nutrients and calories. Extreme calorie limitation will slow the metabolic rate and cause the body to try to conserve energy. Most weight loss at this point will be from water weight and lean tissue, rather than from fat. When the diet ends, the body is still in conservation mode, creating even more fat cells from any excess in calories.[5]

Rollercoaster dieting, or yo-yo dieting (weight loss and regain as a person diets and stops), will also slow metabolism, causing additional weight gain the more often it occurs, and will hamper weight loss when another diet is attempted in the future.[3] Weight gain will cause an increase in fat cell numbers and an increase in fat cell size. Weight loss, however, will only affect fat cell size. This results in an increase number of fat cells in the body, which are there permanently. Weight loss can occur, but is more difficult the more fat cells there are.

There are three types of fat: structural, normal, and abnormal. Structural fat fills the gaps between various organs, acting as a sort of packing material. It performs important functions, such as bedding the kidneys in soft elastic tissue, protecting the coronary arteries, and keeping the skin smooth and taut. It provides the springy cushion of hard fat under the bones of the feet, without which we would be unable to walk. Normal fat is the normal reserve of fuel upon which the body can freely draw upon when the nutritional income from the intestinal tract is insufficient to meet the demand of the body. Normal fat is a substance that packs the highest caloric value into the smallest space for muscular activity and the maintenance of body temperature. Normal reserves are localized all over the body and fat is most economically stored in this form. Structural and reserve fat are normal and, even if the body stocks them to capacity, this can never be called obesity. Abnormal fat is the accumulation of fat from which the overweight patient suffers and wants to lose (belly, hips. thighs, arms, etc). It is also a potential reserve of fuel but, unlike the normal reserves, it is not available to the body in a nutritional emergency.[6]

When obese patients try to reduce by starving themselves, they will first lose normal fat reserves. When normal fat is exhausted, they begin to burn up structural fat. Lastly, abnormal fat reserves will eventually begin to burn. The obese patient usually feels so weak and hungry that the diet is abandoned. They will complain that they feel famished and tired and their face becomes drawn and haggard, but their belly, hips, thighs and upper arms show little improvement by losing the wrong fat. The fat they have come to detest stays on and the fat they need to cover their bones gets less and less. Their skin wrinkles and they look old and miserable. This is one of the most frustrating and depressing experiences a human being can have.

With so many stimulants to appetite, it becomes a challenge to not overeat. Refined carbohydrates, a staple in many diets, cause a spike in blood sugar levels and satiety, soon followed by a low when insulin is released, and triggering a feeling of hunger a short while after eating. Hunger can also be triggered by the time of day, purely due to the habit of eating at the same time every day. The smell of food, and even just a picture of food, can trigger the release of digestive juices and cause a feeling of hunger. When considering what to eat, it is important to include a variety of flavors in one meal. If the desire for 'sweet' hasn't been met during the meal, it increases the likelihood of 'making room for desert'. Adding a bit of fruit to a salad during dinner may be enough to counteract this desire. Alcohol intake impairs judgment on fullness and can cause overeating. Feeling cold and low body temperature also stimulates appetite, as eating helps to raise body temperature.[7]

In addition, the current economic situation results in less expensive foods being consumed. In the average supermarket, the least expensive foods are often the most refined – cereal, white bread, and pasta – the same carbohydrates which will cause a spike in blood sugar levels and a 'crash' shortly after when insulin is released, causing hunger a short time later. Other cheap foods, which are heavy in fat and sugar, are processed deserts, pre-prepared salads, and other 'convenience' foods.

With obesity on the rise, so are the complications of obesity – heart disease, diabetes, cancer, hypertension, high cholesterol, liver and gallbladder disease, respiratory problems, osteoarthritis, and gynecological problems.[1] There is good reason for overweight individuals to seek weight loss options.

The Consequences of Weight Gain

The consequences of weight gain are many, and include and alteration in hormone levels. Excess weight puts a stress on the body, causing an increase in cortisol levels. Cortisol, the 'stress hormone,' has several physiological affects on the body. Most importantly in the case of weight management, cortisol stimulates glucose production while simultaneously decreasing glucose use by tissues. This causes an increase in appetite and cravings for sweets, as cells are not receiving enough glucose. It also causes an increase in blood sugar levels and if persistent, leads to a blood sugar imbalance. Prolonged, elevated cortisol levels can lead to the development of diabetes mellitus. Excess cortisol levels also cause changes in fat metabolism, increasing fat stored in the abdominal area. Increased cortisol causes changes in other hormones as well, including a decrease in growth hormone (GH), testosterone, dehydroepiandosterone (DHEA), and thyroid hormones (which control metabolism).

GH is necessary for bone growth in children, but also has important metabolic regulation functions in adults. It facilitates the transport of amino acids (proteins) to cells, which is used for energy production and to increase muscle mass. GH increases the rate of fatty acid use for energy, and it has a role in maintaining or increasing blood sugar levels by decreasing the use of glucose for fuel. As a consequence, low GH levels cause increased body fat, decreased muscular mass, and decreased energy levels. Studies show that obese people have deficient levels of GH, making it harder for them to lose weight.[8] Studies have also shown that giving low doses of GH help both men and women lose fat while maintaining lean muscle, while also helping to keep the weight off for longer.

Testosterone levels are also decreased by excess cortisol. The main actions of testosterone in the body, aside from its affects on sexual maturation and function in men, are that it promotes protein metabolism, promotes musculoskeletal growth, and influences subcutaneous fat distribution in both males and females. As males have more testosterone than females, men average 50% more muscle mass than women. This leads to an increased metabolism for men. Deficient testosterone levels will cause decreased energy, muscle mass and strength, and feelings of fatigue, depression, and decreased libido.

DHEA is another hormone affected by cortisol levels and obesity. DHEA is a precursor to testosterone. Studies with DHEA have shown some promise in reducing genetic or diet-induced obesity, and have been shown to target fat loss around the abdomen.[9] In weight loss, research has shown that DHEA stimulates enzymes in the liver responsible for thermogenesis, which will increase calories burned.

The thyroid hormones, triiodothyronine (T3) and thyroxine (T4), control metabolism and protein synthesis in nearly all tissues of the body. Deficient thyroid hormone results in a slower metabolic rate, an elevated cholesterol level, a slow-down in the use of fats from adipose (fat) cells, a slow-down in gastro-intestinal function, and a decrease in muscle tone and reflexes. The overall effect of a hypothyroid state is constipation, fatigue, and weight gain.

Another important hormone to consider in obesity is estrogen. Estrogen also has general metabolic functions in both men and women, including regulating fat storage and hypothalamus function (which is involved in metabolic rate control). In menopause, it is not uncommon to see an increased deposition of abdominal fat with the decrease in estrogen levels.

While weight gain can cause hormone level changes, it's also important to know that this process works the other way as well – changes in hormone levels can cause weight gain. Thus there is a similar impact to these same hormones in the aging process. Aging comes with lean muscle mass decreases, body fat increases (which are more difficult to lose), deposits of fat in the central abdominal region, loss of energy, slowing of metabolism, increased illness and risk of age-related disease. Note the similarity of age-related disease to the complications of obesity – heart disease, cancer, diabetes, osteoporosis, Alzheimer's, and dementia. This is why, depending on age and hormone profile, it is sometimes recommended to add hormone replacement therapy (HRT) to the human chorionic gonadotrophin (HCG) weight treatment plan detailed below.

PERMANENT WEIGHT LOSS – A SOLUTION

There are three areas that need to be addressed to achieve permanent weight loss – proper nutrition and supplementation, exercise, and rebalancing the hormones. These are the keys to optimal health. With proper education and support, diet and exercise can be controlled. Rebalancing hormones, however, is not as straight forward, and may require the inclusion of hormone therapy into the weight loss program.

HCG is the hormone produced during pregnancy that promotes the production of progesterone, which allows the uterus to sustain the growing fetus in early pregnancy. HCG levels are the indicator tested for in a pregnancy test. During the pregnancy, HCG protects and nourishes the fetus through the delivery of nutrition delivered from the mother, obtained from the mother's fat stores.

HCG is also used in other medical treatments. For women, HCG therapy is used to treat infertility. HCG will promote the final maturation of eggs and then stimulate ovulation.[10] For men, HCG can be used for the treatment of hypogonadism, or very low testosterone, as it stimulates the testes to produce more testosterone themselves.[11] To convert HCG into a medicine, it is extracted from the urine of pregnant women, tested in a lab for potency, and a sterilization assay is performed.

The use of HCG for weight-loss works by assisting in the removal of stored fat while sparing lean muscle by forcing the body to rid fat through the body's own natural elimination process. HCG targets the abnormal fat – not the normal or structural fat that is targeted by most starvation and low-calorie diets.

HCG was first suggested for use in weight loss in the 1950's, based on its ability to mobilize nutrition from fat cells in the mother's body. Over 50 years ago, Dr. A.T.W. Simeons, MD began treating obese men and non-pregnant women with small daily doses of HCG while placing them on a diet of only 500 calories daily for 6-weeks. The results were staggering.

These individuals lost an average of about one pound per day. Their skin remained fresh and turgid and, gradually, their figures became more normal. Inches were lost around the belly, hips and thighs. The patients lacked the symptoms one would expect from a patient on a very low-calorie diet. For example, they had no headaches, hunger pangs, cravings, weakness, or irritability as long as the low-calorie diet was combined with HCG.

There have been several studies which show no difference in weight loss between HCG and placebo groups on the same weight loss regimen,[12] however, it is not clear whether these studies focused on the measurement of fat loss.[13,14] A study by Belluscio shows that, while weight loss is similar between the two groups, fat loss is higher in the HCG treatment group. Particularly, when combined with a very low-calorie diet, fat loss was experienced in the abdomen, thighs and buttocks. Eight months on from the trial, more of the HCG treatment patients had maintained their weight loss than the placebo group. In addition to fat loss, HCG patients were also shown to feel less irritable and in a better mood during treatment.[15]

In men, the mechanism for weight loss with HCG is two-fold. In addition to its effect on fat mobilization, HCG exerts an action on the testes to create more testosterone, resulting in an increase in metabolism. Men also have more lean muscle than women, generally, so they tend to lose weight more quickly than women. For women, HCG affects hormone levels though the hypothalamus, increasing metabolism.

With 6-weeks of treatment, women can expect to lose about 25-35 pounds (½ to ¾ pound per day), while men can expect to lose an average of 35-45 pounds over the 40 days of HCG injections (about 1 pound per day). This difference is due to several factors. Women of childbearing age tend to lose more weight (30-35 pounds) due to higher metabolic rate and hormone levels than post menopausal women (25 pounds) and those who have had a surgical hysterectomy. Men, on the other hand, have a higher metabolic rate generally, more lean muscle mass, and experience an increased testosterone production which raises the metabolic rate.

Pharmaceutical HCG is available only by prescription and can be administered in three ways. The subcutaneous injection involves a small amount of HCG being injected into the fatty abdominal tissue via a tiny insulin syringe (¼ inch) daily, for a minimum of 21 days and a maximum of 40. The dosage of this injection is between 125 and 200 IUs per day – the exact amount needs to be determined by the physician monitoring the treatment. Sublingual HCG is recommended for individuals that are severely needle phobic. HCG drops are administered orally, under the tongue for 21 to 40 days. The recommended dosage is between 250 and 400 IUs per day. Another option is transdermal HCG with vitamin B-12 for energy at 400 IUs per day, and can also be used if needle phobic. While the subcutaneous injection is recommended due to its greater absorption rate, the sublingual and trans-dermal options have been shown to be effective and give similar results, albeit at a higher dosage. In all cases, the exact dosage levels need to be determined by the physician monitoring the treatment.

HCG is associated with some side effects, these include: mild headache or exacerbation of migraine headache, mild dizziness, irregular menses, and occasional bruising at injection site. These side effects are reversible by adjusting dosage or stopping therapy. The majority of patients do not experience any side effects at all. Adverse reactions to HCG are very rare (none were reported in any of the studies cited in this paper). However, any adverse reactions (allergic reactions, edema of ankles/feet) should be reported immediately.

Can everyone be treated with HCG? No. HCG should not be given to patients who have heart disease, cancer, polycystic ovary syndrome (PCOS), kidney disease, seizures, or respiratory illnesses such as chronic obstructive pulmonary disease (COPD) and asthma. Pregnant women should not be treated with HCG. HCG decreases the effectiveness of ganirelix acetate (Antagon).

Although weight loss on the dietary protocol described below is possible, there are several benefits to adding HCG to the dietary regimen. Its promotes fat loss, spares lean muscle, targets problem areas on stomach, buttocks, thighs, arms and chest, redistributes fat, increases metabolism by raising hormone levels on a small scale, and decreases cravings for sweets. It has also been shown to decrease irritability associated with very low-calorie diets, decrease appetite and the feeling of hunger, and promote a more general feeling of well-being and less fatigue while on a very restricted regime. Weight loss is maintained even after returning to a regular calorie intake, ending the frustration of rollercoaster dieting.[15,16]

The HCG Protocol

Before starting the HCG diet, blood tests, patient history, and a physical examination need to be performed. Lab work should measure are complete blood count (CBC), complete metabolic panel (CMP), and thyroid hormones (TSH/T3/T4). Additionally, women's HCG and estradiol levels are measured. Men should have their free and total testosterone measured. If HRT is to be added to the treatment, a more comprehensive profile must be obtained (Table 1).

Table 1. Detailed Blood Tests

Complete blood count (CBC) with platelet and differential White blood cell (WBC) count Red blood cell (RBC) count Hemoglobin Hematocrit Mean corpuscular volume (MCV) Mean corpuscular hemoglobin (MCH) Mean corpuscular hemoglobin concentration (MCHC) Red cell distribution width (RDW) Platelet Count Mean platelet volume (MPV) Neutrophils Lymphocytes Monocytes Eosinophils Basophils	Chemical-Screen Glucose Blood urea nitrogen (BUN) Creatinine BUN/creatinine ratio Sodium Potassium Chloride Magnesium Phosphorus Calcium Uric Acid	Protein total serum Albumin Globulin Albumin/Globulin ratio Bilirubin total Bilirubin direct Alkaline phosphatase Gamma-glutamyl transpeptidase (GGTP) Lactate dehydrogenase (LDH) Serum glutamic oxaloacetic transaminase (SGOT) Serum glutamic pyruvic transaminase (SGPT) Iron Iron binding capacity Iron % saturation

To be effective, the four parts of the HCG protocol must be followed. Any deviation from the program will alter the results. The steps are as follows:

- HCG administration daily via chosen method for a minimum of 21 to 40 days;
- Specific food chosen from list provided, 800 calories daily intake;
- Daily exercise, walking or other low impact exercise, 30 minutes;
- Pharmaceutical nutrition and supplement regimen.

Phase 1

To prepare for the HCG diet, the patient should eliminate starches, sweets, fried foods, high fructose corn syrup, MSG, diet drinks and fast food. Alcohol, flavor enhancers, artificial sweeteners, preservatives, herbicides, pesticides, and antibiotics, should be avoided. Organic food is highly recommended. The patient should also begin taking a pharmaceutical grade vitamin and mineral supplement, vitamin B-complex supplement, and omega-3 fatty acids.

Phase 2

The HCG diet formally begins when HCG is taken. It must be taken for at least 21 days for the hypothalamus to re-set the body's metabolic rate. Ideally, and for maximum benefit, treatment should last for 40 days. The patient should also take the recommended dietary supplements for optimum energy and overall health, and follow the food guide, maintaining the 800 calories per day. (The calorie restriction is essential to gaining maximum weight loss). Gentle exercise, such as walking, needs to be incorporated into the daily routine, no more than 30 minutes per day. Resistance or weight training is not recommended as it requires a higher caloric intake. 800 calories per day is recommended by the AMA as the lowest acceptable for weight loss, anything less being dangerous to short-term and long-term health.[3,17] The specific protocol is outlined below.

Phase 3

During the maintenance phase, caloric intake increases to 1500 per day for the 3-weeks after the last injection. While proteins, fruit, and vegetables can be chosen and eaten freely, starchy carbohydrates must be avoided. An increase in exercise, adding resistance training, is recommended. The theory is that fat continues to mobilize for another 3-weeks after the last injection – avoiding starchy carbohydrates will maximize this process and final weight loss results.

Phase 4

Maintaining the weight loss long-term is the goal of the HCG protocol. Once the goal weight is reached, the amount of calories needed per day to maintain that weight can be calculated, for example:

- Female, 140 pounds x 13 = 1820 calories per day to maintain weight;
- Male, 180 pounds x 13 = 2340 calories per day to maintain weight.

In order to maximize caloric intake and keep the weight off, the following recommendations are made:

- Avoid more than 1 serving of starch daily, comprising only whole wheat bread, pasta, sweet potatoes, or multi-grain cereals;
- Limit refined sugar;
- Avoid flavor enhancers and preservatives;
- Drink plenty of water;
- Consume organic food if possible;
- Exercise at least 3-times per week.

Diet of Phase 2 in Detail

Day 1 and 2:

- HCG injection (125-200 IUs) in morning;
- Eat complex carbohydrates (starches) to increase fat stores in preparation for diet. Complex carbohydrates to eat include: whole grain bread, pasta and sweet potatoes (avoid pizza, fried food and sweets).
- Drink at least ½ gallon of bottled or filtered water, tea throughout the day;
- Start "Total Body Colon Cleanse" (2 capsules per day for 7 days);
- Follow phase 1 guidelines regarding drinks and condiments.

Day 3 through 40:

- HCG injections daily;
- Maximum 800 calories intake per day;
- Drink water and tea only;
- Food intake should comprise:
  - Protein: 3 x 4oz servings daily – fish, red meat or breast of chicken, two egg whites;
  - Fruit: 3 servings daily – grapefruit, green apple, orange, strawberries;
  - Salad: 3 servings daily – leaf lettuce, may add tomato, cucumber, and celery;
  - Vegetables: 2-3 cups daily – green vegetables only (spinach, asparagus, green beans, cabbage, broccoli, Brussels sprouts).
- Condiments: Use – apple cider vinegar, stevia, lemon juice, fresh herbs, pepper, fresh garlic, fresh onion cooking spray, organic cooking spray. Do not use - salt, cooking oils, butter or margarine.

Daily Diet

Breakfast (1 protein and 1 fruit):

- Drink plenty of tea and bottled or filtered water;
- Eat: 1 fruit (grapefruit, green apple, orange or 6 strawberries) and 2 egg whites.
- Note: Up to 3 fruits per day can be eaten.

Lunch and dinner (1 protein, 1 fruit, 1 vegetable, and 1 small salad):
- Eat approximately 4-5 oz of protein (about the size of the palm of the hand);
- Use an organic cooking spray (do not use any cooking oils, butter or margarine);
- Choose 1 protein from the following:
  - Red meat – filet mignon (the leanest), top sirloin, organic grass fed beef, buffalo, veal (about 180 calories);
  - Chicken – organic preferred or antibiotic free breast of chicken (skinless), white meat only (about 223 calories) ;
  - White fish – examples include: tilapia, cod, halibut, sea bass, sole, flounder, grouper, canned white tuna (low sodium), shrimp, lobster and crab. Any white fish is acceptable. No Salmon (orange fish).
- Eat 1-1½ cups (1 serving) of cooked vegetables. These can be eaten raw, steamed, grilled (without oil). If it isn't green, don't eat it. Examples include: spinach (41 calories), asparagus (43 calories), green beans (44 calories), cabbage (32 calories), broccoli (43 calories), Brussels sprouts (60 calories).
- A salad may be eaten with the meal. Use organic lettuce, tomatoes, fresh onions, and celery. Toppings: Bragg's Organic Apple Cider Raw Unfiltered Vinegar that contains no fat.

Fruit:
- One of the following fruits should be eaten with each meal (breakfast, lunch and dinner):
  - 1 grapefruit   66 calories
  - 1 green apple   125 calories
  - 6 strawberries   57 calories
  - 1 orange   70 calories

Notes:
- There are no fruit substitutes;
- The same protein, vegetable, or fruit should not be eaten twice in the same day if possible;
- Day 41-42 (optional) – the HCG is still in the system for about 3 days after the last injection administered on day 40. The 800 calorie diet can be followed for these 2 additional days, or Phase 3 Maintenance can begin right away on day 41.

Recommended nutritional supplements:
- Pharmaceutical grade multi-vitamin and minerals: Vitamins and minerals are an essential part of any weight loss program. They help maintain and provide adequate nutrients to the tissues, cells, and vital organs in the body. They also help in maintaining energy levels especially on a low-calorie diet regiment.
- Coenzyme Q10 (CoQ10): A powerful antioxidant carrying compound found in every cell within the human body that plays a key role in energy production. CoQ10 promotes weight loss by increasing the body's metabolism. Studies have also shown that CoQ10 can aid in improving cardiac muscle function, blood pressure regulation, and diabetes control.
- Probiotic
- Omega-3 fatty acids: Eicosapentaenoic acid (EPA) and docosahexaenoic acid (DHA) are found in fish such as tuna, mackerel, sardines, and salmon. Many individuals who are overweight suffer from poor blood sugar control, diabetes, and high cholesterol. Clinical studies suggest that overweight people who follow a weight loss program that includes omega-3 fatty acid supplements tend to achieve better control over their blood sugar and cholesterol levels.[18] Other benefits include: increased energy and memory, reduced cardiac problems, improved circulation, and decreased mood swings and depression.

- Vitamin B-complex (B1, B6, and B12): Vitamin B complex plays a leading role in affecting the rate at which calories are burned. Its powerful action of increasing energy levels will help to promote faster weight loss.
- Super fruits and vegetables: Fruits and vegetables are nutrition powerhouses containing the vitamins, minerals, enzymes, fiber, antioxidants, and protein needed for good health. Studies have shown that increasing the quantity of super fruits and vegetables will help aid in losing weight and decrease cravings.
- Total Body Cleanse: This proprietary blend of natural herbs helps to cleanse and detoxify the digestive system. Excess accumulation of toxins may result in stress, constipation, low energy and strong food cravings. Two capsules daily for 7 days will relieve bloating and constipation, improve immune system, function, assist in weight loss, and detoxify the colon, liver, kidney, lungs, lymphatic system, and skin. Total Body Cleanse should be taken from days 1-7 and days 40-46.
- Adrenal Tea Formula: A blend of proprietary herbal ingredients that improves symptoms of adrenal fatigue, often indicated with cortisol imbalance. It is ideal for weight loss at all ages, promoting immune system function, treating insomnia, reducing physical and environmental stress, and increasing stamina and energy.
- Cleansing Tea (Optional)
- MIC injection (also sublingual available): This injection consists of five nutrients (methionine, inositol, choline, vitamin B12, and chromium) that aid in weight loss while following a low-calorie diet. The recommended dosage is once a week during Phase 2 (active HCG treatment), and once a month during phase 3 (maintenance).

Success Stories
Lost 70 pounds in 12-weeks:

Before   After

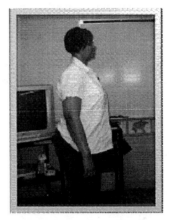 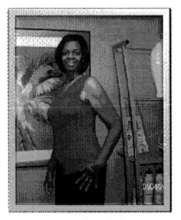

Lost 36 pounds in 40-days:

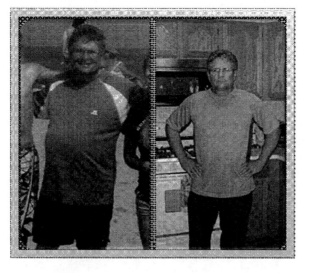

Before   After

Disclaimer and Prescriber Information

The FDA requires physicians that prescribe HCG for the purpose of weight loss to inform their patients the following: "HCG has not been demonstrated to be an effective adjunctive therapy in the treatment of obesity. There is no substantial evidence that it increases weight loss beyond that resulting from caloric restriction, that it causes a more attractive or "normal" distribution of fat, or that it decreases the hunger and discomfort associated with calorie-restricted diets."

REFERENCES

1. Center for Disease Control and Prevention. Obesity and Overweight: Causes and Consequences. Available at: http://www.cdc.gov/obesity/causes/index.html Accessed March 18, 2010.
2. Wadden, TA, Sternberg, JA, Letizia, KA, Stunkard, AJ, Foster, GD. Treatment of obesity by very-low-calorie diet. Behaviour therapy and their combination: a five year perspective *Int J Obes Relat Metab Disord.* 1989;13:39-46.
3. Saris WH. Very-low-calorie diets and sustained weight loss. *Obes Res.* 2001;9 (Suppl 4):295S-301S.
4. Bilsborough SA, Crowe TC. Low-carbohydrate diets: what are the potential short- and long-term health implications? *Asia Pac J Clin Nutr.* 2003;12:396-404.
1. Dieting and the metabolic slowdown. Available at: http://www.weightlossforall.com/metabolic-slowdown.htm Accessed March 18, 2010.
2. Pounds and Inches. (Privately printed, obtainable only from A.T.W. Simeons, Salvator Mundi International Hospital, Rome, Italy.)
3. Kulger J. The Science of Appetite. *Time Magazine* (online). 2007. Available at: http://www.time.com/time/specials/2007/article/0,28804,1626795_1627112_1626670,00.html Accessed March 17, 2010.
4. Kim KR, Nam SY, Song YD, Lim SK, Lee HC, Huh KB. Low-dose growth hormone treatment with diet restriction accelerates body fat loss, exerts anabolic effect and improves growth hormone secretory dysfunction in obese adults. *Horm Res.* 1999;51:78-84.
5. Hansen PA, Han DH, Nolte LA, Chen M, Holloszy JO. DHEA protects against visceral obesity and muscle insulin resistance in rats fed a high-fat diet. *Am J Physiol.* 1997;273(5 Pt 2):R1704-1708.
6. Daya S, Gunby J. Luteal phase support in assisted reproduction cycles. *Cochrane Database Syst Rev.* 2004;3:CD004830. Update in: *Cochrane Database Syst Rev.* 2008;3:CD004830.
7. Porth, C, Matfin G. *Pathophysiology.* Lippincott Williams and Wilkins. 8th Ed. 2009.

8. Lijesen GK, Theeuwen I, Assendelft WJ, Van Der Wal G. The effect of human chorionic gonadotropin (HCG) in the treatment of obesity by means of the Simeons therapy: a criteria-based meta-analysis. *Br J Clin Pharmacol.* 1995;40:237-243.
9. Bradley P. Chorionic gonadotrophin (HCG) and obesity. *Med J Aust.* 1977;2:581.
10. Bradley P. HCG clarification. *Am J Clin Nutr.* 1978;31:3-4.
11. Belluscio, Daniel Oscar, MD, Ripamonte L, Wolansky, M. Utility of an oral presentation of hCG (human Choriogonadotropin) for the management of obesity. Available at: http://www.hcgobesity.org/hcg_obesity_study.htm Accessed March 17, 2010.
12. Asher WL, Harper HW. Effect of human chorionic gonadotrophin on weight loss, hunger, and feeling of well-being. *Am J Clin Nutr.* 1973 Feb;26(2):211-8.
13. Howard AN. The historical development, efficacy and safety of very-low-calorie diets. *Int J Obes.* 1981;5:195-208.
14. Parra D, Ramel A, Bandarra N, Kiely M, Martínez JA, Thorsdottir I. A diet rich in long chain omega-3 fatty acids modulates satiety in overweight and obese volunteers during weight loss. *Appetite.* 2008;51:676-680.

ABOUT THE AUTHOR

Primary author Dr. Brian Wolstein is the Founder/CEO of Infinite Vitality (an exclusive Anti- aging and Rejuvenation Medical Practice that incorporates HRT with diet, nutrition, and exercise), the Founder/CEO of Suncoast Total Healthcare (Multi-Specialty Medical Treatment Centers located throughout the Tampa Bay Area) and the founder/CEO of Vitality Weight-loss centers (specialized weight-loss centers that incorporate weight-loss using HCG and HRT). He has worked with thousands of patients on diet, exercise, and anti-aging. Dr Wolstein received a B.S. in Food Science and Human Nutrition from the University of Florida in Gainesville and a Doctorate of Chiropractic from Life Chiropractic College in Marietta, Georgia.

Chapter 39
A New Approach to Body Fat Reduction by Astaxanthin During Exercise

Eiji Yamashita, Ph.D.

General Manager, Research & Development, Fuji Chemical Industry Co., Ltd.
(Toyama, Japan)

ABSTRACT

Astaxanthin is a naturally occurring carotenoid found in a wide variety of living organisms such as salmon, shrimp, crab, and red snapper. The first study was designed to determine the effect of astaxanthin on endurance capacity in mice. Mice were given orally either vehicle or astaxanthin by stomach intubation for 5 weeks. The astaxanthin group showed a significant increase in swimming time to exhaustion as compared to the control group. Blood lactate concentration in the astaxanthin groups was significantly lower than in the control group. In the control group plasma non-esterified fatty acid (NEFA) levels were decreased by swimming exercise, but in the astaxanthin group NEFA levels were increased with significant differences compared to the control group. Astaxanthin treatment also significantly decreased fat accumulation. These results suggest that improvement in swimming endurance by the administration of astaxanthin is caused by an increase in utilization of fatty acids as an energy source. In a second study we investigated the effects of astaxanthin supplementation in obese mice fed a high-fat diet. Astaxanthin inhibited the increases in body weight and weight of adipose tissue that result from feeding a high-fat diet. In addition, astaxanthin reduced liver weight, liver triglyceride content, plasma triglyceride levels, and total cholesterol levels. The third study was performed to investigate the effects of oral administration of astaxanthin during exercise in obese mice fed a high-fat diet. The suppressive effect on obesity was heightened by combination with exercise. It seems that astaxanthin supplementation may promote lipid metabolism and suppress body fat accumulation. The forth study showed that mitochondrial enzyme activities were elevated by astaxanthin and the activities were more increased by combination of astaxanthin with exercise. The findings of those animal studies were clinically proven by the fifth study; a 6-week long randomized double blind placebo controlled clinical study was performed on 32 healthy women who were divided into two groups, the experimental group (12 mg/day astaxanthin) or the placebo group (0 mg/day astaxanthin). The subjects were instructed to take a walking exercise for 3 times a week according to their own physical strength. After 6 weeks the mean value of body fat percentage was significantly decreased to 26.6% from 27.6% at start with 3.8% reduction in astaxanthin supplemented group compared with no significant difference between before and after supplementation in the placebo. Four weeks after the end of the study, the body fat level returned to the level observed at the start of the study in the experimental group. Based on the studies it is suggested that astaxanthin supplementation might be a practical and beneficial approach for body fat reduction during exercise. We may call the approach "healthy weight management."

Keywords: astaxanthin, anti-fatigue, body fat reduction, weight management, exercise, microalgae, *Haematococcus pluvialis*

INTRODUCTION

Astaxanthin is widely and naturally distributed in marine organisms, including crustacea (shrimps and crabs) and fish (salmon and sea bream). In fact, it is one of the oldest carotenoids to be isolated and identified from the lobster, *Astacus gammarus,* in 1938.[1] Astaxanthin was first commercially used for pigmentation in the aquaculture industry. However, interest in astaxanthin began to grow after the publication of two studies in 1991, which revealed that it possesses potent anti-oxidative properties and has a physiological function as precursor of vitamin A in fish and mammals (rats).[2,3] In 1999, it was reported that astaxanthin does not possess any pro-oxidative properties like β-carotene and lycopene[4] and in 2001, it was found that its potent anti-oxidative property is exhibited at the cell membrane.[5] Astaxanthin has also been found to have anti-inflammatory,[6,7] immunomodulatory[8] and anti-photoaging[9] properties, enhance sport performance and endurance,[10] limit exercise-induced muscle damage,[11] attenuate eye fatigue and improve metabolic syndrome.[12] However there is no study on the relationship between body fat and exercise to date. Here we report four animal studies[13-16] as well as a clinical study[17] to prove the results of animal studies concerning astaxanthin supplementation and aerobic exercise.

The astaxanthin used in all studies is an extract from the microalgae *Haematococcus pluvialis* manufactured by Fuji Chemical Industry Co., Ltd., Toyama, Japan.

STUDY 1: EFFECTS OF ASTAXANTHIN SUPPLEMENTATION ON EXERCISE-INDUCED FATIGUE IN MICE[13]

We designed an animal study to determine the effects of astaxanthin on endurance capacity during swimming as an aerobic physical exercise.

Materials and Methods
Swimming Exercise Test
Four-week-old male ddY mice (SLC, Japan) were allowed to adapt to the laboratory housing for at least 1 week. Forty mice were divided into four groups (n=10 per group). The mice were given either vehicle (olive oil) or astaxanthin in doses of 1.2, 6, or 30 mg/kg body weight by stomach intubation at 10:00 5 d a week for 5 weeks, taking a normal diet (MR stock, NIHON NOUSAN, Japan) and water *ad libitum*. Samples were administrated in a volume of 200 ml. The mice were submitted to weekly swimming exercise supporting constant loads (lead fish sinkers, attached to the tail) corresponding to 10% of their body weight. The mice were assessed to be fatigued when they failed to rise to the surface of the water to breathe within 5 seconds.[18] Another study was performed to compare the effect of astaxanthin (30 mg/kg) to those of other antioxidants such as β-carotene (30 mg/kg), vitamin E (100 mg/kg), and vitamin C (100 mg/kg) under the same condition except for 7.5% of their body weight instead of 10%.

Lactic Acid Build Up and Glucose and Lipid Metabolism During Swimming
The protocol was the same as above except that the mice were made to swim for a predetermined length of time (15 min) supporting loads corresponding to 5% of their body weight. Blood lactate, glucose, and non-esterified fatty acid (NEFA) were measured at 7 times, the beginning and 5-min intervals during swimming exercise as well as 10, 30, and 60 min after exercise after 6 weeks. The following week (at week 7), liver glycogen and adipose tissue weight were measured after the same swimming loads.

Results and Discussion
Effects of Astaxanthin on Swimming Exercise
The 6 mg/kg and 30 mg/kg astaxanthin groups showed a significant increase in swimming time to exhaustion as compared to the control group from the first week. In the 1.2 mg/kg astaxanthin group, a significant increase in swimming time to exhaustion as compared to the control group was evident after 5 weeks (Fig. 1). The significant increase was found in only astaxanthin supplemented group among antioxidant groups such as β-carotene and vitamin E and C (Fig. 2).

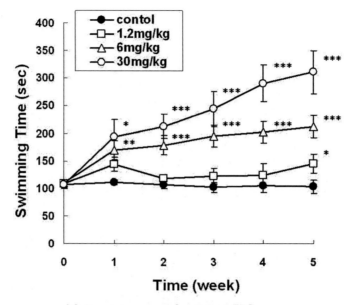

Each value represents mean ± SE.
* : $p < 0.05$, ** : $p < 0.01$, *** : $p < 0.005$ vs. control

Figure 1.   Effects of Astaxanthin on Swimming Exercise

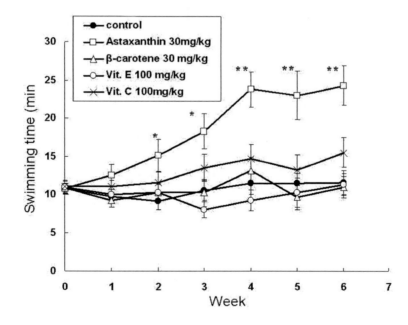

Each value represents mean ± SE. * : $p < 0.05$, * * : $p < 0.01$ vs. control

Figure 2.   Effects of Antioxidants on Swimming Exercise

Effects of Astaxanthin on Lactic Acid Build Up and Glucose and Lipid Metabolism During Swimming

In the astaxanthin groups, blood lactate levels were significantly lower than in the control group (Fig. 3). In the control group, plasma glucose was decreased by 15 min of swimming exercise. After the exercise the plasma glucose was recovered. However, in the astaxanthin 6 mg/kg, 30 mg/kg groups, plasma glucose levels were significantly higher than in the control group. Liver glycogen contents were decreased by swimming exercise. However, liver glycogen contents were significantly higher in the astaxanthin 30 mg/kg groups than in the control group after swimming for 15 min (Fig. 4). Astaxanthin supplementation had no effect on glycogen concentration in the liver (data not shown). As shown in Fig. 5 in the control group, plasma NEFA concentration was decreased by 15 min of swimming exercise. In the astaxanthin 30 mg/kg group, plasma NEFA was significantly increased by swimming exercise. In the 30 mg/kg astaxanthin group, epididymal adipose tissue weight was significantly ($p<0.05$) decreased compared to that of the control group. In the astaxanthin 1.2 mg/kg and 6 mg/kg groups, the epididymal adipose tissue weight tended to be lower than in the control group, but not significantly. However there was no significant difference in body weight between the control group and astaxanthin groups for 5 weeks (control: 42.1 ± 1.0 g, astaxanthin 1.2 mg/kg: 42.9 ± 1.1 g, 6 mg/kg: 42.3 ± 1.2 g, 30 mg/kg: 42.3 ± 1.2 g).

These results indicate that astaxanthin showed anti-fatigue effect enhancing lipid metabolism rather than glucose metabolism.

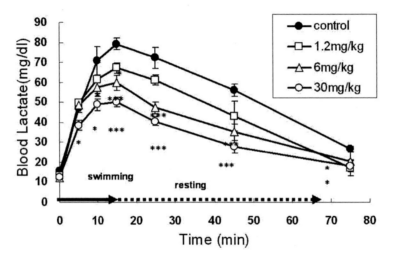

Each value represents mean ± SE. * : p < 0.05 *** : p < 0.005 vs. control

Figure 3.   Effects of Astaxanthin on Lactic Acid Build Up During Swimming.

Blood glucose at week 6

Liver glycogen at week 7

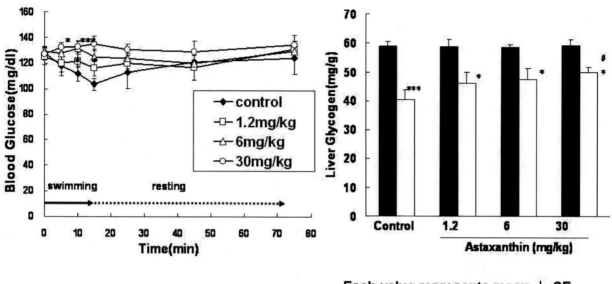

Each value represents mean ± SE.
*: $p < 0.05$ ***: $p < 0.005$ vs. control

Each value represents mean ± SE.
*: $p < 0.05$ ***: $p < 0.005$ vs. pre exercise
#: $p < 0.05$ vs. control (post exercise)

Figure 4. Effects of Astaxanthin on Glucose Metabolism During Swimming

Blood free fatty acid at week 6

Adipose tissue weight at week 7

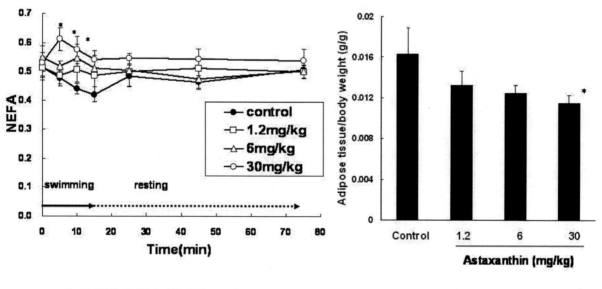

Each value represents mean ± SE.
*: $p < 0.05$ vs. control

Each value represents mean ± SE.
*: $p < 0.05$ vs. control

Figure 5. Effects of Astaxanthin on Lipid Metabolism During Swimming

STUDY 2: EFFECTS OF ASTAXANTHIN IN OBESE MICE FED A HIGH-FAT DIET[14]

We designed a second study to evaluate the effects of astaxanthin on body fat accumulation in mice fed a high-fat diet.

Materials and Methods

Female ddY mice (4 weeks old) were used. After receiving a standard laboratory diet (Oriental Yeast Tokyo, Japan) and water *ad libitum* for 1 week, they were divided into five groups (*n*=8 per group) matched for body weight, one for normal, and the others for high-fat diet. The composition of normal and high-fat diet is shown in Table 1. The high-fat diet fed mice were given either vehicle (olive oil) or astaxanthin in doses of 1.2, 6, or 30 mg/kg body weight by stomach intubation for 60 d for each group. Samples were administrated in a volume of 200 ml. The body weight and the amount of food intake were measured every three days. The weights of adipose tissue and liver, liver triglyceride content and blood triglyceride and cholesterol levels were also measured after 60 d.

Table 1.   Composition of Normal and High-fat Diet

		(g/kg)
	Normal	High-fat
Casein	140	140
Beef fat	40	400
β-Corn starch	465.692	105.692
α-Corn starch	155	155
Sugar	100	100
Cellulose	50	50
Mineral mix	35	35
Vitamin mix	10	10
L-Cystine	1.8	1.8
Choline hydrogen tartrate	2.5	2.5
t-Butylhydroquinone	0.008	0.008

Results and Discussion
Change in Body Weight

Figure 6 shows the changes in body weight during the experiments. The high-fat diet remarkably and significantly increased the body weight compared to the normal diet. However, 6 and 30 mg/kg astaxanthin supplementation significantly reduced the increase in the body weight induced by the high-fat diet. Astaxanthin supplementation did not affect food intake among high-fat diet groups (data not shown).

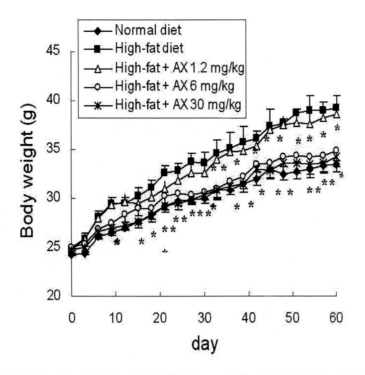

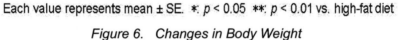

Each value represents mean ± SE. *: $p < 0.05$ **: $p < 0.01$ vs. high-fat diet

Figure 6.   Changes in Body Weight

Weights of Adipose Tissue and Liver, Liver Triglyceride Content, and Blood Triglyceride and Cholesterol Levels

The weights of adipose tissue and liver, liver triglyceride content, and blood triglyceride and cholesterol levels in the high-fat diet group without astaxanthin were significantly higher than those in the normal diet group after 60 days. Astaxanthin supplementation suppressed the increase with a dose dependent manner (Fig. 7, 8 and 9).

These results indicate that astaxanthin supplementation inhibited body fat accumulation in high-fat diet fed mice.

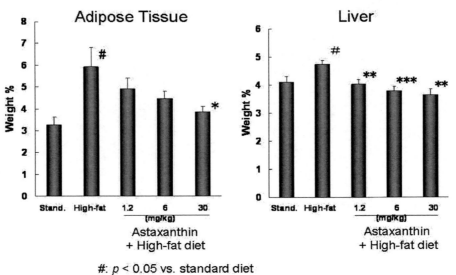

#: $p < 0.05$ vs. standard diet
*: $p < 0.05$, **: $p < 0.01$, ***: $p < 0.005$ vs. high-fat diet

Figure 7. Weights of Adipose Tissue and Liver

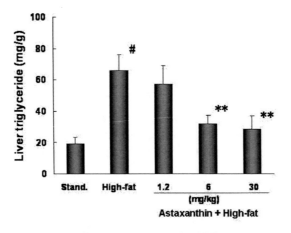

#: p < 0.05 vs. standard **: p < 0.05 vs. high-fat

Figure 8. Liver Triglyceride Content

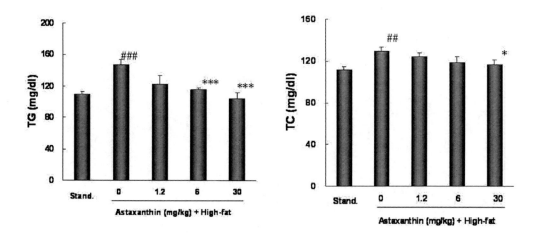

p < 0.05 vs. normal diet *: p < 0.05, ***: p<0.005 vs. high-fat diet

Figure 9. Blood Triglyceride and Cholesterol Levels

STUDY 3: EFFECTS OF ASTAXANTHIN AND EXERCISE, PROMOTING ENERGY METABOLISM AND SUPPRESSING BODY FAT ACCUMULATION[15]

We designed a third study to investigate the effects of astaxanthin during exercise on body fat accumulation in mice fed a high-fat diet.

Materials and Methods

This study was basically performed under the same manner as study 2 described above. Female ddY mice (4 weeks old) were used. After receiving a standard laboratory diet (Oriental Yeast Tokyo, Japan) and water *ad libitum* for 1 week, they were divided into two groups, sedentary and exercise groups, matched for body weight. Each group was further divided into five sub-groups (*n*=8 per group), one for normal and the others for high-fat diet. The composition of normal and high-fat diet is shown in Table 1. The high-fat diet fed mice in sedentary and exercise groups were given either vehicle (olive oil) or astaxanthin in doses of 1.2, 6, or 30 mg/kg body weight by stomach intubation for 60 d, individually. In addition, the mice in the exercise group had a treadmill exercise with a constant speed (20 m/min, 40min) every day for 60 d. The body weight and the amount of food intake were measured every three days. The weights of adipose tissue and liver, liver triglyceride content and blood triglyceride and cholesterol levels were also measured after 60 d.

Results and Discussion
Change in Body Weight

In the sedentary group the same results as study 2 were observed as shown in Figure 10. In the exercise group even 1.2 mg/kg astaxanthin supplementation significantly reduced the increase in the body weight induced by the high-fat diet while no suppressive effect of exercise on body weight increase was found in the normal diet sub-group of exercise group compared to that of sedentary group (Fig. 10).

Weights of Adipose Tissue and Liver, Liver Triglyceride Content, and Blood Triglyceride and Cholesterol Levels

A similar tendency to body weight was observed, and the same results as study 2 were also found (data not shown).

These results indicate that astaxanthin supplementation promoted the energy metabolism and suppressed body fat accumulation.

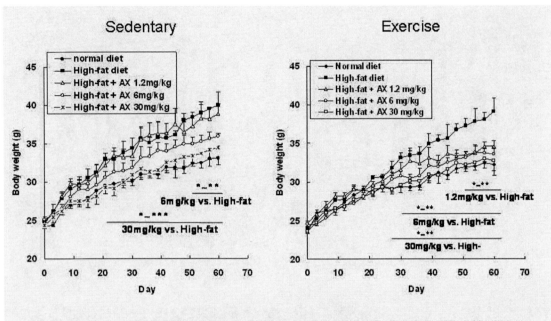

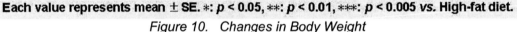

Each value represents mean ± SE. ∗: *p* < 0.05, ∗∗: *p* < 0.01, ∗∗∗: *p* < 0.005 *vs.* High-fat diet.

Figure 10.   Changes in Body Weight

STUDY 4: EFFECTS OF ASTAXANTHIN AND EXERCISE ON MITOCHONDRIAL ENZYMES IN MICE[16]

We designed an animal study to elucidate the action mechanisms of suppressive effects of astaxanthin combined with exercise on body fat accumulation.

Materials and Methods

Male ddY mice were divided into two groups matched for body weight. They were divided into the sedentary and exercise group. Each group was further sub-grouped according to the normal diet group, high-fat diet group and high-fat diet plus astaxanthin 6 mg/kg (*n*=10). The mice were given either the vehicle (olive oil) or astaxanthin in doses of 6 mg/kg body weight by stomach intubation for 60 days. Exercise training of the mice was performed using a treadmill with a constant speed (20 m/min, 40 min) three times for week. Running time was increased gradually from 15 min by 5min daily for 5 day. From 5th day running time was fixed to 40 min. On the final day of an experiment, assays for citrate synthase (1), succinate dehydrogenase (2), and 3-hydroxyacyl Co A dehydrogenase (3) were performed.

Results and Discussion

(1) and (2) activities were elevated by high-fat diet or exercise and those in the high-fat plus astaxanthin group tended to be higher in the high-fat only without significant difference as shown in Fig. 11. (3) activity was also elevated by high-fat diet or exercise. In the either sedentary or exercise condition, in the high-fat plus astaxanthin group it was higher than that in the high-fat diet alone (Fig. 12). It was found from the results that mitochondrial enzyme activities were elevated by astaxanthin supplementation and the activities were furthermore increased by combination of astaxanthin and exercise.

The action mechanism of body fat accumulation suppression by astaxanthin supplementation seems to be to accelerate the β-oxidation-mediated fatty acid oxidation.

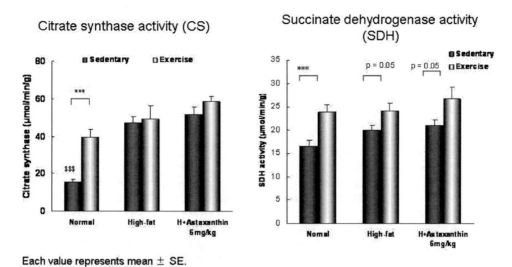

Citrate synthase activity (CS)

Succinate dehydrogenase activity (SDH)

Each value represents mean ± SE.

***: $p < 0.005$. $$$: $p < 0.005$ vs. High-fat (Sedentary)

Figure 11. Effects of Astaxanthin During Exercise on Mitochondrial Enzymes-1

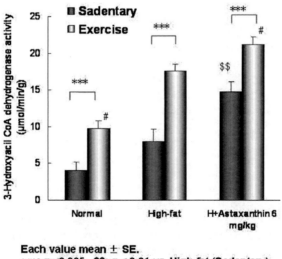

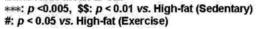

Each value mean ± SE.
***: $p < 0.005$, $$: $p < 0.01$ vs. High-fat (Sedentary)
#: $p < 0.05$ vs. High-fat (Exercise)

Figure 12. Effects of Astaxanthin During Exercise on Mitochondrial Enzymes-2

STUDY 5: ASTAXANTHIN SUPPLEMENTATION AND AEROBIC EXERCISE[17]

We designed a randomized double blind placebo controlled clinical study to substantiate the findings from the former animal studies.

Materials and Methods

The astaxanthin was formulated into a soft gel capsule containing 6 mg astaxanthin and given to the experimental group. For the control group, the identical capsule containing 0 mg astaxanthin was used as a placebo. The study subjects were healthy women aged between 23 and 60 years, selected from those who provided their consent to participate in this study. The 32 selected subjects included tennis club members, sports coaches, and nurses. They were randomly divided into the two groups of 16 participants each for the experimental group and placebo group. The study was under double blind condition. The participants were instructed to take 2 capsules of active supplement (astaxanthin 2 x 6 mg) or identical placebo capsules (astaxanthin 0 mg) after dinner each day for 6 weeks. To assess the health status, all participants underwent a medical examination by a physician at the beginning (week 0) and at the end of the study (week 6) as well as at 4 weeks after the end of the study (week 10); in this examination, blood samples were collected and subjected to hematological and biochemical tests (tested at the clinical laboratory of Suzuka Kaisei Hospital).

Motor function was assessed with an Aeromonitor AE-300S (Minato Medical Science Co., Ltd.,), which consisted of a treadmill (auto-runner AR-200), a respiratory metabolism measuring system (Aeromonitor AE-300S), and an automated sphygmomanometer (EBP-300). Blood lactate levels were measured with a simplified blood lactate test meter (Lactate Pro, Arkray Inc.), and body weight and body fat percentage were measured with a weight scale (TBF-511, Tanita Corp.). At the time of measurement, prior to treadmill exercise, the participants underwent an electrocardiogram and measurements for blood pressure (at rest), body weight, and body fat percentage, and their blood samples were collected for blood tests. Immediately before the motor function test, the blood lactate level (blood lactate level taken before exercise) was measured using the simplified blood lactate test meter, and an exercise test was then performed. We used an all-out exercise test according to the Bruce protocol, with increasing treadmill speed and the tilt angle. Immediately after the participants finished the all-out treadmill test, the blood lactate level (blood lactate level taken after exercise) was measured using the simplified blood lactate test meter. This was performed at week 0 and week 6. During the first 6 week study period, all participants were asked to walk as part of an exercise routine, and the amount of walking was decided according to the percent maximum heart rate of each participant. The participants were instructed to take a 40-min continuous walk 3 times per week at 60–70% of the maximum heart rate for those whose maximum oxygen uptake was 40 ml/(kg·min) or greater and at 50–60% of the maximum heart rate for those whose maximum oxygen uptake was less than 40 ml/(kg·min). The compliance with the instructions for the walking exercise, the ingestion of active supplement or placebo capsules as well as the ingestion of other supplements or drugs, and the health status of the participants were monitored through the weekly submission of a self-monitoring diary maintained by the participants.

A paired t test was used to compare the data of each group obtained at weeks 0, 6, and 10. An unpaired t test was used to compare the 2 groups.

Results and Discussion

No significant difference was found between the 2 groups in average age and body height and in body weight measured at week 0. When average exercise duration for the all-out test for motor function measurements was compared between the times measured at weeks 0 and 6, a slight increase was observed at week 6 in both groups, although the difference was not statistically significant. Moreover, average exercise duration measured at week 6 was not significantly different between the 2 groups. Comparison of the measurements taken at weeks 0 and 6 revealed no significant difference in the average body weight (Table 2), blood pressure, and body mass index of the 2 groups.

Table 2. Supplementation effects of astaxanthin with exercise on body weight (kg)

	Start	6 weeks	10 weeks
Astaxanthin	55.7±5.3	55.5±5.1	55.6±5.4
Placebo	54.3±6.1	54.4±6.3	54.3±6.6

With regard to the body fat percentage, the average body fat percentage of the experimental group decreased from 27.6% to 26.6%. This was a significant reduction of 3.8%. The average body fat at week 10 was 27.4%, which was very close to the value observed at week 0. In the placebo group, the average body fat percentage values at weeks 0, 6, and 10 were 26.6%, 26.8%, and 26.2%, respectively, with no significant difference among the values (Fig. 13).

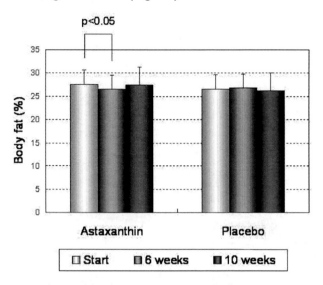

Figure 13. Supplementation Effects of Astaxanthin with Exercise on Body Fat

Motor function was measured by the treadmill all-out test at weeks 0 and 6; the blood lactate level was simultaneously measured before and two minutes after the exercise ceased. At week 0, the blood lactate level taken before exercise was 1.7 ± 0.6 and 2.2 ± 0.9 mmol/l in the experimental and control groups, respectively, and no significant difference was observed between the groups. Moreover, the blood lactate level taken after exercise was 7.4 ± 1.7 and 8.3 ± 2.6 mmol/l in the experimental and control groups, respectively, and no significant difference was observed between the groups (Table 3). On the other hand, when the increase in the blood lactate levels from pre-treadmill to post-treadmill was compared, the increase observed at week 6 was generally higher than that observed at week 0 in both groups. However, no significant difference was found between the increase in the blood lactate level observed at weeks 0 and 6 in the astaxanthin group, whereas the increase observed at week 6 was significantly higher than that observed at week 0 in the control group (Fig. 14). Moreover, the pre-treadmill blood lactate levels observed at week 6 were significantly lower than those observed at week 0 in both the astaxanthin group and control groups, thereby showing the effect of exercise (Table 3).

Table 3. Supplementation Effects of Astaxanthin with Exercise on Blood Lactate Level (Mg/Dl)

	Start		6 weeks	
	Pre	Post	Pre	Post
Astaxanthin	1.7 ± 0.6	7.2 ± 2.6	$1.2\pm0.5^*$	7.5 ± 1.7
Placebo	2.2 ± 1.0	7.3 ± 2.2	$1.2\pm0.4^*$	8.3 ± 2.7

* $p<0.05$ vs. start

357

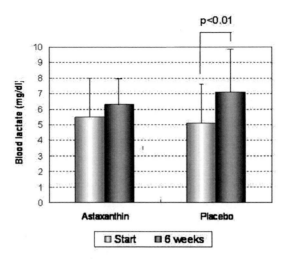

p<0.01

Figure 13. Supplementation Effects of Astaxanthin with Exercise on Blood Lactate Build Up (Each Value Mean the Difference from Pre- to Post-Treadmill Exercise)

All participants underwent a medical examination by a physician at weeks 0, 6, and 10, during which their blood samples were analyzed. Although statistically significant differences were observed in the values of some parameters included in the medical examination at weeks 0 and 6, the difference was considered to be inconsequential (data not shown).

Recent advances in exercise physiology have prompted many studies on the relationship between ingestion of substances that can physiologically influence motor function and their degree of influence on motor function. The generation of active oxygen associated with energy expenditure during exercise is considered to have a great influence on motor function and functional recovery. Elucidation of the relationship of antioxidants that neutralize active oxygen to motor function and prevention or healing of skeletal muscle damage is probably a very important research theme. In the present study, the supplementation effects of astaxanthin, a powerful antioxidant, under exercise stress in daily life were assessed.

Astaxanthin supplementation seemed to contribute to the reduction of body fat, and a significant body fat reduction was observed between weeks 0 and 6 in the experimental group that performed routine walking exercise and received astaxanthin. In contrast, a similar body fat reduction was not observed in the placebo group that performed routine walking exercise alone. Moreover, in both groups, there was no change in body weight between weeks 0 and 6. Thus, it was suggested that astaxanthin supplementation combined with regular aerobic exercise accelerated body fat loss. In the all-out test for motor function measurements, pre-treadmill and post-treadmill blood lactate levels were measured and compared; there was a significant increase in the blood lactate level in the placebo group, whereas the increase in the astaxanthin group was small and statistically insignificant. Thus, combination of astaxanthin with aerobic exercise effectively accelerated the burning of body fat. Further studies are necessary to evaluate the effects of antioxidants in sports that require high energy expenditure in the body.

CONCLUDING REMARKS

Based on the studies it's suggested that astaxanthin supplementation might be a practical and beneficial approach for body fat reduction during exercise. We may call the approach "healthy weight management."

REFERENCES

1. Kuhn R, Sorensen NA. *Ber Deut Bot Ges*. 1938;71:1879.
2. Miki W. Biological functions and activities of animal carotenoids. *Pure & Appl Chem*. 1991;63:141-146.
3. Matsuno T. Xanthophylls as precursors of retinoids. *Pure & Appl Chem*. 1991;63:81-88.
4. Martin HD, Ruck C, Schmidt M, Sell S, Beutner S, Mayer B, Walsh R. Chemistry of carotenoid oxidation and free radical reactions. *Pure & Appl Chem*. 1999;71:2253-2262.

5. Goto S, Kogure K, Abe K, Kimata K, Kitahama K, Yamashita E, Terada H. *Biochimica et Biophysica Acta.* 2001;1515:251-258.
6. Lee SJ, Bai SK, Lee KS, Namkoong S, Na HJ, Ha KS, Han JA, Yim SV, Chang K, Kwon YG, Lee SK, Kim YM. *Mol Cells.* 2003;16:97-105.
7. Suzuki Y, Ohgami K, Shiratori K, Jin XH, Ilieva I, Koyama Y, Yazawa K, Yoshida K, Kase S, Ohno S. *Exp Eye Res.* 2006;82:275-281.
8. Jyonouchi H, Zhang L, Tomita Y. *Nutr Cancer.* 1993;19:269-280.
9. Yamashita E. *Anti-Aging Therapeutics* 2009;11, *in press.*
10. Sawaki K, Yoshigi H, Aoki K, Koikawa N, Azumane A, Kaneko K, Yamaguchi M. *Therap & Med.* 2002;18:73-88.
11. Aoi W, Naito Y, Sakuma K, Kuchide M, Tokuda H, Maoka T, Toyokuni S, Oka S, Yasuhara M, Yoshikawa T. *Antioxid Redox Signal.* 2003;5:139-144.
12. Yamashita E. *Anti-Aging Therapeutics* 2008;10:293-306.
13. Ikeuchi M, Koyama T, Takahashi J, Yamzawa K. *Biol. Pharm. Bull.* 2006;29:,2106-2110.
14. Ikeuchi M, Koyama T, Takahashi J, Yamzawa K. *Biosci. Biotechnol. Biochem.* 2007;71:893-899.
15. Ikeuchi M, Koyama T, Takahashi J, Yamzawa K. *The 21st Annual Meeting on Carotenoid Research* 2007, Osaka, p17.
16. Ikeuchi M, Koyama T, Takahashi J, Yamzawa K. *The 22nd Annual Meeting on Carotenoid Research* 2008, Okinawa, p4.
17. Fukamauchi M. *FOOD Style 21* 2007;11:1-4.
18. Ikeuchi M, Nishimura T, Yazawa K. *J Nutr Sci Vitaminol.* 2005;51:40-44.

ABOUT THE AUTHOR

Dr. Eiji Yamashita is the Global Research & Development Manager for Fuji Chemical Industry Co., Ltd. He completed a pre-doctoral fellowship at the University of Texas Health Science Center and received his Ph.D. from the University of Tokushima. Yamashita's research experience and scientific contributions span nearly 20 years in the study of carotenoids and antioxidants.

Chapter 40
Eye Fatigue (Asthenopia) Relief by Astaxanthin

Eiji Yamashita, Ph.D.

General Manager, Research & Development, Fuji Chemical Industry Co., Ltd.

(Toyama, Japan)

ABSTRACT

Astaxanthin is a naturally occurring carotenoid in a wide variety of living organisms such as salmon, shrimp, crab, and red snapper. Approximately 90% of the astaxanthin in krill is found in the eye. Asthenopia, or eye fatigue, is an ophthalmological condition with nonspecific symptoms such as eye pain, eye strain, blurred vision, headache, and shoulder stiffness. Symptoms often occur after reading, computer work, or other activities that involve visual display terminals (VDT). More recently, the advances of information technology (IT), software, and electronics have led to the widespread and habitual use of VDT resulting in higher visual fatigue complains and more sufferers. There is, however, no effective therapeutic approach to date. Eye fatigue is usually caused by straining the ciliary body, the eye muscle responsible for accommodation. We previously reported a randomized double-blind placebo controlled study using VDT workers (n=25 treated vs. 23 placebo). 6mg/day astaxanthin supplementation for 4-weeks significantly improved eye fatigue measuring ocular accommodation by the objective instrument and subjective individual assessment. Here we report further 4 clinical studies with the different measurements and an animal study. The same source of astaxanthin, extract derived from the microalgae *Haematococcus pluvialis,* was used for all of the studies. The first clinical study was performed under randomized double-blind placebo controlled cross-over conditions using 10 healthy subjects. After a 20-minute near visual task, accommodation contraction and relaxation times were extended in both the astaxanthin and placebo groups. However, accommodation relaxation time in the placebo was significantly longer than in the astaxanthin group, and accommodative contraction and relaxation times after a 10-minute rest in the placebo were also significantly longer those in the astaxanthin group. In the second study, the effects of astaxanthin on accommodative recovery derived from a rest after VDT work were studied using 10 healthy volunteers. 6mg/day astaxanthin supplementation for 2-weeks led to a significant relief in accommodative fatigue induced by 30-minutes of IT work (Nintendo Game Boy). In the third study, 22 middle-aged and elder subjects (mean age: 53.9 years) with complaints of eye strain received 6mg/day astaxanthin. Results showed that the pupillary constriction ratio at week 4 was significantly increased compared to that at week 0. The forth clinical study, using 10 healthy subjects, was performed to investigate the effects of visual fatigue on reaction times. Visual fatigue significantly increases reaction time; however 6 mg/day astaxanthin supplementation for 4-weeks was shown to significantly decrease reaction time. We also investigated the intraocular pharmacokinetics of astaxanthin in an albino rabbit. After 100mg/kg astaxanthin administration in a single dose, astaxanthin was detected in the ciliary body as well as the serum at T_{max} of 24h and 9h and C_{max} of 79.3ng/g and 61.3ng/ml, respectively. Based on the studies it is suggested that astaxanthin supplementation might be a practical and beneficial approach for eye fatigue relief.

Keywords: astaxanthin, eye fatigue, asthenopia, accommodation, ciliary body, microalgae, *Haematococcus pluvialis*

INTRODUCTION

Astaxanthin is widely and naturally distributed in marine organisms, including Crustacea (shrimps and crabs) and fish (salmon and sea bream). In fact, it is one of the oldest carotenoids to be isolated and identified – from the lobster *Astacus gammarus* in 1938.[1] Astaxanthin was first commercially used for pigmentation in the aquaculture industry. However, interest in astaxanthin began to grow after the publication of two studies in 1991, which revealed that it possesses potent anti-oxidative properties and has a physiological function as precursor of vitamin A in fish and mammals (rats).[2,3] In 1999, it was reported that astaxanthin does not possess any pro-oxidative properties like β-carotene and lycopene[4] and in 2001, it was found that its potent anti-oxidative property is exhibited at the cell membrane.[5] Astaxanthin has also been found to have anti-inflammatory,[6,7] immunomodulatory[8] and anti-photoaging[9] properties, enhance sport performance and endurance,[10] limit exercise-induced muscle damage,[11] improve metabolic syndrome,[12] and promote body fat reduction during exercise.[13] Regarding eye health, we previously reported a randomized double-blind placebo controlled study using VDT workers (n=25 treated vs. 23 placebo). 6mg/day astaxanthin supplementation for 4-weeks significantly improved eye fatigue measuring ocular accommodation by the objective instrument and subjective individual assessment.[12] Here we report further 4 clinical studies[14-17] and an animal study.[18]

The astaxanthin used in all studies is an extract from the microalgae *Haematococcus pluvialis* manufactured by Fuji Chemical Industry Co., Ltd., Toyama, Japan.

STUDY 1: EFFECTS OF ASTAXANTHIN ON EYESTRAIN INDUCED BY ACCOMMODATIVE DYSFUNCTION[14]

We designed a randomized double-blind placebo controlled cross-over clinical study to confirm the suppressive effects of astaxanthin on eye fatigue.

Materials and Methods
Subjects

The test materials, study method and other related matters were explained sufficiently to healthy women between the ages of 18-21 years old (average age 20.5 years old) who did not have a previous history or illness that might affect the study. Ten individuals who gave their written consent to participation in the study were selected. Mean values for objective spherical equivalents obtained by autorefractometer in a pre-examination prior to supplementation were -0.34D for the right eye and -0.16D for the left eye, and corrected visual acuity for all subjects for both eyes was 1.0 or higher (decimal visual acuity value). In an accommodation examination, using an infrared optometer (AR3-SV6, Nidek Co., Ltd.), accommodation step response and quasi-static accommodation were also excellent. All subjects were able to clearly recognize three-dimensional images (details are described below) formed by the random-dots stereogram (RDS) used in the experiment, without the occurrence of diplopia with any figure. The hole-in-card test was used to determine the dominant eye of each subject.

Study Design

Two kinds of softgel capsules were used for the study: soft capsules containing 3 mg of astaxanthin and identical placebo capsules not containing astaxanthin. The subjects took two capsules per day after dinner for 14-days. On the 14th day only, the subjects were required to take the capsules after breakfast or after lunch before the tests.

A visual load test was conducted twice, once after astaxanthin supplementation and once after placebo supplementation. The order of supplementation for the group that took the astaxanthin first and the group that took the placebo first was divided randomly for five subjects each by the controller, and a double-blind crossover technique was utilized and the order effects offset based on the supplementation order. The interval between the first load test and the second load test was considered an astaxanthin washout period, and was at least 14-days (Fig. 1).

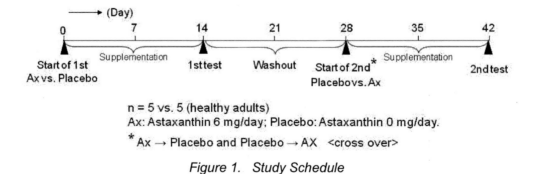

n = 5 vs. 5 (healthy adults)
Ax: Astaxanthin 6 mg/day; Placebo: Astaxanthin 0 mg/day.

*Ax → Placebo and Placebo → AX   <cross over>

Figure 1.   Study Schedule

The visual load test flow is shown in Fig. 2. After the subjects arrived at the test center, they were allowed to rest for 5-minutes in a sitting position in a relaxation room, and then conducted to the test room where ocular accommodation was measured and a subjective symptom survey concerning eyestrain was conducted. A visual load was then applied for 20-minutes. Immediately after termination of the visual load, ocular accommodation was measured again and the subjective symptom survey was repeated. In addition, after measurements following application of the visual load were completed, the subjects moved again to the relaxation room and were given a 10-minute rest. Afterwards, the subjects were again transferred to the test room, and ocular accommodation measurements were taken and the subjective symptoms survey conducted. The value obtained before the load was labeled the Pre value, the value obtained after termination of the visual load was labeled the Post value and the value obtained after ten minutes of rest was labeled the Rest value.

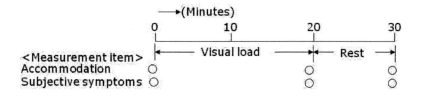

Figure 2. Visual Load Test Process

Visual Load

Visual load was applied using the following method,[19,20] by which an increase in complaints of visual fatigue, as well as accommodative dysfunction, have been clearly determined. A monochrome RDS was shown on a parallax barrier 3D display monitor (THD-10PN3, Sanyo), which subjects perceived as a solid image. Specifically, three RDS figures were prepared: a circle, a square and an equilateral triangle, with the horizontal visual angle set at 4.5°. By utilizing 1.0° of parallax in the intersection property, the subjects were made to perceive these figures as emerging quickly from the center of the 3D display and approaching the subjects. The viewing distance between the 3D display and the subjects was 50 cm. The total visual load period was set at 20-minutes, and during this interval, the circle, square, and equilateral triangle forms were displayed individually and randomly at 5-second intervals. The subjects were instructed to click their computer mouse whenever they perceived a circle figure.

Measurements

Ocular accommodation was checked by measuring the accommodation step response of each subject's dominant eye using the infrared optometer described above. The accommodative stimulation for step response was set at 3D, and as the near target and far target presentation time, stimulation was applied 5-times alternately for 5-seconds for each target. Subjects were instructed to immediately look directly at whichever target appeared on the display, and to maintain their direct viewing condition. The target shape was a star burst at a visual angle of 3° in the optometer. Positive accommodation time (t_1) and negative accommodation time (t_2) were measured from the step response wave shapes obtained (Fig. 3). Positive accommodation time was assumed to be the period from the time the near target was presented until the time when accommodation response ended, and negative accommodation time was assumed to be the period from the time the far target was presented until the time when accommodation response ended.

363

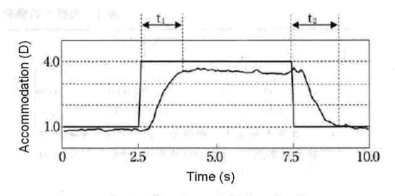

t_1; Contraction time, t_2; Relaxation time

Figure 3.   Accommodation Step Response

Subjective symptoms related to the subjects' eyes were investigated using the standardized questionnaire scoring method.[20, 21] The following 15 items were selected as the subjective symptom items: (1) eye fatigue, (2) eye pain, (3) eye heaviness (4) blurred vision, (5) dim eyesight, (6) double vision, (7) hot eyes, (8) eye dryness, (9) eye tearing, (10) eye irritation, (11) eye itchiness, (12) eyelid twitching, (13) excessive brightness, (14) unusual color vision, and (15) headaches. Five steps were used for the score method, with numerical values assigned to the steps describing the subjects' level of agreement for each item: 1. I do not have this feeling at all; 2. I have this feeling a little; 3. I have this feeling; 4. I have this feeling somewhat strongly; 5. I have this feeling very strongly. To avoid leading the subjects in the subjective symptoms survey, examination interviews were not conducted, and the surveys were completed by having the subjects themselves circle the number of the response corresponding most closely to their present condition.

For the Pre-and Post-values for positive accommodation time, negative accommodation time and subjective symptoms, a paired t-test (two-tailed) was performed for the differences between Pre-and Post-values for the astaxanthin (Ax) group and the placebo (P) group and the Rest value group. A p-value <0.05 was used as the standard to judge a significant difference, and p-value <0.1 was used as the standard for propensity to differ. Because a remarkably unexpected value for ocular accommodation and subjective symptoms was considered unlikely to occur, the investigation results obtained were all assumed to correspond to a normal distribution and the t-test was adopted.

Results
Ocular Accommodation

The results for positive accommodation time and negative accommodation time for both groups are shown in Table 1.

Table 1. Positive Accommodation Time and Negative Accommodation Time

	Positive accommodation time (s)			Negative accommodation time (s)		
	Pre	Post	Rest	Pre	Post	Rest
Ax	1.00±0.08	1.11±0.08	0.98±0.07	1.05±0.07	1.23±0.09	1.06±0.07
Placebo	0.98±0.08	1.20±0.12	1.10±0.09[*1]	1.03±0.07	1.35±0.08[*2]	1.27±0.08[*3]

Ax:Astaxanthin 6 mg/day, Placebo:Astaxanthin 0 mg/day.
Mean±SD:n=10, [*1] p=0.00617, [*2]p=0.0429, [*3]p=0.0004 vs Ax group

Among the changes in the mean Pre- and Post-values, the positive accommodation time increased from 1.00 seconds to 1.11 seconds in the Ax group, and from 0.98 seconds to 1.20 seconds in the placebo group, and in the test between the Pre and Post periods both values increased significantly

(Ax group: p=0.0165, P group: p=0.0111). For negative accommodation time, the mean value increased from 1.05 seconds to 1.23 seconds in the Ax group and from 1.03 seconds to 1.35 seconds in the P group, and the test results were significant for both groups (Ax group: p=0.0008, P group: p=0.0002). Accommodation time increased in both groups after application of the visual load, indicating accommodative dysfunction in both groups.

Based on the results of a comparison between the groups, there was no significant difference in positive accommodation time for either the Pre- or Post-values. In the Rest values after 10-minutes of rest, however, the value for the Ax group was 0.98 seconds and the value for the P group was 1.10 seconds, with the P group showing a propensity to increase (p=0.0617). For negative accommodation time there was no significant difference in the Pre values, but there was a significant difference between the Post values and Rest values. The Post values were 1.23 seconds for the Ax group and 1.35 seconds for the P group, with the increase for the P group being significantly large (p=0.0429). Furthermore, for the Rest values as well, in contrast to 1.06 seconds for the Ax group, the value of 1.27 seconds for the P group was significantly large (p=0.0004).

Subjective Symptoms

Among the total of 15 items, the items for which the rating points rose significantly in the Post survey were "eye fatigue" and "eye heaviness" for the Ax group, and the 4 items "eye fatigue," "eye heaviness," "blurred vision" and "eye dryness" for the P group (data not shown). Among the 15 items, there were no items that had significant difference between the two groups for Pre values, Post values, and Rest values.

Discussion

Accommodation time after visual load increased in both the Ax group and the P group, and ocular accommodation decreased. Based on the change in negative accommodation time, however, accommodative dysfunction was larger in the P group. Based on the change in positive accommodation time and negative accommodation time after rest, the effects of the load remained in the P group, and recovery of accommodative dysfunction from the load was faster in the Ax group than in the P group. The number of subjective symptom rating items related to eyes that had higher points after the load also was smaller for the Ax group than the P group. Based on these results, astaxanthin is thought to mitigate accommodative dysfunction, and to have action on visual fatigue caused by accommodative dysfunction.

Because the three-dimensional image on the 3D display monitor used to create the visual load for this study artificially induces binocular parallax, this created an imbalance in ocular accommodation and convergence function and remarkably forced a load on visual function. In particular, excessive convergence induces a state of tension in ocular accommodation greater than normal vis-à-vis the image presented on the screen that the subjects are to check visually.[22] As a result, gazing at the three-dimensional image causes development of eyestrain from an accommodation modality in the form of inertia of accommodation that increases time required until full focus.[19,20,23] In this study, gazing at a three-dimensional image resulted in a strong visual load because positive accommodation time and negative accommodation time were increased after the load.

In the changes in ocular accommodation after application of the load, negative accommodation time increased to a greater extent for the P group than for the Ax group. Together with accommodation time, negative accommodation time is an examination result that captures the dynamic aspect of ocular accommodation, and especially negative accommodation time, which is the time until full focus when distant focusing was used. This is because the ciliary muscle tension created when near focusing was being used is released, and the ciliary muscle causes the relaxation action. The relaxation time was faster in the Ax group than in the P group because relaxation of the ciliary muscle was stimulated more smoothly in the Ax group. For subjective symptoms as well, although the items for which the rating points rose for the P group after the load included "blurred vision," this subjective symptom is thought to result if the time required to focus when using distant viewing is increased.

There was a clear difference between the two groups after rest. For both positive accommodation time and negative accommodation time, compared with the Ax group, the P group was significantly longer, and recovery was faster for the Ax group than the P group. In addition to far vision, difference with the P group was found for near vision, which caused tension in the ciliary muscle after rest. In the Ax group, the ciliary muscle recovered a smooth action not only after rest but when tensed as well. For reduction or the prevention of eyestrain, having a good effect on recovery is very important. Although the visual load in this study was a strong load that applied an imbalance to visual function, the load was applied for only 20-minutes. The visual load experienced in real life is maintained for longer hours and continues each day. Continuous visual load causes excessive accommodation tension and produces eyestrain.[24] The large recovery in the Ax group is thought to be able to mitigate the load, and its effects remain until the following day, thus suggesting the possibility of a preventive effect against eyestrain. In this study, astaxanthin enhanced the amplitude of accommodation, and this result is consistent with prior reports indicating that astaxanthin is linked to improvement of eyestrain.[12]

In the study reported here, the dynamic aspect of ocular accommodation in the form of accommodation time was captured, and this is a parameter that faithfully reflects the ciliary muscle action. The fact that accommodation time improved means the ciliary muscle was activated – the result being that tension and relaxation were performed more smoothly. This study result indicates objectively that astaxanthin improves accommodative dysfunction and is useful for eyestrain induced by accommodative dysfunction.

STUDY 2: EFFECTS OF ASTAXANTHIN ON ACCOMMODATIVE RECOVERY[15]

We designed a second clinical study to evaluate the effects of astaxanthin on accommodative recovery.

Materials and Methods

Subjects

Ten healthy adults (5 males and 5 females) who satisfied the following selection criteria and did not violate the exclusion criteria were selected. Based on the subjects' statements, 10 dominant eyes were chosen.

Selection Criteria
- Age 30-42 years (as a rule).
- Individuals who are not regularly taking medication or consuming products such as health foods effective against asthenopia (vitamin preparations or tonics containing taurine compounds).
- Without regard to gender.
- Individuals capable of observing the rules to be followed for the study and being tested and examined as set forth in the plan for the study.

Exclusion Criteria
- Individuals with diabetes.
- Individuals with a history of allergy to medicine.
- Individuals who are pregnant, breastfeeding, or might be pregnant.
- Other individuals the physicians in charge of the study find to be unsuitable.

Study Design

The subjects took two capsules (each containing 3mg astaxanthin) per day after dinner for 14-days as the same manner as in Study 1.[14] Examination of the load resulting from IT device work was conducted before supplementation (Day 0) and on the 14th day after start of supplementation. In conjunction with the examination subjects also completed a questionnaire survey.

Measurements

Three items were chosen as examination items. Objective refractivity was measured using an autorefractometer (ARK720 manufactured by Nidek Co., Ltd.). The difference between minimum refraction value and maximum refraction value when accommodative load was recorded at +0.50D – -3.00D (accommodative reaction). The mean value for frequency of appearance of the High Frequency Component in accommodative micro-fluctuation when refraction value is within the range of the difference between the minimum refraction value and 0.00D – -0.75D (the HFC value), were measured using an accommodative micro-fluctuation analyzer (AA-1, Nidek Co., Ltd.). The same individual performed all of the ophthalmic inspections.

The following questionnaire surveys were taken before VDT work, after VDT work, and after rest:

- Questionnaire No. 1 (before work)
  - My eyes become tired very easily
  - My eyes become tired occasionally
  - My eyes don't become tired very often
  - My eyes hardly ever become tired
  - My eyes never become tired
- Questionnaire No. 2 (after work)
  - My eyes became very tired
  - My eyes became tired
  - My eyes became tired a little
  - My eyes did not become very tired
  - My eyes didn't become tired at all
- Questionnaire No. 3 (after rest)
  - My eyes recovered very much
  - My eyes recovered
  - My eyes recovered a little
  - My eyes didn't change very much
  - My eyes didn't change at all
  - My eyes became even more tired

Visual Load

Subjects performed IT device work for 30-minutes (while wearing study glasses fitted with over-corrective lens that placed a -0.75D load on distant fully corrected refraction value). Wires were attached to a hand-held screen game device (Game Boy, Nintendo Co., Ltd.) in a manner that enabled the game device to be fixed in a position 30 cm from the subjects' eyes, and the device placed around each subjects' neck. For the game, a simple descending object game was selected.

Statistical Analysis

All measured values were shown by mean value ± standard deviation. Each comparison was analyzed by paired t-test. The significance level was less than 5%.

Results

After excluding 1 eye that contracted allergic conjunctivitis during the study, 9 eyes were studied.

On the questionnaire survey before supplementation (before work), 1 subject responded "my eyes become tired very easily," 6 subjects responded "my eyes become tired occasionally" and 2 subjects responded "my eyes don't become tired very often," respectively.

Spherical refraction values for the subjects' eyes were distributed between 0.00D – -9.25D. Mean values for objective refractivity prior to astaxanthin supplementation and before work, after work, and after rest were -3.30±3.33D, -3.06±3.43D, and -3.31±3.33D, respectively, and after astaxanthin supplementation were -3.39±3.44D, -3.17±3.61D, and -3.53±3.61D, respectively. Before supplementation, the number of eyes that became myopic, showed no change, or became hyperopic after work compared to before work were 1 eye, 2 eyes, and 6 eyes, respectively; after supplementation there were 0 eyes, 4 eyes, and 5 eyes, respectively. Few eyes showed a change to myopia after work. Before supplementation, the number of eyes that became myopic, showed no change, or became hyperopic after a rest compared to after work were 6 eyes, 0 eyes, and 3 eyes, respectively; after supplementation there were 6 eyes, 2 eyes, and 1 eye, respectively. Many eyes showed a change to myopia after rest.

Mean values for the HFC value, which before astaxanthin supplementation and after work and after rest were 52.09 ± 5.73 and 55.79 ± 9.97, respectively, increased after rest. After supplementation, the values were 54.55 ± 5.05 and 54.23 ± 4.73, respectively, indicating almost no change. The size of the change in the HFC value after a rest compared to after work, which before supplementation was +3.70 ± 6.56, decreased significantly ($p < 0.05$) after supplementation to 0.32 ± 2.60 (Fig. 4). Compared with before supplementation, after supplementation the number of eyes for which the HFC value increased, showed no change, or decreased after rest compared to after work were 1 eye, 1 eye, and 7 eyes, respectively, while after supplementation, the number of eyes for which an increase in the HFC value was found after rest was small (data not shown).

Before astaxanthin supplementation, accommodative reaction after work and after rest was 1.92 ± 0.71D and 1.89 ± 0.65D, respectively, while after supplementation accommodative reaction after work and after rest was 1.80 ± 0.48D and 1.93 ± 0.46D, respectively. Before and after supplementation, accommodative reaction increased for 4 eyes and decreased for 5 eyes – no difference before and after supplementation was found. In contrast to 4 subjects and 5 subjects who responded "my eyes became very tired / my eyes became tired" and "my eyes became tired a little / my eyes did not become very tired / my eyes didn't become tired at all," respectively, on the questionnaire survey after work before supplementation, after supplementation the number of subjects giving these responses were 2 subjects and 7 subjects, respectively. Furthermore, in contrast to 0 subjects responding "My eyes recovered" on the questionnaire survey after rest before supplementation, 2 subjects gave this response after supplementation.

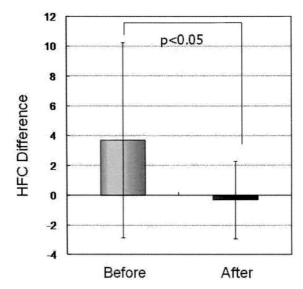

Figure 4. Change in HFC Value after Rest Compared with after Work

Discussion

The accommodative micro-fluctuation frequency component can be divided into a low-frequency component of less than 0.6Hz and a high-frequency component of 1.0-2.3Hz. The low-frequency component originates in accommodative movement, while the high-frequency component originates in vibrations of refractivity of crystalline lens, and is thought to reflect ciliary muscle activity.[25] There is a correlation between accommodative load and the high-frequency component of accommodative micro-fluctuation, and the increase in the HFC value when load on ciliary muscles increases has been clarified.[26] In this study, we investigated what effect supplementation of astaxanthin causes in accommodative recovery by examining objective refractivity, HFC value, and accommodative reaction. Using ocular accommodation before astaxanthin supplementation and after work as a criterion, we performed a comparative study of the extent to which rest aids accommodative recovery after accommodative fatigue is induced by having subjects perform VDT works while wearing overcorrective glasses.

Using an autorefractometer, we found almost no change in objective refractivity before and after supplementation and before work (-3.30 ± 3.33D and -3.39 ± 3.44D, respectively). Compared to before work, the change in objective refractivity after work before and after were +0.25 ± 0.41D and +0.22 ± 0.32D, respectively; although both changed toward hyperopia, neither change was significant. Moreover, the change after rest compared to after work showed a change toward myopia before and after of -0.25 ± 0.60D and -0.36 ± 0.47D, respectively. Compared to before supplementation, where the value returned to the refraction value after rest (change of 0.00 ± 0.48D after rest compared to before work), after supplementation the value obtained after rest was closer to myopia than the value before work (change of

-0.14 ± 0.42D after rest compared to before work). This suggests that astaxanthin worked to stimulate ciliary muscle action, but the change was not significant.

The HFC value after rest compared to after work was observed, the value before supplementation was +3.70 ± 6.56 but declined significantly (p<0.05) to 0.32 ± 2.60 after supplementation. This suggests that prior to supplementation ciliary muscle tension persisted even though VDT work had ended, and that accommodative recovery was not obtained with a 20-minute rest, however after supplementation, accommodative recovery had begun with a rest of 20-minutes.

Accommodative reaction before supplementation and after work was 1.92 ± 0.71D and 1.89 ± 0.65D, respectively, after rest accommodative reaction had declined (-0.03 ± 0.20D). After supplementation, these values were 1.80 ± 0.48D and 1.93 ± 0.46D, respectively; compared to after work, accommodative reaction after rest had increased (+0.13 ± 0.42D), but this was not significant.

According to the questionnaire survey results, after work but before supplementation there were 4 subjects who stated their eyes had become tired because of VDT work, after supplementation this had decreased to 2 subjects. Moreover, after rest but before supplementation there were 0 subjects who responded that their fatigue had improved as the result of rest, but after supplementation 2 subjects responded that their eyes had recovered. Thus, there were examples of improvement based on the subjects' own awareness.

Based on this research, it was suggested that astaxanthin effects ocular accommodation, and particularly that astaxanthin works through the accommodative fatigue recovery process and acts to eliminate fatigue quickly.

STUDY 3: EFFECTS OF ASTAXANTHIN-CONTAINING SOFT CAPSULE ON THE ACCOMMODATION FUNCTION OF THE EYE IN MIDDLE-AGED AND OLDER PEOPLE[16]

We designed a third clinical study to investigate the effects of astaxanthin on the accommodation functions of the eyes in middle-aged and older subjects.

Materials and Methods
Subjects

Twenty-two people who had given written informed consent for participation in this study and met all inclusion criteria, but did not violate any exclusion criteria, described below, were selected to be enrolled in this study.

Inclusion Criteria
- Healthy adult male volunteers aged 45 or over, but under 65.
- Constant eye strain in daily life.
- No eye disease (excluding ametropia).
- Able to keep eyes open without blinking for at least 30 seconds.
- Able to follow the compliance rules described in the study protocol, and to undergo tests and examinations on scheduled days.

Exclusion Criteria
- Presence of a concomitant drug allergy or such history.
- Regular intake of any drugs or health food products effective for asthenopia (e.g. vitamins, supplementary drinks containing taurine).
- Considered unsuited for the study at the discretion of the investigator based on other reasons.

Study Design

A dietary supplement containing 6 mg of astaxanthin in a softgel capsule was used. The subjects took one soft capsule with water once daily after the evening meal. The duration of supplementation was set at 4-weeks.

Measurements
1. Test and time point:
   a. Uncorrected visual acuity was measured before and at 4-weeks after supplementation of the investigational food product, and was converted into logMAR units.
   b. The near response was measured by TriIRIS C9000 before and at 4-weeks after supplementation of the investigational food product.
      i. The vision of subjects was corrected in advance with glasses that would give them clear vision at a distance of 50 cm (shortest distance of distinct vision).
      ii. The visual acuity chart was gradually moved from the 50 cm distance to determine the near point.
      iii. The movement amplitude of the near point + 1 Diopter was set as the accommodation stimulus.
      iv. The visual acuity chart was moved back and forth three times over the distance from the 50 cm point to the "near point + 1 Diopter." During this period, the constricted pupil diameter and the convergence were measured and recorded continuously as the transverse diameter of the central portion and the locus of the central portion, respectively.
      v. The pupillary constriction ratio was defined as [initial pupil diameter (mm) − constricted pupil diameter at the third measurement (mm)]/ initial pupil diameter (mm). The pupillary constriction ratio was compared before and after ingestion of the investigational food product to assess the effects of the investigational food product on the accommodation function.
2. Health interview conducted by physician before and 4-weeks after supplementation to examine the health condition and subjective symptoms during the study.
3. Questionnaire on subjective symptoms for completion by subjects. The following symptoms were examined at 4-weeks after supplementation: 1) difficulty to see nearby objects, 2) difficulty to see far objects, 3) eye strain, 4) ocular pain, 5) blurred vision, 6) eye redness, 7) flashing vision, 8) lacrimation, 9) shoulder and low back stiffness, 10) dull headache. Symptoms that had been present before supplementation of the investigational food product were rated on a scale of 1 to 5, (1= significantly improved, 2= improved, 3= slightly improved, 4= unchanged, 5= worsened) to be compared with the scores before supplementation.

Statistical Analysis
The paired t-test was employed and a significance level of less than 5% was considered statistically significant.

Results
The 22 subjects enrolled in this study were all male, aged between 46 and 65 years with a mean age of 53.9 ± 5.1 years. Nineteen out of 22 subjects were using glasses routinely and no subjects were using contact lenses.

Regarding uncorrected visual acuity (logMAR units) before and after supplementation, the right visual acuity before and after supplementation was 0.85 ± 0.53 and 0.84 ± 0.54, respectively, and the left visual acuity was 0.83 ± 0.55 and 0.76 ± 0.52, respectively, showing no significant changes after astaxanthin supplementation both in the right and left eyes

Prior to measurement, subjects were instructed to not move their jaw and forehead during measurement, and avoid blinking as much as possible. To enable subjects to concentrate on the measurement, we aroused subjects by calling them around the near point to raise their concentration level.

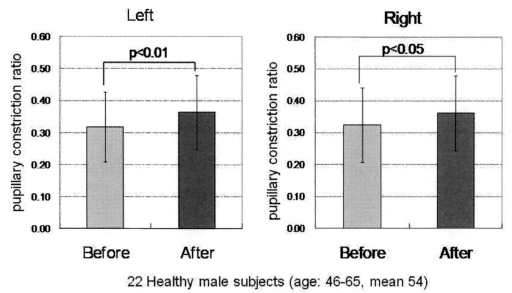

Figure 5. Pupillary Constriction Ratio Before and After Supplementation of Astaxanthin

The pupillary constriction ratio before and after supplementation is shown in Fig. 5. For the right eye, the pupillary constriction ratio before and after supplementation was 0.32 ± 0.11 and 0.36 ± 0.12, respectively, showing a significant increase after supplementation (p < 0.01). For the left eye, the pupillary constriction ratio before and after supplementation was 0.32 ± 0.12 and 0.36 ± 0.12, respectively, also showing a significant increase after supplementation (p < 0.05). The number of subjects in whom the pupillary constriction ratio increased in the right eye after supplementation was 16 out of 22, and that in the left eye was 14, and that in both eyes was 12.

As far as the results of the questionnaire on subjective symptoms are concerned, symptoms about how many subjects had complained before supplementation were as follows: "difficulty to see nearby objects" (20 subjects); "eye strain" (22); "blurred vision" (18); and, "shoulder and low back stiffness" (19). The percentage of subjects who answered "slightly improved" or better for these symptoms after supplementation were 65.0%, 77.2%, 61.1%, and 63.2%, respectively.

Discussion

Previous studies[12,14,15] were conducted in subjects aged from their late 20's to their late 30's, in whom the accommodation ability for focusing the eye is relatively preserved. In this study, middle-aged and older people were targeted and the effects of astaxanthin on their accommodation function and subjective symptoms were investigated. The pupillary constriction ratio was calculated using TriIRIS C9000 to assess the accommodation function, and the effects on subjective symptoms were examined by a questionnaire survey of subjects. Presbyopia is a phenomenon that the accommodation ability to focus the eye declines with aging, making it difficult to focus on nearby objects, and is said to progress gradually from the 40's. Accompanying symptoms include difficulty to see nearby objects, eye strain, shoulder stiffness, dull eye, dull headache, and headache. This study was conducted in 22 subjects aged between 46 and 65 (mean: 54 years) with the following complaints: "eye strain" (all 22 subjects); "difficulty to see nearby objects" (20); "shoulder and low back stiffness" (19); "blurred vision" (18). Based on this, we considered that middle-aged and older people with typical presbyopia were enrolled in this study.

Concerning uncorrected visual acuity, as reported in previous clinical studies that astaxanthin had no effects on it, no significant changes were observed in this study, either.

The accommodation function was assessed by calculating the pupillary constriction ratio using TriIRIS C9000. This device is capable of simply measuring the change in convergence response and miotic response induced by accommodation following near vision, under physiological conditions with both eyes open.[27] In many studies this device has been used for various tests including the presbyopia test (test for accommodation function), the test of abnormal accommodation due to asthenopia induced by VDT operations, etc., and the test for accommodation function before and after eye surgery.[28] Since significant increases were observed in the pupillary constriction ratios in both the right and left eyes, astaxanthin is considered to have positively activated the functions of the constrictor pupillae muscle and dilator pupillae muscle, which are responsible for miosis and mydriasis, respectively. It is estimated that astaxanthin may improve ciliary muscle fatigue, and it is also considered that astaxanthin may improve the constrictor pupillae muscle and the dilator pupillae muscle. The ciliary muscle is composed of a circular muscle and a longitudinal muscle, which are considered to move in coordination with the constrictor pupillae muscle and the dilator pupillae muscle, since these muscles are innervated by the same motor neuron. It is also considered that if the function of the ciliary muscle is activated, the ratio of the pupillary constriction due to the pupil response to nearby vision may be improved.

Concerning subjective symptoms, those for which many subjects answered, "slightly improved" or better were as follows: "eye strain," "difficulty to see near objects," "blurred vision," and "shoulder and low back stiffness." A double-blind study in adult subjects with eye strain, has already shown that "blurred vision" and "shoulder and low back stiffness" were significantly improved after astaxanthin supplementation.[12] It is suggested that improvement in the subjective symptoms might have been achieved by deep depth of focus and ease of focusing that resulted from the active movement of the pupils (increase in pupillary constriction ratio) caused by the action of the constrictor pupillae muscle and the dilator pupillae muscle activated by astaxanthin.

The basic measure for presbyopia is to wear glasses. However, since improvement in both the accommodation function and subjective symptoms was observed in this study conducted in middle-aged and older people with presbyopia, it was suggested that the supplementation of astaxanthin may slow down the progression of presbyopia and myopia associated with focusing on nearby objects and improve asthenopia in middle-aged and older people with advanced presbyopia as well as in younger adults.

STUDY 4: RELATIONSHIPS BETWEEN VISUAL FATIGUE AND REACTION TIMES - EFFECTS OF A REPETITION OF A VISUAL TASK AND LONG-TERM INTAKE OF A SUPPLEMENTATION FOOD INCLUDING ASTAXANTHIN ON REACTION TIME[17]

We designed a fourth clinical study to investigate the effects of astaxanthin on reaction time.

Materials and Methods
Subjects

Ten adults (6 males and 4 females) without visual impairment were recruited as subjects. Their mean age was 24.6 years (range: 22-28 years). A questionnaire survey was conducted in advance to confirm that all potential subjects were routinely engaged in computer operations. All enrolled subjects used the computer for an average of 6.9 hours (range: 4-12 hours) per day. Informed consent was obtained from each subject. Prior to the experiment, all subjects received explanation concerning the safety of astaxanthin and its effectiveness in reducing visual fatigue. However, explanation regarding how reaction times would change in accordance with an increase/decrease in visual fatigue was not provided.

Study Design

A dietary supplement containing 2 mg of astaxanthin in a softgel capsule was used. The subjects took three capsules with water once daily after their evening meal. The duration of supplementation was set at 4-weeks. The subjects were instructed to take the capsules in the same time zone every day. A check sheet was prepared for the subjects in order to confirm their daily intake of astaxanthin capsules as well as for them to record their intake of other drugs or nutritional supplements. The subjects were instructed to enter these data daily. For the experiment, reaction time tests were conducted three times as follows: before astaxanthin supplementation (Day 0), 14-days after supplementation and 28-days after supplementation. Each subject took all of the three tests in the same time zone. Moreover, the subjects were instructed to refrain from performing strenuous exercise and drinking alcohol on the day before the experiment.

Measurements

A personal computer (Dell OptiPlex 260GX) and visual stimulus-generating equipment (Cambridge Research Systems VGS2/5) were used for stimulus generation, management of experiment, and measurement of reaction times. Stimuli were presented on CKT (TOTOKU CV722X). Before the experiment, test stimuli colors were displayed in the full screen of CRT, and brightness in the center of the screen was measured using a luminance meter (Cambridge Research Systems OptiCAL). Stimuli were presented at a distance of 27 cm in front of the subject. The subject visualized a stimulus only with the right eye. The following two tasks were prepared: the pursuit eye movement task which measured the reaction to a light spot displayed during the pursuit of a moving target, and the control task which determined reaction to a light spot displayed during fixed gaze into a static target. Three types of stimuli were presented against a black background (luminance: 0.13 cd/m^2): a red gazing stimulus (x, luminance: 1.7 cd/m^2, 0.8°x0.8°), two circles (○, luminance: 1.7 cd/m^2, diameter 0.8°) and a white light spot (•, luminance: 7.5 cd/m^2, diameter 0.37°). The center-to-center distance between the gazing stimulus and the circle was 5° in a horizontal direction, and the moving speed of the stimuli was 10°/s during the pursuit movement of the eye. In order to confirm that a subject was accurately pursuing the gazing stimuli, an eye tracking system (NAC EMR-8) was used. The sampling rate in the eye tracking system was 60 Hz, and the minimum resolution capacity was 0.1°. To prevent head movement, a jaw stand and bite board (device bitten by the subject to fix the head) were used.

Measurement of visual reaction time was conducted in a dark room. The test was started after 5-minute adaptation to darkness. In the pursuit eye movement test, the gazing stimulus and circles were statically displayed at a horizontal 10° position to the right or left of the screen center. At 300 ms thereafter, the stimulus and circles moved back and forth for a distance of 20° from the center. At a random time point between 1000 and 3000 ms after the start of the back-and-forth movement, a light spot was displayed in the center of one of the two circles. The subject was instructed to visually pursue the gazing stimulus accurately and to press the button corresponding to the position of the light spot as quickly as possible upon its appearance. There were two buttons placed side by side to match the position of the light spot. The interval from the appearance of the light spot to the pressing of the button was recorded as reaction time. When the subject pressed the button, the stimulus disappeared and the next task commenced. A 2000 ms interval was taken between 2 tasks. Fifty tasks were placed into 1 block, and 10 blocks (a total of 500 tasks) were given to the subject. The gazing stimulus and circles always started moving from the right side of the screen center in 5 of 10 blocks, and from the left side of the screen center in the remaining blocks. Before the start of each block, the starting position was told to the subject by a staff member of the experiment. The position of the light spot was random and different between blocks. In the control test, the gazing stimulus and circles were statically presented in the screen center, and thereafter, the light spot appeared in the circle on the right or left side of the gazing stimuli. The task of the subject was the same as that in the previous pursuit eye movement test except that the gazing stimulus was steadily stared at. One block (50 tasks) of the control test was conducted each before (pre) and after (post) the pursuit eye movement test. The tests took approximately 90 minutes to complete. Before the experiment, the subject practiced 50 tasks each for the control and pursuit eye movement tests. After the completion of each block, the subject took a 1-minute break. Reaction times were measured for all tests. During the experiment, eyeball movement was monitored to confirm that the subject was constantly pursuing the stimulus correctly.

Analysis was conducted only for the times of correct reactions (at least 95% of all tasks in all blocks). However, the tasks that took less than 100 ms or more than 1000 ms, that is, the tasks in which the subjects blinked at the moment of target appearance and the tasks in which the subjects did not pursue the circles were excluded from analysis, even if the reactions were correct. In this study, the mean reaction time was calculated for each block (50 tasks) to determine the changes in reaction times as a result of visual fatigue caused by the pursuit eye movement test, which consisted of 500 tasks (10 blocks), and the reaction times were compared between blocks. Furthermore, the mean reaction times were also calculated for 10 tasks (Task 1 to Task 10) after the start of a block of 50 tasks and 10 tasks before the end of the block (Task 41 to Task 50) for comparison.

Results

Figure 6 shows the mean reaction time per block. The reaction times in the pursuit eye movement test were analyzed for variance. Both main effects of the intake period [$F(2,18) = 5.20$, $p < 0.05$] and block [$F(9,81) = 10.86$, $p < 0.01$] were significant, but no significance was found in interactions [$F(18,162)=1.31$]. The effect of the intake period was analyzed by Tukey's multiple comparison test. From the results, the obtained reaction times on Day 0 were significantly longer than those obtained on Day 28 ($p < 0.05$) and tended to be longer than the level on Day 14 ($p = 0.08$). The results of Tukey's multiple comparison test for block effect showed that the reaction times in the second and subsequent blocks were longer than that in the first block ($ps < 0.05$), and that the reactions times in the eighth and subsequent blocks were longer than that in the second block ($ps < 0.05$). The reaction times in the ninth block were longer than those in the third and fifth blocks ($ps < 0.05$). The results reveal that reactions were fast in the first few blocks immediately after the start of the pursuit eye movement test, but became slower as the subjects went through more blocks. The reaction times in the control test were analyzed for variance with [3 (intake period) x 2 (block)]. The main effect of block (pre/post) was significant [$F(1,9) = 48.45$, $p < 0.01$], while that of the intake period was not [$F(2.18) = 0.14$]. Moreover, the interactions were not significant [$F(2,18) = 0.04$]. As shown thus far, the reaction times in the post-pursuit eye movement test were longer than those in the pre-pursuit eye movement test in the control test; however, the reaction times in the pre- or post-pursuit eye movement test were not altered by the duration of astaxanthin supplementation.

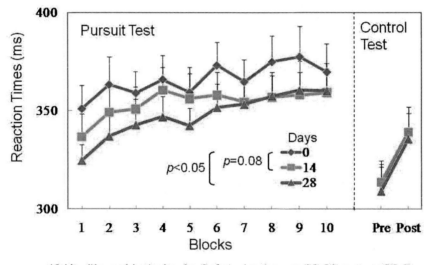

10 Healthy subjects (male; 6, female; 4, age; 22-28, mean; 24.6)

Figure 6. Changes of Reaction Times per Block by Astaxanthin Supplementation

As far as the mean reaction times for the first 10 tasks after the start of block and for the last 10 tasks before the end of block are concerned (data not shown), the reaction times in the pursuit eye movement test were analyzed for variance [3 (intake period) x 2 (order of task) x 10 (block)]. All of the main effects were significant [intake period $F(2,18) = 7.93$, $p < 0.01$; order of task $F(1,9) = 14,38$, $p < 0.01$; block $F(9,81) = 6.36$, $p < 0.01$]. The interactions were not significant [intake period x task order $F(2,18) = 0.36$; intake period x block $F(18, 162) = 0.96$; task order x block $F(9,81) = 0.79$; intake period x task order x block $F(18, 162) = 0.59$]. The effect of the intake period was analyzed by Tukey's multiple comparison test, which showed that the reaction times on Day 0 were longer than those on Days 14 or 28 ($ps < 0.05$). Moreover, Tukey's multiple comparison test on block effect showed that the reaction times in the fourth and subsequent blocks were longer than those in the first block ($ps < 0.05$). The results of the variance analysis of reaction times in the control test with [3 (intake period) x 2 (task order) x 2 (block)] showed that the main effects of task order [$F(1,9) = 20.59$, $p < 0.01$] and block [$F(1,9) = 30.35$, $p < 0.01$] were significant, but that of the intake period was not [$F(2,18) = 0.61$]. The interactions in task order x block [$F(1,9) = 8.43$, $p < 0.05$] and intake period x task order x block [$F(2,18) = 4.12$, $p < 0.05$] were significant, but other interactions in [intake period x task order $F(2,18) = 0.46$; intake period x block $F(2,18) = 0.04$] were not. When sub-tests were conducted on interactions in [task order x block], the effect of task order was significant both for the pre-pursuit [$F_{(1,18)}$ = 5.85, $p < 0.05$] and post- pursuit [$F_{(1,18)}$=28.99, p<.01] eye movement tests. In accordance with the results of the sub-effect tests on interactions in [intake period x task order x block], the effect of task order was significant on Day 0 both for pre-pursuit [$F_{(1,54)}$ = 4.73, $p < 0.05$] and post-pursuit [$F_{(1,54)}$ = 5.55, $p < 0.05$] eye movement tests, and significant on Days 14 and 28 only for the post-pursuit eye movement test [Day 14: $F_{(1,54)}$ = 23.65, $p < 0.01$; Day 28: $F_{(1,54)}$ = 20.35, $p < 0.01$].

Discussion

In the present study, we investigated the effects of visual fatigue on reaction times of subjects who were instructed to repeat reaction tasks. Furthermore, we examined how reaction times would be changed by astaxanthin supplementation. It was clear from the results of comparison of 10 blocks of the pursuit tasks (Fig. 6) that the reaction times were short in the first few blocks and became longer in the latter half. This was similarly observed in the control test, in which the reaction times in the post-pursuit eye movement test were longer than those in the pre-pursuit eye movement test. The comparison within block showed that the reaction times in 10 tasks before the end of block were longer than those in 10 tasks following the start of block in both tests. Nevertheless, when the 10 tasks before the end of each block were compared with the 10 tasks of the next block after intermission (e.g., 10 tasks before the end of Block 1 and 10 tasks after the start of Block 2), the extended reaction times immediately before the completion of block were restored after intermission, and the reaction became faster. These results are consistent with those of previous studies,[29] indicating that reaction times become longer with accumulation of visual fatigue. Significant effects were not observed by astaxanthin supplementation in comparison between or within blocks of the control test. However, the within-block comparison for the pre-pursuit eye movement test on Days 14 and 28 showed that the difference in reaction times between the tasks immediately after start of block and the tasks immediately before completion of block became smaller. In the pursuit tasks, both between- and within-block comparison showed longer reaction times on Day 0 than on Days 14 and 28 after supplementation.

Interestingly, the reduction in reaction times induced by astaxanthin supplementation was only observed in the pursuit tasks and not in the control tasks. In this study, we did not elucidate why the effect of astaxanthin was different between the pursuit tasks and the control tasks. The only difference of the pursuit tasks from the control tasks was that the eyes were tracking the moving target, and the other elements were the same. Therefore, the difference in the observed effects of astaxanthin may reflect the reduction of visual fatigue by a vision-regulating mechanism (e.g. eye muscle) involved in the visual pursuit tasks. However, eyeball movement showed no effect on visual fatigue.[30] As eyeball movement (e.g. drift) was involved even in fixed gaze, it would be difficult to use vision-regulating mechanism in explaining the reason why the effect of astaxanthin was different between the pursuit and control tasks. Moreover, it is also difficult to explain such difference by stating that different muscles of the arm must have been used between the pursuit and control tasks since the same button-pressing responses were required in both tasks. One possible explanation is the difference in the complexity of the performed tasks. In the pursuit tasks, the subject was required not only to react to the light spot but also to move/regulate the sight direction in line with the moving visual target, whereas in the control tasks, the subject was required to provide only the required responses to the visual stimulus. Therefore, the tasks in the pursuit eye movement test were more complex than those in the control test. Previous studies have indicated that the more complex a task is, the more conspicuous is the impact of visual fatigue on performance.[14-16] Therefore, the effects of accumulation and alleviation of visual fatigue may have been more clearly observed in the pursuit tasks than in the control tasks.

Meanwhile, 6 adult males (mean age: 24.33; range: 21-35 years) were newly recruited for a complementary experiment in which they carried out the same reaction tasks on Day 0, Day 14, and Day 28, without any nutritional dietary supplements (Fig. 7). Analysis of variance was conducted for the pursuit tasks [3 (frequency of experiments) x 10 (block)]. Only the main effect of block was significant, the main effects of experiment frequency and interactions were not. From the results of analysis of variance for the control tasks [3 (experiment frequency) x 2 (block)], the main effect of block was significant but those of experiment frequency and interactions were not. The above results indicate that the shorter reaction times in the main test cannot be completely explained by the effect of practice or experience of the reaction tasks and that astaxanthin supplementation might have contributed to reduction in reaction times.

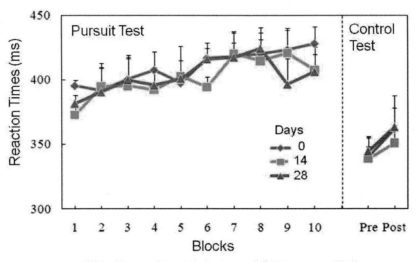

6 Healthy male subjects (age; 21-35, mean; 24.3)

Figure 7. Changes of Reaction Times per Block by Non-Astaxanthin Supplementation

It was found that reaction times to eye tasks were shortened by reduction of visual fatigue, which is a novel finding with regard to the relevance of visual fatigue vis-à-vis reaction times. However, a placebo group was not used in this study, and therefore further investigation is needed regarding the reduction of reaction times by astaxanthin supplementation.

STUDY 5: INTRAOCULAR PENETRATION OF ASTAXANTHIN IN RABBIT[18]

We designed an animal study to investigate the existence of astaxanthin in the eye after oral supplementation.

Materials and Methods
Animals

A total of 24 male New Zealand albino rabbits (NZW: 2.7-3.1 kg) were used in the experiments.

Study Design

A single oral dose (100 mg/kg) of astaxanthin was administered to NZW rabbits, and about 3 ml of blood was drawn from the left posterior ear vein at 0 (before administration), 3, 6, 9, 12, 24, 48, 72, and 168 hours after administration. Subsequently, about 0.2 ml of anterior chamber fluid was collected, followed by eyeball enucleation. Following enucleation, the isolated eyeball was first frozen at -20°C and subsequently thawed within 24 hours. The tissues were then separated, frozen at -80°C or below and preserved until sample treatment.

Measurements

Eye tissues were cut into pieces with scissors in cold phosphate buffer solution (PBS) and homogenized using a Polytron Homogenizer (Polytron, Georgia) while being cooled. The obtained serum was diluted twofold with PBS and directly used as a sample. To the obtained homogenate or serum, 50 U of cholesterol esterase (Wako Junyaku, Japan), 500 U of lipase (derived from *Candida rugosa*; Sigma Aldrich, Japan) and 10 µg of dibutylhydroxytoluene (BHT) were added. After nitrogen filling, incubation was performed for 1 hour at 37°C. The 250 ng/ml internal standard (8'-apo-β-carotene-8'-oate) and the cold EtOH solution containing 10 µg/ml BHT were added in the same volume, followed by vigorous shaking. Fourfold amount of cold methylene chloride was thereafter added, and after nitrogen gas filling, the sample was shaken for 60 minutes at 4°C. Then, a four-fold amount of cold PBS and twenty-fold volume of cold hexane were added. After nitrogen gas filling, the sample was again shaken for 30 minutes at 4°C, and centrifuged for 15 minutes at 4°C and 4,000 rpm to obtain the supernatant. The remaining lower layer was extracted 3 times with methylene chloride-hexane, and then the supernatant was collected. After evaporation to dryness under reduced pressure and nitrogen gas stream, the collected supernatant was re-dissolved in *tert*-butyl methyl ether (MTBE) and then analyzed by high-performance liquid chromatography (HPLC).

The HPLC apparatus and conditions were as follows: Degasser: DGU-20A; pump: LC-20A (Shimadzu, Japan; flow rate: 0.1 ml/minute); auto-injector: SIL20A (Shimadzu; temperature set at 4°C); detector: SPD-M20A (Shimadzu, photodiode array detector: wavelength for measurement at 250-750 nm; 474 nm for quantification, and 630 nm for reference wavelength); column oven: CTO20A (Shimadzu; temperature set at 16°C); analytical column: YMC Carotenoid Column 3S (2.0 x 150 mm, YMC, Japan); mobile phase (Liquid A: MeOH/MTBE/0.1% phosphate (93:5:2); Liquid B: MeOH/MTBE/0.1% phosphate (8:90:2). Gradient elution was performed as follows: Linear gradient elution was started from 100% in Liquid A, becoming 13% in Liquid B at 7.6 minutes, and then to 20% at 13.3 minutes, 50% at 29 minutes, and 100% at 43 minutes. Subsequently, elution was performed for 15 minutes, using Liquid B. The internal standard method was used to determine astaxanthin concentration. Good linearity was shown in the range of 2-1000 ng/ml concentrations. Prior to this experiment, an addition/recovery test was conducted using the iris/ciliary body. To the iris/ciliary body isolated from astaxanthin-untreated animals, astaxanthin was added in the amount that would make 100 ng/ml, and 200 ng/ml internal standard was also added. Extraction was carried out as mentioned above. The recovery rates were 80-110% and 85-110%, respectively. The coefficient of variation for the quantitative values of astaxanthin was 5.4%. Furthermore, the products of reactions such as degradation or geometric isomerization were hardly found before or after extraction, implying that the extraction method used was appropriate for extracting carotenoid from ocular tissues. The lower quantification limits were 2 ng/ml for anterior chamber fluid, 2 ng/ml for serum, and 3 ng/g for the iris/ciliary body.

The non-compartment model was employed for analyzing the changes in astaxanthin concentrations in the iris/ciliary body and serum. C_{max} (ng/g or ng/ml), AUCt (ng·h/g or ng·h/ml), T_{max} (h) and $T_{1/2}$ (h) in the iris/ciliary body and serum were calculated. [C_{max}: maximum tissue concentration; AUCt: area under the concentration-time curve up to the final time point (t); T_{max} (h): time to reach the maximum tissue concentration; $T_{1/2}$ (h): time to reach 50% concentration in tissue]

Results

A time-course increase in the amount and the disappearance of astaxanthin were observed in the iris/ciliary body and serum as shown in Fig. 8. In serum, the astaxanthin concentration reached the maximum (61.26 ± 26.87 ng/ml (mean ± SD), n=5) at 9-hours after administration, and then subsequently decreased gradually and became completely undetectable at 72-hours. On the other hand, the concentration in the iris/ciliary body gradually increased from 6-hours after administration and reached the maximum (79.35 ± 37.35 ng/g (mean ± SD); n=6) at 24-hours, and then subsequently decreased gradually and became completely undetectable at 7-days. In anterior chamber fluid, the concentration was below the quantification limit throughout the observation period. Astaxanthin was not detected in the anterior chamber fluid, serum or iris/ciliary body before oral administration.

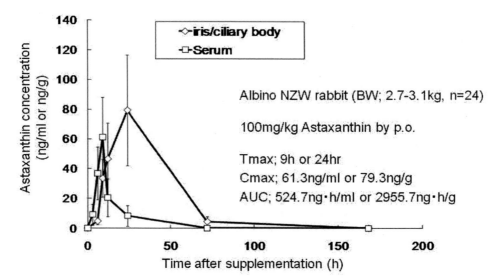

Figure 8. Time-course changes in astaxanthin concentration following 100 mg/kg single oral administration

Discussion

In considering the mechanism of astaxanthin responsible for improving ocular accommodative function, it is important to investigate astaxanthin penetration into the ciliary body as a possible site of action. Here, we attempted to elucidate the intraocular kinetics of orally administered astaxanthin. Measurement of intraocular/serum concentrations of astaxanthin administered as a single oral dose is considered to be one of the basic procedures for establishing the administration method and safety/efficacy of astaxanthin in the eyes, as in the case of ophthalmological drugs. However, to the best of our knowledge, the assay method for astaxanthin in the eyes has not yet been fully investigated. Prior to this experiment, we determined the proper method for establishing the correct procedure for determining astaxanthin concentration in eye tissues. We used the carotenoid extraction method for extracting astaxanthin from eye tissues and HPLC for quantifying astaxanthin, thus enabling the determination of astaxanthin concentration in eye tissues. Based on the results of our investigation of intraocular penetration of orally administered astaxanthin in NZW rabbits, we were able to confirm that astaxanthin can penetrate the iris/ciliary body. In the iris/ciliary body, the astaxanthin concentration gradually increased from 6-hours after administration, reaching the maximum concentration at 24-hours and then gradually decreased afterwards. In serum, the astaxanthin concentration increased up to 9-hours after administration and then subsequently decreased gradually. Considering that the maximum astaxanthin concentration was reportedly reached at approximately 9-hours in human serum,[31] the intraocular kinetics of astaxanthin in the iris/ciliary body of NZW rabbits possibly shows a similar pattern to that of humans. The amount of astaxanthin that penetrated into the iris/ciliary body was higher than that of astaxanthin in serum, and the time in which the maximum astaxanthin concentration was maintained in the iris/ciliary body was longer. The specific reason for this remains unknown. However, since the iris/ciliary body has an abundant vascular structure and melanin pigment, this may be one of the reasons why the astaxanthin concentration remained higher for a longer time in the iris/ciliary body than in serum. The results are considered significant in that astaxanthin penetration into the iris/ciliary body was confirmed and that the effect of astaxanthin in improving ocular accommodative function was demonstrated. Compared with oral antibiotics that reach the maximum blood concentration at 1-2 hours and the ocular maximum concentration at a slightly later time, we found that astaxanthin clearly reached the maximum concentration in blood and eye tissues at a slower rate. This finding must be noted as a major characteristic of astaxanthin. With the spread of IT equipment, VDT work is expected to further increase. In this regard, basic investigations on the intraocular kinetics of astaxanthin are important, since astaxanthin is one of the carotenoids considered to greatly contribute to the improvement of eye fatigue.

CONCLUDING REMARKS

Astaxanthin supplementation improved visual accommodation during eye fatigue, enhanced accommodative fatigue recovery, and accelerated visual fatigue induced reaction times – even in elder subjects with presbyopia and even with complicated visual works. Based on the results of these studies it is suggested that astaxanthin supplementation might be a practical and beneficial approach for eye fatigue relief working in ciliary body.

REFERENCES

1. Kuhn R, Sorensen NA. *Ber Deut Bot Ges*. 1938;71:1879.
2. Miki W. *Pure & Appl Chem*. 1991;63:141-146.
3. Matsuno T. *Pure & Appl Chem*. 1991;63:81-88.
4. Martin HD, Ruck C, Schmidt M, Sell S, Beutner S, Mayer B, Walsh R. *Pure & Appl Chem*. 1999;71:2253-2262.
5. Goto S, Kogure K, Abe K, Kimata K, Kitahama K, Yamashita E, Terada H. *Biochimica et Biophysica Acta*. 2001;1515:251-258.
6. Lee SJ, Bai SK, Lee KS, Namkoong S, Na HJ, Ha KS, Han JA, Yim SV, Chang K, Kwon YG, *et al*. *Mol Cells*. 2003;16:97-105.
7. Suzuki Y, Ohgami K, Shiratori K, Jin XH, Ilieva I, Koyama Y, Yazawa K, Yoshida K, Kase S, Ohno S. *Exp Eye Res*. 2006;82:275-281.
8. Jyonouchi H, Zhang L, Tomita Y. *Nutr Cancer*. 1993;19:269-280.
9. Yamashita E. *Anti-Aging Therapeutics*. 2009;11, *in press*.
10. Sawaki K, Yoshigi H, Aoki K, Koikawa N, Azumane A, Kaneko K, Yamaguchi M. *Therap & Med*. 2002;18:73-88.
11. Aoi W, Naito Y, Sakuma K, Kuchide M, Tokuda H, Maoka T, Toyokuni S, Oka S, Yasuhara M, Yoshikawa T. *Antioxid Redox Signal*. 2003;5:139-144.
12. Yamashita E. *Anti-Aging Therapeutics*. 2008;10:293-306.
13. Yamashita E. *Anti-Aging Therapeutics*. 2010;12, *in press*.
14. Iwasaki T, Tawara A. *J Eye*. 2006;12:829-834.
15. Takahashi N, Kajita M. *J Clin Ther & Med*. 2005;21:43-48.
16. Kajita M, Tsukahara H, Kato M. *Medical Consultation & New Remedies*. 2009;46:89-93.
17. Seya Y, Takahashi J, Imanaka K. *Japanese J Physiol Anthropol*. 2009;14:17-24.
18. Fukuda M. Takahashi J, Nishida Y, Sasaki H. *J Eye*. 2008;25:1461-1464.
19. Iwasaki T, Tawara A. *J Eye*. 2000;17:1719-1725.
20. Iwasaki T, Tawara A, Miyake N. *Acta Ophthalmol Scand*. 2005;83:81-88.
21. Feldman JM, Cooper J, Reinstein F. *Optom Vis Sci*. 1992;69:710-716.
22. Iwasaki T, Tawara A. *J Jap Ophthal Soc*. 2004;108:5-11.
23. Irie S, Furuie H, Matsukuma K. *Med Consul & New Rem*. 2001;38:617-621.
24. Jaschinski-Kruza W. *Ergonomics*. 1988;31:1449-1465.
25. Winn B, Gilmartin B. *Ophthal Physiol Opt*. 1992;12:252-256.
26. Kajita M. *Ophthalmol*. 1998;40:169-177.
27. Hiraoka M, Moroda M. *J Japanese Ophthalmol Soc*. 2003;107:702-708.
28. Asakawa K, Ishikawa H, Shoji N. *J Autonomic Nervous System*. 2007;44:98-103.
29. Yoshimura I, Kanaya K, Mori K. *J Japan Society of Physiol Anthropology*. 1999;4:37-42.
30. Saito S. *Vision*. 1993;5:27-31.
31. Odeberg JM, Lignell A, Pettersson A. *Eur J Pharm Sci*. 2003;19:299-304.

ABOUT THE AUTHOR

Dr. Eiji Yamashita is the Global Research & Development Manager for Fuji Chemical Industry Co., Ltd. He completed a pre-doctoral fellowship at the University of Texas Health Science Center and received his Ph.D. from the University of Tokushima. Yamashita's research experience and scientific contributions span nearly 20 years in the study of carotenoids and antioxidants.

Low-Dose Naltrexone Protocol

Paul J. Battle, PA-C
Barolat Neuroscience (Denver, CO USA);
Boulder Longevity Institute (Boulder, CO USA)

INTRODUCTION

Naltrexone is an opiate antagonist drug, which was FDA-approved for the management of drug addiction in 1984. Naltrexone has been used in chemical dependency clinics to reduce the euphoric effects of opiates. In addition, some practitioners have used it for alcoholic treatment. It is now a generic drug that can be obtained for $15-40 per month. Research suggests that low-dose naltrexone (LDN) may well be a safe, economic, and effective treatment for autoimmune disease and cancer. LDN modulates the deregulation of the immune system with autoimmune disease and inhibits cancer cell growth to help control malignant disease.

The diseases that LDN are most useful for are those involving immunological imbalance with the Th1/Th2 cytokines and/or low β-endorphin levels, e.g. multiple sclerosis (MS), Crohn's disease, and rheumatoid arthritis. It is also useful in the treatment of many types of malignancies. The malignancies that have been treated so far are those that have not successfully been treated by standard cancer therapy. It has been shown that the opiate growth factor (OGF) / opiate growth factor receptor (OGFr) complex that LDN enhances to slow cancer cell growth is a feature in 31 different cancer cell lines.

It is important to remember that the use of naltrexone is only FDA-approved for chemical dependency treatment and the uses described above are off label. There are clinics around the country that include LDN in their integrative cancer care. The beneficial aspects of LDN are that it is very economical at $15-40 per month and that is associated with very few (if any) side effects, therefore the risk/benefit ratio is very low.

TREATMENT PROTOCOL

LDN has to be compounded since the commercially available dose is 50 mg and the drug dosage for the diseases referred to above ranges from 2.0-4.5 mg. It is important that the compounding pharmacy is familiar with the criterion for optimal LDN formulation. There have been cases of decreased efficacy due to the fact that the pharmacy was not following the compounding guidelines. The website www.lowdosenaltrexone.org offers a list of pharmacies around the country that are known to compound LDN reliably. It is important to note that LDN should not be in an extended release form.

Calcium carbonate inhibits the absorption of LDN. Therefore, the filler of the capsule or tablet should be formulated without calcium carbonate. Lactose can be used, although many patients are lactose intolerant, thus lactose is not the optimal choice of filler. Sucrose can be used as a substitute filler for lactose, however Avicell, a cellulose-based filler, is very popular amongst the compounding pharmacies producing LDN.

Dosing

The dose of LDN used to treat autoimmune disease or cancer ranges between 2.0-4.5 mg per day. In the past, it has been recommended that LDN should be taken between 9 pm and 1am. The thought being that LDN would be present in the serum at around the same time of night when the majority of β-endorphin is released in the brain. However, results of several studies by Dr Zagon show that LDN elevates β-endorphin levels for 24-72 hours. Therefore, if a patient has insomnia (which is the most common side effect of LDN) it can be taken during the day. Any sleep disturbances triggered by LDN typically resolves in two weeks, the dose can then be taken in the evening.

The initial dosage of LDN is commonly 1.5 mg to be taken for 2-3 weeks. The dose is low initially to reduce any sleep disturbance side effects. It is then increased to 3.0 mg for another 2-3 weeks, and then increased again to 4.5 mg, which is the maintenance dosage. If the pharmacy makes tablets then a 3.0 mg tablet can be given to the patient, who should be instructed to firstly take half a tablet is used, then a full tablet, and finally one and a half tablets. If the patient feels comfortable at 4.5 mg that should be the maintenance dose. The rate of increase of the dosage can vary depending on the patient's response.

MS patients may have lower dosage requirements. Dr. Tom Gilhooly, a general practitioner in Scotland (which has the highest per capita rate of MS in the world) regularly uses 2.0 mg to treat his MS patients. Thus, for MS patients, it may be better to start with 1.0 mg and then increase by 0.5 mg every 3 weeks to a maximum of 4.5 mg based on symptoms. It is important to note that approximately 10% of MS patients may experience an increase in their symptoms for 1-2 weeks after starting treatment with LDN. According to Dr. M.R. Lawrence in England, spasticity may increase transiently. However, it is very unusual for any increased symptoms to last longer than 2-weeks. Patients who experience increased symptoms should remain at that dose until their symptoms improve and then either titrate up further or stay at that dose for maintenance as long they are taking at least 2.0 mg/day. Many MS patients find that 3.0 mg is a good maintenance dose for them.

The standard dose of LDN for the treatment of malignant disease is 4.5 mg. Intravenous OGF may be used for the treatment of metastatic disease, however the dosage is calculated on an individual basis. Dr. Ian Zagon at Pennsylvania State University can offer more information about the use of intravenous OGF.

Side Effects

Naltrexone has been used for 25 years, and during this time it has proven to be safe in many different settings. Potential side effects of LDN are insomnia, vivid dreams, increased spasticity in MS patients, and reversible liver enzyme elevations. The liver toxicity that has been reported in the past is associated with dosages over the 300 mg/day range. There has not been any reported liver toxicity at 4.5 mg/day or below. There have also been some reports of nausea.

Contraindications

The main contraindication to using LDN is continuing use of opiate-containing compounds. Since LDN is a mu receptor opiate antagonist narcotic agents cannot be used with LDN. Depending upon the type of opiates the patient is using, one should wait at least 2-weeks after the last dose of narcotics before starting LDN. It is up to the practitioner to determine how long to wait for LDN based on the patients other drugs, comorbid conditions, and the presence of any drug with a long half-life, e.g. methadone. If a patient is on LDN and is anticipating a procedure that will require narcotic analgesia, then they should stop taking LDN one week prior to narcotic administration.

Relative contraindications are the use of immunosuppressive drugs, such as high dose prednisone, methotrexate, azathioprine, and interferon. These may diminish or eliminate LDN's effectiveness.

With regards to risk in pregnancy, naltrexone has actually been used in a fertility clinic in the UK since 1985. That clinic has used naltrexone in the higher dose range (50-200 mg/day) and no problems with the children or the women during pregnancy or post partum have been reported.

ABOUT THE AUTHOR

Paul Battle, PA-C received his Physiology degree from University of California, Davis. He went on to complete his Physician Assistant training at Emory University School of Medicine in 1981. He is in practice at Boulder Longevity Institute and Barolat Neuroscience in Denver.

Laser Assisted Lipolysis

Agnieszka Protasewicz M.D., Ph.D.
Specialist in Orthopedics and Traumatology, Hand Surgeon, Laser Lipolysis Physician,
Poznań, Poland

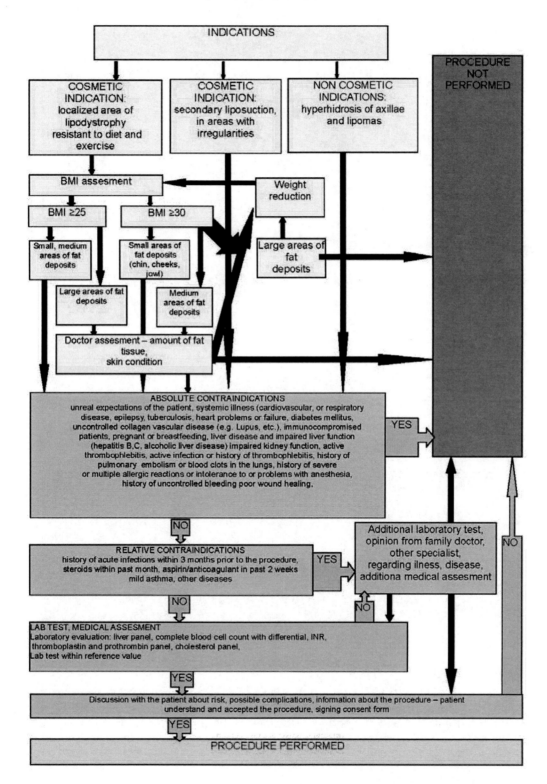

BEFORE PROCEDURE

Discussion with the patient about risk, possible complications, information about the procedure – patient understands and accepted the procedure, signs consent form, patient receives pre and post operative instructions

PATIENT	DOCTOR
Prior to the procedure patient is asked to: stop taking aspirin, or blood thinners 10 days, steroids 1 month prior to the procedure. Consult family doctor before stopping any medication. Try to stop smoking, or keep the number of cigarettes smoked to an absolute minimum. Patient is advised to have a shower in the morning and to wash the areas to be operated on with antibacterial soap.	Before procedure has to prepare and check: **Laser module and equipment** (laser fibre, appropriate cannulas, tips, handpieces, appropriate protective eyewear **Medications** – antibiotic amoxycilin1000, 1 tablet before the procedure then 2 times per day morning and evening) for 3 days. Anesthesia local – for the incisions Lignocain 1% + adrenaline 1:500,000. Anesthesia – Klein Solution – tumescent anasthaesia, (Sodium Chloride 0.9% 500ml, Adrenaline 1:1000 1ml, Lignocane 2% 20ml (average 40ml per patient), Sodium Bicarbonate inj 8.4%), antibacterial ointment (for incision sites), anti-bacterial preparation solution, **Medical equipment:** gloves, surgical gown (for patient and medical staff), drape, 5ml syringe, 30G needles(for injecting local anaesthetic), 50ml syringe +blink infiltration cannula or 20g spinal needle to infiltrate, scalpel No 11 blade, sterile swabs, dressing, steri stips, 50cc syringe for aspiration (if not using suction) or aspirating system (electric or manual),optional: IV sedation, oxygen saturation monitor (O2 Sat monitor) **Other equipment:** surgical marking pen, camera, patient compression garments,

PROCEDURE OF LASER-ASSISTED LIPOSUCTION

Weight and measurement – weight, height, BMI, amount of anesthesia. Pictures, marking the treatment site,
Antibiotics: amoxycilin1000, 1 tablet before the procedure (then 2 times per day morning and evening for 3 days).
O2 Sat monitor is attached to monitor vital signs. Preparation of sterile field and instruments and prepare tumescent anesthesia.
Patient positioning and draping. Local anesthesia to the incision site.
Optional: administer patient sedative.
Make incision.
Infiltrate area to be treated using the wet infiltration technique. Insert the canula with fiber optic or treatment tip – lase area to be treated. During the laser lipolysis procedure the patient and the staff wear protective eyewear.
Recommended volume of tumescent anesthetic solution and amount of energy delivered per treated area:
abdomen (lower) 200-600ml, 7000-24000 j, abdomen (upper) 150-500ml, 3000-12000 j, ankles 50-80ml, 2,500- 5500 j, arms (triceps) 150-350ml, 2500-8000 j, banana (infra-gluteal crease) 80-250ml, 2500 - 7000 j, bra back 100-250ml, 2500 - 7500 j, gynecomastia 200-550ml, 8000 -18000 j, buttocks 250-550ml, 2000 - 12000j, calves 80-180ml, 2500 - 5500 j, cheeks 50-120ml, 2500 - 3500 j, chin 60-180ml, 2500 - 8000 j, flanks 120-300ml, 2500 - 8000 j, knees 80-250ml, 2500 -8000j, love handles 250-550ml, 2500-10000j, thighs outer 200-450ml, 5500-14000 j, thighs inner 200-450ml,
4500-12000 j,
Suction or wound drainage. Dressing. Apply compressive garment. Review post-procedure
instructions with patient. Fill the documents: area treated, energy used, amount optional: tumescent

POST PROCEDURE

Apply compression garment for the advised period, usually. 24-48 hours for treatments on the face and under the chin, and 7/14 days in other areas. Antibiotics are prescribed for 3- 5 days (to prevent infection). Return to every day activity as normal avoiding vigorous activity or sport for 2 weeks. Leakage of fluid from incisions is a normal occurrence within the first 24 hours post treatment. Avoid hot baths or saunas for 7 days following treatment.

RESULTS AND BENEFITS

Less traumatic than the conventional liposuction method -faster healing – smaller incisions mean less bruising, pain, blood loss and swelling due to laser interaction with small blood vessels and using tumescent anesthesia with vasoconstrictors. Most of the patients 55% are very satisfied. 36% are satisfied, notice amount of fat tissue reduction, with good skin retraction. Final results develop within 3 months and final result is permanent. Among the patients who underwent MRI procedure preprocedure and three months after there was an average 17% reduction in fat volume. 25% at the submental area. The higher the total energy delivered the higher the reduction in fat – thus suggesting a dose-response relationship.

POSSIBLE RISK AND COMPLICATIONS

Possible side effects and complications include: postoperative pain, tenderness of the treated area, postoperative edema, swelling (is minimized by using proper postoperative dressings), bleeding, bruising, infection (rare if proper aseptic precautions are followed), seroma, burning, scarring, pigment changes, skin contour changes, irregularities and asymmetry,pulmonary complications, allergic reaction to medication, anesthesia or sedation, tissue hardening, numbness, asymmetry, embolism.

ABOUT THE AUTHOR

Dr. Agnieszka Protasewicz began her work as a hand surgeon in 2002. Dr. Protasewicz earned her medical degree *cum laude* from the University of Medical Sciences in Poznan. She presented her Ph.D thesis in 2006 (in the field of hand surgery) and obtained certification as a specialist in orthopedics and traumatology in 2009. Dr. Protasewicz is one of the most experienced clinicians in laser-assisted lipolysis in Poland, and she provides training and consultancy for other doctors who use laser-assisted lipolysis for fat reduction. Dr. Protasewicz holds the position of aesthetic medicine doctor in private practice. Areas of interest include botulinum toxin and filler injections, laser-assisted lipolysis, anti-aging, hand surgery, and microsurgery.

Anti-Aging Medicine &
Regenerative Biomedical Technology News 2009
Compiled by the Medical Editors of Worldhealth.net
Worldhealth.net is the Official Educational Website of the A4M – www.worldhealth.net

Lifestyle Significantly Influences Risk of Stroke

Four specific health behaviors have now been identified as reducing the risk of stroke in men and women. Phyo K. Myint, from the University of East Anglia (United Kingdom), and colleagues studied 20,040 men and women, ages 40 to 79, with no known stroke or myocardial infarction at the study's start in 1993, following the subjects up to 2007. The team implemented a risk-scoring system to weigh various behaviors and correlate their impact on stroke risk. The researchers found beneficial impact of four specific health behaviors, namely: current non-smoking, not being physically inactive, moderate alcohol intake (1-14 units a week), and having a plasma concentration of vitamin C levels at/above 50 micromol/L (suggesting a daily fruit/vegetable intake of 5 servings a day). All combined, these "four health behaviours combined predict more than a twofold difference in incidence of stroke in men and women," report the researchers. They conclude that: "These results provide further incentive and support for the notion that small differences in lifestyle an have a substantial potential impact on risk."
[Myint PK, Luben RN, Wareham NJ, Bingham SA, Khaw KT. "Combined effect of health behaviours and risk of first ever stroke in 20,040 men and women over 11 years' follow-up in Norfolk cohort of European Prospective Investigation of Cancer (EPIC Norfolk): prospective population study," BMJ. 2009 Feb 19;338:b349 doi: 10.1136/bmj.b349.]

Cardiovascular Risk Linked to Progression of Alzheimer's Disease

Vascular factors including medical history (heart disease, stroke, diabetes, and hypertension), smoking, and prediagnosis blood lipid measurements (total cholesterol, high-density lipoprotein, low-density lipoprotein, and triglycerides) may be predictors for progression of Alzheimer disease (AD). Yaakov Stern, from Columbia University Medical Center (New York, USA), and colleagues studied 156 men and women with AD (mean age of 83 years at diagnosis) for a mean period of 3.5 years. The team found that AD progressed at a significantly faster rate in study subjects with elevated total cholesterol, elevated LDL cholesterol, or personal history of diabetes. HDL cholesterol and triglycerides were not found to have an impact on cognitive decline. The researchers speculate that cholesterol affect AD progression via increased oxidative stress or neuroinflammatory responses that trigger amyloid plaque production in the brain. Diabetes could influence AD through inflammation or by contributing to plaqye and tangle formation, they also explain.
[Helzner EP, Luchsinger JA, Scarmeas N, Cosentino S, Brickman AM, Glymour MM, Stern Y. "Contribution of vascular risk factors to the progression in Alzheimer disease." Arch Neurol. 2009 Mar;66(3):343-8.]

Optimism Promotes Longer, Healthier Life

Researchers from the University of Pittsburgh (Pennsylvania USA) reviewed data collected on 100,000 women, ages 50+, collected since 1994 as part of the Women's Health Initiative Study. Hilary Tindle and colleagues found that optimistic women were 14% less likely to die from any cause (as compared to pessimists), and 30% less likely to die from heart disease after 8 years of follow-up from the study. Optimists also were loess likely to have high blood pressure, diabetes, or smoke cigarettes. Additionally, the team found that women who were "cynically hostile," that is – highly mistrustful of other people, were 16% more likely to die during the study period, and 23% more likely to die from cancer.
[Hilary Tindle, MD, Abstract #1085, "Psychological Traits and Morbidity and Total Mortality in the Women's Health Initiative," presented at the Annual Meeting of the American Psychomatic Society, Psychosocial Predictors of Risk and Mortality paper session, March 5, 2009.

Sister Study Reinforces the Importance of Healthy Living
The long-term Sister Study, sponsored by the US National Institute of Environmental Health Sciences (NIEHS), part of the National Institutes of Health, involves 50,000 women, ages 35-74, and looks at the environmental and genetic characteristics of women whose sister had breast cancer to identify factors associated with developing breast cancer. Christine G. Parks, from the Epidemiology Branch, National Institute of Environmental Health Sciences (Research Triangle Park, North Carolina USA), and colleagues looked at the association between telomere length and the perceived stress levels, and found that stress can impact telomere length. This team observed that: "Among women with both higher perceived stress and elevated levels of the stress hormone epinephrine, the difference in telomere length was equivalent to or greater than the effects of being obese, smoking or 10 years of aging." In a separate study, Sangmi Kim, from the Epidemiology Branch, National Institute of Environmental Health Sciences (Research Triangle Park, North Carolina USA), and team assessed the effect of obesity and weight gain on telomere length. Women who had an overweight or obese body mass index (BMI) before or during their 30s, and maintained that status since those years, had shorter telomeres than those who became overweight or obese after their 30s. This team comments that: "This suggests that duration of obesity may be more important than weight change per se ... Our results support the hypothesis that obesity accelerates the aging process."
[Christine G. Parks, Diane B. Miller, Erin C. McCanlies, Richard M. Cawthon, Michael E. Andrew, Lisa A. DeRoo, and Dale P. Sandler. "Telomere Length, Current Perceived Stress, and Urinary Stress Hormones in Women," Cancer Epidemiol. Biomarkers Prev. 2009 18: 551-560; Sangmi Kim, Christine G. Parks, Lisa A. DeRoo, Honglei Chen, Jack A. Taylor, Richard M. Cawthon, and Dale P. Sandler. "Obesity and Weight Gain in Adulthood and Telomere Length," Cancer Epidemiol. Biomarkers Prev. 2009 18: 816-820.]

Brain Decline Starts At Age 27
Previously, studies have revealed that increased age is associated with lower levels of cognitive performance. Timothy A. Salthouse, from the University of Virginia (USA), and colleagues completed a seven-year study involving 2,000 healthy people, ages 18 to 60 who were tested for mental agility via tests similar to those used to diagnose dementia. In nine out of 12 tests the average age at which the top performance was achieved was 22. The first age at which there was any marked decline was at 27 in tests of brain speed, reasoning and visual puzzle-solving ability. Things like memory stayed intact until the age of 37, on average, while abilities based on accumulated knowledge, such as performance on tests of vocabulary or general information, increased until the age of 60. The team concludes that: "Some aspects of age-related cognitive decline begin in healthy educated adults when they are in their 20s and 30s."
[Salthouse, T.A. "When does age-related cognitive decline begin?" Neurobiology of Aging, 30 (4), p.507-514, Apr 2009.]

Weight Gain Early in Life Leads to Physical Disabilities in Older Adults
Carrying extra weight earlier in life increases the risk of developing problems with mobility in old age, even if the weight is eventually lost, report Denise Houston, from the Wake Forest University School of Medicine (North Carolina USA), and colleagues. The team studied 2,845 American adults, ages 70 to 79 years, enrolled in the Health, Aging and Body Composition Study, collecting and analyzing data on Body Mass Index (BMI) and mobility limitations during a 7-year follow-up period. Men and women who were overweight or obese at all 3 time points of the study had an increased risk of mobility limitation (as compared with those who were normal weight throughout). Further, the researchers found a significant graded response on risk of mobility limitation for the cumulative effect of obesity in men and overweight and/or obesity in women. Concludes the team: "Onset of overweight and obesity in earlier life contributes to an increased risk of mobility limitation in old age."
[Denise K. Houston, Jingzhong Ding, Barbara J. Nicklas, Tamara B. Harris, Jung Sun Lee, Michael C. Nevitt, Susan M. Rubin, Frances A. Tylavsky, Stephen B. Kritchevsky, and for the Health ABC Study. "Overweight and Obesity Over the Adult Life Course and Incident Mobility Limitation in Older Adults: The Health, Aging and Body Composition Study," Am. J. Epidemiol., 15 April 2009; 169: 927 - 936.]

Basic Lifestyle Factors Help to Prevent Diabetes Later in Life

Lifestyle factors play a critical role in diabetes prevention, even for older adults. Dariush Mozaffarian, from Harvard School of Public Health (Massachusetts USA), and colleagues studied 4,883 men and women ages 65+ at the study's start, following them for a 10-year period. For each lifestyle factor considered in the study, one-third to one-half of the study participants was considered at low risk. After adjustment for potentially influencing factors, each low-risk factor was found to be a significant independent predictor of diabetes incidence:

- 26% lower with above average physical activity level (leisure-time activity and walking pace)
- 31% for a dietary score in the top two quintiles for fiber intake, polyunsaturated-to-saturated fat ratio, trans-fat intake, and mean glycemic index
- 23% for having never smoked, quit more than 20 years ago, or smoked fewer than five pack-years total
- 34% for light or moderate alcohol use versus abstinence
- 45% for a body mass index less than 25 kg/m2
- 46% for waist circumference of less than 88 cm (34.6 inches) for women or 92 cm (36.2 inches) for men

All totalled, for men and women ages 65 and older, the team found that a combination of good habits – including physical activity, healthy diet, moderate alcohol consumption, and not smoking, plus monitoring of weight and waist circumference, lowered the incidence of diabetes by a staggering 89%."

[Mozaffarian D, Kamineni A, Carnethon M, Djoussé L, Mukamal KJ, Siscovick D. "Lifestyle risk factors and new-onset diabetes mellitus in older adults: the cardiovascular health study." Arch Intern Med. 2009 Apr 27;169(8):798-807.]

Healthy Lifestyle Key to Preventing Cancer, Diabetes, and Heart Disease

Yet another study confirms that healthy lifestyle factors are effective in reducing relative risk of developing major chronic diseases such as cardiovascular disease, diabetes, and cancer. Earl S. Ford, from the US Centers for Disease Control and Prevention (Atlanta, Georgia USA), and colleagues studied data from 23,153 German men and women, ages 35 to 65 years, who participated in the European Prospective Investigation Into Cancer and Nutrition-Potsdam study. The researchers found that four lifestyle factors -- namely never smoking, BMI of 30 or less, exercising 3.5 hours a week and eating a healthy diet – slashed the risk of cardiovascular disease, diabetes, and cancer by a staggering 80%. The researchers urge that: "The message is clear. Adhering to 4 simple healthy lifestyle factors can have a strong impact on the prevention of chronic diseases."

[Ford ES, Bergmann MM, Kröger J, Schienkiewitz A, Weikert C, Boeing H. "Healthy living is the best revenge: findings from the European Prospective Investigation Into Cancer and Nutrition-Potsdam study." Arch Intern Med. 2009 Aug 10;169(15):1355-62.]

Physical Activity Promotes Longevity, Regardless of Age

While the benefits of physical activity are clear among the majority of the population, there has been little research on its effects in older people. Jeremy M. Jacobs, from Hebrew University Hadassah Medical School (Jerusalem, Israel), and colleagues examined the effects of continuing, increasing, or decreasing physical activity on levels on survival, function, and health status among the very old. In their study involving 1,861 men and women, ages 70 to 88 years, and lasting a follow-up period of 18 years, the researchers found that those elderly men and women who are physically active (4 or more hours of physical activity per day) increase their chances of living longer and maintaining functional independence, as compared to their sedentary peers (less than 4 hours physical activity daily). Among active 70-year-olds, the team found that 15% died over the next 8 years, compared to 27% of sedentary 70-year-olds. Eight-year mortality was 26% for active 78-year-olds, and 41% for sedentary peers. Among 85-year-olds, 3-year mortality was roughly 7% for active individuals as compared to 24% for sedentary counterparts. States Dr. Jacobs: "Controlling for the [major risk] factors allowed us to isolate physical activity as an independent factor in mortality, and not just an indicator of the overall health of the subjects." `

[`Stessman J, Hammerman-Rozenberg R, Cohen A, Ein-Mor E, Jacobs JM. "Physical activity, function, and longevity among the very old." Arch Intern Med. 2009 Sep 14;169(16):1476-83.]

Unhealthy Habits Raise Risks of Memory and Thinking Problems
Previous research has linked declines in thinking and memory skills with unhealthy behaviors such as smoking, sedentary lifestyle, low fruit and vegetable consumption, and other factors. Severine Sabia, from Hopital Paul Brousse (France), and colleagues studied 5,123 men and women enrolled in th4e Whit4ehall II study (United Kingdom), following them for a 17-year period. The team surveyed the health behaviors of civil service office workers in London, when the workers were 44 years (early midlife), 56 years (midlife), and 61 years (late-midlife). After correcting for confounding factors, the researchers found that the more each of the subjects reported engaging in unhealthy behaviors, the greater the risk of cognitive deficit. Those subjects who currently smoked showed the lowest memory, verbal, and math-related thinking and reasoning skills at each survey. Similar findings were noted for those who ate fewer than 2 servings of fruits and vegetables a day. Men and women who did not engage in much physical activity during midlife and late-midlife also showed greater risk for cognitive deficit. Reports the team: "The odds of poor executive function and memory were the greater the more times the participant reported unhealthy behaviors. This study suggests that both the number of unhealthy behaviors and their duration are associated with subsequent cognitive function in later life."
[Sabia S, Nabi H, Kivimaki M, Shipley MJ, Marmot MG, Singh-Manoux A. "Health behaviors from early to late midlife as predictors of cognitive function: The Whitehall II study." Am J Epidemiol. 2009 Aug 15;170(4):428-37. Epub 2009 Jul 2.]

Keep Your Mind Active to Reduce Dementia Risk
In that evidence continues to amass that involvement in leisure activities may reduce the risk of dementia, Tasnime Akbaraly, from INSERM (France), and colleagues studied 5,698 men and women, ages 65 and older, in an effort to elucidate the underlying mechanism of this association. During the four-year study period, the researchers found that mind-stimulating leisure time pursuits, such as doing crossword puzzles or playing cards, exerted a significant protective effect. In contrast, the team did not observe any protective effect from physical, passive, or social leisure activities, such as walking, watching television, or visiting with friends. The researchers conclude that: "Our findings support the hypothesis that cognitively stimulating leisure activities may delay the onset of dementia in community-dwelling elders."
[Akbaraly TN, Portet F, Fustinoni S, Dartigues JF, Artero S, Rouaud O, Touchon J, Ritchie K, Berr C. "Leisure activities and the risk of dementia in the elderly: results from the Three-City Study." Neurology. 2009 Sep 15;73(11):854-61.]

Low Vitamin D Levels Raise Risk of Death
Study of senior women shows that low levels of vitamin D may increase the risk of dying from all causes by 150%. Richard D. Semba, from The Johns Hopkins University School of Medicine (Maryland, USA), and colleagues studied data from 13,331 men and women participating in NHANES III (The Third National Health and Nutritional Examination Survey), to ascertain the role of vitamin D levels (serum 25(OH)D) as contributors to risks of death. The researchers found that women with blood levels of the vitamin lower than 15.3 nanograms per milliliter were more likely to die from causes such as heart disease and cancer, as compared to women with higher levels (above 27 ng/ml). The team observes that: "Older community-dwelling women with low [vitamin D] levels are at an increased risk of death." The team notes that several biologic mechanisms could explain a causal relationship between vitamin D deficiency and mortality, because the active form of vitamin D (1,25-dihydroxyvitamin D) is associated with controlling inflammatory compounds, regulating immune health and blood pressure, and reducing arterial hardening.
[Semba RD, Houston DK, Ferrucci L, Cappola AR, Sun K, Guralnik JM, Fried LP. "Low serum 25-hydroxyvitamin D concentrations are associated with greater all-cause mortality in older community-dwelling women." Nutr Res. 2009 Aug;29(8):525-30.]

Adult Cells Prompted to Become Patient-Specific Stem Cells

Previously, scientists identified four genes that can transform adult stem cells into induced pluripotent stem cells (iPSCs), which have the capacity to differentiate into specialized cells of the body. However, these genes are delivered by a retrovirus, becoming integrated into the DNA and may, over an extended period of time, activate cancer-causing genes. To overcome this issue, Justin K. Ichida, from Harvard Stem Cell Institute (Massachusetts, USA), and colleagues substituted small chemical molecules for two of the genes, successfully demonstrating an alternative for converting one type of cell into another. The team observes that: "By using a non-biased chemical screening approach, we uncovered a previously unknown way to make stem cells. This discovery is exciting because it demonstrates the feasibility of using chemicals to make safer patient-specific stem cells for transplantation medicine." Previously, scientists identified four genes that can transform adult stem cells into induced pluripotent stem cells (iPSCs), which have the capacity to differentiate into specialized cells of the body. However, these genes are delivered by a retrovirus, becoming integrated into the DNA and may, over an extended period of time, activate cancer-causing genes. To overcome this issue, Justin K. Ichida, from Harvard Stem Cell Institute (Massachusetts, USA), and colleagues substituted small chemical molecules for two of the genes, successfully demonstrating an alternative for converting one type of cell into another. The team observes that: "By using a non-biased chemical screening approach, we uncovered a previously unknown way to make stem cells. This discovery is exciting because it demonstrates the feasibility of using chemicals to make safer patient-specific stem cells for transplantation medicine."

[Justin K. Ichida, Joel Blanchard, Kelvin Lam, Esther Y. Son, Julia E. Chung, Dieter Egli, Kyle M. Loh, Ava C. Carter, Francesco P. Di Giorgio, Kathryn Koszka, Danwei Huangfu, Hidenori Akutsu, David R. Liu, Lee L. Rubin, Kevin Eggan. "A Small-Molecule Inhibitor of Tgf-β Signaling Replaces Sox2 in Reprogramming by Inducing Nanog." Cell Stem Cell, 08 October 2009.]

Major Report Addresses Environmental Pollutants and Cancer Risk

A report by the American Cancer Society's Cancer and the Environment Subcommittee encourages the organization's role addressing the relationship between environmental pollutants and cancer risk, and advises the public to minimize exposure to known carcinogens, calling for new strategies to more effectively and efficiently screen chemicals. The Subcommittee's initiative focuses on environmental hazards that have emerged as a result of the industrialization of the early 20th century, with emerging hazards ranging from naturally occurring substances that were first mined for industrial use, such as asbestos and uranium, to products extracted from natural sources such as benzene from petroleum, and newly created substances such as vinyl chloride. Elizabeth T.H. Fontham, national volunteer president of the American Cancer Society and professor and Dean at Louisiana State University Health Sciences Center (USA), explained that while "exposure levels to environmental pollution to the general public are typically far lower than the levels associated with the proven cancer risks shown in occupational or other settings... these low-level exposures do cause us concern because of the multiplicity of substances, the fact that many exposures are out of the public's control, and the potential that even low-level exposures contribute to the cancer burden when large numbers of people are exposed."

[Elizabeth T. H. Fontham, Michael J. Thun, Elizabeth Ward, Alan J. Balch, John Oliver L. Delancey, Jonathan M. Samet, on behalf of ACS Cancer and the Environment Subcommittee. "American Cancer Society Perspectives on Environmental Factors and Cancer." CA Cancer J Clin 2009.]

Living to 100 Linked to Variant of Telomere Enzyme

In that telomeres are the endcaps on chromosomes, and telomeric shortening is thought to govern the number of times a cell can divide, telomeric replication is governed by an enzyme, telomerase. Gil Atzmon, from Albert Einstein College of Medicine (New York, USA), and colleagues studied Ashkenazi Jews, a population group that generally lives well into their 90s and beyond, in a generally healthy condition. The researchers found that participants who have lived to a very old age have inherited mutant genes that make their telomerase-making system extra active and able to maintain telomere length more effectively. For the most part, these people were spared age-related diseases such as cardiovascular disease and diabetes, which cause most deaths among elderly people. The team observes that: "As we suspected, humans of exceptional longevity are better able to maintain the length of their telomeres. [T]hey owe their longevity, at least in part, to advantageous variants of genes involved in telomere maintenance."

[Gil Atzmon, Miook Cho, Richard M. Cawthon, Temuri Budagov, Micol Katz, Xiaoman Yang, Glenn Siegel, Aviv Bergman, Derek M. Huffman, Clyde B. Schechter, Woodring E. Wright, Jerry W. Shay, Nir Barzilai, Diddahally R. Govindaraju, Yousin Suh. "Genetic variation in human telomerase is associated with telomere length in Ashkenazi centenarians." PNAS, November 13, 2009.]

Cardiovascular Fitness Linked to Higher IQ

A Swedish study involving 1.2 million Swedish men reveals link between a strong cardiovascular system in young adulthood and IQ and intelligence later in life. Maria Aberg, from Sahlgrenska Academy (Sweden), and colleagues studied 1.2 million Swedish men, born between 1950 and 1976, who were enrolled in military service. Analyzing physical and IQ test data collected when the men enrolled, the team established a correlation between good physical fitness and better results for the IQ test, with the strongest links found for logical thinking and verbal comprehension. Noting that their findings suggest that only fitness – not strength -- plays a role in the results for the IQ test, the researchers urge that: "These data substantiate that physical exercise could be an important instrument for public health initiatives to optimize educational achievements, cognitive performance, as well as disease prevention at the society level."

[Maria A. I. Aberg, Nancy L. Pedersen, Kjell Toren, Magnus Svartengren, Bjorn Backstrand, Tommy Johnsson, Christiana M. Cooper-Kuhn, N. David Aberg, Michael Nilsson, H. Georg Kuhn. "Cardiovascular fitness is associated with cognition in young adulthood." PNAS, November 30, 2009.]

Adult Stem Cells May Help Repair Muscle Cells Damaged by Heart Attack

\Adult stem cells may help repair heart tissue damaged by heart attack according to the findings of a Phase I study completed by Gary L. Schaer, from Rush University Medical Center (Illinois, USA), and colleagues,. The study demonstrates that stem cells from donor bone marrow appear to help heart attack patients recover better by growing new blood vessels to bring more oxygen to the heart. Researchers say it is the strongest evidence thus far indicating that adult stem cells can actually differentiate into heart cells to repair damage. The team observes that: "The results point to a promising new treatment for heart attack patients that could reduce mortality and lessen the need for heart transplants."

[Joshua M. Hare, Jay H. Traverse, Timothy D. Henry, Nabil Dib, Robert K. Strumpf, Steven P. Schulman, Gary Gerstenblith, Anthony N. DeMaria, Ali E. Denktas, Roger S. Gammon, James B. Hermiller, Jr, Mark A. Reisman, Gary L. Schaer, Warren Sherman. "A Randomized, Double-Blind, Placebo-Controlled, Dose-Escalation Study of Intravenous Adult Human Mesenchymal Stem Cells (Prochymal) After Acute Myocardial Infarction." J. Am. Coll. Cardiol., December 8, 2009; 54: 2277 - 2286. "Study Results Suggest Adult Stem Cells May Help Repair Muscle Cells Damaged by Heart Attack," Rush University Medical Center, December 02, 2009.]

Volunteering Promotes Brain Health

Engaging in volunteer activities may help to promote optimal cognitive function. Michelle C. Carlson, from The Johns Hopkins Bloomberg School of Public Health (Maryland, USA), and colleagues studied women engaged in the Experience Corps, a social service program comprised of volunteer seniors, who tutored young children as part of their assignment. Utilizing functional MRI, the researchers found that after six months of volunteering, the women demonstrated significant increases in brain activity in regions important to cognitive function, specifically the anterior cingulate cortex, left dorsal prefrontal cortex, and left ventral prefrontal cortex. Explaining that: "Neural gains were matched by behavioral improvements in executive inhibitory ability," the team concludes that: "These pilot results provide proof of concept for use-dependent brain plasticity in later life, and, that interventions designed to promote health and function through everyday activity may enhance plasticity in key regions that support executive function."

[Michelle C. Carlson, Kirk I. Erickson, Arthur F. Kramer, Michelle W. Voss, Natalie Bolea, Michelle Mielke, Sylvia McGill, George W. Rebok, Teresa Seeman, Linda P. Fried. "Evidence for Neurocognitive Plasticity in At-Risk Older Adults: The Experience Corps Program." J Gerontol A Biol Sci Med Sci, December 2009; 64A: 1275 – 1282.]